HISTORY OF PHARMACY

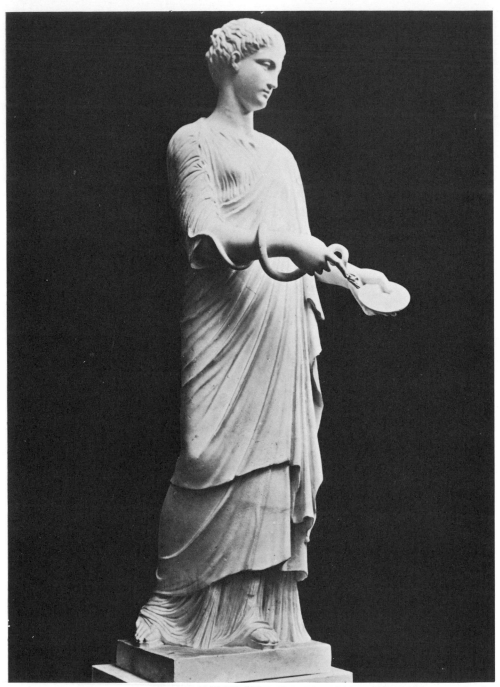

Hygeia, goddess of health in ancient Greece, served beside her father, the great healing god Asklepios. This classical statue in the Wellcome Historical Medical Museum in
London was cast from an ancient original preserved in the Louvre in Paris. Hygeia holds
her traditional adjuncts—a sacred serpent of miraculous powers and a patera or bowl
(containing a healing potion?). As the staff and entwined serpent of Asklepios became
the world-wide symbol of medicine, so the bowl and serpent of Hygeia have become in
modern times an internationally recognized symbol of pharmacy. On the outer spine of
this book the "Bowl of Hygeia" is shown in a modern style recently used by the International Pharmaceutical Federation. (From the Wellcome Historical Medical Museum,
London)

KREMERS AND URDANG'S

HISTORY
OF
PHARMACY

Revised by GLENN SONNEDECKER, Ph.D.

Professor of History of Pharmacy, University of Wisconsin;
Director, American Institute of the History of Pharmacy

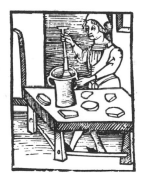

THIRD EDITION　　　95 Figures

J. B. LIPPINCOTT COMPANY

Philadelphia　　　　　　　　　　Toronto

Distributed in Great Britain by
Pitman Medical Publishing Co., Limited, London

Library of Congress Catalog Card Number 63-20827
Printed in the United States of America

Preface

That strand of history formed from the evolving fusion of knowledge and responsibility designed to provide safe, effective drugs and health supplies comprises a significant component of one of man's most basic concerns. An account of this development merits the attention of the general reader. However, we hope more particularly to give the pharmacy student some additional perspective—an informed confidence —to guide his reshaping of traditions and improving of the services and the satisfactions which he expects in the profession.

The history of pharmaceutical science and technology has the cumulative, progressive quality that characterizes the history of science at large; the history of the pharmaceutical profession shows the character of social history, with its unforeseen regressive turns of events, its conflicts of interests, and their resolution by trends and forces that would elude comprehension solely in terms of science, or conviction, or effort, circumscribed by a given time or group.

This sociohistorical view of pharmacy evolving as a profession in the Western world is what we have tried to portray here. The materia medica—and the science and technic that transform it—has not been ignored, but the serious study of pharmacy's history from that viewpoint must be left to another occasion and framework. Likewise, there are large areas of the world—both primitive and highly civilized, in remote and more recent time—whose interesting pharmaceutical endeavors had to be ignored in the task of producing a manageable volume focused on the sources of historical growth that seemed most relevant to American pharmacy.

Despite this limitation of scope, the Kremers-Urdang *History of Pharmacy* has remained since the first edition (1940) the most ambitious work of its kind in English, showing us the truly international character of pharmacy and its development and clari-fying without over-simplifying the context of that development.

In the Preface to the first edition, Edward Kremers observed, "The organization and plan of this *History of Pharmacy* go beyond the merely chronological order which is so common in books of this kind. Facts and events have been grouped in accordance with their organic relationships, thus presenting an integrated picture. . . ." The original concept and arrangement have been proved sound by time, and hence have been retained through the second and this third edition. The main initial difficulties encountered by Edward Kremers and George Urdang likewise have persisted. They found that "material available for the book, while extensive, tends to be scattered and partial. . . . The authors have been faced with the persistent problem of selecting, rejecting, subordinating, and coordinating this mass of material with particular reference to the needs of American students." Secondly, it was "necessary constantly to keep in mind the varying pedagogic demands to be made on the book"; as a result, the organization permits it to be "used for courses of different lengths by omitting certain chapters or portions of chapters."

This challenge of selecting and presenting a systematic account that would best serve a pharmacy student's needs—to help satisfy the urge we all share to know something about where we came from—has continued to dominate the work through two revisions. At the same time, trying to fill a broad gap in the English literature of pharmacy, the authors could not ignore the mature practitioner, or the reference needs of libraries, or the layman or historian seeking a lead to information on some pharmaceutical development. The original authors therefore tried to give the book dual service as a reference volume by including (beyond normal textbook requirements) precise detail in the narrative, careful documentation, and an encyclopedic supplement, and, in the second edition, by taking the first step in a plan for broadening geographic coverage.

These reference features were welcomed by those whose interests required more than a textbook; yet, teaching experience and reports from elsewhere convinced me that the scholarly weight of the book was not being too happily sustained by the average student, nor the scope readily encompassed in the normal course. To make the book more palatable to the student and yet retain as much of the reference value as possible, considerable textual detail has been moved to the "Notes and References" of the respective chapters, where it can still be consulted. Some detail (such as the original section on the U. S. Pharmacopeia) and the chapter on Spain have been omitted, reluctantly. Many dates have been either deleted as unimportant or placed in parentheses (but a good sense of time is important to keep one's thinking about the past orderly and sequential). Some material of particular reference value has been made into appendices. New illustrations have been added to enliven the narrative. The encyclopedic supplement elaborating the text (Appendix 7) has not only been brought up to date but has been pruned of entries tangential in topic or unessential in a textbook.

More important, an attempt has been made to bring the entire text into accord with historical findings since the second edition appeared, to take into account events and consequences on the pharmaceutical scene during the intervening years, to correct whatever errors came to my attention, and to edit the text with the aim of communicating effectively the development of the pharmacist's role through the sweep of history.

Anyone who has examined this rather monumental historical structure, brick by brick, must be respectful of the grand design and the heroic effort of Kremers and Urdang, which gave a solidity and successful expression to pharmacy's heritage unprecedented in English. How did it come about?

In his Preface of 1940, Edward Kremers explained that for years he "had the desire and intention of writing a history of pharmacy. Well meaning friends have prodded him on to the task. . . . The manifold and insistent duties of the author's teaching work left little leisure for the sustained effort necessary. Moreover, much detailed study and collecting of material has been essential in preparing such a history of pharmacy. The collecting and coordination of source material has been a primary interest to the author," he said, during his entire professional life. This collection has been characterized as unique in the United States and seldom equaled in Europe. It may therefore be permissible to consider Madison, Wisconsin, the natural birthplace of the history of American pharmacy.

One of the great American pharmacists, Kremers had the intellectual grasp of history to create the volume before us, but— not himself a professional historian—he could not meet the insatiable demand for time and concentration to give his dream reality. At the end of his career, however, Kremers had the satisfaction of bringing to Madison one of the great European pharmacists, a pharmaceutical journalist who had become the first in Germany to earn a doctorate on the basis of historical studies centered about his own profession. At the University of Wisconsin, without official position at first, Urdang dedicated himself to giving fulfillment to Kremers' long-standing plans for a *History of Pharmacy*.

"The effective stimulus leading to the actual writing of the book was the presence and help of a colleague, Dr. George Urdang, whose entire time could be devoted to the work. The general plan and organization of the book are the senior author's," Kremers noted, "while the actual composition, documentation, etc. have been done by Dr. Urdang, to whom full credit should be given for the manner in which this difficult and arduous task has been performed."

In his preface to the second edition (1951), Urdang commented, "Shortly after the publication of the first edition, in 1941, Edward Kremers, the man who gave the initiative to the writing, died, and the responsibility of making the present revision was assigned to his coauthor. The author of this revision is glad that there was no need for a change of the arrangement, with its attempt at a sociologic integration in stead of a mere chronologic narration. . . . This new book has been changed in its content but not in its spirit and its goal. It has remained 'a guide and a survey,' to be used for teaching as well as for reading, as a book of reference so far as data and dates are concerned, and a book presenting and evaluating concepts."

As had Urdang in Germany, the present pharmacist-writer had been a pharmaceutical journalist who became the first in this country to earn a doctorate on the basis of historical studies centered about his own profession. Those studies were nearing completion when Urdang penned the above lines and added some kind words about his "friend and assistant, Glenn Sonnedecker, whose never-failing readiness . . ." had— one is now tempted to add—provided an apprenticeship on some of the more tedious aspects of that first revision!

In 1960 the second of the book's remarkable original authors died. To try to carry forward the working center for pharmacy's history that these two had established at Madison, including the preparation of this third edition, has been my privilege. It will be obvious and understandable that the structural soundness of the original conception left no need for major remodeling.

There has been much talk of the need for ensuring that a man professionally educated be a man generally educated also— in pharmacy, a practitioner equipped for a high level of citizenship within the profession and within his community. One natural bridge between the humanistic and the technical is formed by the profession's own history, which seems essential to an adequate understanding and philosophy of the pharmacist's role in society. For such reasons, a majority of the schools devote a course or a substantial part of a course to the historical development of pharmacy,* and it appears as a required subject in all course patterns shown in the influential study, *The Pharmaceutical Curriculum* by Lloyd E. Blauch and George L. Webster,† on the ground that "no subject so readily lends itself to developing in the pharmacist the orientation he should have as a professional person, to producing in him a sense of appreciation for, and pride in, his profession."

To provide an introduction to the knowledge and the values furthering that purpose, and as a basis for discussion and more specialized reading, the *History of Pharmacy* was written.

ACKNOWLEDGMENTS

During preparation of this third edition, Professor David L. Cowen of Rutgers, The State University of New Jersey, has been generous above all others in providing information and advice (especially for the chapters on the American colonies, the Revolution, and legislative standards). Among European colleagues, particularly valuable guidance concerning the chapters on their own countries was generously given by Dr. Maurice Bouvet and Dr. H. Bonnemain (France), Professor Wolfgang Schneider (Germany) and Dr. T. Douglas Whittet (England).

Besides appreciation to authors whose work has been drawn on and cited in the footnotes, special thanks are due to the following men for personal help either through revision material and suggestions or through critical reading of portions of the proof: Professor George E. Osborne of the University of Rhode Island, George B. Griffenhagen of the American Pharmaceutical Association (especially for Appendix 5 on museums), Professor Alex Berman of the University of Texas, and Professors Robert W. Hammel, Ernst W. Stieb and Dale E. Wurster of the University of Wisconsin.

Dean A. H. Uhl of the University of Wisconsin kindly volunteered to relieve me of a teaching responsibility for one semester to further completion of the work. Cleo Sonnedecker provided sympathetic understanding and beyond that, thinking as well as typing that proved to be of major assist-

---

* Amer. J. Pharm. Educ. *16*:16, 1952.

† Washington, D. C., 1952, pp. 162-3, 213-4, 235-5.

ance. As in most such ventures, librarians and libraries provided essential collaboration, but space restricts specific mention to the University of Wisconsin Library and the Pharmacy Librarian in particular, Miss Dolores Nemec.

Publishers and organizations who have permitted quotations, answered queries, or provided illustrations have been thanked privately, but their collective contribution deserves recognition here also.

Any standard work that goes through repeated revisions becomes increasingly an amalgam of the thought and the work of so many individuals that it is hard to iden-tify, much less adequately recognize their contributions. Among these are the collaborators mentioned in the Preface to the first and the second editions as particularly helpful, a service that continues to merit recognition of Mr. Howard Bayles, Dr. M. Bouvet and M. Louis Irissou, Profs. Guillermo Folch Jou and Rafael Folch Andreu.

As George Urdang dedicated the second edition to "the memory of his friend Edward Kremers," so I dedicate this edition in the same spirit to both of them, with the high respect and grateful memory shared by so many pharmacists everywhere.

GLENN SONNEDECKER

Contents

Part Three: Pharmacy in the United States

SECTION ONE. THE PERIOD OF UNORGANIZED DEVELOPMENT

Notes and References

Appendices

Part One

Pharmacy's Early Antecedents

1:   Ancient Prelude

Wherever civilization arises we find "pharmacy," because it fulfills one of man's basic needs. This effort to grasp from nature whatever might shield us from affliction became old as a service before it was new as a "profession." Its origins have disappeared into the veiled millennia—perhaps as much as a million years—that hide the origin of man himself.

Various opinions about pharmacy's origin continue to be put forward, because speculation is tempered only by logic and analogy when there is not much real evidence. More is known about prehistoric man's diseases, for many traces of damage were written indelibly into bones that awaited the archaeologist's shovel. But the earliest random and desperate efforts to use natural resources as "drugs" left scarcely an enduring trace.

For prehistoric man, we would suppose that therapy would not be first of all drug therapy. Disease came upon him with such mysterious ways and frightening forces that, as an imaginative and rational being, he must have concluded that "supernatural" countermeasures were called for—measures that for *him* were a part of the ordinary natural world. The "magic" thus invoked ultimately was reinforced by a custom of using plants and other objects in ways that brought their friendly spirits to bear on the evil powers manifested by disease. Even if only a blind empiric groping over many tens of thousands of years should be postulated, it would be understandable that by the time of the earliest written record, about four thousand years ago, the materia medica already included quite a number of substances which we call pharmacologically active, as well as substances having only the higher spirit-powers (what we call inert). This trend of speculation about the origins of pharmaceutical endeavor seems reasonable in the light of the pharmaco-magical beliefs of millions of our contemporaries.

Clearly, magic and empiricism each played an important role in the finding and the employing of remedies. Yet, it can be said that "neither empiricism nor magic stands at the beginning of the internal employment of remedies by men but the animal function, the instinct."[1] Instinct was affirmed or denied by an increasingly self-conscious empiricism. This empiricism became the foundation of our medical and pharmaceutical "science" as observations were systematized and constantly purified by inductive and deductive reasoning. In the whole field of medicine so much remained beyond ordinary observation, explanation or control that for thousands of years magical-religious practices tended to pervade medical practices, and only in our own millennium have they been placed gradually in a separate category.

This is not the place to argue whether the great civilizations of the ancient Far East or of the Middle East were the earliest and the most original, pharmaceutically speaking. The linguistic problems of comparative study are so challenging and the dating of ancient evidence is so often speculative that we remain uncertain about the locus of many medical and technologic innovations of antiquity, and the directions in which their influence ran.

The Far Eastern civilizations hold great historical interest for their early achievements and their imperfectly understood influence on Western culture, especially as mediated by the ancient Greeks and the medieval Arabs. Interesting accounts of premodern pharmacy in the Far East, and its rich materia medica, now may be read in Western languages to a certain extent, such as in the English writings of G. P. Srivastava, an Indian pharmacist.[2]

However, pharmacy in the West sees its early antecedents most clearly in the river valleys of the Nile, the Tigris and the Euphrates. Today's ruins once throbbed with magnificent civilizations as remarkable in their own time as the westerly cultures that they helped to shape.

BABYLONIA-ASSYRIA

In a southern Babylonian kingdom of city states, in the region of today's Iraq, the Sumerians developed a system of cuneiform writing by about 3000 B.C., thereby entering the historical period. They and the heirs of Sumerian civilization—Babylonia and, later, Assyria—left thousands of clay tablets in the ruins of their remarkable civilizations. Their history remained locked in the clay until about a century ago, when a few men recaptured enough of the "lost language" to make serious attempts at translation. Today we have a fairly clear picture of the general development of this part of the ancient world, although research still goes on and adds continuously to our knowledge. However, our knowledge of medicine and pharmacy in Babylonia-Assyria remains fragmentary.

General Therapeutic Concepts

The ideologic fundamentals of Babylonian-Assyrian medicine have been described as follows:

. . . as a consequence of the persistent hold maintained by the belief in signs of all kinds, disease became primarily an omen, the interpretation of which on the part of the priest as diviner supplemented the efforts of the priest as exorciser; while the priest as healer availed himself of both these aids to supplement his efforts in the direct treatment of the disease. These three aspects of Babylonian-Assyrian medicine—exorcism, divination and medical treatment—blend together to form a composite picture in which it is not always possible to distinguish the different strains.[3]

Illness was a divine punishment, and healing a purification. With this, medicine had its fixed place in the religious ideology, in the immemorial purification from sin through penance, called "catharsis." This concept of catharsis, which entered into various religions, found its most famous expression in the sacrifice of Jesus Christ, who gave his life to purify sinful mankind. The fact that medicine in antiquity (i.e., in Babylonia-Assyria, Egypt and, partly, in Greece) stood within the ideology of "catharsis" categorizes it as "archaic" medicine.[4]

This interests the pharmacist specifically because it explains the original meaning of the Greek word *pharmakon* (see Appendix 7), from which we have made the term "pharmacy" and its derivatives. From the religious ideology of catharsis there emerged the word and the concept *pharmakon*, in the sense of a means of purification through purging. This idea—first spiritual, then pharmacologic—finds a still more direct expression in the term "cathartics" for especially effective purgatives.

Ancient cultures always must be considered from the standpoint of their time, that is, the outlook on life afforded by their own spiritual, geographic and economic conditions. Thus it would be unfair to accept as proof of an "unscientific" spirit the fact that Babylonian-Assyrian, ancient Egyptian, and the early part of Greek medicine contained a great deal of "magic." For these peoples, magic was a part of systematized "science." It went hand in hand with empiric discoveries[5] and was no doubt harmonized with the latter.

Drugs

We find a comprehensive materia medica in these times of "archaic" medicine. R. Campbell Thompson examined many hundreds of the clay tablets from the library of King Assurbanipal of Assyria.[6] He succeeded in identifying 250 vegetable drugs and 120 mineral drugs. He also found that alcoholic beverages, fats and oils, parts of animals, honey, wax and various milks were then being used medicinally.

Many, if not all, of the minerals mentioned by the Greek Dioscorides in his famous book on materia medica (1st century after Christ) were apparently already known and used by the Assyrians. Excrements likewise played a part in the Babylonian-Assyrian therapy. Filth was expected to disgust the evil spirit that had invaded the body of the patient and cause it to leave forthwith.[7]

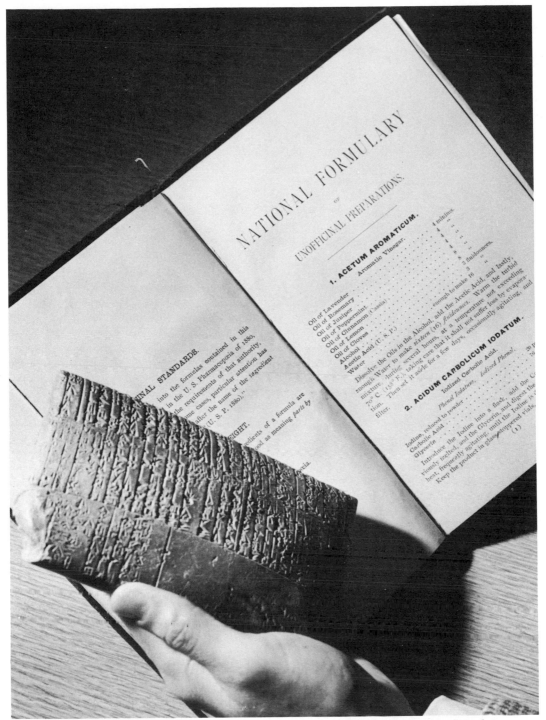

Replica of the first formulary known, cast from the original in the University of Pennsylvania Museum. Believed to be the oldest pharmaceutical document the contents of which are known, this clay tablet has been dated toward the end of the third millennium B.C. An unknown Sumerian wrote the drug formulas on the small slab of soft clay with a reed stylus, then baked the tablet hard. It is one "leaf" among thousands of tablets dug up at Nippur, representing part of man's earliest written records. It is being held against the background of a first edition of the National Formulary (1888).

Among the drugs of vegetable origin we find pine turpentine, styrax, galbanum, hellebore, myrrh, asafoetida, calamus, ricinus, mentha, poppy-opium, glycyrrhiza, mandragora, cannabis, crocus, thymus.

As to the modes of administration, we find mention of medicated wines, draughts, mixtures, ointments, embrocations, cataplasms, enemas, poultices, plasters, lotions, infusions, decoctions and fumigations.

The oldest pharmaceutical document now known tells how the Sumerians prepared some of these drugs, perhaps about 4,000 years ago. It contains a series of drug formulas such as the following:

"Pulverize the seed of the 'carpenter' plant [perhaps *Gymnosporia serrata* Loes], the gum resin of the markasi plant, [and] thyme; dissolve it in beer; let the man drink."[8]

Mesopotamian drug formulas such as this one typically were not quantitative (although their Egyptian counterparts were). This is especially curious, since the system of weights and measures invented by the Babylonians has been considered to be one of their contributions to civilization.

Their materia medica "includes substances which presuppose a broad acquaintance with many chemical operations," Sumerologist Martin Levey observes, "and elaborate procedures are implied in the text in order that the substances listed may have been obtained."[9]

Incantations and magic were so much a part of Mesopotamian culture that it may be sheer accident that they form no part of the earliest formulary known. After all, it is a single clay tablet, only partly legible, which probably was one "page" of a longer document. Later records illustrate how incantations gave drugs their healing power or enhanced it. Probably some substances eventually were recognized to have inherent healing power that made them useful without priestly intervention.[10] However, many centuries passed before a new interpretation of the causes of disease (abandoning the supernatural) removed the magico-religious core of pharmaceutical and medical practices as exemplified in both ancient Mesopotamia and Egypt.

A class of preparers of remedies and cosmetics is said to have arisen, called "pasisu," but we find no details about the time of its documentary appearance and its position in relation to medicine. In Sippar at the time of the great Babylonian king Hammurabi (about 2111 B.C.), the retailers of drugs seem to have plied their trade in a special street.[11]

Mythology and the Healing Arts

The Babylonian-Assyrian gods mentioned most frequently in the incantations often interspersed among drug formulas are Ea and Gula. Of special interest is the fact that the serpent cult and the use of the serpent as a symbol appear already in Babylonian-Assyrian mythology. There was a medical god, Ninazu, "the lord of physicians." His son Ningischzida functioned as messenger of the gods. The symbols of both were the rod and the serpent, reminding us of the modern symbol of medicine, although that comes to us from the later Greek culture. The Babylonians venerated Sachan "as a symbol and as a healing god."[12]

In Babylonia observation of the planets and the stars laid the groundwork not only for the science of astronomy, but simultaneously for the pseudoscience of astrology, which had pharmaco-medical applications in its claim to determining a relationship between the course and the constellation of the stars and life on earth.

EGYPT

The Babylonian-Assyrian and the ancient Egyptian cultures were closely related. Both had a theocratic foundation, and theurgic medicine prevailed in both of them. On the whole, Egyptian medicine appears to have been less dominated by metaphysical concepts. Nevertheless, there is an obvious similarity between the Assyrian and the Egyptian medical texts,[13] and there were epochs during which the magic elements in Egyptian medicine gained in prominence.

Not until the early 19th century was a beginning made in deciphering the ancient Egyptian hieroglyphics. In 1799 the famous "Rosetta stone" was found near the

Rosetta mouth of the Nile. It bore a tri-lingual inscription in hieroglyphics, demotic characters (simplified hieroglyphics in use since about 700 B.C.) and Greek. This gave the Frenchman J. F. Champollion the first clue toward deciphering hieroglyph-ics, the mysteries of which hid many glories of the ancient Egyptian civilization. In spite of much progress in the meantime, the correct interpretation of the documents concerned—not least of all the puzzle of identifying drugs referred to in medical papyri—remains a difficult problem.

Medical Papyri

There are eight medical papyri thus far translated and commented on. All of them were written between about 1900 and 1100 B.C.[14] Much of the knowledge contained in them probably is far older than the textual copies that have come down to us.

The Papyrus Ebers (bearing the name of a German Egyptologist, Georg Ebers) contains the greatest number of drugs and formulas, but the medical papyri as a group testify to the extensive attention accorded the preparation and the use of drugs.

Thorough analysis of the entire material by Grapow (beginning in 1935)[15] has done much to recapture a picture of ancient Egyptian medicine; meanwhile other highly specialized studies have added pieces to the mosaic.

Ebers Papyrus. Containing remnants of many different books, but complete as written and more than 20 meters long, the Ebers Papyrus has attracted scholars again and again to its challenging and rewarding text. The work is so difficult that it has been said of even the most recent translation[16]:

> The identification of many names of diseases, symptoms and drugs by Ebbell is the result of long labor . . . yet even on superficial reading of the translation, one becomes doubtful as to the reliability of these identifications. In most cases they are mere conjectures . . .[17]

The text is dominated by drug formulas and, when taken with other evidence, sug-gests that the pharmaceutical side of medi-cal care received more attention than it did in ancient Greece later on when medical concepts left a relatively large place for

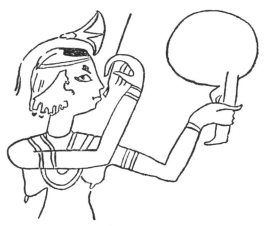

An ancient Egyptian artist caricatures a girl who holds a mirror in one hand and, with the other, applies red-ochre rouge to her lips (about 1200 B.C.). She knew other cosmetic devices such as eye and face pigments, perfumes, hair dye, wigs, cleansing unguents and elaborate make-up kits. The Papyrus Ebers in-cludes cosmetic as well as therapeutic formulas, and artifacts testify that even before the earliest written history human vanity had established the importance of cosmetics. (From the Oriental Institute, Univ. of Chicago *in* Hughes, G. R.: J. Soc. Cosm. Chem. *10*:159-176, 1959)

dietetics. In crude and basic form, the Egyptians knew most of our modes of ad-ministration by 1500 B.C., notably except-ing parenteral drugs. They used gargles, snuffs, inhalations, suppositories, fumiga-tions, enemas, poultices, decoctions, infu-sions, pills, troches, lotions, ointments and plasters. In the Ebers Papyrus alone, these various forms have been found, embracing more than 700 drugs in more than 800 pre-scriptions.

The drugs were drawn from the plant, the animal and the mineral kingdoms, but botanic drugs predominate for internal use —such as acacia, castor bean, wormwood, date, fennel, fig, garlic and poppy seeds. There appear to be references to such min-eral substances as alum, iron oxide, lime-stone, sodium carbonate, salt and sulfur. Excrements of various animals were used occasionally, as we noted in Babylonia-Assyria. Beer, milk, wine and honey were popular vehicles. Honey and wax were often used as binding agents in the formulas.[18]

A representative formula reads:

Another to clear out purulency:

Hyoscyamus	2 ro
Dates	4 ro
Wine	5 ro
Ass's milk	20 ro

are boiled, strained and taken for four days.[19]

The quantitative formulas favored by the ancient Egyptian practitioners—and usually lacking in Babylonian formulas—customarily specify measures rather than weights, even for dry substances.[20] As seen in the above formula, a "ro" is about 15 ml. The 4 days specified as the course of treatment occurs commonly in Egyptian pharmaco-therapy and may originate in magic

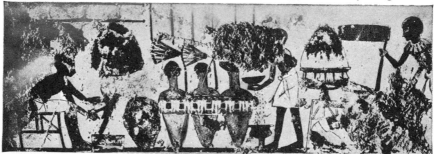

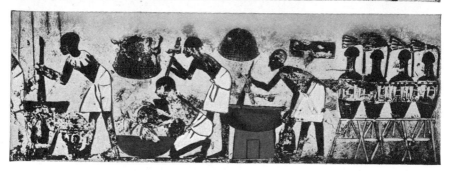

Egyptian ointment kitchen portrayed in a tomb painting of the 18th dynasty. The time is prior to 1400 B.C. (The original painting is here divided, the upper reproduction being the left half of the original and the lower, the right half.)

Interpretation of this picture is not entirely certain, but comparison with contemporary paintings shows that this is no common kitchen. Using classical representations of ointment kitchens for comparison, the following interpretation is presumably correct:

A man (lower left) is crushing oil fruits, in a mortar, which have been taken from baskets. A workman near the table bearing the mound of finished ointment (upper right) is comminuting a drug, possibly frankincense or myrrh. The ointment cook (right center, below) melts some of the drug with animal fat (suet) in the kettle on the hearth, to impart the proper consistency. Finally, a kneeling man (left center, below) shapes the cooled ointment into round lumps.

Treatment of wine with rosin, called rosinizing, seems to be illustrated also. Two of the three jugs (left center, above) are closed with clay stoppers, and on the third a bowl has been placed. A man seems to be holding a sieve through which the liquid is flowing into the container underneath. Perhaps he is straining the rosin which was added to the wine to give it the peculiar taste relished even today in eastern Mediterranean countries.

The man at the extreme upper left appears to be hewing a log or plug. Before him are baskets which probably contain some crude ingredient used by these ancient preparers of medicines. (After Walter Wreszinski, *Atlas zur altaegyptischen Kulturgeschichte*, Plate 356.)

formula rather than in clinical observation.

Mortars, hand mills, sieves and balances were commonly used in technologic operations such as pharmaceutical compounding.

Copies of the drug formulas were handed from one practitioner to another and from one generation to the next. Sometimes a scribe, ignorant of medicine, would simply combine in his copy a number of simple ingredients listed originally as individual prescriptions. "This procedure," says Chauncey Leake, "may have contributed to the rise of polypharmacy."

The straightforward formulas occupy so much space in the Ebers Papyrus that the generally applicable incantations of the introduction tend to be subordinated. Although the Egyptologist Ebbell prefers to look on them merely as "evidence of the piety of the Egyptians,"[21] it appears that they were intended for use whenever a remedy was applied or a bandage loosened, and that they were intended, not surprisingly, to reinforce the drugs with divine power against "afflictions [caused] by a god or goddess, by a dead man or woman, etc."

Edwin Smith Papyrus. A treatise that revealed the surgical side of Egyptian medicine has been considered to be equally as important as the Ebers Papyrus commented on above and, perhaps, still more impressive because of its organization, wealth of information and freedom from magical elements. Since the publication of the text, the translation and the commentary by the pioneer American Egyptologist James Henry Breasted (an erstwhile pharmacist), respect for the medicine achieved by so ancient a people has increased considerably. The distinguished medical historian Henry Sigerist has called the work of Breasted "one of the most accomplished editions that has ever been made of an ancient text."[22]

Egyptian Medicinal Plants

The opinion has been expressed that there were not many indigenous medicinal plants in ancient Egypt due to topographic peculiarity. The country was bounded on the east by the Arabian desert and on the

west by the Libyan desert, thus restricting the populace to the valley inundated by the Nile. This hypothesis seemed to be probable. On the other hand, Theophrastus (4th century B.C.), quoting the verses of Homer, praises the many and efficacious medicinal plants of ancient Egypt; Dioscorides (1st century A.D.) mentions the Egyptian origin of 80 vegetable drugs that he described. Dawson[23] states that the pomegranate was not indigenous to Egypt but must have been cultivated extensively there about 1100 B.C. We may suppose that the ancient Egyptians also cultivated other plants originally not indigenous to their country and used them medicinally.[24]

Mythology

The specialization of pharmaceutical activities found its expression even in Egyptian mythology. The tasks of the divine house of medicine and of the chamber of embalmment were assigned to a special god, Anepu (called Anubis by the Greeks), who thus might be regarded in one respect as the pharmacist of the gods.[25]

As in other ancient countries governed or influenced by theocratic rule, medicine in Egypt was supposed to have originated with some mythologic deities of the country. In Egypt, notably Thoth, Osiris, Isis, Horus and Imhotep play this role. Gradually, Imhotep became more and more the divine representative of medicine in Egypt. Imhotep was a real personage, one of the earliest of known physicians. He lived about 3000 B.C. and was deified 2,500 years after his death. The Greeks reportedly saw in Imhotep (whom they called Imouthes) a representation of their own god of the healing arts, Asklepios.[26] According to Egyptian mythology, Isis, the wife of Osiris, revealed to her son Horus the secret of pharmacy.

The Practice of Medicine and Pharmacy

We have noted in ancient Babylonia-Assyria a group of preparers of medicine, of whom we have no detailed knowledge. However, they did not play an important part in the development of medicine and pharmacy. The variety of preparations used in Egyptian medicine requiring professional skill implies a more definitely distinguished group of preparers of medicine, and we find that such a group did exist.

The exact character and refinement of "pharmacy" at such a remote time eludes us. To present any systematic account of pharmaceutical practice requires scholarly conjectures and assumptions based on single passages or even a half-understood phrase in the ancient hieroglyphics.

With this in mind, we present a free translation of the conclusions put forward by the medical Egyptologist, Frans Jonckheere:

The personnel of pharmacy included two echelons, in Egypt: a group of specialist-functionaries and a complex of technical services, the first being hierarchically above the latter.

In the category of well-informed pharmaceutical workers we should place especially the "chief of the preparers of drugs" and the "conservator of drugs," perhaps associating with them a "priest-herbalist."

In the group of technicians, one perhaps distinguishes "collectors of drugs" and "laboratory aides."

Here, then, carrying or not a particular name, are those who form a class of "pharmacists," so to speak.

The evidence duly attesting to this medical auxiliary—not physician and not layman—reduces to nothing the notion that medical prescriptions were executed in a laboratory annexed to the temple, by "priest-physicians."

On the other hand, it forces the partisans of the idea of pharmaceutical work being in the hands of physicians alone to correct their point of view, and it invites them to accept, at the side of the man of healing art, the presence of an assistant charged with the preparation of remedies, a task that he at times fulfilled in the home of the patients.

In conclusion, the classic opinion ought to be erased that the place is in Rome—and in part of the 4th century solely—for the first appearance of a specialist, the *pigmentarius*, for preparing and delivering the prescribed products, in view of our "preparer of remedies," a lower echelon of a veritable pharmaceutical organization of which we have been able to catch only a glimpse in the complex administrative cadre.[27]

To what extent do these views clash with what Henry Sigerist had written before Jonckheere completed his wide-ranging critical study? Sigerist wrote:

There was no pharmacist in ancient Egypt. The physician himself compounded his remedies or his servants did it under his supervision, just as he and his assistants probably gathered the necessary ingredients and stored them in the house. . . . Drugs imported from abroad were probably stored in royal warehouses, whence the physicians could obtain them.[28]

The two views are not as incompatible as they may seem to be at first. What meaning should we expect of the term "pharmacist" as applied to conditions in Egypt 3,500 years ago (or for that matter, America 100 years ago)? In any event, both scholars see a probable assistant, or associate, of the physician with special responsibility for pharmaceutical work. For drugs imported or brought from the remote countryside by the "collectors of drugs," the pharmaceutical associate may well have depended on stocks held by Sigerist's "royal warehouse." Jonckheere's evidence holds a counterpart in the "House of Life" (medical training center at Saïs?), where apparently drugs were both collected into storage (under the "conservator of drugs") and prepared, at least in certain instances, by "those who fabricate the medicaments." When we note that there was a designation for "chief of those who fabricate the medicaments," quite distinct from medical functions, it must also be noted that at least in the House of Life this "chief" was also chief of the royal physicians, among various other titles.

Indeed, in reading recent studies of individual papyri it is hard to escape the feeling that the person who practiced medicine often practiced pharmacy also, even though pharmaceutical work may have been more distinct and distinctive—at least at the more centralized level—than we once believed.

In positing pharmaceutical activities in medical care distinct from priestly ministrations and temple "laboratories" (yet not denying a theurgic foundation), Jonckheere and Sigerist stand together against past views. If tomorrow the Egyptian sands yield additional documents, the picture of our early antecedents may be unified or, more probably, it may be diversified into several different, clearer pictures, by supplying evidence of how different medical practices were in different periods of Egypt's long history.

For example, Hermann Grapow[29] believes that ancient Egyptian medicine, revealing a "scientific character," reached its full development before 1600 B.C. but, in the time of the New Kingdom, degenerated into sorcery.

This statement offers an explanation for the differences of opinion as to the "magical" or "rational" character of medicine in ancient Egypt. In the more than 3,000 years of the empire's changing destiny, there were periods of cultural blossom in which rationalism reached a high degree, and others in which the dogmatic fetters were drawn tighter. However, there was never a time in which the theocratic regime and the theurgic ideology accompanying it lost their grip. Hence, even in periods of comparatively rational medical practice, there still remained the "archaic" superstructure.

With all due respect for the high standard of the ancient Egyptians' medicine and therapy under a theocratic system, for further developments we look to the astonishing culture achieved by the Greeks about a thousand years after the Egyptians reached their zenith.

GREECE AND ROME

Pharmacy in ancient Greece and Rome shows few differences, since the Romans adopted most of their customs from the Greeks and from them largely drew their ideas regarding medication.[30]

The Greeks, living on both sides of the Aegean Sea and on its islands, received many outside stimuli from both Mesopotamia and the Nile valley. Hence, if we compare the drugs and the forms of medication used by the ancient Egyptians with those used later on by the Greeks, we find that the differences are neither very great nor very important. The rise of the oldest and best known medical schools, Cos and Cnidos, on the main sealanes to the Orient facilitated a fruitful connection between ancient Egyptian and Greek medicine.

It is pertinent to recall the special character of ancient Greek civilization, which impressed itself so indelibly on the Western world and created what we call European culture. In contrast with the ancient Oriental peoples with their disregard of the individual, the Greeks (Attic and Ionian especially) based their culture on individuality. With the appearance of famous physicians different opinions were presented by the several schools. These varying viewpoints were defended in public. As a result, secrecy and mystery were replaced gradually by communication and critical discussion.

Mythology and Temple Medicine

A penchant for natural explanation and critical examination of old dogmas did not make the Greeks intolerant of religion or its place in healing. Rather, we find our own "modern" view that lay medicine must pursue diagnosis and treatment of disease within the framework of natural science, yet must not deny that the supernatural may have a separate place in the patient's resources. At this stage medicine still had a severely limited scope of effectiveness, and it was a scientific merit of the best Greek physicians that they did not claim overmuch. Such modesty could not have been very satisfying to a desperately ill patient. Hence, we are not surprised at the popularity of the unlimited possibilities offered by several deities and demideities to whom healing qualities were attributed —for example, Apollo, among others. Prometheus was especially referred to as a preparer of remedies.

Beginning in the 7th century B.C., Asklepios gradually superseded Apollo as the greatest of healing gods. In his legend we find that the centaur Chiron taught Asklepios his pharmaceutical knowledge about drug plants growing in the Thessalian plains. Sanctuaries devoted to healing the sick were erected all over Greece, wherein dwelt the kindly but powerful spirit of Asklepios, aided by his two daughters, Hygeia and Panacea. What happened there finds an analogy in places of pilgrimage today. The image of Asklepios embodied so many of the finest qualities of medicine that he became a divine ideal for lay physicians, and the "staff of Asklepios" still remains the official symbol of medicine all over the world.[31]

Beside this Greek version of temple medicine, there flourished a lay system of medical practice, the finest exponent of which was the Hippocratic school. It rejected a theurgic conceptual basis for dealing with disease. Though by that time concepts and therapeutics usually found their explanation in the natural world, they eventually were shaped considerably by speculative philosophy, from which "science" could not yet be extricated.

Philosophy and Its Influence on Medical Concepts

Greece originated the systematized reasoning about phenomena of the universe and the place of the human being in it that we call philosophy. The very term "philosopher" has been derived from the Greek words *philos* (friend) and *sophia* (wisdom). Through the Greeks, wisdom has become available to everyone who seeks to be its friend.

Most of the philosophers were eager to explain nature and its phenomena in a rational way. They dealt likewise with the healing arts and even sometimes practiced them. The most important problem facing these early philosophers was this: What rational explanation can be found both for the origin of the kind of world that human beings are living in and for the diseases that are their lot? Above all, it was the nature of matter that asked for an investigation. The most alluring idea was that of one essential and fundamental substance from which everything in nature developed. Four Greek philosophers in turn conceived one fundamental principle after another. Finally, the fourth of these men not only

suggested one not advocated before but also linked it with the three fundamentals of earlier origin, into one conceptional unit.

Thales of Miletus (639-544 B.C.) considered water to be the one fundamental substance from which everything is derived; Anaximenes of Miletus (570-500 B.C.) suggested air (which he called *pneuma*); Heraclitus (556-460 B.C.) selected fire. Empedocles (b. 504 B.C.) added earth to these three primary principles and pronounced the theory of the so-called four elements, namely, water, air, fire and earth as the components of all matter, including the animal (hence human) body.

According to Empedocles, health was the result of equilibrium of these four elements in the body, and disease was the result of a disequilibrium. In their application to health and disease the four elements yielded the first rational medical theory.

The question naturally arises, why were the four elements eventually called "Aristotelian" elements in preference to "Empedoclean"? The answer is that Aristotle, a strong proponent of the four-element theory, was so famous as a philosopher and a natural scientist that he overshadowed by far all the other Greek philosophers working in the same field. For thousands of years—up to our time—he has been regarded (to quote the Italian Renaissance poet Dante) as "the Master of those who know." His writings present "an extraordinary accumulation of facts relating to the structure and functions of various parts of the body,"[32] and his influence on the entire development of European intellectual life, including medicine, was enormous.

Another Greek philosopher whose influence on medicine and pharmacy makes it necessary to mention him at this point was Pythagoras (580-489 B.C.). Generally known as the father of the so-called Pythagorean proposition and as the founder of a special philosophical-religious sect, he was also in all probability the first to discover a relation between musical pitch and the length of vibrating cords that can be expressed in definite numbers. This discovery was regarded by the Pythagorean sect as a confirmation of the Babylonian-Assyrian mystical evaluation of numbers. The number seven was considered especially significant, as expressing the idea of a relationship between the seven then-known planets (each of them assigned to and symbolizing one of the gods) and the seven metals that had been identified. In the Greco-Roman time the order was as follows:

Planets	Jupiter	Mars	Mercury	Moon	Saturn	Sun	Venus
Greek Gods	Zeus	Ares	Hermes	Selene	Cronos	Helios	Aphrodite
Roman Gods	Jupiter	Mars	Mercurius	Luna	Saturn	Apollo	Venus
Metals	Tin	Iron	Mercury	Silver	Lead	Gold	Copper
Symbols	♃	♂	☿	☾	♄	☉	♀

It was assumed that through the planets the gods exerted their influence on happenings on earth. This influence gradually became attributed to the planets themselves; hence, the factors revealing these influences at work were sought in the position of the stars at a particular time. On this basis the pseudoscience of astrology (from the Greek words *astron* (star) and *logos* (sense, reason, word)) developed.

In regard to pharmacy, it meant that the time when plants were to be collected and even when some preparations were to be compounded had to be chosen according to astrologic consideration.

One Greek idea—an atomic theory—about two thousand years later found a revival and verification, although very much modified. It was conceived in a speculative way by Leucippos and Democritus (about 440 B.C.). According to these philosophers, the world consists of indivisible small corpuscles that differ in shape and position but not in substance. The antique theory of atomism gave a boldly mechanistic explanation to motion and qualitative change.

Hippocratic Medical Writings

It was after the development of the theory of the four elements that Hippocrates entered the scene. This man posterity has termed "father of medicine." He was born about 460 B.C. on the island of Cos and died about 370 B.C. in Thessaly. However, "nowadays scholars have given up the use of the word Hippocrates as denoting an historical person who was the author of at least some of the books that are contained in the Hippocratean Corpus."[33] Probably not a single book in this Corpus, collected at Alexandria during the 4th and 3rd centuries B.C., can be associated definitely with Hippocrates.[34] The fact that these books were written not by one individual genius but by a number of physicians of the Hippocratic school of thought proves that the high scientific and ethical level evidenced in these writings was not achieved by one great man only. Rather, it was representative of Greek medicine in the 5th through the 3rd centuries B.C.

Hippocratic "Humors." In the Hippocratic Corpus the concept of the harmony of the four elements (of which the body was supposed to consist) was replaced by the concept of the harmony or disharmony of the "four humors" as the cause of health or sickness. These four humors paralleled the four elements. To the authors of the Hippocratic Corpus this concept remained an explanatory theory and did not become a binding doctrine. They were empiricists, believing in the healing power of nature and believing that the task of the physician is to help nature to help herself. "The great Hippocratic group imply the doctrine of humors in their phraseology and outlook on symptoms, but it is in the background, and nowhere are the humors described."[35]

Drugs and Therapeutics. Although the regulation of diet occupies the most important place in the Hippocratic Corpus, we also find many drugs, mainly of vegetable origin. Wootton[36] lists 195 drugs; other sources record as many as 400. The pharmaceutical processes mentioned in the Corpus are manifold and include the preparation of fomentations, poultices, gargles, pessaries, pills, ointments, oils, cerates, collyria, looches (i.e., lohochs), troches and inhalations. Narcotics were known and used (juice of the poppy, henbane seeds and mandragora). The frequent references to purgatives, sudorifics, emetics and enemas are due to the Hippocratic theory that the first requirement of medical treatment has to be the purification of the body from illness-producing humors.

This purification represented a bodily catharsis and led to a change in the concept of the word *pharmakon* from the original meaning of a charm, whether a healing or a poisonous one. The word *pharmakon* in the Hippocratic Corpus means a purifying remedy and, later, became the general designation for remedy.

Simplicity, freedom from irrationalism and, especially, the idea that each individual represents a unit that has to be treated as such are regarded as main features of the Hippocratic theory and therapy. For this reason, throughout the ages, whenever medicine had lost itself too much in complexities and disregard for the individual patient, the battle cry could and can be heard: "Back to Hippocrates!"

Hippocratic Oath. If the name Hippocrates is "a name without writings" or, more correctly, a collective name for various writings by different unknown authors, who then wrote the famous "oath of Hippocrates"?[37] Only recently has this question been answered satisfactorily, at least as to the time of the conception and the spiritual origin of this first-known and most significant manifestation of professional medical ethics.

Apparently the oath was composed shortly after the death of Hippocrates, not later than "the fourth century B.C." However, it expresses not ideas then dominant but those of the Pythagorean philosophical-religious sect. Therefore, it must have been adherents of this sect who composed the oath. Since it mirrored the ideas of a Greek minority, it did not become popular until the end of antiquity, when "a new religion [Christianity] arose that changed the very foundation of ancient civilization." The similarity of the Pythagorean concepts to those of Christianity, together with the desire of Greek physicians in Rome to maintain their exclusive rights, gradually made the Hippocratic Oath generally recognized.

The School of Alexandria

The victorious sweep of Alexander the Great through the Eastern world brought in its wake the spread of the Greek way of thought over this enormous area. The founding of Alexandria in 331 gave this *Magna Graecia* a new cultural center that soon overshadowed in importance the old seat of Greek wisdom, Athens.

Under the Greek dynasty of the Ptolemies there developed the famous library where, for instance, the Hippocratic Corpus was preserved. A medical school there not only replaced but outshone its predecessors at Cos and Cnidos. At Alexandria different medical sects developed. The most important sects became known as "empiricists" or "experimentalists" and as "methodists."

"Empiricists" followed the Hippocratic idea of therapy based primarily on experience, allowing its adherents conclusions but not speculations. Its main representative was Herophilus (about 300 B.C.) who was a more ardent advocate of the use of drugs than the Hippocratic physicians were.

The "methodists" followed a special "method" propagated by Themison (about 300 B.C.) and elaborated on by Soranos (about A.D. 100). This method was based on a theory that disease resulted from too strong or too weak tension of the walls of the ducts in the body or, as they called it, the *status laxus* or the *status strictus*. The former condition called for strengthening by physical exercise and irritating drugs; the other called for relaxation and soothing drugs. Since this theory was based on the "solids" rather than the "humors" of the body, it is termed one kind of solidar pathology.

Pharmaceutical Botanists

Before, during and after the time of Hippocrates there was a group of experts in medicinal plants. Their group name, *rhizotomoi* (from the Greek word *rizoma*, the mass of roots of trees), points to frequent use of roots in Greek therapy. Tschirch characterizes this group of people as follows:

The *rhizotomoi* were erudite pharmacobotanists whose writings, if they had come to us, would probably fill the niche between Homer and Hippocrates and would show where the representatives of the Hippocratic period got their knowledge of medicinal plants. The fragments, which we know, are not less valuable than the writings of Dioscorides and contain the very earliest descriptions of medicinal plants.[38]

The rhizotomoi collected the indigenous vegetable roots and sold them. In addition they themselves often practiced medicine. Probably the most important representative of these rhizotomoi was Diocles of Carystos (4th century B.C.). He is considered to be the source for all Greek pharmacotherapeutic treatises between the time of Theophrastus (d. 286 B.C.) and Dioscorides (fl. A.D. 60). Another famous rhizotomist, Crateuas (first century B.C.), left us the earliest known illustrated herbal.[39]

Theophrastus, friend and pupil of Aristotle, was primarily a botanist, so distinguished that he is often called the "father of botany." Historians agree that the herbal of Theophrastus was not one of the sources used by Dioscorides, the man who is remembered in history as the first to deal with medical botany as an applied science —that is, as the first real pharmacognosist.

It is not certain whether or not Dioscorides practiced medicine. However, it is known that he accompanied the Roman armies through Asia Minor and also traveled in Italy, Greece, Gaul and Spain, collecting information about plants of possible use in medicine. He not only described the drugs of his time and explained their effect but also arranged his descriptions systematically. This made him the first teacher of materia medica and his treatise the most important and most used source in this field. Many later authors (up to the 17th century!) tried to identify the plants in their native countries according to the descriptions given by Dioscorides for Mediterranean plants, which caused many mistakes. However, they are the best proof of the high authority accorded Dioscorides.

Dioscorides' *De materia medica libri quinque* was translated into English (1655) and today is still kept in print[40] as a classic representing an intellectual milestone in the development of pharmacy and botany. The contents of the five books are arranged as follows: Book I: aromatics, oils, ointments, trees; Book II: living creatures, milk and

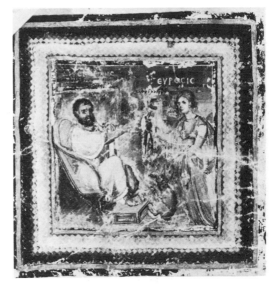

The miniature shown was painted into a manuscript copy of Dioscorides' work on pharmacy and applied botany early in the 6th century. This antique cornerstone of pharmaceutical science appears to be the oldest illustrated work of its kind that has survived. The artist depicted a sage (intended to be Dioscorides, seated) receiving a forked mandrake root (center) from a female figure (Eurasis, right). The magical power of the mandrake has forced the dog (bottom, center) back on its haunches in a paroxysm of agony, which reflects one of the superstitions about this solanaceous drug that commanded awesome respect up to modern times. (Codex Vindobonensis, Med. Gr. 1, f. 4r., Austrian National Library, Vienna; from MacKinney-Smith Fund Collection of Medical Miniatures, University of North Carolina)

dairy products, cereals and sharp herbs; Book III: roots, juices, herbs; Book IV: herbs and roots; Book V: vines and wines, metallic ores.

Dioscorides knew the preparation of leadplaster from fats and lead oxide. He mentions the processes of purifying woolfat, of making extracts by maceration followed by evaporation (e.g., extracts of glycyrrhiza) and of expressing the fresh juice of plants and concentrating it by exposure to the sun. He knew the difference between various gums, such as acacia, tragacanth and the gums of cherry, plum and almond. He explained the usual adulterations and suggested means of discovering them. His remarks on the collection of drugs are excellent. His directions for storage, since they are the first known and formed the basis for many later writers, may be quoted:

Flowers and sweet-scented things should be laid up in drug boxes of lime wood; but there are some herbs which do well enough if wrapped up in papers or leaves for the preservation of their seeds. For moist [liquid] medicines some thicker [impermeable] material such as silver, or glass, or horn will agree best. Yes, and earthenware if it be not thin [permeable] is fitting enough, and so is wood, particularly if it be box-wood. Vessels of brass will be suitable for eye-medicines and for liquids and for all that are compounded of vinegar or of liquid pitch or of Cedria, but fats and marrows ought to be put up in vessels of tin. (Translation by John Goodyer.)

Galen

As personified by Hippocrates, Greek medicine of the 5th and 4th centuries B.C. gave the world the spirit of real medicine; to Dioscorides it is indebted for fundamentals of materia medica and to Pliny for a summary of ancient knowledge. What entitles Galen to be added to this illustrious group? Galen was born in Pergamon (ca. A.D. 131), practiced and taught medicine extremely successfully in Rome and died (ca. A.D. 201) in his native town. What carried his name through the ages was the fact that he created a system of pathology and therapy that ruled western medicine for 1,500 years. This was possible because of the logic of his system, the reverence for his authority and the lack of experimental methods that would readily reveal the fallacies embedded in his brilliant writings.

Galen drew from all available sources whatever he thought worthwhile (mostly without giving any references). "His habit," says Albutt, "was to mention not those he copied but those he attacked."[41] There was at least one exception: Hippocrates. Galen regarded himself as the one whose task it was to complete and systematize the work

ascribed to "the father of medicine," and it was, indeed, "essentially in the form of Galenism that Greek medicine was transmitted to after ages."[42]

The school of Hippocrates had formulated the theory of the four humors (paralleling the four elements), the correct balance of which meant health, while every disturbance of this balance spelled disease. To the authors of the Hippocratic Corpus this concept had been only a convenient theory. Galen made a stringent rule out of it. There were the four humors: blood, phlegm (supposed to come from the brain), yellow bile (supposed to be secreted from the liver) and black bile (supposed to come from the spleen and the stomach). Each one of these humors had definite qualities. Blood was moist and warm; phlegm, moist and cold; yellow bile, warm and dry; black bile, cold and dry. Furthermore, there was a definite connection between predominance of any one humor in the metabolic system and an individual's temperament. The diagram (p. 17) gives an idea of the relations concerned.

The drugs were classified accordingly into those having in various degrees (four) one or more of the qualities of warm, cold, moist or dry. Hence they could be applied whenever a deficiency or excess of the one or the other humor made a counteraction desirable, in whatever degree or variation. Drugs supposed to have only one quality were classified as "simples," while those with more qualities were considered "composites." Finally, there were the so-called "entities," drugs with specific effects that did not fit one of the regular systematic categories. Examples of these are emetics and purgatives, poisons and antidotes, which were said to be effective through their "whole substance."

Galen prepared his medicaments himself and had a very high opinion of the efficiency of well chosen and prepared remedies. He had not only an *iatreion*, the usual room of the Greco-Roman physicians for the preparation of remedies, but also an *apotheca* or storeroom.

Galen described 473 drugs of vegetable, animal and mineral origin. In addition, a profusion of drug formulas is found in his medical treatises. Three remedies in particular, though in use before Galen, gained a world wide reputation for a millennium and a half because of his recommendation, namely, *hiera picra* (holy bitter), *terra sigillata* (sealed earth) and *theriaca* (treacle).[43] Galen originated the formula for a cold cream essentially similar to the official Unguentum Aquae Rosae.

Retail Trade in Drugs

In Greece as well as in Rome the necessity of well organized medical care was gradually recognized. There developed a system of providing community-paid physicians who, however, were allowed to charge wealthy people. Since these physicians were supposed to take care of the pharmaceutical part of the treatment likewise, there was no similar official recognition and regulation of pharmaceutical activities although there were quite a few groups of drug preparers and sellers in existence.

Indeed, it had become common comparatively early for Greco-Roman physicians to have these specialists do compounding for them. Pliny complained about this tendency,[14] and Galen admonished his colleagues very sincerely to do their drug compounding themselves and not to leave it to the pigmentarii. In any case, the physician remained the one who applied or gave the medicaments to the patients under his care, and it was his responsibility to see that the drugs had been prepared properly. The division of labor and responsibility between the physician as the prescriber and the pharmacist as the legitimate agent for filling the prescription and dispensing the medicaments to the patient still had not become a recognized concept, still less an accepted reality.

The preparers and sellers of drugs and

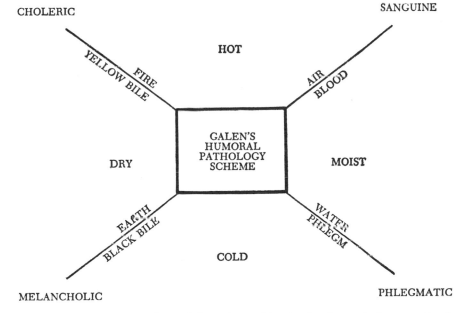

A diagram clarifies and simplifies relationships in the theoretic framework of humoral pathology. The *four humors*, whose balance and distribution were fundamental to the living organism, are given below the diagonal lines. Each of the *four elements* comprising all matter is adjacent to its analogous humor (over the line). Above and beneath each diagonal are the two *qualitative characteristics* associated with each elemental substance. *Temperament,* as well as one's health, reflected the humoral state, hence the designations at the end of each diagonal line. The etymology of each term of temperament reminds us of its ancient association with one of the humors.

cosmetics were known in Greece as *rhizo-tomoi, migmatopoloi, pharmakopoeoi, phar-makopoloi, myropoeoi* and *myripsoi;* in Rome as *pharmacopoli, circumforanei, sellularii, seplasiarii, unguentarii, aromatarii, pharmacopoei, medicamentarii, pharmacotritae, pharmacotribae* and *pig-mentarii.* (For explanations, see the Glossary: Appendix 7.)

Limited by meager evidence, it has been hard to perceive or assess whatever significant changes in the structure and the administrative arrangement of pharmaceutical services had arisen in the "golden age" of Greek culture as compared with the Egyptian zenith reached 1,500 years

before in a quite different intellectual climate. Perhaps more important for the future of pharmacy was the potential created by striking advances in the knowledge of drugs and the refinement of technics and by the embryonic scientific methods that now characterized the best medical thought and practice.

While theurgic concepts had long since been thrust aside, apparently the rational technics were not yet sufficiently complex nor was medical care sufficiently mature to split pharmacy and medicine into two distinct specialties. Some practitioners served as both physician and pharmacist, others had a pharmaceutical assistant, and

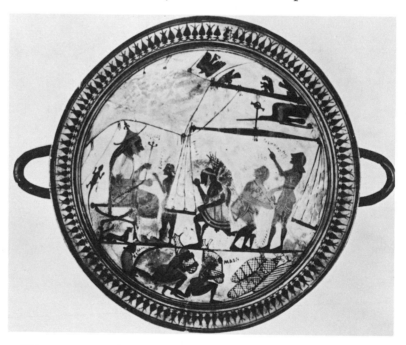

This scene on a shallow Greek bowl (about the 6th century B.C.) has been called the oldest known representation of the packing of drugs. A crude botanical drug, silphium, is being put aboard ship for export from Cyrene, a great trading center of that time and capital of a Spartan colony on the Libyan coast. From a yardarm the beam of a large balance (far right) has been suspended for weighing the drug. A quantity already weighed is being packed in large flexible containers which the workmen (below) then stow in the ship's hold. King Arkesilas (far left) is depicted overseeing these operations, since a royal monopoly controlled the export of silphium—a pharmaceutical cargo said to have been literally worth its weight in gold. (Bowl in Cabinet des médailles, Bibliotèque Nationale, Paris. Illustration from Am. Inst. Hist. Pharm. calendar, 1959; text after Tschirch: 188, 460, 528 of vol. 1, and Schmidt, 61)

still others were relying more and more on special dealers to prepare certain compounds as well as gather, as of old, the crude drugs needed.

Certain groups may have been little more than collectors or dealers in herbs (such as the *rhizotomoi*); others were merely street-corner quacks (the *pharmakopol* had that reputation). Some (the *seplasiarii*) settled down in permanent shops to vend remedies. If at first they specialized in cosmetics, they later branched out into medicinal salves and plasters. In any event, the very fact that these different groups existed shows that during Greek and Roman antiquity there was no distinct profession or class comparable with the pharmacist of later periods.[45]

With Galen the Greco-Roman epoch of medicine and pharmacy reached its climax. For a long time it was essentially Galen's treatises on anatomy and clinical medicine and those of Dioscorides on materia medica —in innumerable copies and extracts, under the names of the original authors or disguised—that disseminated medical and pharmaceutical wisdom throughout the Western world.

FOUR ROMAN MEDICAL AUTHORS

Medicine in Rome was almost monopolized by Greek physicians. With examples of Roman writers of great pharmaceutical and medical influence we include Pliny, because medicine found a place within his great encyclopedic work on everything in natural history.

An Influential Medical Encyclopedia

Chronologically the first treatise is that of Aulus Cornelius Celsus. Like his great contemporary Pliny, he was in all probability not a physician but a learned and medically experienced encyclopedist. As part of a large encyclopedic work, he wrote the book *De Medicina*. The great influence that his treatise had since it appeared in print late in the 15th century is due on the one hand to an accident and on the other hand to two distinguishing qualities. The accident was that Pope Nicholas V found the entirely forgotten treatise among some ancient manuscripts, and he had it printed at a time (1478) when no other classical book on medicine or medicaments was available in printed form. The two qualities distinguishing the book were the excellent Latin in which it was written and the fact that Celsus had translated many Greek medical terms into Latin, and so offered not only a list of synonyms but a Latin medical nomenclature that has been widely adopted. W. G. Spencer[46] gives a list of the medicaments discussed by Celsus and his weights and measures.

Recently it has been contended that Celsus' *De Medicina* represents mainly a translation into Latin of a book written late in the 1st century B.C. by a Sicilian physician, Titus Aufidius. This man wrote in Greek and, in spite of his Latin (or Latinized) name, was apparently a Greek. This would only testify to the fact that original genius and work in medicine and pharmacy during the period of Roman world domination was still Greek and not Roman. It does not negate all credit owed to Celsus. Being an encyclopedist and not a physician, he was expected to be able to select with knowledge and to present with grace what he had found in available sources rather than to produce original work of his own.[47]

The First Dispensatory?

A work which may be regarded as a kind of precursor of the later pharmacopeias is the *Compositiones* of the Roman physician Scribonius Largus, written about A.D. 43.[48] A great part of the preface of this early dispensatory is a defense of a thorough and plentiful use of medicaments, opposing the medical nihilism which existed even in those early days. Scribonius Largus says:

We have to condemn all those who intend to deprive medicine of the use of remedies, the name "medicine" being derived not from healing (*a medendo*) but from the power and efficiency of the medicament (*medicamentum*). All those should be praised who try whatever is possible to save the sick patient.

The formulary of Scribonius Largus contains only a few simples (*simplicia*), most of his formulas representing compounded medicaments *(composita)*, with many ingredients. Scribonius describes the preparation and gives the first definition of opium, insisting on the use of immature poppy capsules as the source of opium (reserving the designation *meconium* for the inspissated juice of poppy leaves). He warns against the substituting of the juice of the leaves for the juice of the unripe capsules, "as the *pigmentarii* prepare it in order to make a profit."[49]

All Science His Province

Pliny was a Roman general, admiral and diplomat with a passion for collecting and compiling the entire scientific knowledge of his time. He was a contemporary of Dioscorides, writing in part on the same subjects and often using the same sources. While Singer[50] gives Dioscorides full credit, stating that he has "practically determined modern plant nomenclature both popular and scientific," he characterizes Pliny as follows:

Pliny is the compiler par excellence, the learned collector who will put down anything he is told or can read without verification. Scientifically the work is, therefore, worthless. Read throughout the ages, alike in the darkest as in more enlightened periods, copied and re-copied, translated, commented on, extracted and abridged, a large part of Pliny's work has gradually passed into folkkeeping.

Nevertheless, the work of Pliny holds immense value because most of the books that Pliny used have been lost (he himself spoke of more than 2,000!). The reflection of a vast lost library that can be found in Pliny's encyclopedic *Natural History* has attracted study by a number of historians.[51]

End of an Epoch

This group of Greco-Roman medical authors is completed chronologically with Paulos Aegineta (7th century), whose *Seven Books on Medicine* represent essentially a critically selected compendium, with commentary, composed of the writings of earlier authors, principally Dioscorides, Galen and Oribasios of Pergamon.[52] Paulos Aegineta gives a complete picture of Greco-Roman medication. He lived at Alexandria when the Arabs took possession of this old stronghold of Greek science and remained there under the Arabian government. He therefore obviously represents, in his person as well as in his activity, the transmission of Greco-Roman medical wisdom to the Arabs.

In Babylonia and Egypt, in Greece and Rome, we have glimpsed some of the foundation stones on which the Arabs and, later, medieval Europe were to build a more distinctive "pharmacy." In this ancestral sense, as an "ancient prelude," these early civilizations capture our interest. However, we value them properly only if we think of them as rather an astonishing climax after eons of brutalized life and of primitive reaction to the profound mystery of disease.

2: The Arabs and the European Middle Ages

THE ARABS

The conquest of a great part of the ancient civilized world in the 7th and 8th centuries by a group of Semitic tribes called Arabs is one of the miracles of history. Suddenly this primitive people became the heir and the administrator of the surviving remnants of Greco-Roman culture. The literature found by the Arabs in Alexandria, especially translations of Greek manuscripts into Syriac and Arabic mainly by the Nestorians, provided a basis for the Arabic civilization.

Nestorius, patriarch of Constantinople, had been condemned by the Council of Ephesus (431) for maintaining that the divine and the human nature were not merged in one person in Christ (who was God in man) and, hence, that it was wrong to call the virgin Mary the mother of God, though she might be called the mother of Christ. Banned by the official church, the "Nestorians" who held this belief established themselves in Persia, Syria, India and other oriental countries. Among these sectarians were many scientists, who took into exile their books and their wisdom and became teachers of the world into which they immigrated. Their schools (Nisibis, Edessa and Gondêschâpûr) became famous. When the Arabs entered the politico-cultural scene, this special kind of Greco-Oriental synthesis offered itself to them.

The Arabic civilization was at bottom the Hellenized Aramaic and Iranian civilizations as developed under the aegis of the caliphate and expressed through the medium of the Arabic tongue.[1] . . . The academies of the Arabians were true imitations of the famous Greek school of Alexandria.[2]

From the 9th to the 13th centuries a flood of books written in Arabic testified to this flourishing of culture on the basis of a marriage between the Greek and the oriental spirit. However, especially as far as medicine was concerned, it was by no means the exclusive product of people of pure Arabic stock.

The term Arabian does not necessarily imply an Arab, for the Persians and Nestorians in the East, and the Spaniards and Jews in the West, took the principal part in the development of medicine which was expressed in the Arabic language . . . the language of the learned in the Empire of Islam just as Latin was the linguistic medium of the educated in Western Europe.[3]

Some Important Authors

Mesuë, Sr. The first medical scientist of importance, Jûhannâ Ibn Māsawaih (in the West, called Johann Mesuë Senior, 777-857) one of the earliest physicians who wrote in Arabic, was a Nestorian Christian. He is known less for his formulary, which has not come down to us, and for his assumed authorship of the earliest known systematic Arabic treatise on ophthalmology than for the theft of his name by the so-called Mesuë Junior.

To a pupil of Māsawaih, Hunain Ibn Ishāq (809-877), a Nestorian like his teacher, goes the credit of having been one of the earliest and most effective translators of Greek writings: the works of Galen, the Hippocratic authors, Aristotle and Dioscorides. "The translations prepared by Hunain and his school were the foundation of that Muslim canon of knowledge which dominated medical thought almost to modern times."[4]

The most outstanding figures in the Arabian medical world were Al Rāzi (called Rhazes; d. ca. 932) and Ibn Sīnā (called Avicenna, 980-1037). Both were Persians.

21

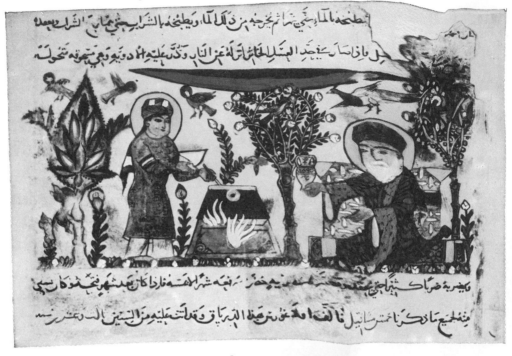

This colorful miniature was painted in an early 13th-century Arabic manuscript based on Galen's treatise concerning electuaries. It depicts the preparation of drugs in terms of the artist's own time rather than the Greco-Roman period in which Galen wrote. A liquid remedy is being mixed over a fire in the open air, where flora and fauna serve to exemplify the pharmaceutical bounty of nature. The bearded figure (right) holds out an ornate ceramic drug container.

Rhazes. The work of Rhazes was important, and much used in the European world.[5] His *Kitab-al-hāwī* (translated into Latin under the title *Continens Rhazes*) represents a comprehensive view of ancient Greek and early Arabic medical knowledge, which was further increased by the author's own experience.

Rhazes describes the most effective as well as most palatable methods of administering medicaments—in which preference is given to the pill form—and gives recipes, many of them very complicated, against specified diseases. In these mention is made for the first time of [preparations similar to] brandy and arrack.[6]

Rhazes was instrumental in introducing the extensive use of mercurial ointment both among the Arabians and in the Western world.[7] A pioneer of scientific chemistry, his writings departed from the merely symbolic and allegoric style of alchemy, to provide a model for all chemical treatises of a practical and factual nature.[8]

Rhazes was the first to start an introduction into "alchemy" with an entirely sober and rational description of the substances and apparatus, and to deal with the chemical operations mentioned in systematic sequence. In his book, "The Secrets of the Secrets," he not merely lists but explains the secrets.[9]

Avicenna. About one century after Rhazes appeared "the most famous scientist of Islam and one of the most famous of all races, places and times."[10] Ibn Sīnā (called in the West Avicenna) was a physician, philosopher and diplomat, to whom even his contemporaries attributed the title "prince of physicians." He wrote (among many other books on philosophy, natural history and medicine) the *Qānún fi'l tibb* (translated into Latin under the title *Canon medicinae Avicennae*).

To summarize Avicenna's contribution:

The entire theoretical and practical medicine, with all its special branches, is brought into a unified system. A perfectly uniform product is created without an equal of its kind in the entire history of medicine. The impression on the medical world in Orient and Occident was, therefore, enormous, surviving all other works. It continued to be used as guide and authority nearly to the 17th century.[11]

Of the five books into which the *Canon* is divided, the second is devoted to the simple drugs *(simplicia)* and the fifth to the compounded remedies *(composita)*. The arrangement is alphabetic. This treatise of Avicenna supplemented that of Galen. Adopting and even elaborating on Galen's humoral pathology, Avicenna well deserved his cognomen "Arabian Galen." The author also used Dioscorides, many other Greek medical writers and his Arabian predecessors, especially Rhazes. Parts of the *Canon* dealing with medicinal uses of

metals show extensive similarity to Dioscorides. Entire parts of the *Canon* prove to be more or less literal translations of this Greek author.[12] Avicenna speaks of silvering and gilding of pills and is said to have introduced this practice into pharmacy.

Haly Abbas. Another great medical author of Persian stock was Alī Ibn Abbas (called Haly Abbas, d. 994). He wrote a medical encyclopedia, *Kitāb al-Maliki* (translated into Latin under the title *Liber regis, regalis dispositio*). Parts of this book became the first witness of Arabic science to be transmitted to the western world.

Abulcasis. The famous "Arabians" of Persian origin who wrote on medical and pharmaceutical subjects were followed by authors born in the Western Caliphate (largely the Spanish peninsula). Abū-l-Qāsim al-Zahrāwī (called Abulcasis; d. 1013) became famous largely through the popularity of his treatise on surgery.

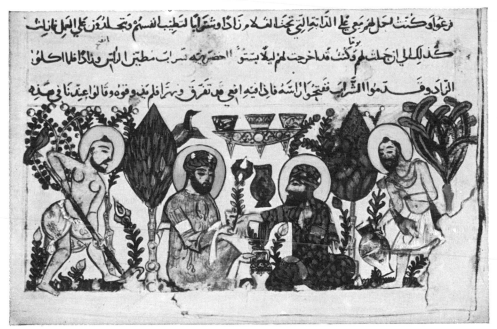

This miniature, a companion to the illustration on the facing page, shows the preparation of theriac, a complex antidote that Galen's recommendation helped to raise to the level of an internationally renowned panacea. Between and above the two central figures are various drug containers from which they are measuring the ingredients. Two assistants (extreme left and right) are depicted obtaining supplies of crude drugs for the compounders. (Ms. in Austrian National Library, Vienna.) (From Zekert, O.: Chem. and Druggist *120*:728, 1934)

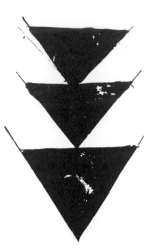

الاردت ال برورسى يمر المطوحات .
المطوح الاصول والرونا
والواسول والسكليح
واصا والكاح رتاسر
المطوح ادا رعت
طعها ومرتها صينها
اولا بحل شعرم دحل المرواو
عمما يحمل ٢ حمرا يموس
الاوسط دا ٢ وسطس
الاكبر يكمل ٢ لا صهر
مرليف الجارادا لخل سوينا
اومرتنوا لجل يختويا
نرلهما المرواو ركهل
كها اما سهبده مافطر
م مصس المروا والاعل
البرى هوا صوا لبرى فيها لليفها لمطوح وبركه مده ما برل موعمران
مستد فامه مرل نرا الولا الما ٢ فى بوالنبرا ٢ الما لنان اننرا الهراودر
نانيال المطوح ولم يبرمنه سى نا حرم ما فيه واعماه مالما من
الا انمال مردا لمطوح ودعه مرروق بلاموال مهليه دك نصرعله
لالا برلا لمطوح اجم مرور الانمال رسهرا لمطوح فيا نرب

Among the earliest drawings of pharmaceutical equipment for instructional purposes known is this one of a triple strainer, which is found in a late medieval Arabic manuscript of the famous 28th treatise of Abū-l-Qāsim al-Zahrāwī of Cordova (10th century). A decoction poured into the top strainer filtered through successively finer strainers arranged underneath. Such strainers often were woven of horsehair. (Veliyuddin ms. 2491 (copied 1265 A.D.), f. 39 v. and 40 v.; from Süleymaniye 'Umūmī Kütüphanesi, Istanbul. See Hamarneh, Sami K.: J. Am. Pharm. Ass. (Pract.) 21:91, 1960)

Pharmacy has known Abulcasis best for his 28th treatise (*Liber servitoris*), which is devoted largely to medicinal chemistry. Osler regarded it as "primarily a manual for apothecaries, generations of whom battened on its rich polypharmacy . . . the most marvelous production of its kind."[13] Since the research of the pharmacist-historian Sami Hamarneh, we know that a large majority of the 30 treatises in Abulcasis' complete *al-Tasrīf* also are heavily

pharmaceutical. They comprise a highly objective and comprehensive encyclopedia that appears to have been the first of its kind produced in Arabic Spain.[14]

Ibn al-Baitār. The work of the Spanish-born Ibn al-Baitār (b. 1197) offers the most comprehensive list of drugs. Baitār mentions in his *Kitāb al jāmi* (Book of Simple Drugs) 145 mineral drugs, 130 drugs from the animal kingdom and about 1,800 vegetable drugs.

[The *Kitāb al jāmi*] is not only a very methodical and critical compilation, but it contains also a good number of personal observations. It does not deal only with drugs, but also with various species of food. . . . Practically the whole of Dioscorides' and of Galen's knowledge on the subject was incorporated in the Jāmi, but many other authors were quoted, some 150 in all, among whom were twenty Greeks.[15]

Maimonides. A Spanish Jew, Abū 'Imrām Mūsā ibn Maimūn (1135-1204; called Maimonides), perhaps influenced the European world more through his philosophy than through his medical works. His dietetic rules became especially famous. Although his glossary of drug terms is remarkable and still useful historically,[16] Maimonides is known widely today in pharmacy largely through a mistaken identity! In the 19th century a so-called oath or prayer of "Maimonides" became known. It was then thought to be an original contribution to medical ethics by the great physician-philosopher. Since then it has been proved to be a compilation in the "tone and spirit of Maimonides" by one of his German admirers (late 18th century), which then was translated into Hebrew by another. Though it was neither written by Maimonides nor designed particularly for pharmacists, the language expresses aspirations of the health professions so beautifully that it remains popular among American pharmacists as well as physicians.[17]

Great as has been the influence of these various authors on Western pharmacy and chemistry, it was surpassed by the works of two unknown writers, to whom we now turn.

Borrowed Names and Fame—
Pseudo Mesuë and Geber

Mesuë Junior and Jābir (Latinized as Geber) now are known to have belonged to the 13th century and probably were Europeans. While this does not change the role and the influence that their writings had, it does mean that—having lived at least 2 centuries later than it was supposed —they would have been able to copy from others the discoveries that have been attributed to them.

In both cases, the names adopted by the unknown authors were ennobled by previous fame, namely by the books of two authentic medieval Arabs, Mesuë Senior and the mysterious Jābir Ibn Hajjan.

Sudhoff contends that the main treatises of pseudo-Mesuë (his *Antidotarium* or *Grabadin*) were written in upper Italy, probably in Bologna or Padua. "It remained obviously unfinished, hence Peter of Abano and Francis of Piedmont, both authors worthy of note, concluded the work."[18]

The *Grabadin* of the pseudo-Mesuë was for centuries the authority on the composition of medicaments. Not only was the book in use in practically every European pharmacy, but also it became a basis for later official pharmacopeias. The *Grabadin* is "the pharmacological quintessence of Arabian therapeutics," and contains the entire armamentarium of compounded medicines that we owe to the Arabians. The arrangement is like that of the later pharmacopeias. The compounded medicines are divided into groups according to their forms—for example, confections, juleps and syrups. The monographs contain directions for the preparation of the products and notes on their medicinal uses.

The case of the works of pseudo-Jābir is still more complicated. There were writings (philosophical, religious and scientific) thought to have been written by Jābir Ibn Hajjan about A.D. 800. These writings, according to Julius Ruska and Paul Kraus,[19] were produced and distributed more than a century later by an Islamitic sect (i.e., in the early 10th century and *after* the appearance of Rhazes' fundamental work). The objective was to justify the theologic and philosophic ideology of the sect by proving that it was in harmony with the scientific knowledge of that time. These writings, displaying a considerable amount of chemical knowledge believed to antedate Rhazes, were held in the highest esteem by the medieval alchemists. Therefore it is not surprising that someone eventually tried to take advantage of this fame by attaching the name of Jābir to recent writings of his own.

In the late middle ages Latin writings appeared that were supposed to be translations of treatises by the mysterious early Arab, Jābir. No Arabic originals of these writings have ever been found, and they or their contents were not mentioned in the books of the great European 13th century naturalists Albertus Magnus and Roger Bacon, who were closely following and taking advantage of the Arabic sources becoming available at this time. Hence these assumed "Jābir" (Geber) writings are believed to have been produced in Europe in the late 13th century.

Today a doubt no longer exists that these books are late Latin scripts which were attributed for their better recommendation to the great Geber quite as other writings were attributed at about the same time to Aristotle and Plato or to Rhazes and Avicenna.[20]

Seen in this light, all the processes and the chemicals mentioned in the Latin "Jābir" writings have to be regarded not only as early Arabian wisdom but as European chemical knowledge of the late 13th century. Their author must have been one of the earliest scientific chemists in Europe.

Alchemy

The apocryphal "Jābir" writings were for centuries the holy books of the alchemists, as they sought to make gold from baser metals and to discover the elixir of life.[21] However, "alchemy" itself was much older. It was in the period of decay of the Greco-Roman empire and the religious and philosophic syncretism of the 4th and the 5th

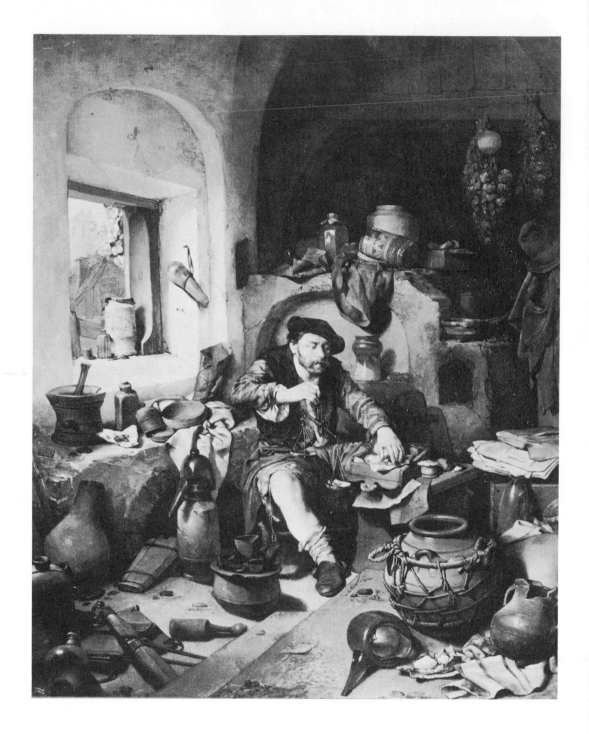

A needy European alchemist sits among a litter of equipment, weighing out a chemical for one of his experiments in making gold, in this 17th-century painting by Cornelis P. Bega of The Netherlands. The brushes of a number of painters have been attracted by the fascination of alchemy. A traditionally secret and nonscientific art, alchemy remained foreign to both the spirit and the methods of modern pharmacy or chemistry. Although no forerunner of the pharmacist, the alchemist transmitted or invented equipment and technics of value to modern pharmaceutical development. (From the Fisher Collection, Fisher Scientific Company, Pittsburgh)

centuries of the Christian era that the peculiar mixture of religious and philosophic ideas with chemical experimentation, called alchemy, found fertile soil. As to the origin of an alchemical theory, Ruska says:

That the application of chemical experience is many thousands of years old, hardly needs to be stated. The oldest speculations about the possibility of a transmutation of metals, which might be regarded as the beginning of a chemical theory, have their origin, however, in the valley of the Nile, in the Hellenistic Egypt of the late Roman emperors. We still possess in precious manuscripts all that could be collected and preserved by Byzantine philologists, around the year 1000, of the literature on the subject during about four centuries. For Occidental alchemy, however, which came into its own somewhat later, not these Greek writings but Arabic compilations have been the exclusive sources.[22]

Unfortunately Arabic alchemy from the 10th to the 13th centuries lost the factual character that it had achieved through Rhazes and Avicenna. The contents of the alchemistic writings of that period are more or less fanciful literary inventions. On European soil, these outgrowths became perfect nonsense as they passed through the hands of generations of ignorant copyists.

The ideologic basis of alchemy was two ancient concepts: Assyrian-Babylonian and Pythagorean astrology, and the idea of perfection and purification. It is significant that the book attributed to "Jābir" (Geber) that exerted the greatest influence here the title *Summa perfectionis*.

The Practice of Pharmacy

The great attention paid to the science and the art of pharmacy by the medical authors of the Arabic world was bound to influence the practice of pharmacy. The drug armamentarium became enlarged considerably. Persian and Indian drugs unknown to the Greco-Roman world—camphor, cassia, cloves, cubebs, musk, nutmeg, rhubarb, sandalwood, senna and tamarind, to name only a few—were described by authors writing in Arabic. Of equal importance were new modes of drug therapy that

required considerable skill on the part of the preparer—for example, confections, conserves, juleps and lohochs.

These advances in pharmaceutical knowledge and technic on the one side and medical knowledge on the other, in connection with a growing recognition of governmental responsibility for the health of the people in the Arabic world, fostered a division of labor between pharmacy and medicine and, finally, the creation of a public welfare system in which the profession of pharmacy was given a definite place of its own.

Before the 8th century, medical care remained largely the "Medicine of the Prophet," especially hygienic rules and pre-Islamic folk medicine. Then, during the century of the Umayyad dynasty, beginning about 4 decades after Muhammad's pilgrimage to Mecca, a growing emphasis on the health field and a professionalized medicine can be discerned. Representative of the early, rather elaborate attention that medical practitioners gave to pharmaceutical technics, forms and resources was the great Arabic compendium written at some time before A. D. 709 by Theadoq, a Christian.[23]

Probably soon afterward in the early 8th century a "state hospital," much as we understand the term, was founded in Damascus—perhaps the first hospital in Islam.[24]

Under the caliph al-Mansur, Baghdad became a dazzling capital city (in the years following 762), a center of learning as well as of administration.

The vigorous development of intellectual life and health facilities makes it understandable that drug shops which we dare call pharmacies had appeared by the early 9th century.

One of the earliest mentions we know of "al-Saidalani" (still today a term denoting a qualified pharmacist) is associated with the name Abū Quraish 'Isā al-Saidalani. A rather needy practitioner near the caliph's palace in Baghdad, he survives in history as a man catapulted into a court position when he successfully predicted a male offspring by examining the urine of the caliph's wife. This incident about a presumed pharmacist supposedly occurred sometime be-

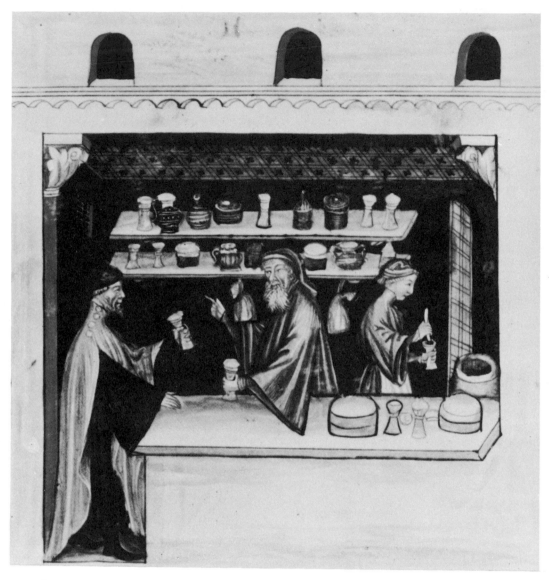

This Italian pharmacy in a miniature painting from the end of the 14th century reminds us of its Arabic antecedents in some of its features. It is typically small and open to the street, with a counter that folds up at night to help to close off the pharmacy from both the elements and intruders. Its shelves hold drug containers made of glazed ceramic, for which both the process of manufacture and the geometric ornamentation came out of the Middle East. The manuscript *Tacuinum Sanitatis* in which this scene appears probably originated near Venice, at that time a principal center for the trade in drugs and other spicery from the Arabic world. (Austrian National Library, ms. n. s. 2644; from Art and Pharmacy, II, Deventer, Netherlands, De Ysel Press, 1958)

tween 775 and 785, yet certain inconsistencies in surviving accounts leave us uncertain. Perhaps we must move on to the first half of the 9th century to find firmer evidence of the emergence of a more independent and professionalized pharmacy.[25]

Here we find practitioners operating small drug shops open to the street, as well as hospital pharmacists, distinguishable from the alchemists, the physicians, and the "al-Attar" (who also dealt in drugs but traditionally specialized in aromatics).[26]

A certain analogy appears between the "seplasiarii" of ancient Rome, who settled down in shops and expanded in scope from fragrant cosmetics to a wider range of pharmaceutical products, and the "al-Attārīn" found in the medieval Arabic world. However, in the elaboration of pharmaceutical technic and knowledge and in the acceptance of responsibility by a pharmaceutical class within an ordered health system, the Arabs made a distinctive place for pharmacy going well beyond pharmaceutical function either as a sideline of a medical practitioner's offices or as technical commerce of ordinary marketplace vendors.

This Arabic development helped to establish and shape Western pharmacy as we know it.

TRANSIT WAYS OF KNOWLEDGE

Sicily and Spain especially served to channel Greco-Arabic medicine into the Latin West (the 7th to the 12th centuries). Sicily was a center of Arabic culture from the time Syracuse fell to the Arabs (878) until the Normans conquered the island (completed 1091). In Spain, Cordova became a cultural capital as well as the political capital of Islam's Western caliphate (by the 10th century). Of the Spanish centers where scholars were busily translating out of the Arabic, Toledo especially yielded an exciting outpouring of Arabic learning that was soon widely absorbed and discussed among Western scholars. Much of this knowledge had its roots in classical Greece.[27]

Greek science returned to Western Europe by three routes: through the continuous tradition of Southern Italy, through the Eastern (Byzantine) Empire and through the Arabians as well. Until the period of the Renaissance, the most important of these was the Arabic route. It was the main current even in Salerno, where the three streams met.

With Salerno, we are on European soil.

We shall now consider what was happening to European medicine and pharmacy meanwhile, during the period between the rise of Islam and the time of the Renaissance—that is, during the Middle Ages.

MEDIEVAL EUROPEAN PHARMACY

The conquest of the ancient Roman Empire of the West, especially of Italy, by German tribes (the Vandals, the Longobards, the Visigoths and the Ostrogoths) found only a shadow of Rome's old glory and culture. Italy had been haunted for centuries by civil war, hostile invasions and epidemic diseases that depopulated and demoralized the country. In such a situation, the disparagement of earthly life and wisdom which was the significant trend of early Christendom not only found broad acknowledgment and success but often led to the destruction of works of pagan art and science.

The German invaders now continued the work of cultural destruction. They were all the more prone to do so because their increasing belief in the healing power of faith and relics of saints could not be harmonized easily with some of the scientific wisdom of antiquity. Thus, the first tutelary saints for medicine and pharmacy, which in a measure replaced the old pagan deities of medicine, began to appear about the 5th century. Cosmas and Damian, Arabian Christians, were martyr twins killed in the persecutions under Emperor Diocletian during the 4th century. They became the most celebrated patrons of medicine and pharmacy in all the countries of Christendom. Later on other saints were added to replace or to supplement Cosmas and Damian as guardians.

Monastic Medicine and Pharmacy

Individuals with some knowledge of the old intellectual treasures tried to rescue at least those parts that had practical value. The most important of these men was Marcus Aurelius Cassiodorus (490-585), a learned Roman and chancellor of the great Ostrogothic king Theodoric, in Ravenna (Northern Italy). Cassiodorus induced the

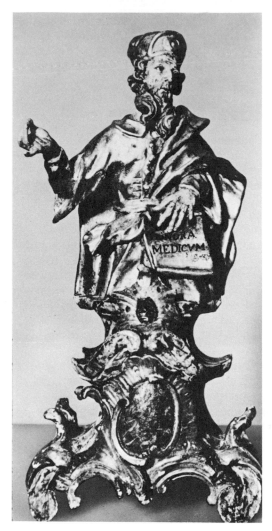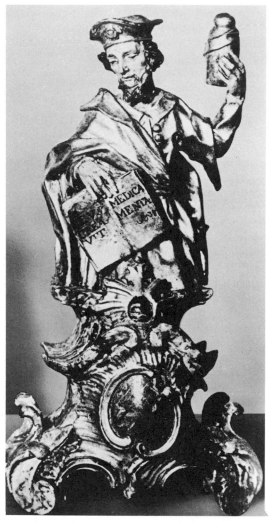

Pharmaceutical work has been conducted under the protecting hands of diverse religious figures; in Christendom, it has been associated above all with the saints Cosmas and Damian. Their martyrdom and legendary feats of healing inspired works of art from at least as early as the 11th century until these small wooden figures were carved by Ferdinand A. Hiernle of Lower Bavaria in the 18th century. Saint Damian (*right*) is shown holding a book open to the aphorism, *God has created drugs*, while, in his other hand, he holds aloft a drug container. The twin brothers from ancient Aegea seem to symbolize the twinship of medicine and pharmacy; Saint Damian particularly has been considered to be guardian of both pharmacy and surgery. (From Verbandstoff-Fabriken Paul Hartmann AG: Kostbarkeiten aus der Apotheke, Heidenheim/Brenz, 1952; photographs by Maximilian Doerr)

king (who was himself familiar with ancient culture through his education at Byzantium) to create a magistrate especially empowered to safeguard relics of classical antiquity.[28] Cassiodorus himself founded a kind of classical academy in which the cultivation of medicine and pharmacy played an important part. In his *Institutiones*, a "fundamental book of medieval science,"[29] Cassiodorus established the rule that the monks who acted as physicians were required to consult Dioscorides, read Latin translations of the works of Hippocrates and Galen and study the work of Caelius

Aurelianus, a Roman medical compiler of the 1st century.[30] Thus, the activity of Cassiodorus was basic to monastic medicine as well as to the survival of such independent scientific medical life as could exist during the period from the 5th to the 10th century.

What results did Cassiodorus get? The great medical historian Henry Sigerist says:

Conditions developed in Ravenna and other centers that were very similar to those in Alexandria. And granted that there, too, the medical men may have been chiefly members of the church, their medicine was anything but monastic. The medical literature of the period is entirely Latin. . . . By the end of the 6th century a fairly large number of classical books had been translated into Latin.[31]

This "fairly large number of classical books" represented, naturally, only a very small part of ancient medical wisdom. Moreover, it was used almost exclusively by a small group of persons. Then the empire of Theodoric the Great disappeared, and new swarms of barbarian invaders put an end to that modest attempt toward a cultural renaissance. In those times of perpetual war, bloodshed and destruction, study was "almost exclusively restricted to the clergy, because only the church was a safe asylum provided for the studious. . . . Thus was born monastic medicine."

Medicine, after having played a most important part in Roman civilization, withdrew into the shadow of the church and became, under the influence of Christian dominance, a dogmatic medicine in which the first and most important point was faith. Faith alone could cure the body and the soul of the sufferer and was the essential point in the help of the sick.[32]

Therefore, no opportunity was provided for the development of science or for the enlightenment of men by science. In many monasteries monks heeded the advice of Cassiodorus that they collect and use the old manuscripts. But only the few Latin treatises that the monks had rescued could be studied and used, principally "those of Celsus, Scribonius Largus, Pliny the Elder (to a slight degree only), and Caelius Aurelianus."[33] The Greek manuscripts that they had collected and preserved for posterity they could not use, "being unable to read Greek." These manuscripts did become important several centuries later in the time of the Renaissance, when scholars eagerly searched all the cloisters of Italy and the West for original manuscript copies of the Greek medical writers. They found copies in a number of institutions.

What happened meanwhile in a small sector in which there was a possibility of the cultivation and the practice of scientific medicine in the Middle Ages?

What was mostly needed was short treatises, abstracts, epitomes, giving brief instructions for practice. A new literature arose, consisting of short treatises on urine, pulse, fever, dietetics, prognostic, bloodletting and, above all, endless prescriptions were written. These treatises sometimes were given the form of epistles or of dialogues, or of catechisms. They were anonymous, many of them falsely bearing the great names of Hippocrates, Galen, Democritos, Apuleius to give them more authority. . . . This literature lasted, unchanged in character, until the 11th century. The turning point in the literary development was made by the translations of Constantine of Africa. They started a new movement, inaugurated a new literature, which from now on invariably had traces of Arabian influence.[34]

The light of science in the Middle Ages burned only gloomily. It was oxygen of Arabian origin that made it bright again.

Before the invaluable translations of Constantine of Africa, the European scientific world had available the work of Dioscorides; parts of the treatises of Hippocrates, Galen, Celsus, Scribonius Largus, Pliny the Elder, Caelius Aurelianus, Oribasios and Alexander Trallianus; and some anonymous and pseudonymous abstracts. Searching Italian libraries, Sigerist[35] encountered "over and over again" two such abstracts, which he therefore considers to have been "undoubtedly the most popular treatises for many centuries, . . . the Passionarius Galeni and the herbal of Pseudo-Apuleius."

The *Passionarius Galeni* probably was compiled in Salerno (the 8th or the 9th century) from fragments or extracts of treatises by Galen and from compilations by authors (the 6th and the 7th centuries) based on Galen and other famous Greek physicians. The Pseudo-Apuleius, once called "a futile work with its unrecognizable figures and incomprehensible vocabulary," represents an illustrated herbal, taken mainly from Dioscorides.[36]

Such was the materia medica of the Middle Ages until the infiltration of the Greco-Arabic medical literature into Europe: some second-, third- and fourth-hand compilations brought together from the incidentally extant remnants of antiquity; a very few fragments of original ancient medical literature,[37] written in or translated into Latin and, here and there, Anglo-Saxon, Irish, French or German books or lists containing descriptions of indigenous vegetable drugs and directions for their medicinal use. Of the last-mentioned type of treatise, the Anglo-Saxon "leech books" are the most famous representatives.

Irish and English scientists "contributed in a large measure to the preservation of civilization during the Dark Age."[38] For example, the Anglo-Saxon Bede, called "the Venerable" (680-735), wrote a book entitled *De natura rerum*, in which he frequently refers to the encyclopedia of Isidore of Seville and to the scientific and medical knowledge of that time, such as it was. This manuscript was eagerly distributed by Irish and English scholars wandering through France, western Germany, Switzerland and as far as northern Italy.[39]

The monastic medicopharmaceutical literature reached its climax in the Latin poem about herbs entitled *De viribus herbarum*, or *Macer floridus*, probably produced toward the end of the 11th century by Odo of Meune, abbot of Beauprai, and in the treatises *Physica* and *Causae et curae* of the abbess Hildegard of Bingen (1098-1179). The *Macer floridus* has been called one of the most popular books and the first independent herbal to be produced in the medieval West.[40] However, its author used older Latin sources. Perhaps he also drew on Arabic authors through the writings of Constantine the African; certainly Hildegard did.[41]

The School of Salerno

By their very nature, monastic medicine and pharmacy were dogmatic, their first and most important element being faith. At the same time, a growing tendency developed among the clergy to discover traces of Christian ideas in some Greco-Roman philosophers and physicians and, later on, even in Arabian masters, and thus they rationalized the use of pagan wisdom in a Christian world. This tendency paved the way for the systematic reconquest of lost antique knowledge from Arabian sources and later on from the Greek originals that became available.

The 7th to the 12th centuries saw Islam and Christianity in intimate contact in Spain and Sicily. Hence, it was mainly these two areas from which the Latin West drew on Greco-Arabian knowledge (see page 29); and a little seaside town, Salerno near Naples, was destined to play an important part in this development.

The famous School of Salerno dates from about the 8th century. The fact that the town was the seat of an archbishop and a cloister led to the assumption that the school had an ecclesiastic origin. According to F. Garrison, that cannot be accepted, "for the whole character of the school was that of an isolated laical institution, a *civitas Hippocratis*, in the midst of purely clerical foundations, and there is significant silence about Salerno in the ecclesiastic chronicles."[42] Gradually Salerno became the seat of a guild of physicians, attracting not only patients but also students.

Arabic influence there continued to increase. An "antidotarium" by a Jewish physician called Donnolo (913-970) was based on Arabic sources.[43]

After Constantine the African had come to Salerno (middle of the 11th century) these infiltrations became both consequential and fundamental. In him we have the first of the Western Latin translators of Arabian manuscripts. He "translated everything that came into his hands without picking the valuable from the meretricious, often forgetting to give the name of the author whose works he was translating."[44]

The most important work of Constantine was the free Latin arrangement of the *Liber regalis* of Alî Ibn Al-'Abbâs'. He impressively called it *pantegni*, the entire art in theory and practice, and issued it without naming the real author. Constantine influenced the European medical world enormously.[45] Instead of mere fragments of ancient wisdom, there were suddenly available systematic and complete works that opened entirely new vistas. The effect became obvious within and outside Salerno.

Even the famous book of materia medica called *Circa instans* (the opening words of the book) may be basically a treatise by Constantine, as revised and enlarged by Mathaeus Platearius (mid-12th century).[46]

Another drug book renowned in the late Middle Ages, the *Antidotarium magnum*, apparently drew heavily on the Arabic drug formulas that Constantine had translated. It also transmitted late classical and early Byzantine drug formulas. A copy of this "Large Formulary," which was found and deciphered by Lutz, had been written in a Swiss monastery about 1190. It contains about 1,100 formulas, some quite complicated, with marginal annotations about them by Mathaeus Platearius. This rich store of pharmaceutical lore was overshadowed later by what seems largely a modified extract of the *Antidotarium magnum* just mentioned. The small formulary (140 formulas in the mid-13th century) became identified with the name Nicholas (several editors by that name eventually complicating the genealogy of the treatise). The *Antidotarium Nicolai* was translated into various languages; by the late 13th century it had become the official textbook on materia medica at the University of Paris, and it continued to influence pharmaceutical literature strongly until the 18th century.[47]

Another famous book closely associated with Salerno is the *Flos medicinae*, or *Regimen sanitatis*, which contains dietetic and pharmaceutical rules in impressive verses. Probably most historians would agree with the statement that the *Regimen sanitatis* came about when "Arnald of Villanova composed a small selection of some 360 verses using old medical poetry from Salerno, from other Italian places, and France, and added a commentary in prose[48] which, in the earlier editions, was always printed with the verses." It was translated into all European languages, frequently with comments and additions, about 300 editions in all.

The presumed author, Arnald of Villanova (1235-1311), was one of the most progressive physicians of the late Middle Ages. He taught medicine at the University of Montpellier for more than a decade. Naturally influenced, like his colleagues, by Arabic medical science, he was one of the first European scientists who turned against meaningless subtleties of Arabian authors and against the strained interpretations that monastic authors placed on them. He was one of the first physicians in Europe to recognize the importance of chemistry for medicine. However, he leaned in the direction of alchemistic speculation and mysticism. The process of distillation, which was already well known to the Arabs, was introduced into European pharmacy mainly through Arnald of Villanova.

Translators

Outside of Salerno, the effect of the activity of Constantine became obvious in two directions: (1) in the employment of his translations in medical practice and instruction, and (2) in a series of further translations, for the most part produced on Spanish soil.

For example, Latin translations of Arabic manuscripts from Toledo, Spain, provided the basis for famous works by the so-called *Doctor universalis*—a German bishop who taught and wrote on natural history—Albertus Magnus (1206-1280), and the so-called *Doctor mirabilis*, Roger Bacon, an English monk and natural philosopher (ca. 1214-1292).[49]

The relation of Constantine's work to that of some other translators whose work served pharmacy and medicine distinctively has been noted by Joseph Hariz as follows:

1. Gerbert of Aurillac, who later became Pope Sylvester II, visited Spain about 967. He

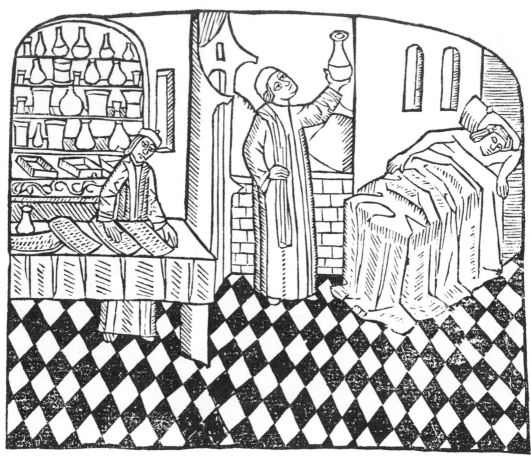

A late-medieval artist carved on a block of wood this remarkable scene showing a pharmacist at work (left), while a physician examines a urine sample (center) from the patient in bed (right). It may be the earliest depiction of the concept of the "triad of medical care" to appear in an English book. The illustration introduces Book 7 (medical counsel largely derived from Constantine the African) of the encyclopedia *On the Properties of Things,* by Bartholomew the Englishman, which came off the press at Westminster about 1495. Bartholomew probably wrote his great work between 1230 and 1240. (From the Univ. of Wisconsin)

introduced the Arabic numerals into Europe and brought the knowledge which he acquired in Spain first to Germany, later on to Rheims, then to Chartres and finally to Rome. He can be considered the renewer of the scientific studies in the monasteries at the end of the 10th century and the first transmitter of Arabian wisdom to northern Europe.

2. Constantinus Africanus is the second transmitter of Arabian science and the first translator of Arabian medical treatises into Latin (11th century).

3. Gerard of Cremona, doubtless one of the most intelligent men of the Middle Ages, surpassed Constantine by far. He translated Avicenna, Rhazes' "Lumen Luminum," Albucasis, Serapion junior, and treatises of Hippocrates and Galen (12th century).

4. The Jewish physician Faraj Ibn Sálim (Fararius or Faragut) completed his translation of the "Continens" of Rhazes in 1279.

In summary:

Arabian medicine was the means of connecting ancient Greek medicine with modern medicine, initiated in the period of the Renaissance. It was first Chartres and Rheims, then, through the influence of Salerno, Paris and Montpellier, which gave Arabic medicine a dominant part in the development of French medicine. During nine centuries Arabic medicine led the way for French medicine.[50]

What Hariz states for France can be said for the entire European world. This is illustrated by the fact that the pharmacists of Basel (15th century) were required to have the books of Pseudo-Mesuë, Avicenna, Serapion, Dioscorides, the *Macer floridus*, the *Circa instans*, the *Synonyma medicinae* of Simon of Genoa (Symon Januensis, died 1303) and the *Antidotarium magnum et parvum Nicolai* in their libraries.[51]

All these books are of Arabian origin or more or less based on Arabic sources, with the exception of Dioscorides and perhaps of *Macer floridus*. The book of Symon Januensis gives the best possible evidence of the amalgamation that took place, representing a dictionary of the Greek, the Latin and the Arabian terms for medicinal herbs to be found in the literature.

This triumphant return of antique wisdom in an Arabic garb makes it understandable why the Europeans Pseudo-Mesuë and Pseudo-Geber thought it advisable to disguise themselves as Arabs. There is no doubt that in the late Middle Ages writings of presumed Arabian origin enjoyed more authority than those of European origin.

The invention of printing greatly extended Arabian influence on European medicine. Among the first dated medical books off the press we find the *Grabadin* of the Pseudo-Mesuë, the *Antidotarium Nicolai* and the *Liber servitoris* by Abulcasis, all printed as early as 1471. Works by Serapion (1473), Rhazes (1480), Avicenna and others soon followed.[52]

The Establishment of European Professional Pharmacy

With the transmission of Arabian medicine and polypharmacy to Europe, conditions that caused the creation of public pharmacies in urban centers of the Middle East likewise produced similar institutions in European states. In the 11th century, perhaps even earlier, public pharmacies began to appear in Southern Italy and Southern France, and probably in other places.

Thus, pharmacy, with its beginnings in the instinctive defense against disease by primitive peoples, had developed under several diverse influences. It was part of the work of priests at first; later it fell among the duties of lay practitioners of medicine and pharmacy combined. It found its own form and expression in the culture of Greece and Rome and took a further step in Byzantium. However, only under the influence of the Arabic wisdom and pattern did pharmacy take firm root in European soil as a distinctive institution of public welfare, to be respected, regulated and further developed.

Part Two

The Rise of Professional
Pharmacy in Representative Countries of Europe

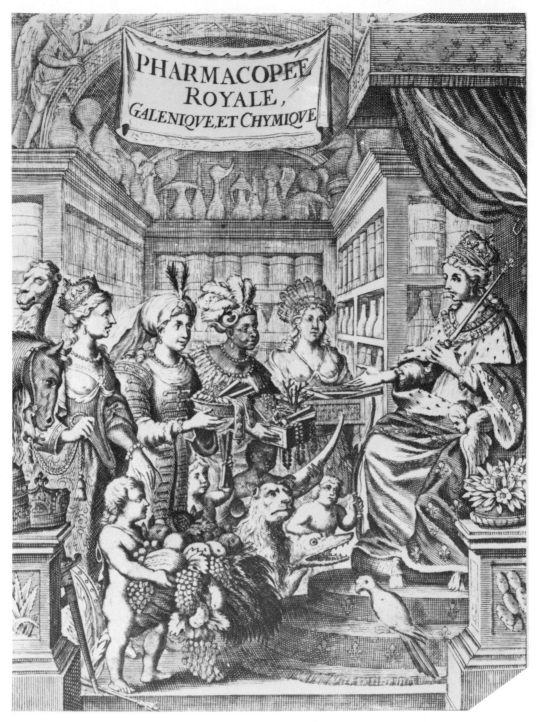

The medicinal bounty of nature has always impressed pharmacists and laymen alike. On the allegorical title page shown here, angels (top) hang out a banner proclaiming that it ornaments the Royal Pharmacopeia prepared by the French pharmacist Moise Charas (1672). Below, the royal profession of pharmacy on her throne receives the products of the animal, the vegetable and the mineral kingdoms from representatives of the continents (l. to r.) Europe, Asia, Africa and the Americas. (A humanized camel, far left, is more interested in looking critically at the reader!)

3: Concepts and Medicaments Become Modern

THE BIRTH OF EUROPEAN PROFESSIONAL PHARMACY

Sometime before February 1240 the German Emperor Frederick II issued an edict that was to be the Magna Charta of the profession of pharmacy.[1] Although promulgated by an emperor of the Holy Roman Empire of the German nation, the edict applied only to that part of his realm called the kingdom of the Two Sicilies.

Three regulations of the edict created pharmacy as an independent branch of a governmentally supervised health service. They won nearly universal application in the centuries that followed. Two additional regulations were highly consequential in the development of pharmacy in most of the countries coming under German politico-cultural influence.

The three essential regulations are:

1. *Separation of the pharmaceutical profession from the medical profession.* This rule, transgressed now and again by both parties, nevertheless constituted the charter of pharmacy as an independent profession. This separation acknowledged the fact that the practice of pharmacy required special knowledge, skill, initiative and responsibility if adequate care of the medicinal needs of the people was to be guaranteed. Forbidding any business relation between physician and pharmacist, the law tried to establish the ethical principles that the only function of the healing professions should be professional service, and that the sick should not be exploited.

2. *Official supervision of pharmaceutical practice.* Thus was acknowledged the importance of pharmacy as a public health service for the protection of the public.

3. *Obligation by oath to prepare drugs reliably, according to skilled art, and in a uniform, suitable quality.* This requirement acknowledges the necessity, not only of reliable remedies, but also of their uniform preparation. Thus it might be considered the first European legal reference to a pharmaceutical standard, a harbinger of later pharmacopeias.

The two sections of the law that did not find general application (especially not in the Anglo-Saxon countries) were:

1. *The limitation of the number of pharmacies*
2. *Governmentally fixed prices for remedies*

The provisions and the context of this legal milestone in the history of pharmacists suggest that a fairly well developed system of public pharmacies must have emerged already in the 13th century. Whether these pharmacies developed from the monastic dispensaries or from general stores in which the trade with drugs became more and more specialized has been debated. In the history of the period both trends can be discerned. However, the clerical dispensaries, open to the general public and therefore competitors of the private pharmacies, were transferred to private owners at a relatively late period. In the case of the Swiss city of Basel, "monastic and private pharmacies existed for a long time side by side. . . . Only the discontinuance of the monasteries after the reformation about 1528 caused the monastic dispensaries to disappear."[2] In countries that retained or restored the Catholic faith, as in Bavaria and Austria, such public monastic pharmacies existed until the early 19th century.[3] However, no doubt the first European nonmonastic pharmacists, like the nonmonastic physicians in the Middle Ages, owed most of their scientific knowledge and practical skill to their clerical predecessors.

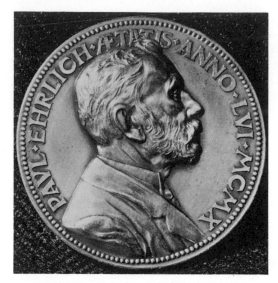
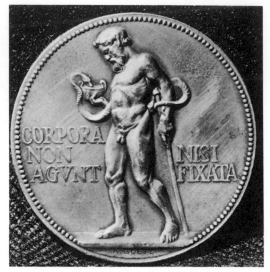

Both the methods and the results of Paul Ehrlich's work—most notably, chemotherapy—have played key roles in transforming drug therapy during the 20th century. The commemorative medal shows Ehrlich as he looked at the height of his fame; while, on the reverse side Asklepios is shown bringing medicinal help (the symbolic bowl and serpent) to the afflicted. The Latin inscription quotes a guiding principle that Ehrlich "tried to turn to practical account" over a quarter of a century, namely, that substances do not work unless they are taken up by the organs concerned. (From the Philadelphia College of Physicians and Surgeons, medal No. 1039 in the collection; medal by K. Goetz)

Monasticism has eternally to its credit that it afforded to culture a sanctuary in the midst of barbarism and with far reaching result sowed the seeds of civilization simultaneously with those of the healing art where the Roman legions had never penetrated.[4]

UNIVERSITIES EMERGE

"Monasticism . . . in the midst of barbarism" became more fruitful when, comparatively early, the medieval clerics detected—or persuaded themselves that they could detect—traces of the belief in one God and of Christian thought and principles in the wisdom of Greco-Roman antiquity. It was for the most part teachers at the clerical schools or *scholae* (hence the term "scholasticism") who renewed the study of ancient philosophy and science. They aimed either to prove or to disprove classical knowledge from the point of view of dogmatic Christianity. We saw in the example of Jābir that a similar tendency prevailed in the Mohammedan world, and Arabic and medieval Christian scholasticism were equally guilty

of mistaking hair-splitting subtleties for research. Thus, what has been called medieval Western scholasticism was mainly the grandiose attempt of the Christian Church to arrive at a dogmatic system in which science and philosophy—as inherited from antiquity and more recently developed—were harmonized with religious thought. "The doctrines of medical science were a finished book—just as the authorities of the Church were final—they might be commentated, expounded, interpreted . . . but not contradicted nor seriously questioned."[5]

Though under such conditions real scientific progress could not be expected, yet there was an urge for knowledge that expressed itself in the development of places of higher learning. These "universities," although, up to the 15th century and sometimes even later, under the influence of the Church, were open to the layman for education in the arts and sciences. True, these universities were the main seats of scholasticism, but they were simultaneously the places where new ideas originated and were nurtured when the time was ripe. By the early 13th century, European institutions of higher learning had been founded at Salerno (medical school, 848; university, 1180), Parma (1025), Paris (university, 1110-1113; with medical school from 1205), Bologna (1110-1113), Oxford (1167) and Cambridge (1209). During the 13th century, 13 more universities were founded (7 in Italy, 2 each in France, Spain and Portugal). The 14th century brought the first Germanic universities (Prague, 1347; Vienna, 1365; Heidelberg, 1385). Before the Renaissance, pharmacy had not become sufficiently independent as a profession to find a special academic place, except as expressed in materia medica courses of early medical schools.

THE IDEA OF THE "RENAISSANCE"

The Renaissance meant a return not only to the original writings of the Greeks but also to Greek spirit, to the esteem of Attic Greeks for individualism and, with this, to their liberty of thought.[6] It meant that fetters imposed on European intellect by the Arabian and clerical scholasticism were removed. It meant the rebirth of independent thought, with the promise and the challenge to the imagination that it offered. It opened new worlds of thought, discovered new horizons, created unexpected possibilities. The discovery of America in 1492 gave to this spirit opportunity for actual physical expansion and expression. Those who followed Columbus did so with the creative vigor demanded of them by the richness and the promise of the new world. Vasco de Gama found an all-water route to the East Indies 6 years later in 1498, and the treasures of the Far East were brought closer to eager hands by the discoverers. The introduction of printing with movable type, which came at about this time, brought the knowledge of the new discoveries, inventions and ideas within quick and easy reach.

Now began that admirable intellectual competition of European individuals and peoples which made Europe, small though it was, the dominant continent in the world.

As in all fields of science, so in medicine and therapy the new developments fathered a number of varying ideas or systems that followed one upon the other. Many of these systems gained international acceptance, influencing the materia medica and, through it, pharmacy.

PARACELSUS, THE ICONOCLAST

In 1530 Nicolaus Copernicus completed his famous book (*De revolutionibus orbium*), wherein (contrary to the then current belief) he stated that the earth moves around the sun. As to medicine and pharmacy, the Swiss physician Theophrastus Bombastus von Hohenheim, called Paracelsus (1493-1541), did an analogous revolutionary deed in exploding old theories and opening the doors to new findings.

Before Paracelsus, various modifications of two main hypotheses concerning pathologies played their part again and again: the humoral and the solidar pathologies (see pp. 13 & 16). Paracelsus introduced instead the concept of the body as a chemical laboratory. As a result of advocacy by Paracelsus, the internal use of chemicals, which had been started sporadically before him, was made a matter of principle and study. He coined the famous phrase that "it is not the task of alchemy to make gold, to make silver, but to prepare medicines."

In his own speculation on the basic nature of matter he did not drop the idea of the four "Aristotelian" elements as such. However, Paracelsus considered them as "also consisting of the , *tria prima*."[7] These three primary principles, "sulphur, mercury and salt" were by no means simply identical with the substances generally understood by these names. Sulfur represented the principle of combustibility, mercury that of liquidity and volatility; salt, being permanent and resisting the action of fire, represented that of stability. In Paracelsus' own words, "all that fumes and disappears in vapors is Mercury; all that burns and is consumed is Sulphur; all that is ashes is also Salt."

Paracelsus opposed the concept of humoral pathology and, especially, the sys-

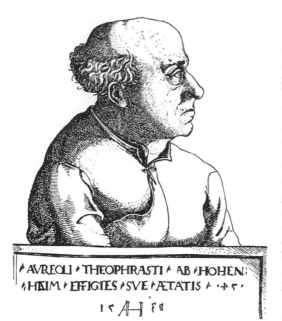

· AVREOLI · THEOPHRASTI · AB · HOHEN ·
· HEIM · EFFIGIES · SVE · ÆTATIS · · ♃ ♄ ·

ıſ AH ɛ8

This portrait of Paracelsus conveys the rugged, bold quality of his thought and action. It is a copper engraving made (1538) toward the end of Paracelsus' life, probably based on sketches of Paracelsus himself by A. Hirschvogel. Below the portrait is his autograph, reproduced from a letter, which may be translated, "Theophrastus von Hohenheim, the dedicated writer and likewise medical doctor." (From Stillman, J. M.: Theophrastus Bombastus von Hohenheim called Paracelsus, p. 162, Chicago, Open Court)

tematization into which it had been pressed by Galen and Avicenna. He is said to have burned the books of these two main representatives of Greco-Roman and Arabic medicine and pharmacy—in all probability a fable. If he did not actually burn the books, he certainly did it figuratively. In every way possible he tried to deprive them of the esteem in which they were held. In 1527 he started his lectures at Basel with a startling attack against the medical tenets of his time.

"Only a few," he said, "practice medicine successfully. Too closely did we cling to the words of Hippocrates, Galen and Avicenna, as if they were oracles. It is not the adornment by titles, eloquence, linguistics and book wisdom that makes the physician, but the knowledge of the secrets of nature." Paracelsus promised to read about practical and theoretic medicine according to his own notes, which he assured his students he did not "beggarly collect out of Hippocrates and Galenos," but had taken "from the best possible teacher, to wit, from my own experience and experimentation." He declared that "there will be no reference to complexions and humors which, while thought to be the cause of all diseases, have widely prohibited the understanding of them, their origin and their critical course."[8]

Pharmacy was enriched by Paracelsus, not only by the introduction into internal therapy of quite a number of chemicals, but also by his endeavor to extract the real "essential" from the more or less inert substances in which he thought it to be hidden. This idea led Paracelsus to prepare alcoholic tinctures and extracts, essences and —supposedly the most essential products— the so-called "quintessences." According to the Paracelsian concept, tinctures as well as extracts originally were considered to be "chemicals" or, to use a more descriptive early synonym, as "spagyric" products— from the Greek words *spao* (to separate) and *ageiro* (to assemble).

However, of what use were these "essentials" if they did not exert some particular power, if they did not provide a specific means of achieving a specific purpose? The idea that there must be, or could be prepared, a particular remedy for each particular disease directed the therapeutic thinking of Paracelsus. All of the chemicals that he recommended and all of his *arcana* (Latin *arcanum*, "sacred secret") were thought to be specifics.

In this light, his often ridiculed revival of the old theory of "signatures" becomes understandable. Paracelsus was a faithful believer, to whom a benevolent Providence was an indisputable dogma. He was not surprised to find Nature hinting at the therapeutic bounty of her store of raw materials, signified by characteristics of their outer appearance (e.g., turmeric to be used against jaundice). What else were these but specifics "signed" by the Lord himself, with direct designations as to their specific usefulness? Far from being strange to the Paracelsian way of thought, the theory of "signatures" offered him a welcome divine confirmation of his thinking.

To call Paracelsus the father of iatrochemistry, as often has been done, does not conform with historical truth. On the contrary, he rejected the system of Galen and Avicenna without replacing it with another theory. That made him hated and feared by the friends of fixed schemes, who saw him as the propagandist of chaos, and it made him the champion of those who saw in this breaking away from any scheme the first step to a new beginning. Paracelsus did not only open doors: he left them open.

While Paracelsus' relation to the rise of pharmaceutical chemistry is complex and easily oversimplified, it can be said that he did influence tremendously the transformation of pharmacy from a profession based primarily on botanic science to one based on chemical science. If Paracelsus himself was not the most important innovator, it was he who inspired the "Paracelsians" of the subsequent century to bring to therapy a whole new outlook by the chemical procedures that they developed and by the definition of chemical drugs that thus were created.[9]

IATROCHEMISTRY AFFECTS PHARMACY

Paracelsus was a mystic as well as a revolutionary empiricist. He not only believed in the doctrine of the signatures, but assumed the presence of a mysterious vital force. He called it *archaeus*, endowed with the power of dominating all processes of life. This idea of a vital force and the concept that sickness reflects chemical changes in the body produced by a morbid mood of the *archaeus* are expressed still more definitely in the medical system of the great

Flemish physician Jean Baptist van Helmont (1577-1644). He is famous as the discoverer of carbonic acid, which he called *gas sylvestre*, thus originating the concept and the term "gas." However, the real founder of iatrochemistry was François de le Boë Sylvius (1614-1672). His theory was a kind of compromise between humoral pathology and the ideas of Paracelsus.

The vantage point of De le Boë Sylvius' theories is what he called "fermentation." He believed that food is transformed through saliva and a ferment secreted from the pancreas, and that blood becomes the life-maintaining substance he thought it to be through certain ferments carried into the bloodstream from the gall bladder and the lymph glands. These continuous transformations, influenced by the body temperature (*calor innatus*) and the spirits of life (*spiritus*), result in either alkaline or acid end products. If both are in the right proportion qualitatively as well as quantitatively, the person concerned is healthy.

Disease, on the contrary, is caused by an "acrimony" or excess of either the acid or the alkaline substances, or their being at a wrong place. According to iatrochemical theory, this acrimony leads to a change in the blood, the bile or the lymph. Hence all diseases were subdivided into those based on alkaline or an acid acrimony. The drugs used in treating them had to be of a contrasting nature, either acid or alkaline.

This medico-chemical theory became naturally the basis for the preparing of new chemical drugs. It was welcomed still more as a convenient guide for selecting from among a myriad of drugs already known and as an explanation of their empirically observed effects. This felt need for an adequate explanation of known effects attracted a number of physicians of the 17th and the early 18th centuries to another hypothesis, the iatrophysical or mechanical theory, developed some decades before De le Boë Sylvius' hypothesis by the Italian physician Santorio Santorio (1561-1636). It was based on the concept of the body as a kind of engine, following mainly physical laws.[10] This outlook led Santorio to invent the first instrument intended to measure

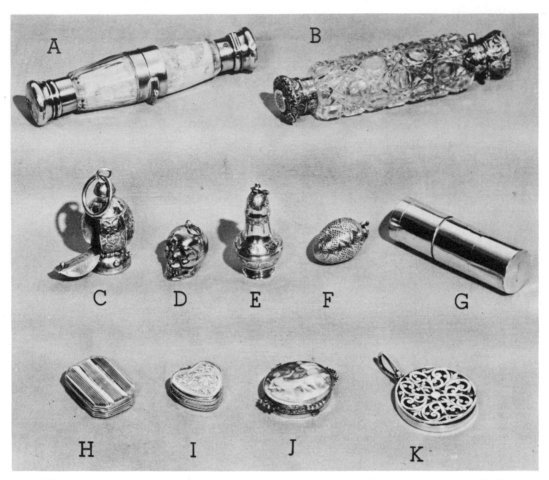

Elegant containers may have made more impressive the old drugs whose actual effects were usually doubtful or nonspecific. Supposedly anti-infective aromatics intended to neutralize the "ill air" were carried in containers such as the multicompartment pomander (C) which held ambergris (16th century) and other pomanders (D, E, F) of later vintage; the vinaigrettes (H, I, J), which were small silver boxes that held a bit of sponge charged with aromatic vinegar (early 19th century); and the camphor locket (K). The silver pill box (G) is a rare example (ca. 1800), but pocket "pill boxes" have never gone completely out of style even though pills have. Bottles (A, B) for smelling salts (ammonium carbonate with lavender-scented ammonia water) were popular when swooning was fashionable. (Artifacts from the Drake Collection, Academy of Medicine, Toronto, Ont.; *see* Drake, T. G. H.: J. Hist. Med. *15*:31-44, 1960; photograph from University of Wisconsin.)

body temperature, a predecessor to our clinical thermometer, and to make the first systematic attempt to explain by as exact means as possible what we call metabolism.

A CENTURY OF SPECULATIVE THEORIES

The 18th century brought new men and theories that were certain to be speculative and debatable, since the health professions still lacked experimental technics for establishing the site and the mechanism of drug action. A new kind of solidar pathology was announced in Halle by Friedrich Hoffmann, the famous inventor of many remedies (1660-1742). According to him life depends —as the ancient Soranos assumed—on a normal tension of the solid parts of the body. However, unlike Soranos, Hoffmann taught that these solid parts are not the ducts but the fibers.

He assumed a hypothetical ether-like fluid acting through the nervous system upon the fibers and keeping them in a state of partial tonic contraction, and also keeping the humors of the body in the motion necessary for life.[11]

This materialistic theory had its antipode in the ideology of Ernst Stahl (1660-1734), at Halle. His concept of illness and therapy was named *animismus*, because Stahl considered the soul (Latin: *anima*) the highest principle of life, balancing all bodily functions by a distinct rhythmic movement. This movement produced a certain tension called tonus. The individual was ill if this tonus was not normal. The task of remedies was to help the anima to restore normal tonus.

Similar to the animism of Stahl was the "vitalism" of the Frenchman P. J. Barthez, in which the soul was replaced by the so-called vital principle (1778).

In England two theories in particular gained wide acknowledgment. (1) William Cullen (1710-1790) postulated that all bodily functions are regulated by a so-called nervous principle, which in cases of illness tries to restore normal conditions by convulsion or by atony. Therefore, the remedies had to be either irritating or emollient. (2) The hypothesis of the Scotch physician John Brown (1735-1788), a pupil of Cullen, was that not the nervous principle itself but the stimuli that set it in motion are the decisive factors for health or sickness. Normal life is a harmony between excitability and the incessant external and internal stimuli acting on the body; all diseases have their final cause in a disproportion between the excitability of the organism and the stimuli (too strong or too feeble) that affect it.

BACKGROUND TO MODERN PHARMACY

Pathologic anatomy focused medical thought during the first half of the 19th century on the localized changes revealed by careful observations and the advancing technics of microscopy. A brilliant line of investigators begins with Morgagni (1682-1771) of Bologna, continues with Corvisart (1755-1821) and Laennec (1781-1826) of Paris and is brought to its culmination by Rokitansky (1804-1878) and Skoda (1805-1881) of Vienna.[12] According to this school of thought, maladies were localized in the ill parts of the body and made obvious by anatomic changes. There were generalized diseases too, their habitat being the blood. Nevertheless, even these general diseases were supposed to have a tendency to localize themselves. Thus there were no sick individuals but only distinct, anatomically demonstrable pathologies. The natural consequence of this theory was to relegate therapeutic efforts more and more to the knife of the surgeon and to condemn or at least to deprecate internal medication that was of necessity more general in its effects. By mid-century this spirit of skepticism became an actual therapeutic nihilism.[13]

The man whose work crowned the development of solidar pathology was Rudolf Virchow (1821-1902), the founder of cellular pathology, which has continued to dominate medical biology to the present day. His theory, briefly stated, is as follows: The cell is the bearer of life. Disease is the reaction of the cell to abnormal stimulation. According to Virchow's own statement, "the organism is not a unified but a social arrangement." The influence of the work of Virchow

. . . enabled doctors to realize that the point of onslaught of remedies in the organism are not the organs in general but the cells. We now know that there are peculiar affinities between particular cells and particular chemical substances.[14]

On this ground pharmacy and drug therapy took on renewed meaning and purposefulness. Once all but annihilated by the Viennese school, internal therapy again commanded respect. As cellular pathology was joined with the new chemistry and bacteriology, experimental pharmacology began to chart the world of drug therapy during the second half of the 19th century in terms that we understand today.

Immunology and Medical Bacteriology

The scientific basis for massive conquests of disease during the past century had a remarkable empiric beginning in the field of immunology.

The idea of artificially induced immunity against contagious diseases was outlined by the English physician Edward Jenner. Leaning on earlier empiric observations and his own experiments, he reported (1798) on his success in inducing in humans the harmless cowpox, which he found to be a reliable prophylactic against smallpox. This courageous deed received scientific support with the discovery of the laws of bacteriology and their practical application by the French chemist Louis Pasteur (1822-1897) and the German physicians Robert Koch (1843-1910) and Emil von Behring (1854-1917). To Pasteur we are indebted for the methods of employing cultures of weakened bacteria, the vaccines; for his demonstration of the existence of sickness-producing germs in the air and, especially, for the discovery of sterilization and pasteurization. These discoveries in turn made possible the introduction of antisepsis (through the use of disinfectants in the treatment of wounds) by the English surgeon Joseph Lister. Finally, this was followed by asepsis. In addition to the discovery of a series of morbific agents, we owe to Koch the modern technic of bacteriology; to Behring we are indebted for the knowledge of how to produce antitoxins in the blood serum of animals by immunizing them with specific toxins.

What this development means to pharmacy becomes evident from the fact that the so-called biological products—serums, vaccines, toxins, antitoxins, etc.—have become one of the important parts of the responsibility and the service of the pharmacist. Moreover, it is now difficult to imagine the practice of pharmacy or medicine without the variety of medicated and sterilized gauzes, cottons and other surgical materials, and of sterile parenteral medications, the manufacture and use of which are based on the laws of antisepsis and asepsis.

Chemotherapy Ascendant

During our own century drug therapy has been unfolding largely under the banner of "chemotherapy," which rests on the theory of relationships between chemical constitution and pharmacologic action.

In a figurative sense, chemotherapy climaxes the triumph of Paracelsus over Galen. We see in Paul Ehrlich (1854-1915)[15] the pioneer of a new way of work and line of development (albeit unthinkable without the headlong scientific advances during the century preceding him).

From 1906, when Ehrlich took up atoxyl for tests against experimental spirillosis, until 1910, when arsphenamine went into widespread clinical trial, Ehrlich and his co-workers had persisted in an organized, planned program. Arsphenamine ("606") was the 606th compound they prepared and tested, with the objective of finding a chemical that would seek out in the body and destroy the spirochete causing syphilis.

This direct attack on morbific agents in the body by means of chemicals, without doing unbearable harm to the cells containing the microbes and to the body at large, was called "chemotherapy" by Ehrlich. There is now a tendency to extend use of the term, originally meant only for internal treatment, to include external attack on microbes as well. The discoverer of penicillin, Alexander Fleming, favored (1946) the use of the term chemotherapy "to cover any treatment in which a chemical is administered in a manner directly injurious to the microbes infecting the body. In this latter sense antiseptic treatment comes under chemotherapy—call it local chemotherapy if you like."[16]

After a frustrating quarter century, during which the concept and the methods of Ehrlich could not be made to yield another major breakthrough, the announcement came from Gerhard Domagk in 1935 of the curative action of Prontosil (4-sulfonamid-2',4'-diaminoazobenzol) against streptococcal infection in man—a success foreshadowed 3 years earlier by tests in mice.[17] Like arsphenamine, this compound was a chemotherapeutic specific. After this specific action became identified with the sulfonamide group, a series of related compounds converted the character of other areas of therapy from symptomatic to curative; the sulfonamides opened a new frontier of conquest among the acute bacterial infections. In America by 1955 the official compendia contained no less than 13 sulfonamides, not counting simple variations of the basic drugs.[18]

Repeated success in the "sulfa era" is important not only for the specific diseases brought under control but for the tremendous stimulus and the hints it gave to research workers and the resultant industrial optimism that led to heavier investment in pharmaceutical research.

Despite optimism and progress concerning theories of structure-activity relationship, the role of empiricism and quasi-accidental discovery have been displaced only slowly from pharmaceutical research since the time of Paul Ehrlich. Evidence in point may be seen in the massive random screening programs which were set up following the sulfanilamide discoveries. This effort, especially directed toward finding effective antimalarial and anticarcinogenic compounds, has yielded valuable results.

The fruitfulness of chemotherapy as originally conceived pointed the way toward additional discoveries and understanding of drug action that have been achieved since the 1930's (even though many of these are used beyond the area of infectious diseases at which Ehrlich was aiming his "magic bullets") such as the new diuretic, antihypertensive and psychotropic drugs.

Meanwhile, newer theoretic concepts have illuminated the probable relationships between chemical structure and biologic activity, but their predictive value has not excited research workers at the bench. In fact, it has been said authoritatively that recent major discoveries in medicinal chemistry owe little to such concepts.[19] One of the most dramatic illustrations of this disconcerting circumstance can be found in the antibiotic drugs.

The story of the exciting accident and the perceptive observation through which Alexander Fleming discovered penicillin (1928) is a well known one. Equally remarkable was the wait until other Britons (Chain, Florey and Heatley in 1939) sensed the import of the discovery clearly enough to take up a vigorous investigation, which brought the drug into therapy—with an important assist from American pharmaceutical industry—in time to meet urgent military demands of the early 1940's.

Less well known is the fact that the term (and the vague notion) of "antibiosis" occurred to the Frenchman Paul Vuillemin as early as 1889. Twelve years earlier still, Louis Pasteur himself mentioned the phenomenon of antagonism between living organisms. A whole series of half-forgotten observations of antibiotic action among micro-organisms came out of European laboratories before the turn of the century; even the effect of a *Penicillium* mold is said to have been recorded by an Italian named Bartolomeo Gosio (1896).[20] However, it was the observation by Fleming that proved to be consequential, in that it gave the Oxford group headed by Florey and Chain the direct lead they needed to isolate the little penicillin that was given to a London policeman on February 12, 1941.

Penicillin represented the most startling advance in medicine and pharmacy since the initial success of Ehrlich. However, unlike his work, it represented no systematic attack on the problem within a stated concept. This fact is underscored by the frantic testing of thousands of antimicrobial substances in the ensuing decade, of which less than ten found noteworthy use in therapy.[21] However, the practical value of these few antibiotics has improved the life chance of the human race, first notably extended by the American discovery of streptomycin by Selman Waksman in 1944 and then within a decade by the wider resource of broad-spectrum antibiotics, which is still being explored.

It has been said that "chemotherapy" is a revival of the "iatrochemistry" of old— inaugurated by Paracelsus and systematized by François de la Boë Sylvius, but this certainly is not the case. De le Boë Sylvius' system was another attempt at a scheme of comprehending and trying to explain the whole of medicine. Above all, it was a medical speculation, although using the contemporary chemical concepts as its basis.

Ehrlich's chemotherapy (unlike iatrochemistry) was restricted to a special area of chemico-biological attack, in which chemical considerations play the dominant part. The term "chemotherapy" itself points to the distinction, giving chemistry precedence over therapy, just as the term "iatrochemistry" gives preference to iatros (the physician), i.e., to the medical side of the concept thus designated.

The cellular pathology of Virchow, which provided the ground on which chemotherapy developed, may be regarded as a European attempt to formulate a general explanation of the fundamental nature of health and sickness and, by implication, to give a guidepost for therapy. However, recent years have brought several more specific medical, medico-chemical and biologic theories and discoveries which, like the aforementioned immunology and medical bacteriology, have a great influence on therapy and, hence, on pharmacy.

Vitamins and Hormones

Among the modern discoveries, the avitaminoses—diseases caused by a lack of some of the substances found in food (substances which we now know under the name of vitamins)—and, furthermore, the regulative effect of the hormones hold prominent places.

The word "vitamin" derives from the Latin vita (life) and amine, the chemical class to which the inventor of the term (1912) erroneously considered the vitamins to belong. The many-branched research on the vitamins came largely only in our own century, because the earlier blinding revelation of medical bacteriology had made it difficult to grasp in all its far-reaching consequences the concept of disease as caused by the *absence* of something rather than by the presence of infectious organisms. Since 1913, the United States and England have contributed the most to newer knowledge of the vitamins. The vitamins have been found in foodstuffs of both vegetable and animal origin and have been synthesized in ever growing numbers.

The word "hormone" is taken from the Greek, meaning "to excite." The hormones, products of the glands of internal secretion, became of practical importance in therapeutics only after the experiments of a Franco-American in the 1880's, the physiologist C. E. Brown-Séquard. With the unfolding of endocrinology, a few endocrine extracts (e.g., suprarenin and thyroiodin) were made already in the 19th century, but, like vitamin therapy, effective hormonal therapy is mainly a research child of our own century. A cornerstone was the discovery of insulin by the Canadian physician F. G. Banting, in collaboration with McLeod, Best and Collip in 1922. Its manufacture on a large scale was made possible by the far-sighted assistance given to these scientists by an American pharmaceutical firm, Eli Lilly and Company. This concern developed the processes for mass production and put the experience thus obtained at the disposal of other manufacturers who agreed to meet established standards and to submit the products to controlling tests. Thyroxin was isolated from the thyroid gland in 1915 (E. C. Kendall of the Mayo Foundation). More recently, the so-called "sex hormones" have gained therapeutic importance. The first naturally occurring androgenic hormone to be obtained in crystalline form was isolated from male urine in 1931 (Butenandt and Tscherning). The hormones from animal sources have been, like the vitamins, synthesized in increasing number.

Homeopathy—Original but Wrong?

In addition to these theories and discoveries, a peculiar pharmacologic system was proposed in the beginning of the 19th century by the German physician Samuel Hahnemann (1755-1843). Somewhat later, this found wide acknowledgment and sectarian cultivation, particularly in the United States.

Hahnemann established the general therapeutic principle that disease is cured by such remedies as call forth symptoms which resemble the disease in question. More than this, the remedies were to be used in very weak concentrations. The treatment was thus based on the principle "similia similibus" and Hahnemann called his theory homeopathy (from the Greek word *homoion*—similar) in contrast to the principles of the ancient therapy "contraria contrariis" (contrasting symptoms and remedies) and which Hahnemann consequently called "allopathy" (from the Greek word *alloion*—different).[22]

This concise statement by Sigerist requires some supplementation from a pharmaceutical point of view.

The "Simile" Principle. The general idea of homeopathy is to incite the defense mechanisms of the body by adequate irritation, rather than to attack the disease as such. This leads to the *simile* theory: The similarity (if not the identity) of the symptoms produced by certain drugs, when tested on healthy individuals, to the symptoms signifying a particular disease, indicates which drugs should be used to mobilize the defense mechanisms of the body.

Minute Doses. This irritation concept also provides a rationale for the use of very minute doses in homeopathic practice. In the late 19th century this application of very small doses for the purpose of irritation found support in the so-called "biologic fundamental law" promulgated by the German physicians Rudolf Arndt and Hugo Schulz. This "law" states that "minute stimuli initiate the activity of living organisms and those of medium strength promote it, while strong stimuli slow it down and very strong ones stop it." Naturally, the question concerns the degree of "minuteness" that still allows for an inciting effect, and it is understood that dilutions transgressing the limits drawn by modern chemistry and physics are beyond scientific evaluation and hence beyond consideration.

In his prescriptions Hahnemann himself insisted on the use of only a single active drug at a time. His followers often have been less rigorous in regard to the prescribing of mixtures and compounded drugs. Another pharmaceutical principle required that the homeopathic tinctures be made from fresh crude drugs (not dried). Because of such special requirements,[23] homeopathic drugs in the United States are often dispensed by homeopathic physicians themselves or, in metropolitan areas, through special pharmacies.

Writing of the heyday of homeopathy, the medical historian Erwin Ackerknecht concludes:

At least Hahnemann's system offered a fairly innocuous alternative to the heroic and often fatal orthodox therapeutic methods of the age, which still consisted of extensive bloodletting, purging, large doses of toxic drugs, and induced vomiting. The dogmatism of his system has separated it from the main stream of scientific development, and it now lives on as a cult with a relatively small following.[24]

THE MATERIA MEDICA CHANGES

Every change in medical concepts that influenced therapy made itself felt in the practice of pharmacy. The question is how far did these influences extend?

Therapy (hence pharmacy) is based mainly on empiric or experimental observations. But even without new observations changing medical theories could still alter the combinations of remedies. They could influence physicians in their choice of drugs. Finally, through the medical profession, theories could deny the usefulness of drugs altogether. However, new drugs could hardly be found in the wake of new theoretical concepts not based on or followed by experimental work.

The consequences to be derived from this fact are obvious: There was no real change of medication until the development of the respective basic sciences. Chemistry first, and bacteriology later, furnished the broad substantial and experimental possibilities for the creation of new kinds of drugs, and experimental physiology and pharmacology finally offered a new way of testing, checking and verifying the assumed effects. Until the late 18th century, there were continuous, more or less haphazard additions to the official materia medica, but hardly any deletions.

It has often been overlooked that the masses of the medical practitioners were more indifferent toward the changes in theories than the heated discussions published by the medical elite seem to indicate. Only some of the physicians followed new speculative theories for which there

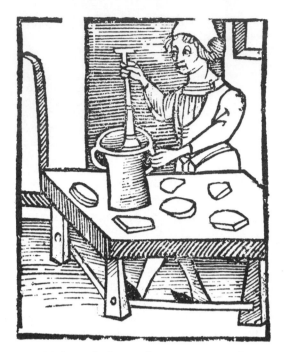

Medicinal chemicals came into wider use internally with the Renaissance. This woodcut from a famous drug book of that time shows a contusion mortar being used to grind up "Armenus," a variety of cupric carbonate then obtained particularly from Armenia. (*Hortus Sanitatis*, Chap. 13, Strasbourg, about 1507; from the American Institute of the History of Pharmacy; University of Wisconsin Library)

could not yet be experimental tests. Furthermore, many of these—and even the creators of the theories—were by no means fanatical adherents. Thus we know that François de le Boë Sylvius, for example, made liberal use of the old and tried remedies that had no justification according to his own chemical theory.[25] This conflict between theory and practice we meet again and again, and it always ends with the victory of practice.

A case in point is offered by the conservative medical teachers, bound to Galenic theory, at the University of Paris in the 17th century. Leaders in the fight against iatrochemistry, with its presumed specifics against certain diseases, they likewise were antagonized and confounded by the arrival of new drugs coming from America.

These were herb preparations which like the chemical preparations exerted violent, in fact specific, effects without the addition of other materials. Foremost of them was quinine [at that period not the alkaloid but the cinchona bark]. "An impertinent innovation," it was called by Guy Patin, but its effect in malaria was too apparent to allow any of its opponents to hold out against its use for long. Even the Paris faculty had to admit it shamefacedly.[26]

Even if the "Galenists" had to admit drugs of the new school in the codes appearing under their authority, they retained those of old.

Still another factor played its part in preventing the disappearance of useful drugs merely because they did not fit into a medical system. Even during periods dominated by certain medical theories there always were great and highly esteemed eclectic physicians who went "back to Hippocrates," i.e., who aided the healing power of nature with all reasonable and available means regardless of theory. Such physicians were the famous English medical practitioner Thomas Sydenham[27] (1624-1689), whom his grateful contemporaries called the English Hippocrates; the Dutch physician and teacher Hermann Boerhaave (1668-1738),[28] and the German C. W. Hufeland (1762-1836).[29] These men exerted great influence on the practice of medicine.

The common people, conservators of folk medicine, also held fast to traditionally proven remedies and continued to use them. Sometimes drugs that had lost official acknowledgment because they were not in harmony with the dominant medical theory were preserved by popular use and, later on, with the rise of a new and more satisfactory theory, were again officially approved. The best example is cod-liver oil.[30]

From the early 19th century on, the development of scientific chemistry progressively replaced botanic drugs by better chemical drugs and even threatened to eliminate the former entirely by a modern materialization of the Paracelsian idea of the "essential." The vegetable drugs, insofar as their usefulness was too obvious to be denied, were investigated chemically, in order to isolate and identify their active constituents and, finally, to synthesize them. Alkaloids, glucosides, vitamins and hormones are among the important results of this development.

As pointed out above, iatrochemistry and, still more, chemotherapy were "medical" theories mainly with regard to their application to medicine. However, they were based on chemical concepts. Sylvius was not only a physician but, within the limits of his time, an excellent chemist as well. It was his knowledge of chemistry that made him conceive a medical system in which chemical concepts played an important part. Ehrlich, the founder of chemotherapy, passed the medical examinations but, throughout his life, practiced chemistry, not medicine. He did not take his ideas from medicine and support them by chemical knowledge; he took them from chemistry and transferred them to medicine. From the effect in vitro, both men assumed a like or similar effect in vivo.

The empirico-experimental root of medical chemistry, growing up from the soil of pure chemistry and sending its branches into the air and the area of medicine, made possible the fruits that we are enjoying today. Furthermore, the origin of medical chemistry explains why, in this epoch of therapy, pharmacists have played such an important role in the finding of new remedies—for example, such men as the discoverer of morphine, the German Sertuerner, and the discoverers of quinine, the Frenchmen Caventou and Pelletier.

As the requirements in methods and facilities grew, much of this investigative basis of modern therapy has been elaborated elegantly and fruitfully in the laboratories of pharmaceutical industry.

It has been pointed out above that in the pharmacopeias the authorities had for a long time merely added the new drugs to the old ones. Thus the first edition of the *Pharmacopoeia Augustana* (1564) contained about 1,100 medicaments.[31] Yet that "number is relatively small when compared with that of the official and unofficial pharmacopeias of the 17th century resulting from the union of Galenical and chymiatric remedies."[32] One of the best-

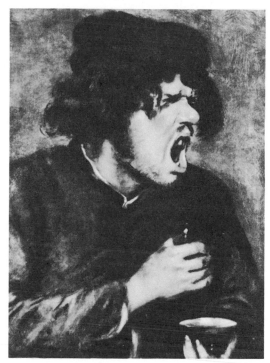

This 17th-century painting by Adriaen Brouer is titled "The Bitter Medicine." It conveys vividly the reaction of a rustic patient to the copious, unpleasant draught that one could expect to receive from a pharmacist before investigations had yielded the active constituents of drugs in more concentrated, palatable and reliable forms. (From A. I. H. P. Archive, Madison, Wis.; 1941 calendar of the Nederlandsche Maatschappij ter Bevordering der Pharmacie. Original canvas at Frankfort on the Main)

reputed pharmacopeias of the 18th century (*Pharmacopoeia Wurtembergica,* 1741) contains 1,952 different drugs and formulas.

When in 1746 the Royal College of Physicians of London published a "purified" revision of the *Pharmacopoeia Londinensis,* purged of a number of outmoded drugs, it considered itself "to be the first medical society in Europe which shall have duly undertaken this reformation."[33] After the acceptance of the chemical theories of Lavoisier, such "purifications" of pharmacopeias (i.e., the omission of many old formulas containing dozens of ingredients) became more general. When the first *Pharmacopoeia Borussica* appeared (1799), decisively influenced by the great pharmacist-chemist M. H. Klaproth, medical as well as pharmaceutical practitioners complained about its radically simplified materia medica so vehemently that some of the omitted drugs were again included in the 1827 edition of the Prussian standard.

In addition to the official standards, there has always been an unofficial literature dealing with drugs not admitted to the official books. That literature grew with the increasing trend to purification and simplification of the pharmacopeias. Many of the complicated preparations, sanctioned more by tradition and fading belief than by effect, disappeared altogether. However, a greater number remained and formed, altered or unaltered, the contents of the unofficial books. Thus the "extra" pharmacopeias (England), the *officines* (France), the *Ergänzungsbücher* (Germany), the "dispensatories," the "national formularies" and the "recipe books" (America) came into being.

The development of therapeutic thought and practice, as explained above in its relation to pharmacy, has been common to Western civilization in general. Was that the case likewise in regard to the more particular development of scientific and professional pharmacy in the most important cultural centers of Europe, in Italy, France, Spain, Germany and England? As a matter of fact, it was not.

4:   The Development in Italy

Italy is the classic soil of European pharmacy as it is that of most of the European professions and arts. The law of the German ruler of the Two Sicilies, Frederick II (see page 39 and Appendix 7), although promulgated in Italy and for Italian territory, was born more out of the German than out of the Italian spirit. The first real Italian legal regulations of the duties of both physicians and apothecaries, of which we have knowledge, are the Venetian *statuta* promulgated in 1258.[1] Although they resemble the edict of Frederick II, the *statuta* mention neither a limiting of the number of pharmacies nor governmentally fixed prices for remedies. It is of interest to note that the statutes not only forbade the practice of medicine by the pharmacist in general terms but also stated strongly that he was not allowed to examine the urine of patients, which up to the 17th century was one of the most important means of medical diagnosis. Official supervision of the drug trade, including wholesalers as well as retailers (the latter called *speziarii* and *aromatarii*) had existed in Venice as early as the 12th century.[2]

ORGANIZATION INTO GUILDS

Italian professional pharmacy and apothecary shops were not created by governmental edicts but existed long before legislation dealt with them. Consequently, they had found their natural place within the framework of the guild system—an organization that had a special dignity and task, particularly in Italy.

We know of guildlike associations already in ancient Rome. The somewhat peculiar predecessors of the pharmacists, the *seplasiarii* (see page 17 and Appendix 7), are said to have been united in such a guild.[3] These associations bore the designations *ars collegium, schola* or even *universitas,* to which an occupational designa-

tion for each guild was added. (The names were adopted in part by later medieval guilds.) These names by no means imply that the guilds had primarily an educational purpose. They were founded mainly for social and welfare purposes, and the regulating of conditions of trade.[4] In wartime they could be mobilized for military purposes.

The organization of merchants and craftsmen into guilds, according to the kind of goods sold or the kind of wares manufactured, is one of the most significant features of the Middle Ages. During the period of feudalism the guild system created a bourgeoisie regulating both production and distribution.[5] However, there were great differences in the manner in which the guilds in the several countries fulfilled their task. In France, England and Germany the guilds were restricted largely to the internal organization, regulation or administration of their special occupation. In Italy, much more than elsewhere, they were also political, important cogs in the governmental machinery of the city republics up to the 17th century.

In Florence, physicians and pharmacists combined in the same guild, together with some others, toward the close of the 12th century.[6] When, in 1236, the principal trade corporations of Florence were divided into two divisions, i.e., the seven major arts and the fourteen minor arts, the distinction was one both of technic and of class.[7] As group six, the guild of physicians and pharmacists belonged to the major arts, the arts of higher esteem.

In the membership lists of the various guilds (1297 to 1444) about 70 different callings were represented. Among these the pharmacists and the wholesalers of drugs outnumbered all the others. This is understood readily if we recall that at this time Italy (more particularly Florence, Genoa and Venice) governed the entire European trade in oriental drugs and

53

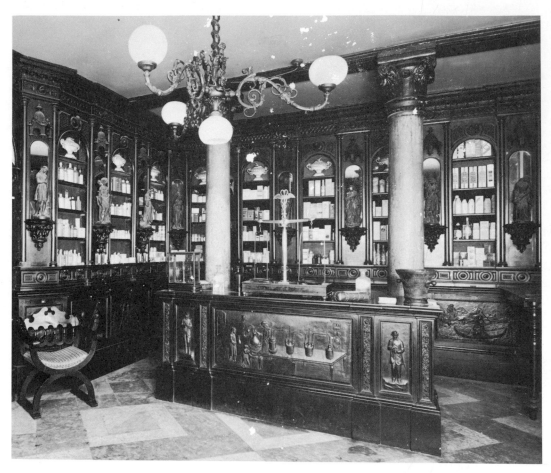

The beautiful old Farmacia Daniele Manin, at Campo San Fantin, still serves the populace of Venice. The terra-cotta sculptures that watch over the work of Pharmacist Guiseppe Zaini and his associates are thought to be the work of the brothers Zandomeneghi, of the 19th-century school of Cannova. (Photograph copyrighted by Foto Giacomelli, Venice.)

spices.[8] Guild statutes (1349) mention no less than 206 different articles as belonging to the monopoly of the pharmacists or spicers. Their trade extended to many products that at this time were rare and costly. The sale of books was in their hands. They had the monopoly of wax candles. Even funerals, especially those of the wealthier citizens, were conducted by the pharmacists.[9] Supervision was rigid. Once a year the pharmacies were inspected by a commission of the guild. Drugs not meeting the requirements were confiscated and the culprits excluded from professional practice for variable periods.

The part played by the guild of physicians and pharmacists in Florence is well characterized in this brief sentence: "And a great guild it truly was . . . it yielded to none in the loftiness of its aim and in the splendor of its achievements."[10]

In various other Italian cities, guilds of pharmacists—either separate or together with physicians—first appear in records of the 13th and subsequent centuries.[11]

The oldest Italian pharmaceutical guild still existing is the *Nobile collegio chimico farmaceutico*, founded as *Universitas aromatariorum* in time immemorial and solemnly renewed in 1429 by a special edict (*bolla*) of Pope Martin V under the title *Nobile collegio degli aromatari*.[12] The tasks of the guild were (1) the care of poor and sick members, (2) the "immatriculation and location" of all pharmacists who have passed the examinations, (3) the regulation of the distance between pharmacies, (4) the regulation of the prices for remedies, (5) the collection of taxes, to be delivered to the government and (6) the supervision of the producers and the retailers of food, liquors, pastries and medicinal herbs. These tasks can be regarded as those traditional for the Italian pharmaceutical guilds.

Of course, pharmaceutical conditions were not uniform in the different states established on Italian soil between the 13th and 19th centuries. Thus, there were variations in the important provision for separating the medical and the pharmaceutical professions. While all commercial association between the professions was forbidden (although this was not always rigidly enforced) in Southern Italy, Rome, Pisa and many other Italian states,[13] the Florentine statute (1313) allowed the pharmacist to employ a physician in his shop and the physician to employ a pharmacist. A similar regulation appears in the

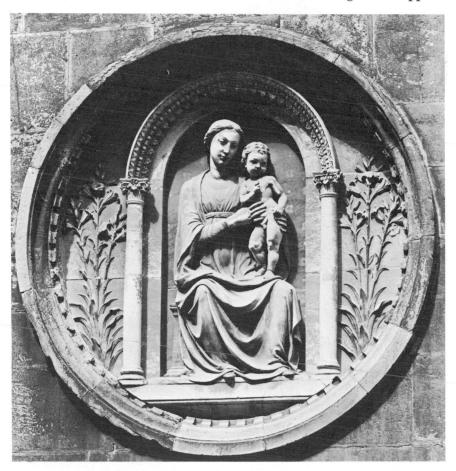

The lustrous guild of physicians and pharmacists in Florence, Italy, commissioned the sculptors della Robbia to execute their emblem (above) as a polychrome medallion, one of a series dedicated by various professions and practical arts (15th century). Its superb composition, serenity and grace may still be admired today high on the south gable of the church Or San Michele. Other churches likewise bear mute evidences of the patronage of the rising class of early modern pharmacists. (Photograph from Ed. Alinari, Florence.)

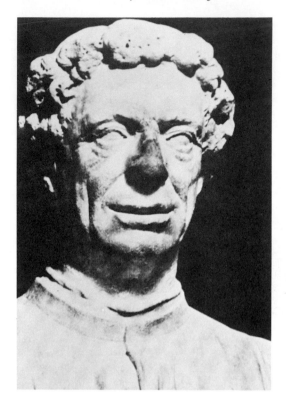

This marble bust of an Italian pharmacist which looks out across a gallery of the Bargello National Museum at Florence is treasured not only because of its excellence as 15th-century sculpture, but also because Matteo Palmieri earned honor in his time as a statesman and a gifted humanist. A memorial tablet on the modern pharmacy standing where Palmieri once practiced reminds passersby of this simple but many-sided man, whose strong personality was caught in stone by Antonio Rossellino (1468). (Adapted from Illustrierter Apotheker-Kalender, Deutscher Apotheker-Verlag, 1959.)

Mantuan statute of 1303. In Pistoia, physicians and pharmacists founded a commercial company; the pharmacy was common possession, and the profits were shared. Similar arrangements later became customary in Florence. The pharmacist was forbidden to reimburse the physician for individual prescriptions; however, the physician was allowed to own a share of the entire establishment of the pharmacist.

In most Italian towns it was customary for the physician to see his patient in a pharmacy, or at least to be available through the pharmacy.

Until the close of the 16th century the cultural influence of the powerful city-states made their institutions a model for other parts of Italy. From the 12th to the 16th centuries Italy was once more the cultural center of the world. Pharmacists of Northern Europe, as well as physicians who desired a better education than they could acquire at home, came to the renowned Italian universities (especially Padua, Bologna, Pisa and Ferrara). This cultural development rested on the wealth acquired by the city-states. Their merchant princes, such as the Medici of Florence, not only controlled the oriental spice trade but were international bankers as well. The Italian trade, including drugs,[14] extended from Constantinople, Damascus, Alexandria and Tunis to southern Germany, France, London, Lisbon, Antwerp and Bruegge in the north.[15]

EARLY LARGE-SCALE MANUFACTURING

The Italian drug trade was supplemented very early by the development of a chemical industry, which was the first on European soil. In 1294 Venice was producing corrosive sublimate and cinnabar and, somewhat later, sugar of lead, borax, soap, sal ammoniac, Venetian talc and Venetian turpentine.[16] A very important pharmaceutical export was Venetian treacle (from Latin, *theriaca*, an antidote, q.v. Glossary). Another was the famous Venetian troches of vipers, legally required in some European states for the local preparation of treacle.[17]

In Italy we also observe for the first time industrial pharmaceutical activity by the monasteries. Thus the monastery of the church of Santa Maria Novella in Florence was famous for distilled waters and cosmetics that the monks prepared and sold.

RANK IN SOCIETY

The important role played by Italian pharmacy and pharmacists in the political and social life of the country found one expression in public esteem as well as in the equipment of the pharmacies. The Italian pharmacist was always considered a patrician. In Venice the profession was officially recognized as an *arte nobile;* pharmacists were granted the right to marry Venetian ladies of noble rank. During the middle of the 14th century, the Florentine pharmacist Matteo Palmieri was ambassador of his country to the court of the King of Naples.[18] Up to the present there has always been a great number of pharmacists active in Italian politics and represented in the literature of their country. Even in the military service the social and professional recognition of the calling found an early expression, putting the pharmacist on an equal level with the physician. This has been true from the establishment of the modern Italian kingdom up to our time.

The Italian pharmacies of the Renaissance period were often rooms of architectural beauty, with equipment that even today is highly valued by connoisseurs of Italian art[19] and is the pride of many museums and private collections.[20] The development of pottery from a simple handicraft to an art was especially stimulated by Italian pharmacy. Private pharmacists, hospitals and the high nobility competed with each other in adorning their shops or pharmaceutical workrooms and storerooms with precious faïence jars, jugs and vases to hold precious drugs.

FROM GUILD TO GOVERNMENT RULE

Italian trade and wealth declined after the discovery of America and, more particularly, of the all-water route to the East Indies. As early as 1501, King Manuel of Portugal wrote to the Venetian government that there was no longer a reason for Venetian merchants to send ships to Egypt (and the Levant), and he suggested that they should rather buy their oriental goods in Portugal.[21] The time of the Italian intermediate trade was a thing of the past. The drugs of the Orient were brought directly to Europe by the Portuguese and, later, by the Dutch; the drugs of the New World were made available first by the Spaniards and then by the English. In the unhappy Italian situation of the 17th century, "Venice and Genoa were on the road to decadence, Lombardy was pillaged by the Spanish, French and Germans, the small Italian states were tormented by the fights of princes."[22]

The political importance of the guilds declined with the declining wealth and political power of the Italian municipalities. However, under government authority they retained a certain internal authority within their own occupational fields.

Conditions changed in the 18th century, which was characterized politically by interference on the part of Austria, the rise of Savoy in the North, and the re-establishment of the southern Italian kingdom as the Kingdom of Naples. It was Austrian regulations *(Piano di regolamento per le farmacie della Lombardia austriaca,* 1778) that gave the impulse for progressive pharmaceutical legislation in Italy as a whole. One of the most important innovations was the limitation of the pharmacies, allowing one pharmacy to 5,000 inhabitants in the Northern Italian territory then under Austrian rule. However, the organization of pharmacy in the various Italian states existing before 1870 differed greatly. In some of them the number of pharmacies was not limited; in others one pharmacy was allowed to 3,000 inhabitants, as in Rome, or a certain distance was required between the pharmacies, as in Naples.[23]

The new Italian Kingdom established in 1870 gradually reduced these variations to a uniform system. Then, in 1888 a law was passed permitting registered pharmacists to practice the profession in all parts of Italy, and allowing the unrestricted opening of pharmacies. Unfortunately, the new pharmacies opened under this law were for the most part in the large cities. Severe competition destructive of standards developed in the metropolitan districts, while in the country the need for well distributed pharmacies was not met. The unrestricted and uncontrolled establishment of new pharmacies thus proved of no advantage either to pharmacy itself or to the public.[24] In 1913, a new set of restrictions replaced the freedom of the law of 1888. Since that time the government has determined where a new pharmacy shall be opened. The privilege of establishing and operating such a pharmacy is awarded competitively to the best applicant. These privileges or concessions cease with the death of the concessionaire and are neither salable nor hereditary. Upon the death of the owner the vacant concession is again subject to competition.

A pharmacy thus acquired is conducted on the basis of a license given by the governmental authorities to the licensee for his lifetime only. The old ratio of 5,000 inhabitants to one pharmacy, introduced by the Austrians in 1778, has become general, supplemented or in some cases replaced by a compulsory distance of at least 500 meters between an old pharmacy and a new one to be established.

A semiauthoritative pharmaceutical organization, the *Federazione Ordini dei Farmacisti Italiani* (F.O.E.I.), with headquarters in Rome, works in close contact with the governmental authorities. There is an *Ordini dei Farmacisti* in every province, as a branch of the government and under the authority of the provincial governmental administration.

The official fees to be paid for the establishment of a new pharmacy are rather high. The law provides governmentally fixed prices, but for only a rather small number of drugs enumerated in an official list.[25]

DEVELOPMENT OF EDUCATION

The studies and the preparation for pharmacy during the earlier period of organized pharmacy in Italy may be exemplified by the Venetian statutes (*Collegio degli speziali Veneti*, 1565). A student of pharmacy had to serve 5 years as an apprentice and another 3 years as a clerk; finally, he was required to pass a rather rigid examination, after which he became a pharmacist fully qualified to operate a pharmacy of his own.[26] Such requirements were more or less general for a long period.

It was the above-mentioned Austrian legislation of 1778 regulating pharmacy in Northern Italy (Lombardy) that made academic study and examination a requirement for pharmacists in this area. In 1805 (during the short-lived Napoleonic Kingdom of Italy) this regulation was legally extended to the whole peninsula. Pharmaceutical education was thereby taken away from the pharmaceutical guilds and transferred to the universities, a development, here as elsewhere, never reversed by later political events.

The present educational requirements for a license are:

1. *Preliminary education*: graduation from a lyceum (a high school approximately equivalent to 2 years of college)

2. *Professional education*: a 4-year university course

3. *Professional experience*: 1 year of probation in an especially authorized pharmacy, after completion of the university studies

4. *Examinations:* (a) after completion of the university studies, a written, a laboratory and an oral examination in the studies pursued; (b) after the year of probation, a practical examination including laws and regulations

After the close of the 17th century the Italian pharmacists as a class no longer contributed very much to the advancement of the pharmaceutical sciences. This was in spite of the high standards for the practice of pharmacy and the social rank of the pharmaceutical practitioner. Whereas in France and Germany a constellation of pharmacists went on to attain high standing as scientists and, therefore, recognition for their profession, the attainments of Italian pharmacists went scarcely beyond the compilation of treatises for the practice of their calling. A possible explanation may be that, throughout the triumphant development of chemistry from the latter part of the 18th through the 19th century, progress came largely from researches conducted in France, Germany, England and Sweden. The great scientific achievements of the Italians lay rather in the spheres of physics and medicine.

PHARMACEUTICAL TREATISES AND JOURNALS

Italy made its main contributions to the art of pharmacy in the late Middle Ages and the Renaissance. As in all other countries of the Western World, the first authors of pharmaceutical interest were from the ranks of medicine.

Of greatest influence on the practice of pharmacy among early Italian works was the *Compendium aromatariorum* by the physician Saladin de Asculo,[27] written in the middle of the 15th century. Especially written for the information of pharmacists, the book gives advice for collecting, preparing and preserving drugs and, in question and answer form, it explains pharmaceutical terminology and drug names. Furthermore, the book describes the behavior which, in the author's opinion, befits the true pharmacist. The directions given by Saladin for different kinds of containers for the preservation of drugs correspond in large part with those of the Greco-Roman Dioscorides. This book has been called "the first real treatise on pharmacy in a modern sense . . . which became the model for all later textbooks of pharmacy and for centuries was the indispensable vade mecum [reference book] of the apothecary."[28]

Mention should be made, among other similar books, of the *Lumen apothecariorum* (The Light of the Pharmacists), by the physician Quiricus de Augustus de Dertona;[29] the *Luminare majus* (The Greater Luminary), written toward the end of the 15th century by the pharmacist Joannes J. Manlius de Bosco,[30] which "until the middle of the 16th century was the official guide in several countries and cities, e.g., in Nuremberg"[31] and of the *Thesaurus aromatariorum* (The Treasure Chest of the Pharmacists), written by Paulus Suardus in the first decade of the 16th century. With Bosco and Suardus, both of them practicing pharmacists, pharmaceutical authors of pharmaceutical treatises enter the scene. Whether or not the treatise by the Spanish pharmacist, Petro Benedicto Mateo was written before that of J. Manlius de Bosco is an open question.

Among Italian books of the next 150 years the most notable was the *Nuovo et universale theatro farmaceutico* (1662), written by pharmacist Antonio de Sgobbis da Montagnana, owner of the famous Ostrich Pharmacy in Venice. This book contains comprehensive and noteworthy directions for the management of a pharmacy. It describes and illustrates all pharmaceutical processes and apparatus of the period and contains much biographical material. Here we see a real pharmaceutical encyclopedia, in some respects foreshadowing the later "universal pharmacopeias."[32]

After the close of the 17th century, scientific pharmaceutical treatises by Italian pharmacists and physicians seldom acquired renown beyond the borders of Italy.

The earliest Italian pharmaceutical journal, the *Giornale di farmacia, chimica e scienze affini,* was founded in 1824 (by Antonio Cattaneo in Milan). Later Italian journals have become well known in the scientific world.[33]

OFFICIAL PHARMACOPEIAS

In 1499 the medical members of the Florentine guild of physicians and pharmacists (*L'arte dei medici e speziali*) issued a pharmaceutical formulary entitled *Nuovo receptario.* Since this book was made obligatory for pharmacists by their guild, it often has been considered the first European pharmacopeia. Lack of precise agreement on what constitutes a "pharmacopeia" makes it a moot point. Recent research suggests that the Florentine book (88 leaves), like that of Barcelona 12 years later, could be characterized as containing the drug standards authorized by the guild. (The later Nuremberg dispensatory of 1546 received government sanction and support, which places its pharmacopeial status beyond question.)[34]

The *Nuovo receptario* followed the spirit of Arabic therapy, as we should expect. More than a half century passed before Mantua (1559) and later, other Italian city-states[35] followed Florence's lead in issuing their own drug standards. Across Europe, the sequence and the circumstances

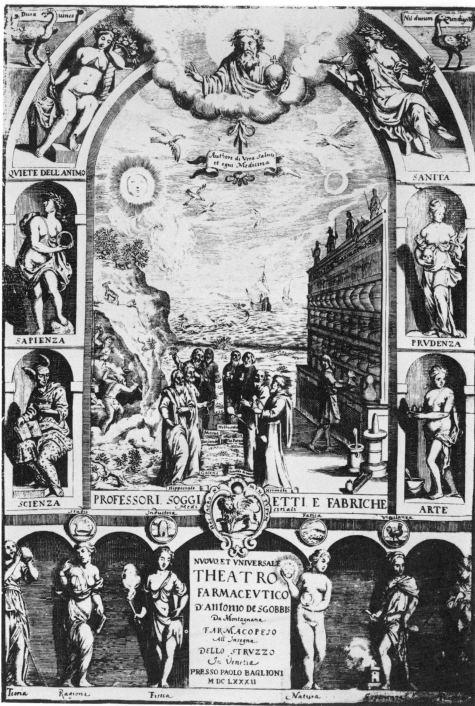

Pharmaceutical books before the 18th century often had artistic title pages, sometimes including riotous symbolism, as in this title page of an Italian book by Pharmacist de Sgobbis of Venice (see text). In the central panel a pharmacist (right) envisions the colloquy that his pharmaceutical studies give him with sages of the past. Ships bear exotic drugs to him, through waters infested with sea serpents. The hill (left), with miners underground and flora and fauna above ground, represents the resources of the three natural kingdoms. These the pharmacist can put in the service of mankind if he possesses the virtues and the knowledge represented by allegoric figures in the border.

of the founding of these early local pharmacopeias tend to reflect the standard of pharmacy and the nationalistic tendencies in the various political units. It will be noted that the title *"Pharmacopoea"* was not used as such in Italy until 1580, at Bergamo, following an example set by the French physician Jacques du Bois (Sylvius) in 1548. However, Sylvius' *Pharmacopoeae libri tres* was a private book and not "official."

Not until 1892 did the government of the new kingdom of Italy (established 1870) issue the first official pharmaceutical standard for the entire country, the *Farmacopoea ufficiale del regno d'Italia*.[36]

PHARMACOGNOSY AND BOTANIC GARDENS

So far as is known, the first chair at a European university for pharmacognosy (*lettura dei semplici*) was established in Padua (1533), and others soon followed.[37] The well known botanist Ghini taught there. One of his students, Pietro Andrea

Mathioli of Siena (1501-1577), physician-in-ordinary to the German Emperor Maximilian II, published (1544) a famous commentary on Dioscorides that was translated into many languages. It continued in use through numerous editions as the encyclopedia of herbal materia medica of the Renaissance.

By the 14th century, plots of medicinal herbs, theretofore notable as an adjunct of monasteries, had appeared as part of private gardens. One of the earliest known belonged to the famous author Matthaeus Sylvaticus at Salerno, who wrote a dictionary of simple drugs and their uses (*Pandectae . . .*, ca. 1317). Similar gardens flourished about this time at Castelnuova and Naples. In 1545 the famous botanic garden at Padua was established, which might be called the first in a modern sense.

Italian pharmacists and their apprentices frequented such gardens or maintained their own, for their learning in botanic science was one hallmark of their calling and its ascendant repute.

5:   The Development in France

Italy cradled European professional pharmacy, but almost simultaneously a similar development took place in France. Pharmacy had emerged in a form we can recognize by about 1300 and, during the preceding century or so of maturing, legal regulations separating pharmacy and medicine and setting other requirements reminiscent of the edict of Frederick II had become effective in Montpellier, Arles and Marseille. Indeed, the requirements at Montpellier antedate the others in Southern France and Italy. Perhaps as early as 1180, the preparer of drugs (the especiador) obligated himself in many ways when taking the professional oath after a qualifying examination.[1] It is suggestive that these three French centers of early professional structuring all lay on the Mediterranean, geographically exposed to interaction with Italian and Arabic influences.

There has always been a close connection between Italy and France. During the last centuries of the Roman Empire, Ancient Gaul (the Gallia of the Romans) was more a Roman province than a colony. Thus France felt itself to be and, indeed, was a legitimate heir to Roman civilization, almost to the same extent as was Italy. One fundamental difference influenced the political and cultural development of both peoples, i.e., the difference in the elements composing the populations of the two countries. The original Italians did not amalgamate appreciably with the northern peoples who overran them for longer or shorter periods. In all their dominant features, they remained a Mediterranean people. In France, on the contrary, the pre-Roman inhabitants (Aquitani, Celtae and Belgae), then the Romans, then the several Germanic tribes who overran the country (Visigoths, Burgundians and Franks) and, finally, the Normans, blended into a new and almost homogeneous people. The French are one of the most striking examples of amalgamation of different peoples into a single nation, united by the same customs and language, the same aims and thoughts. In 486 Clovis, a chief of the Franks, definitely put an end to Roman rule in the north of France, and settled a German tribe on French soil. For a time, France and Germany constituted a united empire. However, this unity was political only. The division of France from Germany in 987 was but the recognition of their different racial and cultural developments.

ORGANIZATION INTO GUILDS

The intermediate cultural position of France between Germany to the north and Italy to the south finds an obvious expression in the evolution of French pharmacy. In France, as in Italy during the Middle Ages, pharmacy found its place in the guilds. However, unlike the great Italian guilds, these French associations were non-political. They were professional or commercial organizations, based on decree of royal, parliamentary or local authorities.[2]

The fact that until the reign of the House of Bourbon (1589) many feudal lords governed their territories like sovereigns and that, later on, until the great revolution (1792), the individual municipalities enjoyed wide administrative independence, did not prevent a rather uniform development of pharmacy throughout France. The guilds were given far-reaching self-determination in all matters concerning admission to the profession, education of apprentices and their examination, the limitation of the number of pharmacies, and the care of poor colleagues and their widows and orphans.[3] In general, wise use was made of the right of self-government.

There were three kinds of regulation of pharmaceutical life: by the central government, by local authorities and by the pharmacists themselves (that is, by their asso-

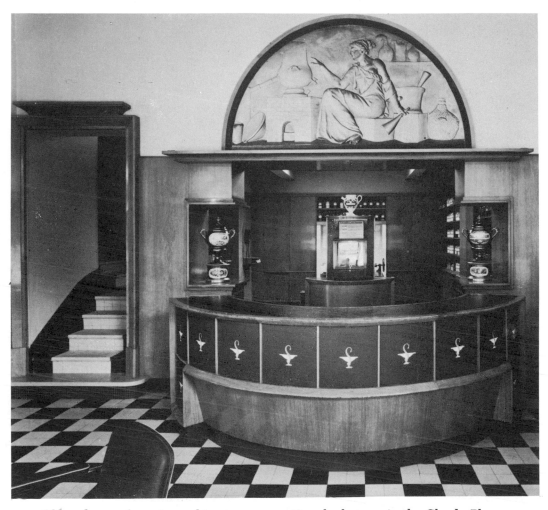

Old and new elements combine to preserve French elegance in the Claude Pharmacy at L'Aigle (Orne). The graceful curve of the main dispensing counter is ornamented by rhythmic repetition of pharmacy's symbol, the Bowl of Hygeia; the bas-relief overhead probably represents the goddess Hygeia herself, sitting among antique pharmaceutical equipment. (Photograph from A. I. H. P. Archive)

ciations). The last type of regulation was the most common.[4]

By the 13th century the field of pharmacy had developed sufficiently, here and there, to generate a group consciousness and identity. A century or two earlier we find only traces of individual practitioners, the pharmacist's forerunner sometimes called "pigmentarius" (e.g., Angers in 1093; Poitou in 1123).[5] The first guildlike association known in French pharmacy arose in Avignon (1262), where sellers of drugs joined with an association of spicers. At Dijon, also in

the late 13th century, we know that pharmacists owned a kind of association-headquarters building (*domus apothecariorum,* 1281).[6] In Paris, at least as early as the middle of the 13th century, pharmacists had an association together with spicers and others in more or less related callings.

To this association King Philip IV entrusted (1312) the control of weights and balances used by all retailers, thus making the pharmacists and spicers the appointed custodians of the standard weight. (The ordinance refers to all merchants as *d'avoirs de poids,* meaning dealers selling their merchandise by weight.[7] Here we apparently have the etymologic root of the term "avoirdupois" for a certain kind of trade weight.) Outside of Paris similar regulations were issued, most of them making the pharmacists the appointed guardians and inspectors of the balances and the weights used by all retail merchants.

In communities in which the number of physicians was not large enough to form a special medical group, they were united with the pharmacists. At times, surgeons, pharmacists and barbers were in the same corporation. However, the special pharmacy guilds were predominant. Of 199 guilds in which pharmacists are known to have participated, 103 were exclusively pharmacy associations.[8]

By means of these guilds, the pharmaceutical profession in France gained and maintained a high standard. As measured by the values of that time, the requirements for entrance into the profession were high and strictly enforced.

The applicant had to be of legitimate birth and of the Roman Catholic faith; he had to know sufficient Latin to read intelligently the formularies and the prescriptions; in addition, the guildmasters often asked whether the applicant's family was wealthy enough to enable him to buy a pharmacy later on.

Most of the apprentices were recruited from the rich bourgeoisie of the towns, very often from the apothecaries' families. The son succeeded the father, the nephew the uncle. That explains the numerous dynasties of apothecaries. In Rouen, for instance, a widow Chandelier practiced [the profession] in 1214 and eleven members of the family practiced pharmacy in that town from 1600 to 1786.[9]

The statutes of many guilds restricted the number of apprentices. Generally, only one apprentice was allowed for each pharmacy.[10] Even the number of pharmacies was very often limited, sometimes by statute as in Nancy and Nice,[11] sometimes by other means—for instance, by the requirement that each pharmacist coming from another district pass a local examination.

Apparently, in a number of cases the limitations—restricting membership in French guilds to certain cliques—went too far. The famous edict of Villers-Cotterets (1539) improved the situation by means of the drastic remedy of banning the *confréries de gens de métier* (guilds of trades and professions) as they then existed.[12] Subsequently, many new guild statutes based on a model statute approved by the king were issued in the late 16th and early 17th centuries.

PHARMACISTS AND SPICERS

In the Parisian *Livre des métiers* (book of trades and professions, written by Etienne Boileau in 1270), the term *apothicaire* appears for the first time. However, members of the profession of pharmacy were at that time more commonly called *épicier* (spicer).[13] The fact that the designation *apothicaire* did not become general until about 1400 proves that until that time neither the public nor the governmental authorities had seen much difference between the apothecary and the spicer.

Due to the lack of sharp distinctions of rights and privileges, there had never been much love lost between the two groups. Each accused the other of trespassing; each required and had enacted legislation for its benefit, dealing particularly with the situation in the capital, Paris.

An edict issued by Charles VII in 1484 forbade the practice of pharmacy by spicers.[14] Another ordinance (1514) separated the small spicer from the apothecary-spicer. The small spicer was forbidden to practice pharmacy, which, according to the ordinance, "requires much art, science, experience and knowledge of drugs as well as of the compounding of prescriptions which enter into the human body." However, the apothecary (pharmacist) was permitted to practice both professions simultaneously.

Contending ambitions and fluid boundaries of function—which would continue to haunt pharmacists in other centuries and circumstances—made pharmacy's privilege unstable. Within a generation pharmacists too had to choose between the two callings (1553). Then the king reunited the hostile groups within the same guild (1560). Repeated amendment of the ordinances governing the competing groups into the 18th century reflects the conflict of interest and the friction between them.[15]

The attention paid to the spicers and the consideration given them by the French authorities until the early 18th century find explanation in the economic importance of these tradesmen, especially the importers and wholesalers (and often retailers) of spices and drugs from the Orient and later from America. Their influence in certain French cities along the changing routes of import (until the end of the 16th century mainly Marseilles and Lyons, and later Bordeaux, La Rochelle, Nantes and Rouen) was so great that at times professional pharmacy was overshadowed by the spicers.[16]

The definite separation of the pharmacists and the spicers of Paris was brought about by a royal declaration in 1777 that replaced the old guild with the quite different *Collège de Pharmacie*. This declaration allowed to the spicers the wholesale trade in drugs, the retailing of a few specifically enumerated drugs and trade in all herbs and roots in their natural state, requiring no preparation or compounding.

In the provinces, quarrels between the pharmacists and the spicers were exacerbated by, rather than the result of the fact that the hostile groups were often members of the same guild (e.g., Lille, Abbeville). The disagreements were not peculiar to France, but occurred in all countries and still occur today among pharmacists, herbalists and merchants. The French quarrel with the herbalists culminated in the famous law of Germinal (1803), which stabilized the situation. After having proved their knowledge by examination, the herbalists were given a certificate entitling them to sell indigenous crude drugs. New licenses no longer are being granted to herbalists, and, when the owner of an old herb shop dies, the doors are closed.[17]

FROM "APOTHICAIRE" TO "PHARMACIEN"

The social status of the French apothicaire from the 14th to the 18th century was doubtless that of a patrician. His social position was maintained in spite of the fact that his duties included not only the preparation but the administration of medicated clysters (enemas), which were a therapeutic fad from the 15th to the 18th century. Louis XIII received no less than 312 clysters within a year! Only when the apothecaries became the target of ridicule on the part of the poets, especially Molière (a development which fortunately coincided with the passing of the fad), did they become aware of the unworthiness of this practice.

It is sometimes overlooked that Molière, in his famous play *Le malade imaginaire*, scoffs at physicians and apothecaries in quite the same manner and that, for him, the *apothicaire's* involvement with clysters was only a welcome occasion for added ridicule. At any rate, in French public opinion the designation *apothicaire* gradually became associated with the ridiculous picture drawn by the caricaturists. Hence we can well understand why members of the profession preferred the new name *pharmacien*, which made its appearance in the 17th century and became official with the establishment of the *Collège de Pharmacie* in 1777.

It has to be stated that the giant syringe used for the application of clysters was too good a motif not to be taken advantage of by caricaturists long after clysters, and especially their application by *apothicaires*, had ceased to be a matter of fashion. The great master of French politico-satirical graphics, Honoré Daumier, used this motif several times during a period in which people with pharmaceutical background, especially Jean Baptiste Dumas (1880-1884), played an important part in French politics.

The attacks of Molière and his literary contemporaries were to a large extent directed against the high prices charged for remedies.* In France prices fixed by the government were never a general institution, and we know of pharmaceutical invoices which, indeed, seem to be very high.[18]

---

* E.g., introductory scene to *Le malade imaginaire*.

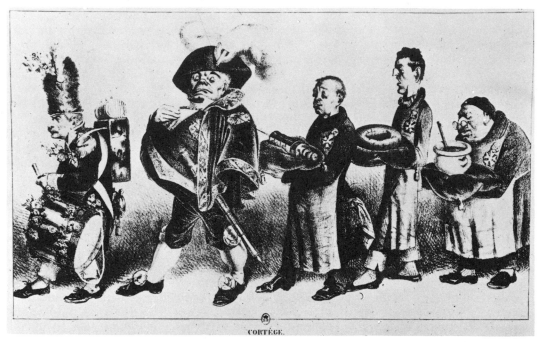

CORTÉGE.

The French pharmacist's erstwhile duty of administering clysters stirred the polemical imagination of the great caricaturist, Honoré Daumier. On the surface, his "Cortége" (above) purports to show "the commanding General of the Pharmacists, prince Lancelot of Tucamule, upon his entry into the chamber of Peace." Who, in reality, is this officious and vacuous general with a huge enema-syringe instead of a sword, followed by aides bearing auxiliary equipment? Actually, the barb was thrown at General Mouton (Count Lobau), who had offended by ordering fire-hoses turned on public demonstrators (1831) and, immediately afterward, had received his field-marshal's baton and a peerage. (From *La Pharmacie & la Médecine dans l'Oeuvre de H. Daumier*, Les Pharmaciens Bibliophiles, Paris, 1932, Plate 12; photograph from A. I. H. P.)

PHARMACISTS AND PHYSICIANS

Pharmacists and physicians, who are so closely associated in their professional life and are the common target of sarcasm, nevertheless often have had conflicts, possibly because of their close relationship. However, nowhere did these quarrels reach such a degree of malice as in France.* As early as 1271, the medical faculty of Paris admonished the apothecaries not to trespass on the field of medicine; on the other hand, we know that some French physicians in their turn sold medicines as late as about 1470.[19] Besides, the lack of learned physicians sometimes forced the pharmacists to practice medicine. For example, in 1724, a royal ordinance permitted the pharmacist to visit the sick if no physician was available.[20]

The literary quarrel between the professions, launched by the physician Symphorien Champier in the early 16th century, gained notoriety the world over. Vitriolic treatises were met by countertreatises. Translated into other languages, the most telling verbal attacks were quoted wherever someone wanted to find fault with pharmacists. In Germany and in England, echoes of these French publications[21] were heard later, a classic source of barbs to be hurled at pharmacists on the one hand, or against physicians on the other.

In another quarrel about 70 years later, medical authors used the old arguments but tried new means as well, with the

---

* Philippe's *Histoire des apothicaires* proves this in its contents as well as in its entire tenor.

clearly expressed intention of ruining the pharmaceutical profession as a whole. Guy Patin, the famous head of the faculty of medicine at the University of Paris and a conservative clinician, was campaigning against the use in medicine of what he considered to be dangerous chemicals. He and his friends wanted pharmacists to refuse to dispense prescriptions containing chemicals. The pharmacists' answer that they felt obliged to fill all prescriptions was considered a declaration of war.

In 1625 a low-priced book appeared that instructed the public concerning common pharmaceutical processes and ways of procuring raw materials, so that everyone might prepare needed medicaments himself! The revised edition of this so-called *Médecin charitable*, which had been written by the physician Ph. Guibert, has been called "a genuine treatise on popular pharmacy which lived through numerous editions in French, and was translated into other languages, together with the other works by Guibert."[22] As a result, Guy Patin could write (1649) that the pharmacists of Paris had been ruined, the only clients remaining being strangers.

Nevertheless, the quarrel ended with common sense triumphant over hatred, prejudice and presumption. In 1666, the Faculty of Medicine at Paris admitted the use of the controversial antimony (in the form of wine of antimony) "as a purgative," and the Parlement de Paris even gave governmental blessing to this decision.

ORGANIZATION OF FRENCH PHARMACY SINCE 1777

The Royal Declaration of April 25, 1777 ushered in modern French pharmacy. By establishing the *Collège de Pharmacie* as an administrative as well as an educational institution, the declaration replaced the old guild, and strictly stated the tasks and the rights of professional pharmacy. Thus a definite borderline was drawn between activities considered to be pharmaceutical, and hence reserved to pharmacy, and those open to everyone, including the herbalists. The declaration forbade the selling of drugs by religious hospitals and societies (a practice which had been rampant before),[23] and it authorized pharmacists to educate their rising generation without interference arising from medical jealousy.

The French Revolution changed little more than the name of the tested institutions—after a short, painful trial of "free" pharmacy, which meant pharmacy thrown open to anyone, without educational requirements. A decree (March 2, 1791) had declared everyone entitled to practice any profession or trade! One immediate result was that uneducated owners established numerous stores called pharmacies everywhere in France, especially in Paris. This put an end to revolutionary enthusiasm for liberty in the field of pharmacy. A month later, a new decree (April 14, 1791) announced the return to the customary regulation of the practice of pharmacy.

In 1796 former members of the *Collège de Pharmacie* set up a new association called the *Société libre de Pharmacie de Paris*. A *Société de Pharmacie de Paris*, founded (1803) to provide scientific interchange and stimulus, gained an illustrious reputation. Analogous local societies were founded in other scientific centers of French pharmacy.[24]

The defense of the commercial interest of pharmacy was left to other and younger associations,[25] (especially *L'Association* [now *Fédération*] *générale des syndicats Pharmaceutiques*, founded in 1876).

Meanwhile, the organization of French pharmacy has been changed entirely. The above-mentioned royal declaration of 1777 and the law of 1803, after having formed the legal basis of French pharmacy for about 140 years, were replaced (September 11, 1941; modified May 23, 1945). Since 1945 there has been an all-inclusive pharmaceutical association called *L'Ordre des pharmaciens*. Membership is compulsory for (a) community pharmacists, (b) pharmacists responsible for the manufacture of pharmaceutical proprietaries, (c) pharmacists in pharmaceutical wholesale and distribution, (d) pharmacists not belonging to groups a, b or c—for instance, hospital pharmacists. It has to be kept in mind that in

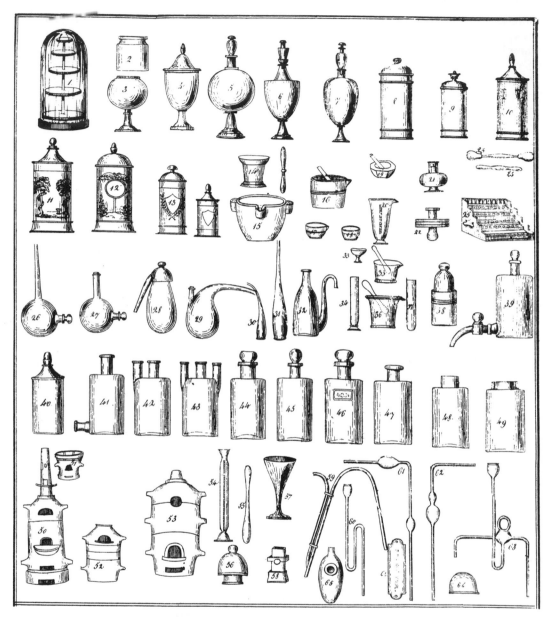

The character of French pharmacies and their small laboratories in about the middle of the 19th century is almost tangibly conjured up by this parade of equipment, reproduced from a price list of a Paris dealer. The numbered items (left to right) are: (1) Mahogany display rack with cylindrical glass cover; (2 and 3) leech jars; (4) jar for medicaments; (5, 6 and 7) show-window bottles (globe-shaped, urn-shaped and egg-shaped); (8, 9 and 10) conserve jars with convex, Paris-market and Chinese cover styles, respectively; (11, 12 and 13) ceramic pharmacy jars, with Chinese, acorn and convex cover styles, respectively; (14) cast iron mortar, with pestle; (15) marble mortar; (16) serpentine mortar; (17 and 18) small serpentine mortars, with and without lip; (19) agate mortar with pestle; (20) graduated measure; (21) lamp for spirit of wine (i.e., ethyl alcohol); (22) bulb of barometer; (23 and 24) pestles of guaiac and of boxwood; (25) reagent box; (26) long-necked, round-bottom flask with ground-glass stopper; (27) same without tube; (28) cucurbit (i.e., boiler) with distillation head; (29) tubulated retort with ground-glass
(*Caption continued*, bottom of facing page)

France large-scale manufacture of pharmaceuticals, as well as pharmaceutical wholesale and distribution activities are regarded as "pharmaceutical practice" and are by law under the control of registered pharmacists. Anyone not listed as a member of the *Ordre* and active in one of the capacities enumerated is practicing pharmacy illegally and is subject to punishment. The aims of the *Ordre* (*ordonnance*, May 1945) are "to assure respect for the professional duties, [and] to assure the defense of the honor and the independence of the profession." The *Ordre* is given a certain professional jurisdiction which, according to official interpretation, makes its councils [one for each of the four groups named and regional councils for the community pharmacists forming group (a)] "guardians of morale." They are supposed "to ferret out violations of a professional nature, which only too often escape the jurisdiction of the common courts and are sanctioned by the latter."[26]

The *Société de pharmacie de Paris*, which had replaced the old *Société libre*, has changed its name (governmental decree of September 5, 1946) to *Académie de Pharmacie*, thus underlining still more the purely scientific character of this institution and putting it on the same level with the time-honored *Académie de Médecine*.

While French law has not restricted the number of pharmacies severely, compared with some other countries, it does try to ensure fairly even distribution of pharmaceutical service and sets some limit to their number. In the country as a whole, a little more than 3,000 persons are served by each pharmacy. Besides other conditions to be met, a new pharmacy may open only where the number of inhabitants per pharmacy would be at least the ratios shown below for localities in the three population categories:

3,000 to 1, for populations of more than 30,000

2,500 to 1, for populations of 5,000 to 30,000

2,000 to 1, for populations of less than 5,000[27]

A list of localities not having the maximum number of pharmacies is kept current for the guidance of registered pharmacists who wish to apply in one or another district for a permit to open their own pharmacies.

DEVELOPMENT OF THE PHARMACEUTICAL SHOP

Up to the late 16th century, the French pharmacies were mostly open to the street; the pharmacist worked in the public gaze. The equipment gradually became more elegant. However, with few exceptions, only the pharmacies of hospitals or religious societies equalled the luxury of Italian pharmacies of the Renaissance. In the 17th century, faïence jars and jugs from French potteries (Nevers, Rouen, Moustiers) greatly improved the appearance of the pharmacies. After the close of the 18th century, drug containers from French porcelain manufacturers also went onto the shelves. In this connection it is of interest that the discovery of the kaolin of St. Yrieix by the pharmacist M.-H. Vilaris of Bordeaux made the French porcelain industry possible.

Products of French pottery were even used as distinguishing signs of pharmacy.

stopper; (30) curved adapter or coupler; (31) straight adapter or coupler; (32) Florentine receiver; (33) eye cup; (34) footed cylinder; (35) mortar of twice-baked porcelain; (36) glass mortar with pestle; (37) test tube; (38) disinfecting bottle; (39) bottle with stopcock, for syrup of ether; (40) undecorated conserve jar with Chinese-style lid; (41) Woulf flask with one tube below; (42 and 43) Woulf flasks with two and three tubes above; (44, 45 and 46) glass-stoppered bottles, one with glass-label; (47) necked bottle for distilled water; (48) salt-mouth, short-necked bottle; (49) wide-mouthed bottle for plants; (50) furnace with cupeler; (51) furnace with basin; (52) tube furnace; (53) reverberatory furnace; (54) alkalimeter; (55) spatula; (56) cupping glass; (57) glass for experiment; (58) ingot mold; (59) siphon; (60) S-tube; (61) pipette; (62) blowpipe; (63) burrette; (64) oval cupping glass, English; (65) infant feeding-bottle; (66) drawer label. (Photograph, University of Wisconsin, *from* a brochure of Ancienne Maison Acloque, Vimeux Vieillard & Cie, successors)

The so-called *chevrettes*—specially shaped jugs for syrups, medicinal honeys and oils —"constituted the pharmaceutical jar par excellence." Their display was forbidden to all but pharmacists.[28] A Parisian ordinance forbidding the spicers to use the so-called *pots à canon* (containers of cannonlike shape for ointments, electuaries, etc.) gave this type of container likewise a pharmaceutical distinction.[29]

As these embellishments suggest, the French pharmacy is often well appointed, and is always devoted primarily to professional activities. Legally limited to 21 categories of stock, the more commercial subsidiary lines of a pharmacy include perfumes, insecticides, special dietary aids and the like.[30]

Since each pharmacy serves about the same population, on the average, as a pharmacy in the United States, the much more uniform professional appearance and specialization of French pharmacies seems striking to American pharmacists. While factors accounting for this are complex, it is important to recall that physicians do not pre-empt any significant part of the pharmacist's practice and, secondly, that well-trained pharmacists have biologic (clinical) analysis as a second professional function. About 70 per cent of all such laboratories were directed by pharmacists in 1950, and pharmacies that do not conduct testing may obtain commissions for forwarding specimens to such a laboratory and handling the test reports. While physicians are divided in their attitude toward this function of French pharmacy as a public service, pharmacists tend to see clinical laboratory work as a means of utilizing their scientific education more fully in a second professional sense, despite a countercurrent of industrial and economic change within the practice of pharmacy itself.[31]

Pharmaceutical Inspection

During the first centuries of professional French pharmacy, the supervision either was entirely the responsibility of the physicians or was dominated by them. In 1336 the faculty of medicine in Paris was charged with the inspection of the pharmacies. Then an ordinance (1353) created a commission consisting of the head of the pharmacist's guild, two master pharmacists appointed by the municipal authorities and two members of the medical faculty. Mixed commissions of this type appeared everywhere, although medical dominance over pharmacy was maintained. Supervision by pharmacists exclusively was rare.[32]

The above-mentioned law of 1803 made the supervision of the pharmacies the business of commissions elected from the staffs of the schools of medicine and pharmacy in Paris and of the departmental councils of hygiene in the provinces. After another century, a new law (1908) established the supervision by pharmaceutical inspectors not only of the pharmacies but of the entire drug trade. "Pharmacy was thus freed from a servitude which has lasted too long and which could only injure its reputation by illusory control and repression."[33] Present legislation provides for full-time and part-time inspectors appointed by the Ministry of Health.

LARGE-SCALE MANUFACTURING

In the development of the French pharmaceutical industry pharmacists played a large and important part. One of the first in France to manufacture chemicals and galenics on a large scale was the pharmacist Antoine Baumé, the inventor of a number of technical improvements, which he proved in his own manufacturing laboratory and generously made known to his colleagues. His price list (1775) shows about 2,400 preparations, among them about 400 which can be considered chemical.

Some of the early French discoverers of alkaloids, for instance Joseph Pelletier (quinine) and P. J. Robiquet (codeine), made their discoveries the basis of large-scale manufacturing. Furthermore, in the 17th and the 18th centuries, community pharmacies contributed most to the proprietary industry and continued to do so. For it has been characteristic of the French proprietary industry that, beyond a few very large drug manufacturers, there stand "countless small manufacturers, each of whom specializes in one or two remedies," and that "fully 50 per cent of the licensed pharmacists in France are engaged in this business, most of them in a small way."[34] From this group of practicing pharmacists emerged Stanislas Limousin, the inventor of the apparatus for administration of oxygen, of wafer capsules and, above all, of parenteral ampuls.[35]

Around the middle of the 19th century, French pharmacists created the first cooperative of national scope covering pharmaceutical industry and commerce. The similar venture undertaken by London apothecaries in the early 17th century (see page 97) was only local in scope and restricted to the members of the Society of Apothecaries of London. Initiated and steered through its infancy by F. L. M. Dorvault (1815-1879) this cooperative, the *Pharmacie centrale de France,* whose shareholders are exclusively French pharmacists, has developed into one of the world's largest pharmaceutical manufacturing and wholesale enterprises. It affects practically all aspects of the life of French pharmacists.[36]

DEVELOPMENT OF EDUCATION

During the time of the guilds, as we noted, the applicant for apprenticeship had to meet high social, financial and educational requirements. To become a master he had to pass difficult examinations. In Marseilles such examinations were required as early as the 13th century. A Parisian ordinance in 1484 stated that the candidate had to prove his knowledge of drugs and of the compounding of medicaments by undergoing a protracted and difficult examination and, lastly, had to perform his "masterpiece," by preparing galenics requiring special technical skill and scientific knowledge. This masterpiece became a general requirement throughout France up to the 18th century, of which a modern counterpart may be seen in American "practical" examinations by state boards. The number of the required preparations varied from one (Nancy before 1624) to six (Amiens in 1567) or more.[37] The prospec-

tive pharmacist also usually had to serve a certain time as *compagnon* (clerk) before he could become a candidate for mastership. The entire time thus spent varied from 2 to 8 years as apprentice, to a total time of 4 to 10 years as apprentice and clerk.[38]

Academic studies were introduced comparatively early and gradually became general. Already in 1536 an ordinance of Parliament required apprentices of pharmacy to attend two lectures each week relating to the art of the apothecary. These lectures were given by a member of the faculty of medicine. In Poitiers (1588) only those candidates who had attended lectures on the art and the science of pharmacy for 1 year could become masters of pharmacy.

In the famous University of Montpellier the doors were always open to the students of pharmacy of the entire world. In 1558, the pharmacists at Montpellier requested and eventually established, at their own expense, a course in the pharmaceutical sciences. The master pharmacist who gave this course, Bernhardin de Ranc, was the first practicing pharmacist to become officially a member of the teaching staff of a European university. There pharmacy matured academically in successive steps: Henry IV created at Montpellier a chair for surgery and pharmacy (1601). The famous master pharmacist Laurent Catelan lectured on medicinal herbs and demonstrated the art of pharmacy (1605). Finally, Louis XIV created a chair of pharmaceutical chemistry at Montpellier (1675).[39]

In Paris the *Jardin des apothicaires* (founded by the pharmacist Nicolas Houel on the basis of a special ordinance of Henry III, October 1576, and preserved and enlarged during several centuries by the pharmacists' guild) provided general scientific instruction for the apprentices of pharmacy. Other courses were given primarily at the Garden of the King (founded 1635).[40] These courses were supplemented by private courses on pharmaceutical chemistry given by some of the famous pharmacist-chemists, such as Lefebvre and Lémery in the 17th century and Rouelle and Baumé in the 18th century.

It was necessary for these courses to be a private undertaking, because the several attempts of the Parisian guild to organize official academic instruction met with the same lack of fair professional sentiment on the part of physicians that has been noted earlier. Official courses twice launched (1705 to 1723, and, again, 1753 to 1765) had to be abandoned because of opposition by the Paris faculty of medicine. They were resumed after replacement of the guild by the so-called *Collège de Pharmacie* (1777) and were continued during the lifetime of this institution. The successor of the *Collège*, the *Société libre des pharmaciens de Paris* (founded in 1796) established an *Ecole gratuite de pharmacie* (free school of pharmacy).[41] This developed into the *Ecole supérieure de pharmacie de l'Université de Paris* and more recently into the present *Faculté de pharmacie de Paris*.[42]

The legislation of 1803 provided six higher schools of pharmacy for the education of pharmacists of the first class, who were permitted to practice pharmacy throughout the nation. It also provided committees for the examination of pharmacists of the second class, who were allowed to practice only in the district where they passed their examination.

These regulations have been changed several times. The present educational requirements (since the abolition of second-class pharmacists in 1909) are as follows:

1. *Preliminary education:* the "baccalaureate" in secondary schooling, perhaps equivalent to 2 or 3 years of American pre-professional college studies

2. *Professional experience:* a 1-year internship with a pharmacist who has been authorized officially to provide this kind of practical instruction

3. *Professional education:* a 4-year course in pharmacy at the university level[43]

4. *Examinations:* first, an examination on the technic of pharmacy, following the apprenticeship or internship and, secondly, a comprehensive examination during the final year covering the entire curriculum *(examens probatoire)*. This searching test of qualification has three divisions, the last divided into two parts. In effect, then, there are four examinations—each with an oral part and a practical part—corresponding to the following categories:

    a. Physicochemical sciences (inorganic chemistry, mineralogy, organic chemistry, analytic chemistry, physics)

    b. Natural sciences (botany, cryptogamy, zoology, parasitology)

    c. Biologic chemistry (hygiene and public health, toxicology, hydrology, microbiology)

    d. Chemical pharmacy, galenical pharmacy, materia medica, pharmacodynamics, legislation[44]

DEVELOPMENT OF A LITERATURE

The professional spirit so evident in the entire development of French pharmacy likewise found expression in a professional literature. Until the end of the 16th century, the works of Arabian authors and their European followers naturally constituted the libararies of the French pharmacists. To these treatises were added occasionally such books as the *Grand herbier*, a very free translation of the *Circa instans*. In the 16th century, books of French origin increased—at first written mainly by physicians.[45] In 1561 the first book in French written by a pharmacist on the art of pharmacy appeared. It was a manual of technic for pharmacy students *(L'Enchirid ou manipul des mirapoles)* by Michel Dusseau of Paris.[46] During the following century the profession continued to generate its own literature.[47] Of particular influence on the practice of French pharmacy were the writings of Jean de Renou (1608), providing a formulary, a textbook and a guide to the preservation of drugs, the use of pharmaceutical equipment and to the rules of professional ethics. A similarity to instructions given by the Italian Saladino d'Ascoli in the 15th century can be discerned frequently.

After the middle of the 17th century the number of books by French pharmacists increased markedly, including among the authors such famous names as Moise Charas, Nicaise Lefebvre, Nicolas Lémery, Antoine Baumé and E. F. Geoffroy.[48] The chemical side of the literature began to be transformed after the late 18th century when Lavoisier—no pharmacist himself, but a pupil of the pharmacist Guillaume François Rouelle—published his famous experiments concerning the role played by oxygen in combustion. He thereby established the basis of the "new chemistry," the chemistry of our own time—and hence of scientific pharmacy.

Pharmacopeias

The first local pharmacopeia or formulary of France appeared early in the 17th century (Lyons, 1628) and was followed by others.[49] The local approach to unifying drug standards was not superseded entirely until the first edition of the *Codex medicamentarius seu pharmacopoeia Gallica* became obligatory for the whole of France in 1818.

Journals

The excellent men who formed the *Société libre des pharmaciens de Paris* created only a year later (1797) the first French pharmaceutical journal, the *Journal de la société des pharmaciens de Paris*. Two years later it was consolidated with the *Annales de chimie* (founded 1780), which had had several famous French pharmacists on its editorial staff. This initiated a rich journal literature that branched out diversely in the 19th century, reflecting the professional and scientific vigor of French pharmacy.[50]

Representative of the present century are the *Annales pharmaceutiques françaises*, its distinguished scientific antecedents dating from 1809 (and serving the Académie de Pharmacie since its founding in 1946), and the *Bulletin de l'Ordre des Pharmaciens* (since 1947) as a professional journal. An early and remarkable cultural offshoot of French pharmacy—the first journal of its kind—is the *Revue d'histoire de la pharmacie* (beginning in 1913 as the *Bulletin*).

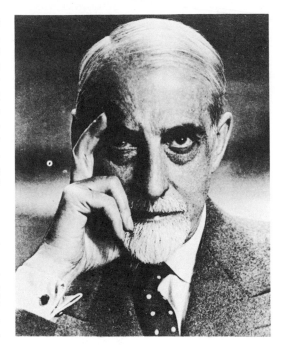

Ernest F. A. Fourneau (1872-1949), who owned a pharmacy for many years, rose to international fame as a brilliant investigator in pharmaceutical chemistry. For 30 years he directed the chemotherapeutic laboratory of the Pasteur Institute, whose research paved the way for sulfonamide products, produced pioneer antihistaminic agents and yielded other significant discoveries. When Fourneau sent the above picture to George Urdang (1947), he inscribed it on the back, "With cordial homage from a pharmacist."

PROMINENT PHARMACISTS

Thirty-two pages of the history of French pharmacy written by André-Pontier[51] and 48 pages of Bouvet's history[52] are devoted to a brief enumeration of famous French pharmacists from the 17th century to the present. These men intensively and often decisively promoted scientific progress in the different branches of the natural sciences. While so doing, some of them served their country in prominent positions with remarkable success. Some names have already been mentioned. A few further examples (for whom biographic notes may be found in Appendix 7) are Balard (1802-1876), Bayen (1725-1798), Caventou (1795-1877), Parmentier (1737-1813), Pelletier (1788-1842), Proust (1754-1826), Robiquet (1780-1840), G. F. Rouelle (1703-1770) and his brother H. M. Rouelle (1718-1778), Sérullas (1774-1832), Soubeiran (1797-1858) and Vauquelin (1763-1829). Bouvet tells us that 13 pharmacists were members of the French Academy of Science before 1803, 6 pharmacists were members of this academy in 1936 and 11 pharmacists are at present members of the French Academy of Medicine.[53]

HOSPITAL AND MILITARY PHARMACY

Modern hospital pharmacy was born in Paris in the early 19th century. As a specialty, it constituted one of the unique features in the development of pharmacy in France and was without precedent in other countries, even in Germany where French pharmacists encountered their most formidable scientific and professional rivalry.[54]

The role of the hospital pharmacist in this period has been characterized and distinguished from both monastic and lay predecessors as follows:

For one thing, he was a lay practitioner and not a member of a religious order. Unlike the English hospital apothecary of the 18th and early 19th century, he did not assume the dual role of pharmacist and minor medical practitioner. The Parisian hospital pharmacist was a municipal employee, selected on the basis of a competitive examination (*concours*) and, after 1814, recruited from those having completed an internship in hospital pharmacy. The internship became more and more important during the course of the century, not only for staffing hospital pharmacies but also in stimulating young pharmacists to become scientists. This new hospital pharmacist was generally oriented toward research and was often an excellent analytical chemist working in the fields of biochemistry, toxicology, and hygiene. Thus, with the passing of the years, a tradition of scientific eminence was established, and we see the hospital pharmacists of Paris acquiring

advanced degrees, becoming members of learned societies and professors in the various Faculties, making original discoveries, and publishing in learned journals.[55]

As in the community pharmacies, clinical laboratory work has been an important function of hospital pharmacists, but at present its volume and complexity make it difficult for the hospital pharmacist to fulfill his traditional role of joint director of the pharmacy and the medical biochemical services.

Hospital pharmacy holds a special place in military service, and there we find the French pharmacist first mentioned in 1630.[56] From the beginning he was placed on the same footing with the surgeon. The permanent office of "apothecary-major of the battlefields and the armies of the king" was created in 1766. However, the usual designation was abridged to "apothecary-major general."[57] To accord with the title of *médecin inspecteur général* held by the leading military physician, this title was replaced (1824) by the designation *pharmacien inspecteur général*. The French military pharmacists have enjoyed (since 1928) ranks equal with those of the army physicians, from that of *pharmacien sous-lieutenant* (pharmaceutical second lieutenant) to that of *pharmacien-général* (brigadier general).

In the pharmacists' effort to avoid subordination to military medicine, "the most significant factor was the impressive display of their scientific accomplishments—a display without precedent in pharmacy of the English-speaking world, and unmatched by military pharmacy in other European countries at that time."[58]

Many of the best-known French pharmacists have seen service in the army. The pharmacist-general of the so-called *Grande armée* of Napoleon I, Ch. Laubert, enjoyed the special confidence of the Emperor. After the siege of Moscow in 1812, Napoleon planned a mint to stamp coins out of the gold and the silver that the French had found in the conquered city. When asked whether he knew someone who could set up and operate a mint, the Emperor answered, "Don't we have our pharmacist-general? I commission him with everything!"

French pharmacists have retained their participation in the development of the sciences. The following opinion expressed by the famous chemist and statesman, Jean-Baptiste Dumas, in his capacity as Secretary of Agriculture, apparently still prevails in France:

To produce several eminent chemists, it is necessary to educate many. It is pharmacy which trains them. For this reason I have long ago been led to regard the learned profession of the pharmacist as a national asset which it is necessary to preserve without alteration and to restore little by little to the healthy conditions of its normal existence.[59]

6:   The Development in Germany

THE BEGINNINGS

The first pharmacies in Germany may have appeared during the 13th century, although surviving records leave us uncertain. It can be discerned that from an early time

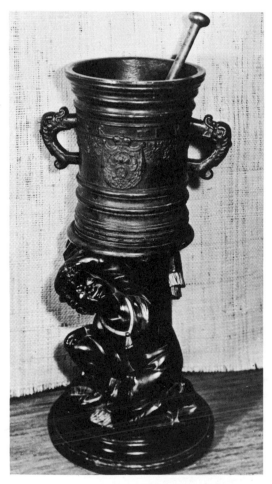

A crouching Moorish boy serves as a stand for this heavy bronze mortar with dolphin handles (made in 1704). On the front, the mortar bears the coat of arms of the prince-bishop at Mainz, in whose court pharmacy it stood. (Photograph from Verbandstoff-Fabriken Paul Hartmann AG, Heidenheim/Brenz)

in Germany—unlike such countries as Italy and France—the pharmaceutical profession was regulated by government rather than being self-governing. During the Middle Ages, the number of pharmacists in German communities was too small to make pharmaceutical guilds or guildlike associations possible. Since some cities in Germany (and the German-speaking part of Switzerland) did not allow tradesmen not belonging to a guild to operate businesses, pharmacists were forced at times to join a guild of another calling.

There were highly esteemed guilds, e.g., the *Hansegrebenguild* in Kassel and the Guild of Safran (saffron) in Basel, comprised of leading commercial groups and members of the intellectual professions.[1] In both of these, pharmacists not only were guild members but often were elected to office. In general, the German pharmacists objected to becoming members of the guilds of ordinary retailers, and in such a "marriage of convenience" only the commercial side of the pharmacist's activity was subjected to guild regulation.[2]

SYSTEMS OF PHARMACEUTICAL OWNERSHIP

Controls guaranteed to merchants and craftsmen by their guilds—for example, the "closed shop" and the monopoly of sale and of manufacture—were accorded to pharmacists by the ruling authority through a *privilegium,* that is, special privileges granted on the basis of particular duties carefully stipulated in a signed and sealed document carrying full legal power.

Such a contract—typical of the feudal system, especially in Germany—was bestowed on the apothecaries by an individual ruler or an aristocratic governing body of a principality of the Holy Roman Empire. This *privilegium* was of various types. It might concern the building in which the pharmacy was established; in this case, the buyer of the "privilege" would have to buy the building. Another type of *privilegium* might contain a proviso that it would end with the grantee's death or that it would be hereditary. It might be granted by a ruler without restriction, and the pharmacist could sell at any time this exclusive right to operate a pharmacy in the area specified.[3] An "exclusive" right—by no means rare up to the 17th century—excluded the establishment of another pharmacy in the community or the area concerned no matter how large the population might grow.

Concession System

Either with or without the "exclusive" right, privileges remained the usual legal basis of pharmacies in Germany until the early 19th century.

From then on, no new "privileges" were granted, generally speaking, although the old ones were not invalidated. The arbitrariness and the unlimited authority reflected in the old feudal mechanism were replaced by a competitive system of granting a government "concession" to operate each pharmacy serving a specified segment of the population. The concession system recognized a new time, without abandoning the German values of regulated order, dignity and quality in pharmaceutical development.

If we ignore minor differences in provisions among the various German states, the procedure may be summarized as follows: The town, or area in a town, where a pharmacy is to be established issues a public announcement. Interested pharmacists are invited to apply. A commission compares the qualifications of the applicants, but, in general, the right to operate the pharmacy (the concession) tends to be awarded to the employed pharmacist who has been longest in practice.

These concessions could be neither sold nor inherited in some German states. However, in the largest state (Prussia), a concession holder could nominate his successor ("right of presentation")—which, in practice, was almost equivalent to the right

of sale and hereditary transmission. The government could say "no" to a nomination, but did so in only a few cases. Since the ability to purchase the "concession" for a pharmacy practically assured a large and prosperous professional practice, this salable form of concession was a sought-after property of high value, and was called a "real-konzession."

It was symptomatic that these salable concessions became subject to investment speculation, especially during the long period of prosperity in Germany before World War I. Certain pharmacists (called among colleagues *Apothekenschächer!*) bought and sold pharmacies as speculations rather than as places to practice their profession.

However, the granting of concessions carrying the "right of presentation" was discontinued even in Prussia beginning in June 1894. Concessions then conformed to the pattern of awarding a permit for a new pharmacy or a vacated old pharmacy by competitive selection among applicants. This type is termed a "Personal-Konzession" because the selected pharmacist had the right to operate the pharmacy only during his lifetime.[4] Unlike the "real" concession, the "personal" concession changed hands on payment of the value of the stock and equipment only, and possibly a certain amount for any capital improvements made by a predecessor.

Until after World War II German pharmacists operated under any one of three types of permit; for, when one of the German states modified its permit system, the action was not retroactive. Hence in some pharmacies rights that had been granted in a remote time persisted:

1. *Privilegia* could be disposed of quite as the owners might desire.

2. *Real-konzession* could be transmitted by sale or inheritance, but government confirmation of each transfer was required.

3. *Personal-konzession* gave the right to the operation and the income of a particular pharmacy, awarded for a person's lifetime on the basis of professional merit and, especially, of length of service as an employed pharmacist. Being a concession to

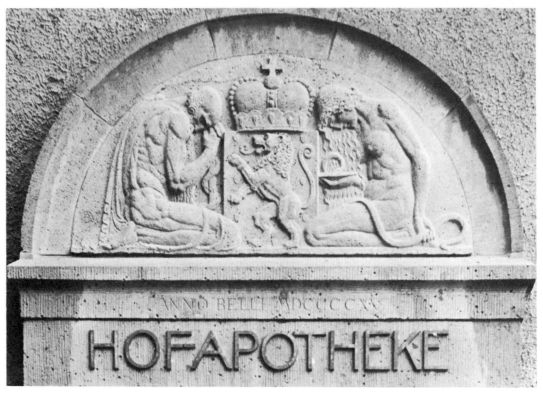

The kinship between pharmacy and medicine is symbolized by this bas relief (cut into basalt) over the entrance to the old court pharmacy at Lich, Germany. In a classical spirit, the sculptor Augustus Heumann (1915) shows the great healing god Asklepios (left) leaning on his staff entwined by a serpent (symbolic of medicine), and his daughter Hygeia with bowl and serpent (symbolic of pharmacy). Between the figures is the coat of arms of the sovereign under whose patronage the pharmacy was once operated. (Photograph from Ludwig Weber)

a particular pharmacist, it could not be sold or inherited.

Various exceptions to these categories were usually pharmacies owned by communities, organizations or the old aristocracy.

Municipal and Princely Pharmacies

Until after World War II, a few pharmacies in certain German states were owned by the government or by former sovereigns. Most of these descended from the 16th and 17th centuries, when they were established as the court pharmacies of German princes.[5] Here were vestiges of an early time of German pharmacy, when pharmacies often were established by the larger municipali-

ties also. Such pharmacies were found especially in the imperial cities, which possessed the same governmental sovereignty as the German princes of the time and were subordinate only to the Emperor himself.[6] Significantly, the municipalities did not derive the advantage from their pharmacies that they had expected. Consequently, they first leased and then sold them. In modern times communities in some of the German states (Anhalt, Baden, Hessia and Thuringia) were given governmental permission to establish pharmacies in places where the government considered them to be needed. These pharmacies were leased to pharmacists who were selected in the usual way by public contest, in which the length of service as an employee in pharmacies played a decisive part. In Hessia there were, in 1934, 23 such communal pharmacies among a total of 128.

As was the case with the early municipal pharmacies, the first German attempt at socialized pharmacy—that is, pharmacy as an institution of the state, conducted by pharmaceutical officials—proved to be a failure, at least from a financial point of view. The Duke of Brunswick tried the experiment as early as the second half of the 18th century. He bought the pharmacies in his country and created a central pharmaceutical administration, a central laboratory and a central department for the purchase of all drugs and supplies. After 20 years, during which neither the expected profit was achieved nor better service rendered to the public, the pharmacies were sold to private individuals.[7]

All of these different systems of regulation found in the history of German pharmacy agree in one decisive principle: the limitation of the number of pharmacies. This principle was abandoned in Prussia for only one year (1810), with the introduction of the general liberty to practice any calling *(Gewerbefreiheit)*. Another exception, for almost a century, was Hamburg—a city influenced by England as a result of its location and trade; here anyone who could prove his pharmaceutical knowledge was permitted to open a pharmacy. However, in 1818 the difficulties of maintaining professional standards and order brought a limitation on the number of pharmacies in relation to the population served.

The general tradition of controlling the number and the distribution of pharmacies—at a certain price in freedom of opportunity and decision—did achieve a high and unusually uniform level of professional practice, appearance and pride in the German pharmacies, all of which have been devoted exclusively to health-related and technical services.

Limitation Overthrown

A fundamental turn away from the traditional limitation on the number of pharma-

cies first came at the close of World War II. The four military occupation zones of Germany became regulated under different concepts and circumstances. The American zone introduced the freedom of establishing pharmacies; the British and French zones remained in principle with the "concession" system; while in the Soviet zone the pharmacies gradually came under government operation. This process continued until a new regulation was issued after the founding of the West German republic. Next, the unregulated freedom of location of pharmacies in the American occupation zone was abandoned for all practical purposes.

Then came court proceedings culminating in the "Karlsruher Urteil," a decision under the constitution that made freedom of location of pharmacies general after 1959 throughout the West German republic. To be sure, the special pharmaceutical rights and privileges were not rescinded, but they were made worthless by a wholly new situation, which permits new pharmacies to mushroom from the German land. Whereas in 1951 there were about 5,000 community pharmacies operating in West Germany, a decade later there were nearly 9,000. This means that the average number of persons served by each pharmacy had dropped to about 6,000, or only about twice as many per pharmacy as in the United States. Naturally, this is a "historical development that calls for vigilance, lest the high professional standing of German pharmacy is lost."[8]

The president of the Hamburg Chamber of Pharmacists, Werner Klie, says:

German pharmacists themselves have no uniform idea of what the future regulation of the German pharmacy system should look like. They are unanimous only in one point, and that is that they all oppose an unrestricted Right of Settlement [freedom of location] law. . . . The past experiences in Germany and in other countries abroad clearly indicate, that this road should not be attempted again. The high ethical standards set by the German pharmacists are founded primarily on the protection

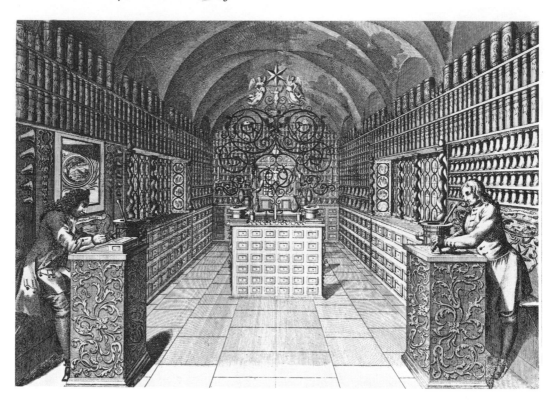

German pharmacies, old or new, set a high standard of professional character. The Pharmacy of the Golden Star in Nuremberg as it appeared in the early 18th century is contrasted with the Angel Pharmacy of Merck (opposite) as it appeared in mid-20th century.

In the Star Pharmacy, the chief pharmacist (at the desk on the left) is bringing his records up to date, while one of his associates (on the right) seems to be preparing a dispensing container. The main prescription counter stands in the center of the pharmacy, surmounted by ornamental rococo grillework. Matched sets of stock containers fill the shelves. Below waist-level the pharmacy is lined with small drawers. (Copper engraving by H. Bohrmann, 1710)

which the government has granted to the profession.[8a]

MONOPOLY, FIXED PRICES, "DROGERIEN"

Most of the *privilegia* issued between the 14th and the 18th centuries contained detailed instructions about the management of the pharmacy and enumerations of the goods that were monopolies of the pharmacist. Among products that others were forbidden to sell, we often find such articles as sugar, spices, liquors, wine, tobacco, coffee and chocolate. Some of these were used in medicine and were costly substances. However, the main reason for reserving them for sale by pharma-

cists was a presumed need to assure a livelihood to an essential group whose professional function was too limited quantitatively. For example, a privilege granted a pharmacist named Kestner, in Landsberg a.W., in 1585, explicitly states that he must be given a monopoly in the trade in spices, wine and liquors, because it would be impossible for him to earn his livelihood from the sale of medicaments only.[9] We find the same idea expressed in many laws, ordinances and edicts. In the ordinance of the Count of Schleiz in the 17th century, the town authorities were admonished to protect the pharmacy from illegal competition by ordinary retailers lest "this precious jewel so very useful for town and country becomes damaged or even perishes!"[10]

Later on, naturally, the monopoly rights of the pharmacists became restricted more and more to medicaments. Nevertheless, the fundamental concept of governmental obligation to protect the pharmacies in behalf of the public welfare has not been changed.

A consequence of the German principle of maintaining a just balance between the rights and the duties of the people by legal regulation was that the governmental limitation of competition had to be supplemented by governmental protection of the people from an abuse of this restriction. This concept caused the early introduction (e.g., the legal system of Frederick II of Hohenstaufen) of regulated prices for remedies sold by pharmacists granted *privilegia*. It gave rise to carefully elaborated lists of governmentally fixed prices that still regu-

late commercial relations between the pharmacists and the public to the benefit of both, in Germany and in those countries under German cultural influence.

We know of more than 500 such German governmental price lists *(Taxen),* from the 15th century until the present time. The earliest was printed in Dresden in 1553.[11] In 1905 the price lists of all the smaller German states and the individual towns,[12] which with a few exceptions had gradually disappeared in the 19th century, were replaced by the first *Arzneitaxe für das Deutsche Reich* (governmentally fixed drug prices obligatory for the entire German Empire). New editions have been issued periodically (usually annually except in times of war and postwar confusion), with prices in accord with changes in wholesale prices.

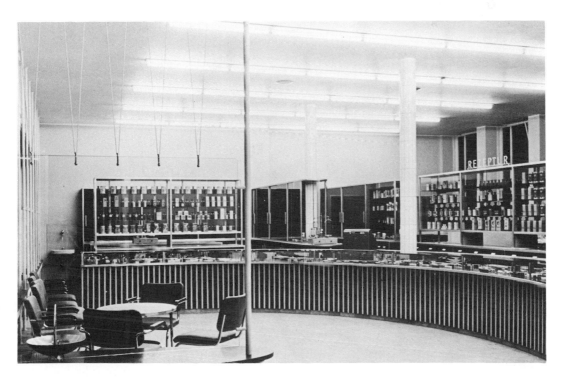

The Merck pharmacy is the modern version of the same pharmacy in Darmstadt out of which grew the great manufacturing laboratory. (The American Merck is an offshoot of the latter, which became independent.) The main area for prescription work in this pharmacy is to the right (Rezeptur). The section on the left reflects the curious survival of homeopathy in sufficient strength to warrant a special department. Modern pharmacies such as this one—like those of preceding centuries—have several other rooms besides the public dispensing room shown in these photographs: an office with reference books, a laboratory, a specialties room and stock rooms, including cold storage. (Photograph by Apotheken von Mayer, 1954)

The *Arzneitaxe* not only fixes prices for drugs, but also sets fees for the pharmaceutical work done in filling prescriptions, in accordance with the amount of time required and the technical skill involved.[13]

As stated above, the monopoly rights of pharmacists gradually came to be limited to remedies. There was a continuous quarrel, naturally, between the pharmacists and would-be competitors. A large part of the many edicts and laws concerning pharmacy which were issued through the centuries was devoted to this subject.[14] Again and again, the various governments stated the kinds of products reserved to pharmacies and those that might be sold elsewhere.

The original tendency to reserve all dispensing of remedies to pharmacists underwent a gradual change. Concessions had been made to the *Materialisten*, a combination of retail grocer and hardware dealer. Further concessions were made by opening the retail trade in spices and cosmetics to everyone. In 1872 the first of a series of Imperial edicts was issued. This took out of the pharmaceutical monopoly all unprepared and unmixed drugs—with the exception of a number of very potent ones—and all preparations sold avowedly for use as cosmetics, foodstuff, dietetic aids and preventives, even those with healing or mitigating properties. One result was a new art of advertising, developed to remove from the pharmaceutical monopoly as many remedies as possible by labeling them cosmetics or dietetic aids or, above all, as preventives. Nevertheless, such products continued to be recommended for their primary use as healing agents.

Inasmuch as the edicts did not enumerate what was allowed for free trade but only stated the kinds of preparations reserved to the pharmacies, many possibilities for interpretation were left open. Gradually a distinct class of shops developed called *Drogerien,* specializing in the sale of technical chemicals, cosmetics, dietetic aids, spices, candy, dyes, toiletries, varnishes and all those drugs and remedies that were not restricted to pharmacies, or that could be so interpreted.

These shops (in superficial appearance like below-average American drugstores, but without any potent drugs or prescription service) are operated by *Drogisten* (literally "druggists," but in no respect being or considered to be pharmacists). The owners of the *Drogerien* have had since 1872 a quite separate and very active organization. While the number of such shops has tended to decline in recent decades, there are still more *Drogerien* than there are *Apotheken* (pharmacies).

Having achieved their position on the basis of a contention that no special pharmaceutical knowledge is needed to sell "harmless" drugs, the *Drogisten* later changed their tune. Since the early 20th century they have clamored for official recognition as a kind of second-class pharmacist (with certain privileges not permitted general storekeepers), and as part of this move they organized special schools for their apprentices.

After World War II the *Drogisten* widened the scope of their efforts, seeking permission to deal in all drugs not requiring a prescription. However, they have had no success. Neither the pharmacy law of 1960 nor the drug law of 1961 shrank the area over which the German pharmacist has responsibility. The drug law has sharpened stipulations concerning the claims made for drugs, their manufacture, the special registration of proprietary specialties, the distribution of drugs and the safeguarding and the control of their use.[15]

DEVELOPMENT OF EDUCATION

During the early period, the professional education of the German pharmacists[16] was not so well regulated as it was in France. Lack of cooperative self-determination left the regulation of pharmaceutical education to circles outside of pharmacy. Thus until the end of the 17th century the numerous decrees concerning pharmacy contain but vague remarks concerning professional education.

An apprenticeship of 6 years was customary during that period. A satisfactory knowledge of Latin was a general requirement. From an edict of the Duke of Bavaria (1595) we learn that the examinations had to be written, oral and practical.[17] The examiners were physicians. Aside from the required preliminary Latin instruction—needed to read the books of the time as well as prescriptions—no fixed course was outlined. Therefore, in general, German pharmacy in the 17th century could scarcely rise above the level of technical skill.[18]

However, this situation was changed in the course of the 18th century. Obligatory examinations based on definite requirements, first introduced in Prussia in 1725, gave the German pharmacists a place among the representatives of the scientific professions. Thereafter, in Prussia, two classes of pharmacists existed.

Those of the second class, who were permitted to practice in small towns only, were not required to study academically. They had to serve their apprenticeship, usually of 5 years' duration, and a clerkship usually of 6 years, and then pass an examination before their provincial *Collegium medicum* (medical board). The pharmacists of the first class were required to serve at least 7 years as clerks after their apprenticeship and had to attend a course at the higher *Collegium medicum* in Berlin, an institution mainly for the scientific education of military physicians and surgeons. This course consisted of lectures in chemistry and botany, discourses on the chemicals used in remedies, their preparation and "the chemicophysical reasons" for the several kinds of preparations and, lastly, practical pharmaceutico-chemical instruction. The first professor of pharmaceutical chemistry at the higher *Collegium medicum* was the pharmacist Caspar Neumann (1683-1737); the last one was the pharmacist M. H. Klaproth (1743-1817), who later on became the first professor of chemistry at the University of Berlin. The division of the Prussian pharmacists into two classes disappeared in 1854.

During the last third of the 18th century the German pharmacists themselves began to raise their educational standards. A series of private institutes, devoted to the education of pharmacists, was established. Some of these institutes became famous far beyond the German frontiers. For example, the institute of the pharmacist Johannes Bartholomaeus Trommsdorff in Erfurt (1770-1847) had many students from foreign countries. The Prussian government acknowledged the education acquired in this institute as equivalent to the study "at Berlin or at universities."[19] In 1808, Bavaria made study at a university obligatory for pharmacists. The other German states soon followed.

The present educational requirements for German pharmacists (law of April 1, 1935) are as follows:

1. *Preliminary education:* a certificate of graduation from one of the secondary schools that prepare for university studies, called Gymnasium, Realgymnasium, or Superior Realschule, corresponding roughly to 2 or 3 years of preprofessional college studies in the United States

2. *Professional experience:* 2 years of apprenticeship, previous to admission to a university, in a pharmacy (the proprietor of which must be officially authorized by a highly selective procedure to receive apprentices); then 1 year of probationary practice after the completion of the university studies.

3. *Professional education:* a 3-year university course

4. *Examinations:* (a) After the 2 years of apprenticeship, written, oral, and laboratory examinations test the practical skill of the applicant and his knowledge of the professional fundamentals. (This examination entitles one to work as a so called *vorexaminierter* clerk in a pharmacy, with somewhat restricted responsibility and for a limited time.) (b) After completion of the university studies, comprehensive written, laboratory and oral examinations cover the entire range of the curriculum. These include general chemistry, botany, pharmacognosy, physics, galenical pharmacy, bacteriology and history of pharmacy. During the 3 years of study, the student also must complete courses successfully in pharmaceutical law and economics, pharmacology and toxicology, hygiene, sterilization and homeopathy, the

fundamentals of which may be included in the examinations.[19ᵃ]

Before World War II one half of the year of probation following the diploma examination was to be served in a town having only one pharmacy and with a pharmacist who was unable to pay a professional assistant (called *Landhalbjahr*). Remuneration was restricted to free room and board. The eligible owners of such pharmacies were enumerated in a list revised annually.

SUPERVISION OF PHARMACY

For a long period the inspection of German pharmacies was generally the duty of physicians. By 1642 an edict issued for the town of Brandenburg officially admitted the cooperation of a pharmacist. There followed a delay of more than 80 years before this local regulation became general for the entire Prussian kingdom. In some other German states the supervision of pharmacies was placed in the hands of pharmacists only (as in Hessia, Saxony and Thuringia).

However, the Prussian system of cooperative inspection by a medical official and a pharmaceutical practitioner persisted and, since 1935, has been obligatory for the entire German Reich.

According to the regulation, the pharmacist participating in the inspection is co-ordinate with, not subordinate to, the physician. He has a 5-year term as an honorary official (with the title *Pharmazierat* or in special cases even *Oberpharmazierat*).

The inspection of the retail trade in drugs outside pharmacies, hence the inspection of the *Drogerien*, is the responsibility of pharmaceutical practitioners. Naturally, the owners of these stores resent this "interference" and demand that their places of business be inspected by officials appointed from their own ranks.

SOCIAL STANDING

Socially, the position of the German pharmacist has been similar to that of his French colleague. He has been a typical representative of the middle class. Throughout the centuries, representatives of pharmacy have been awarded all the honors which ordinary civil life has to offer.[20] Again and again we find pharmacists as municipal deputies, senators, mayors and, later on, as members of parliament.[21] There were three reasons for this social esteem: (1) the fact that the pharmacist for the most part belonged to the well-to-do class; (2) often there were "dynasties" of pharmacists active for generations in the same place;[22] (3) they were the most available and sometimes the only representatives of natural science within their communities, and they used their knowledge for the benefit of their fellow citizens.

As a classic illustration of the scientific and social standing of German pharmacy at the beginning of the 19th century, one of the greatest Germans, the poet and statesman Goethe, may be quoted. Goethe stated (1822) that "in Germany the pharmacist enjoys a highly esteemed position within society. . . . The German pharmacists cultivate science. They are aware of its importance and endeavor to utilize it in practical pharmacy."[23]

This scientific endeavor of the German pharmacist at times made him a target of literary derision.[24] He has always stood between trade and science and, particularly in Germany, with its precise class distinctions sharply differentiating socially between tradesmen and scientists, this hybrid condition created tragicomic situations.

In the 17th century the pharmacies in Germany began to mirror the social position of their owners. Among 16th century *Apotheken* we know only one architecturally beautiful building still serving pharmaceutical purposes. It is the *Ratsapotheke* in Lemgo, Westphalia. This is one of the most characteristic edifices of the Renaissance period that has come down to us. During the 17th and the 18th centuries the German pharmacists tried to make their homes and shops places of dignity and of artistic culture.[25]

In response to a growing demand, indigenous faïence production developed, which spread over the whole of Germany after the 17th century; thus, most pharmacies obtained elegant equipment previously restricted to the few who could afford to import Italian, French or Delft shelfware.

The fact that, from the beginning of their professional service in the armed forces, pharmacists were given rank and pay comparable with that of commissioned officers testifies to the social as well as the professional level that they had achieved. The German military pharmacists (in rank up to colonel) have been entrusted not only with strictly pharmaceutical work but also with hygienic and chemical warfare tasks, and they have been given the responsibilities of well-educated natural scientists.[26]

SCIENTIFIC PHARMACEUTICAL LITERATURE

As in all European countries, the first scientific pharmaceutical knowledge came from Arabian sources via Italy. The first German original literature dealing with subjects of pharmaceutical interest, and influencing pharmacy, was of a special kind: books on general natural history that included pharmacy. There were also so-called *Arzneibücher* (books dealing with remedies and their application), the *Destillierbücher* (books on the art of distillation) and the *Kräuterbücher* (herbals). Most of these books were written in German and in a popular style.[27]

Both the distillation books and the herbals often contained more than their names implied. In the herbals not only herbs but also animals and gems and their assumed medicinal effects are described. Thus the large *Hortus sanitatis* describes 392 animals and 144 gems, besides 530 herbs. In Braunschweig's large book on distillation we find not only detailed instructions on distillation, enhanced by numerous illustrations, but also the herbs used, the products obtained and their medicinal effects. These books, written mostly by physicians, were intended to serve the colleagues of the authors as well as the pharmacists and, last but not least, the laymen. For example, the illustrations are to inform the illiterate, says Braunschweig in the preface to his small *Destillierbuch!*[28]

Besides his distillation books, Braunsch-

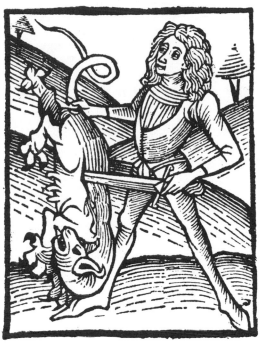

Early printed herbals were embellished with woodcuts showing the sources of drugs, animal as well as vegetable. Reflecting late medieval folklore, a dragon, "greatest of all serpents and beasts," is shown impaled on the sword of its conqueror. If a dragon's tongue can be obtained, make a decoction of it in wine to anoint the body against various ills. (*Hortus sanitatis*, Strasbourg, about 1507, Chap. 48; from the University of Wisconsin Library)

weig wrote a renowned formulary on inexpensive prescribing for the poor (*Thesaurus pauperum*), to which there were many successors. Otto Brunfels wrote one of the most used herbals, as well as a book on the equipping and the managing of pharmacies (*Die Reformation der Apotheken*), similar to the book of the Frenchman Renou (see page 72), which in turn was based on Saladin de Asculo. The famous commentary on Dioscorides by Mattioli was published in German (*Neu deutsch Kreuterbuch*, 1563).[29]

Still in the 16th century, there appeared encyclopedic books that covered the entire scope of pharmacy, the ambitious counterparts of which still appear on pharmacists' shelves today. In 1561 the physician J. J. Wecker of Basel issued his *Antidotarium Generale,* which contains a comprehensive formulary, instructions on the art of filling prescriptions, directions for preparing galenics and for preparing the chemicals of that time.[30]

However, the universal textbook of German pharmacists for at least a century was another book, *Pharmacopoea medico-physica,* by the physician Joh. Christian Schroeder (1600-1664).[31] In the 17th century an important book in botany also appeared, written by a pharmacist, Basilius Besler of Nuremberg, describing and cataloging the botanic garden in Eichstaett (*Hortus Eystettensis,* 1613).

Among the most important pharmaco-chemical books of the 17th century were three by German physicians: the *Basilica chymica* of Oswald Croll (1560-1609), an ardent Paracelsist; the *Pharmacia moderno saeculo applicanda* (Pharmacy Applied to Modern Times) of D. Ludovici (1625-1680); the *Pharmacopoea spagyrica* of Joh. Rudolf Glauber (1604-1670), one of the first German chemists whose work helped to lay the foundations for German chemical industry.[32]

Joh. Christoph Sommerhof is credited with the first book on pharmaceutical subjects by a German pharmacist—his excellent *Lexicon pharmaceutico-chymicum* (1701). From the mid-18th century on, the number of such books by pharmacists increased extraordinarily. Almost without exception they set a high standard.[33] German scientific pharmacy had come of age.

The great number of prominent scientists coming from the ranks of German pharmacy since the middle of the 18th century explains why most professors teaching chemistry at German universities, up to the first third of the 19th century, came from pharmacy and, ofttimes, even instructed students in their pharmacies.[34] In the appointment of K. G. Hagen as professor of chemistry at the University of Königsberg, in Prussia, the circumstance that he was the owner of "a well-equipped *Laboratorium chymicum*" was decisive.[35]

Representative of the remarkable scientific productivity of German pharmacy are the following men (not already mentioned in the text or footnotes), for whom brief biographic notes may be found in the Glossary, Appendix 7:

A. S. Marggraf (1709-1782), E. W. Martius (1756-1849), Fr. A. C. Gren (1760-1798), A. F. Gehlen (1775-1815), K. L. Willdenow (1765-1812), J. W. Doebereiner (1780-1849), F. W. A. Sertürner (1783-1841), J. A. Buchner (1783-1852), Ph.L. Geiger (1785-1836), Th.F.L. Nees v. Esenbeck (1787-1837), F. F. Runge (1794-1867), H. W. F. Wackenroder (1798-1854), H. H. J. Hager (1816-1897), C. F. Mohr (1806-1879), Fr. A. Flückiger (1828-1894), E. Schmidt (1845-1921), E. Beckmann (1853-1923), H. Thoms (1859-1931) and A. Tschirch (1856-1939).

The laboratories of German pharmacies were to a remarkable extent the precursors not only of the later university chemical laboratories but also of the large-scale pharmaceutical industry.[36] The names of E. Merck, Schering and Riedel, to mention only a few, have become known all over the world. There is ample evidence that the rapid development of scientific and industrial chemistry since the end of the 18th century has been due in great measure to the rivalry of French and German pharmacists in this field of science.

GERMAN AND AUSTRIAN PHARMACOPEIAS

The first official pharmacopeia in Germany was the *Dispensatorium* of Valerius Cordus, issued in 1546 and made official for the imperial city of Nuremberg.[37] Many consider it to be the first true "pharmacopeia" anywhere in the world, since it was enacted specifically as legally binding on all practitioners in the Nuremberg area, whereas the famous earlier book in Florence (1499; see page 59) was made an authoritative standard only by the considerable power of the Florentine guild of physicians and pharmacists (rather than by documented enactment by civil authorities).

The Nuremberg book was followed

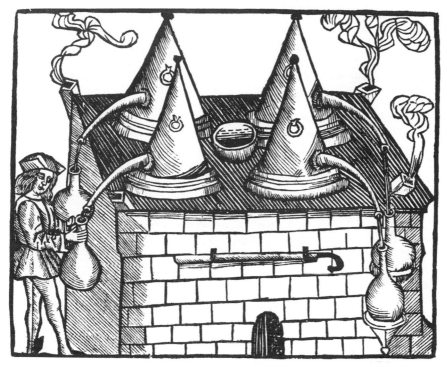

Medicinal distillates gained wide popularity after the early 16th century when this woodcut was published. Distillate is being collected from four cucurbits, each with a conical air-cooled alembic. An inner rim collected and guided the distillate to the delivery tube. At the corners of the furnace are four small chimneys, and in the center is a funnel for filling the water bath. This illustration comes from a book by Braunschweig, a Strassburg surgeon, whose works were enormously influential in making distillation technic an important part of pharmacy. In the next generation, Paracelsus gave this part of the "spagyric art" further importance by his emphasis on separating the "quintessence" from the dross and the impurities of crude drugs. (Photograph, University of Wisconsin, from Die Distellacien en Virtuyten der Watere, Brussels, 1517; *see also* Forbes, R. J.: . . . Art of Distillation)

within 20 years by pharmacopeias for Augsburg (compiled by Adolf Occo in 1564) and for Cologne (1565).[38] These three earliest German pharmacopeias represent three types of official books that recur later elsewhere. A good and concise compilation of old formulas, in a critical and progressive spirit but without elaboration, is the approach of Cordus. A more comprehensive approach was taken by Occo, with the added feature of a legal regulation that required pharmacists to keep in stock all drugs marked with an asterisk in the pharmacopeia. Most comprehensive of the three

is the *Dispensarium Coloniense*, providing not only an official formulary but also a textbook type of information about the drugs. This latter concept became predominant among European pharmacopeias up to the end of the 18th century.

At the end of the 17th century, the *Dispensatorium Brandenburgicum* (1698),[39] the first official pharmacopeia for a larger German political unit, appeared.

In Austria, one of the most important parts of the German Empire until 1806, a peculiar situation existed. The medical faculty of the University of Vienna had compiled a *Dispensatorium pro pharma-copoeis Viennensibus* (1570), which was to be obligatory for the pharmacists in Vienna. At that time no book could be printed without permission of the sovereign, and for some unknown reason, this permission was not obtained. Thus this pharmacopeia, although official, was never printed; the Viennese pharmacists were forced to copy such parts as they thought necessary! Eventually (1618) the *Pharmacopoeia Augustana* became the official standard not only for Vienna but also for the Austrian provinces. From 1729 on, various pharmacopeias appeared in Austria, culminating with the first edition (1812) of the present *Pharmacopoea Austriaca*.[40]

Besides the Prussian-Brandenburgian dispensatory, the *Pharmacopoea Wirtembergica* was the official book of its time most esteemed and used, even beyond the German frontiers. A special section gave good descriptions of the simple drugs. Thus it represented the combined textbook and formulary style, the prototype of which was the *Dispensatorium Coloniense* of 1565. It was one of the most comprehensive formularies, supplying information about all drugs, new and old. The edition of 1771 still contained 107 drugs of animal origin. Both of these official books (Prussian-Brandenburgian and Würtembergian pharmacopeias) reflect the victory of the chemical or Paracelsian school of thought. The names of Arabian physicians, of Pseudo-Mesuë, and those of their European followers (Nicolaus, Fernel and Occo) have been dropped from the titles of the compounded formulas of which they were the real or supposed authors. Instead, the Brandenburgian-Prussian pharmacopeia (1698), in addition to the name of Paracelsus himself, cites the names of various paracelsists (Becher, Craanen, Croll, Ludovici, Mynsicht, Quercetanus, Rolfink, Sylvius, Wirtz and Zwelffer). In the *Pharmacopoea Wirtembergica* of 1771 this list of names is augmented by those of other chemically minded men (Camerarius, Dippel, Minderer, Schroeder, Stahl, Wedel and others).[41]

In consequence of the new theory of Lavoisier concerning the role of oxygen in combustion, the authorship of the German pharmacopeias underwent a decided change. The first *Pharmacopoea Borussica* represents an important milestone in the history of German pharmacopeias (1799). This book was one of the first official pharmaceutical formularies based on the new chemical theories, and was the first one in Germany prepared primarily and influenced decisively by pharmacists and not by physicians.[42] This was because the German development of chemistry, and more particularly of pharmaceutical chemistry, had been fostered by pharmacists since the middle of the 18th century. Their opportunity had come and it had found them ready. Thus they could not be overlooked or ignored. It was the triumvirate, M. H. Klaproth, S. F. Hermbstaedt and Valentin Rose, Jr., who elaborated the pharmacopeia, with the assistance of other pharmacists and the collaboration of physicians.[43]

The preparedness of German pharmacists proved to be of consequence in the next decisive stage in the history of German pharmacopeias. During the middle sixties of the 19th century, the general as well as the pharmaceutical situation in Germany demanded some kind of unification. Before the German political unification (not including Austria) became a reality in 1871, the German pharmacists anticipated it by presenting to the German professional world a *Pharmacopoea Germaniae* (1865), elaborated exclusively by pharmacists under the sponsorship of their association.[44] This book became official only for Saxony, but it paved the way for a pharmaceutical standard obligatory throughout the reunited Germany and showed how necessary such a standard was. Indeed, one of the first governmental acts of the new German Empire was to create such a standard. Only one year after the establishment of the new Empire, the first *Pharmacopoea Germanica* appeared (1872).[45] This book, as well as all later editions (published since 1890 in German instead of Latin), was elaborated by representatives of all interested professions and groups, but the decisive influence of the pharmacist has prevailed.

PHARMACEUTICAL PERIODICALS AND ORGANIZATIONS

The first periodical devoted exclusively to pharmacy was German born: the *Almanach oder Taschenbuch für Scheidekünstler und Apotheker,* an annual founded in 1780 by Johann Goettling.[46] It was followed by the first pharmaceutical publication appearing at more frequent intervals, hence having more the character of a journal, *Trommsdorff's Journal der Pharmacie* (1794). Since then a large number of scientific pharmaceutical journals have made their appearance.[47] Among independent journals (not affiliated with or supported by an association), the *Pharmaceutische Centralhalle* became best known (founded by Hermann Hager in 1859 and still being published). A new journal on drug research appeared in 1950 *(Arzneimittelforschung).*[48]

Of the independent journals devoted to professional pharmacy as a whole—ethical and commercial aspects as well as scientific—mention should be made of the *Pharmazeutische Zeitung* (founded in 1856 by Hermann Mueller) and the *Süddeutsche Apotheker-Zeitung* (founded in 1861 as *Pharmaceutisches Wochenblatt).*[49] The *Pharmazeutische Zeitung,* a victim of the Nazi regime toward the close of 1937, was revived in 1947 (uniting in 1953 with the *Apotheker-Zeitung*). The *Süddeutsche Apotheker-Zeitung* (revived 1946) merged into the *Deutsche Apotheker Zeitung* (1950). A counterpart journal of general circulation in the Soviet zone of Germany, *Die Pharmazie,* has appeared since 1946.

Organizations

Besides the independent journals, others appeared as the official organs of pharmaceutical associations. The first German organization of considerable size and importance was founded in 1632 at Nuremberg,[50] and at least three other local societies appeared by the beginning of the 19th century.[51]

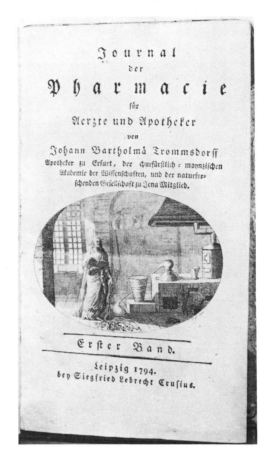

The earliest regular journal of pharmacy having a scientific character was issued between 1793 and 1834. Its Pharmacist-Editor, J. B. Trommsdorff, had a teaching laboratory for practical chemistry associated with his pharmacy, which may not have been unlike the pharmaceutical laboratory shown (above) on the title page of Volume 1. (From the University of Wisconsin)

A more comprehensive organization for northern Germany (Apothekerverein im noerdlichen Teutschland, founded in 1820) combined in 1872—promptly after the national federation of the German states—with the south German society (Süddeutscher Apothekerverein, founded in 1848), to form the national Deutscher Apothekerverein.[52]

This was replaced during the Nazi period

(1933-1945) by a totalitarian association, the only one permitted to represent the professional and commercial interests of German pharmacists during those years.[53]

To promote pharmaceutical science and research specifically, the Deutsche Pharmazeutische Gesellschaft had been organized in 1890 (on the initiative of Hermann Thoms).[54]

Both the Deutscher Apothekerverein (professional) and the Pharmazeutische Gesellschaft (scientific) have issued their own publications. In addition to the *Archiv der Pharmacie*, the Apothekerverein since 1886 had published the *Apotheker-Zeitung*.[55] The Pharmazeutische Gesellschaft, since its founding (1890), published the *Berichte der Deutschen Pharmazeutischen Gesellschaft*, which consolidated with the *Archiv der Pharmazie* (1924). Since then it has borne the dual title, *Archiv der Pharmazie und Berichte der Deutschen Pharmazeutischen Gesellschaft*. (Discontinued at the downfall of the Nazi regime, the *Archiv* was revived in 1950.)

The journal of the Arbeitsgemeinschaft Pharmazeutische Industrie is *Die Pharmazeutische Industrie* (first issued in 1934, suspended after the Nazi downfall, then revived in 1950).

Employees' Organization. Attempts have been made repeatedly (since 1818) to organize associations of pharmaceutical employees, and they have met with some success. A lasting and very active association of this kind was founded (1904) by Ehrlich and Wiskirchen under the name Verband Konditionierender Apotheker für das Deutsche Reich and, after 1910, was known as the union or the alliance of German pharmacists (Verband Deutscher Apotheker). Gradually this came to include the majority of pharmaceutical employees. (From 1905, the Verband issued the *Zentralblatt für Pharmacie*.) In 1934 this employees' association and its journal were absorbed by the new totalitarian pharmaceutical association.

Official Organizations. Apart from the associations already mentioned—for the most part voluntary—there were and are

official bodies. The first of this type was the "gremium" (first organized in 1842 in Bavaria),[56] in which membership was compulsory for all owners of pharmacies in each governmental district. The gremiums were administrative bodies auxiliary to state regulation. The gremium was required to report to the government about conditions, abuses and desirable changes in the field of pharmacy, either on request or on its own initiative. In addition it took care of the social welfare of its members, and established and supported welfare institutions. The Apothekerkammern, founded later on, served essentially the same purposes but, in addition, were given disciplinary power over unethical acts of their members.[57]

During the Nazi period this type of organization was given a totalitarian form (under the title "Reichsapothekerkammer") which had far-reaching power over pharmacists, politically as well as professionally (see reference 57). After World War II the district offices became nuclei for the "Landesapothekerkammern," which more and more became regulative bodies concerning drugs and chemicals in the individual German states. Groups representing the West German states have come together in an "Arbeitsgemeinschaft Deutscher Apothekerkammern" ("Bundesapothekerkammer").

Each "Kammer" is a corporate body under public law and cannot properly undertake administrative tasks on behalf of pharmacists' private interests. For such a purpose, beside the "Kammer" in each state stands a professional society (*Apothekerverein*, as a continuation of the earlier *Deutscher Apothekerverein* and its successors).

As a roof organization uniting German pharmacy there was created after 1948 the "Arbeitsgemeinschaft der Berufsvertretungen Deutscher Apotheker" (often abbreviated "ABDA"). This ties together and coordinates the management of the Bundesapothekerkammer (regulative affairs) and the Deutscher Apotheker-Verein (professional affairs).[58]

Pharmacy in Germany since World War II unfolds various facets of fundamental change—unprecedented freedom to open pharmacies, a wider opportunity for the individual mixed with a threat to professionalism and, across the zonal boundary, a socialization of the pharmacies; important new laws, including both a national pharmacy law and a law on drugs, new organizational concepts, as exemplified by "ABDA." Thus German pharmacy appears to be forging a new chapter in its history that will be much more than a new expression of the old.

7: The Development in Britain*

THE PECULIAR BRITISH SITUATION

A striking feature marks the history of British pharmacy: A profession based entirely on the art of pharmacy, with the purpose of developing the professional and social standards of its members, did not exist in England, Wales and Ireland before the 19th century and in Scotland before the 18th century. In this respect Britain differs significantly from the other large European cultural zones—such as the Italian, the French and the German.

Naturally, in Britain as well as on the Continent, there were early dealers in drugs. Moreover, the terms designating them were the same as those used on the Continent. However, while the creation of the calling of the continental pharmacists was based principally on the early separation of the medical and the pharmaceutical professions, either by law or by regulations and privileges, in Britain this separation was not the beginning but a recent result of the development.

In all European countries, transgressions of the legal boundaries of both professions were frequent; the complaints on both sides belong to the history of continental pharmacy as well as of medicine. Nevertheless, the principle of separation was in general considered to be beyond all dispute. At times, even in Europe, the transition from one profession to the other was not difficult. In the 17th and the 18th centuries many persons on the European continent had passed the examinations both in pharmacy and in medicine and, therefore, were entitled to practice both professions. Moise

Charas, the author of the famous *Pharmacopée royale* (1676), Nicolas Lémery, the author of the first *Pharmacopoeia universalis* (1697) and many other Frenchmen were simultaneously pharmacists and physicians. In Germany this dual education was even more common and caused many conflicts.[1] However, England, Wales and Ireland were the only European countries in which an entire calling gained the legal recognition of its ambition to practice in a neighboring field and became part of another profession without—and this is the irony of the situation—resigning completely the rights of the first profession.

The reason for this peculiarity is found in the insular and the topographic character of Britain, which isolated it from continental Europe. Of its aboriginal inhabitants, the Celts (who were closely related to the French Celts), only those who lived in Wales and Scotland or were able to flee into these areas survived the conquest of the country by Germanic tribes (about 450). Throughout the centuries, there was not much harmony between the people of Wales and Scotland and those of England. The amalgamation between the Anglo-Saxons and the later conquerors of the islands, the Normans, who came over from France (Normandy) and dominated the country after the battle of Hastings (1066), took place very gradually.

Consequently, until the Elizabethan period (in the 16th century), conditions in Britain were not sufficiently stable to cast professional life into uniform and rigid moulds. Even later the proportion of educated people was relatively small. As a result, the way had to be free for each to make the most of opportunity. Indeed, this freedom of every Briton to seek adventure and success inside and outside the British Isles created the wealth and the power of England. On the other hand, this system of *laissez faire*—which found its theoretical

---

* While an effort has been made to characterize the pharmaceutical development in Great Britain, the limited space available in a textbook, and not historical circumstances alone, places England in the main focus of discussion and prevents all but cursory mention of differences and similarities elsewhere in the British Isles (such as in Northern Ireland and Ireland).

basis in Manchester liberalism and was formulated in the thirties of the 19th century
by the Manchester school of economics—has
often retarded the steady, uniform development and balance within and for the to-
tality of the people. Such may be achieved
only by stating and protecting definite
principles and regulations.

PHARMACEUTICAL BEGINNINGS

The social circumstances thus help us to
understand the erratic course that must be
taken to follow the pharmaceutical path
from its faint beginnings in the late Middle
Ages onward. T. D. Whittet points out:

In Saxon England and in the early Norman
period there was no difference between physician, apothecary or surgeon. The practitioners
known as leeches performed the functions of
all three. During Norman times the trade in
drugs and spices was eventually handled by
the mercers (a term which originally simply
meant a merchant who dealt in small wares).*

From France a few spicers and pepperers
may have carried their trades across to the
British Isles as early as the 11th century.
Their number multiplied, and within a century or so they had taken over much of
the drug trade—the pepperers as wholesalers, the spicers as retailers. The main
stock in trade of both was "spicery," which
G. E. Trease characterizes as substances
"mainly of vegetable or animal origin; almost invariably derived from the East or
the Mediterranean; of high value in relation to their weight." This variety of substances of course included spices.[2]

Some of the more knowledgeable and
skillful spicers specialized increasingly in
dispensing and compounding medicines. By
the late 13th century some were being
called spicer or apothecary interchangeably. This undoubtedly was a transitional
period, a period of maturing for an ambitious group that would become distinctively
"apothecaries."

Meanwhile, the pepperers (wholesalers
and shippers of spicery, etc.) changed the
name of their guild to the Grocers' Company; in it, at least from the 14th century
on, the apothecaries obtained guild benefits as a special section until they finally
seceded in 1617.[3]

In 14th-century England, Chaucer could
write in his Physician's Tale, "Ful redy
hadde he hise apothecaries to send him
drogges."

We are not surprised that, in the absence
of legal regulation, the functions of medicine and pharmacy remained poorly separated. The 16th-century "apothecary" has
been referred to not only as an assistant to
the physician, but also as an independent
preparer and dispenser of drugs who not
infrequently took a hand in medical practice.[4] In the time of Henry VIII, the long
contention between apothecaries and physicians over the division of function of
medical care had begun, and in 1511 the
king issued the first regulations for the English practice of medicine and pharmacy,
ordering that

. . . no person could lawfully practise medicine or surgery in the City of London, or
within seven miles of it, unless he had been
first examined, approved, and admitted by the
Bishop of London or the Dean of St. Paul's,
who were to be assisted in the examination of
candidates by four doctors of physic and of surgery, or other expert persons in that faculty.[5]

To have a bishop as chairman of a medical board of examination is not so peculiar
as it might seem. The chairman should be
impartial (not a physician), and he had to
be a master of the Latin language. A significant proof of English conservatism is the
fact that persons were licensed by English
bishops to practice medicine within their
dioceses as late as the middle of the 18th
century.

The system of bishop's licenses eventually was extended to the provinces and to
Wales. The College of Physicians (later,
"Royal College")—founded soon after the
first medical regulation and licensing—was
empowered in 1540 to "search, view and see
the apothecary wares, drugs and stuffs."

Thereby the continental practice subject-
ing apothecaries to medical supervision
was introduced into England. In an act of

---

* From essay in Archive of the American Institute
of the History of Pharmacy, Madison, Wisconsin.
(Mimeograph)

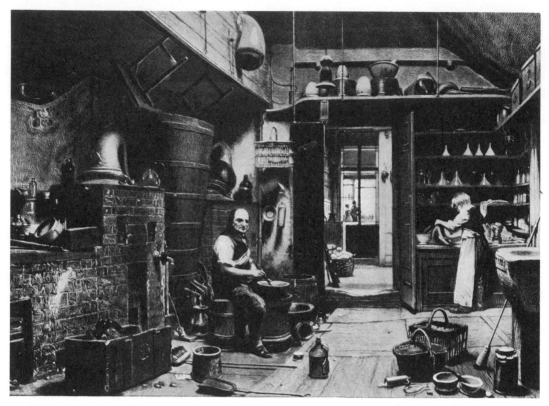

The back-room laboratory of a mid-19th century pharmacy in London typifies practice before large-scale industrialization of operative pharmacy. A furnace (left) is fitted at the top with a distillation head, which probably is attached to a condensing worm running through the large wooden vat beside it. Through the doorway can be seen a corner of the front dispensing room. A shop-boy is busying himself (right) beneath shelves laden with various funnels and bottles. A large marble mortar can be seen in the extreme right foreground. Here, at 225 Oxford Street, practiced John Bell, father of Jacob Bell who was a founder of the Pharmaceutical Society, founder and editor of the *Pharmaceutical Journal* and owner of this shop after the death of his father in 1849. The firm later developed into a large-scale manufacturing laboratory. (Engraving from a painting by W. Hunt, 1840; *see* Kassner, E. W.: J. Am. Pharm. Ass. *20*:236-246, 1931)

1618 the new powers of the college were stated more specifically. Four members were authorized to survey and examine the stocks of "apothecaries, druggists, distillers and sellers of waters and oils, and preparers of chemical medicines." This enumeration gives a complete picture of the different groups that were in any way active and officially recognized in the field of pharmacy.

Evolving law tended to make the practice of medicine the monopoly of physicians licensed as such. But physicians were more zealous in defending their rights than their small number and the urgent need of medical help, especially in the open country, warranted. Therefore, a new act was passed (1543) confirming the right of "every person being the King's subject having knowledge and experience of the nature of herbs, roots and waters to use and minister, according to their cunning, experience and knowledge."[6] This act is a typical instance of *laissez faire*. It paved the way for everyone who had "cunning, experience and knowledge," leaving the decision as to the possession of these qualities entirely to the individual claiming them. However, it related only to medicaments for external application and "Drinks for the Stone, Strangury, or Agues."

By this act the numerous irregular practitioners were protected and they were legally tolerated. It could hardly have been otherwise as these formed the ordinary "doctors" or professors of the healing art at the disposal of the general public throughout the kingdom. . . . These unincorporated practitioners were the forerunners of the incorporated "Apothecary" of the first Stuart King of England.[7]

THE SOCIETY OF APOTHECARIES AND ITS LABORATORY

When King James I first gave privileges to the apothecaries (1607) as a section of the powerful Grocers' Company, he did not give them independence. The more ambitious apothecaries were neither content nor complacent, and, after many dissensions, the King (influenced by his court physicians Theodore Mayerne and Henry Atkins, and by Gideon de Laune, Apothecary to the Queen) granted them independence in a new charter. Thus was founded on December 6, 1617 a separate City Guild called the "Master, Wardens, and Society of the Art and Mystery of the Apothecaries of the City of London."

This charter conferred upon them the monopoly of keeping an apothecary's shop, and rendered it unlawful for the grocers or any persons, "to make or sell, to compound, prepare, give, apply or administer any medicines or medicinable compositions, viz., distilled waters, compounds or olea chimica, apozemata, sirrups, conserves, eclegmata, electuaria, condita, medicinalia, pilulas, pulveres, troches, olea, unguenta, emplastra, or by any other way to use or exercise the art, faculty, or mystery of

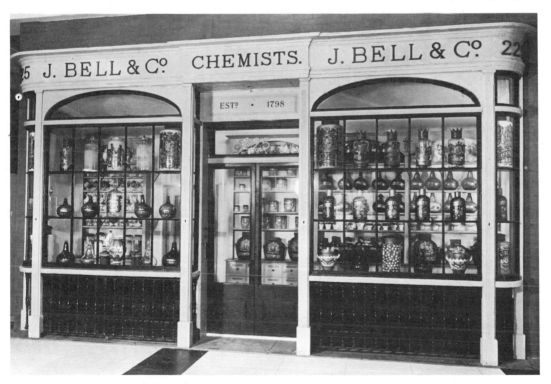

The front of Bell's shop may be seen today in a reconstruction at the Wellcome Historical Medical Museum on Euston Road, London. When the old shop front was torn down (1909), it was purchased by the erstwhile American pharmacist, Sir Henry Wellcome, a founder of Burroughs Wellcome & Co. The windows contain objects from Bell's pharmacy and contemporary shops. See also illustration on facing page. (Photograph copyright, Wellcome Historical Medical Museum)

an apothecary or any part thereof, within the City of London and the suburbs or within seven miles of the City."[8]

Naturally, the grocers protested. Nevertheless, the king held to his original decision, stating that the grocers were but traders, having no professional skill.

In 1618 the new "Dispensatorie Troy weights," having remained the English apothecaries' weights, were recognized by

law, and their use was made obligatory for the members of the new society.

In the 17th century, after the founding of the Society of Apothecaries, the wealth and the esteem of the calling increased. The guild hall, which they acquired in 1632 (rebuilt after the Great Fire, which destroyed the largest part of London) stands even today as a witness of the old glory.[9] The good financial condition of the Society

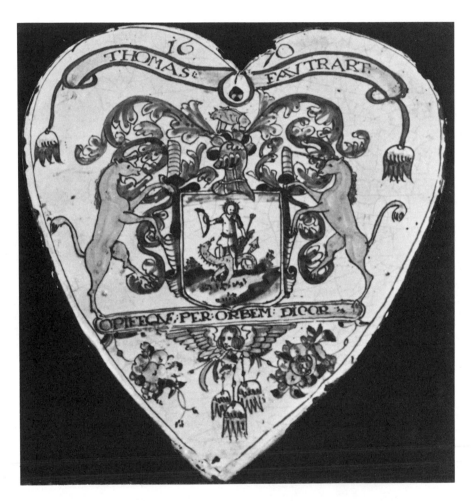

The pill tile bears the coat of arms of the Worshipful Society of Apothecaries of London, with its Latin motto, "Throughout the world I am called helpbringer" (polychrome English delft, 1670). Such tiles were hung on the wall (note hole, top center) and, perhaps, were as much a sign of membership and a symbolic ornament to the pharmacy as they were useful for prescription work. Between the two unicorns in the heraldry, Apollo (the ancient Greek medical god who fathered Asklepios) is vanquishing the dragon with bow and arrow, his traditional weapons. (Original, about 11 inches high x 9½ inches wide, in the collection of the Pharmaceutical Society of Great Britain, London)

was not so much based on membership fees as on its manufacturing and commercial undertakings. Early in its history, the Society started to prepare galenics and chemicals. In 1682 this cooperative acquired the status of a regular commercial company. The laboratory had become a real chemical plant, and in 1703 the Society was granted a renewal of the monopoly of supplying the English navy with drugs. Later (1766) the East India Company also decided to buy huge amounts of drugs and medicines annually from the Society of Apothecaries.[10]

The Pharmacie Centrale in France (founded in 1852), comprised of the pharmacists of the entire nation, has been referred to as the first national cooperative pharmaceutical undertaking. The "companies" of the London Society of Apothecaries, although organized on a local basis, are the first known example of a pharmaceutical cooperative operated on a larger scale.

APOTHECARIES BECOMING MEDICAL PRACTITIONERS

Only a few decades after the founding of the Society of Apothecaries of London the new group found itself in a fight on two fronts: against the physicians, to defend the assumed rights of "apothecaries" as minor medical practitioners in addition to pharmaceutical duties, and against the "druggists" and "chemists" who, in spite of the monopoly of the apothecaries, continued to multiply and flourish.

The merchants and druggists, being a section of the grocers' company, merely sold articles in the raw or unprepared state, and the chemists (who were not incorporated) took upon themselves the duty of preparing those medicines which required the aid of fire and which were chiefly, if not entirely, minerals, earths, or preparations of the metals.[11]

The struggle against the physicians was difficult and lengthy but finally victorious. Both words and actions were involved, and the struggle lasted more than a century. Without any doubt, apothecaries practicing medicine trespassed on territory not belonging to them. Yet, they had gradually gained a large number of clients who depended on them, and they had proved themselves useful in their medical role in a time of need, during the Great Plague (1665-66). At that time, when the majority of the physicians in London either had died or had fled, "the friends of the sick were obliged to call in the aid of the apothecaries, who readily forsook their shops to visit the sufferers at their bedsides."[12]

The battle of words, each side using the arguments already reviewed in the similar French quarrel (see p. 66) found its most famous expression in "The Dispensary," a poem in mock heroic verse by a well-known physician Samuel Garth (1699).[13] The apothecaries on their part, in a tract titled *Pharmacopolae justificati* (The Justified Apothecaries) based their defense on the thesis "that an academical education is nowise necessary to qualify a man for the practice of physic."[14]

So far as action was concerned, the quarrel centered on the opening of dispensaries by members of the College of Physicians, and on the prosecution of apothecaries practicing medicine. While the first-mentioned undertaking of the physicians was successful and harmed the apothecaries— Pitt stated in 1703 that "the Dispensaries of the College now make up 20,000 prescriptions,"[15]—the other, the prosecution of the apothecaries, led to the defeat of the physicians! At first, a judgment of the Court of Queen's Bench decided (November 10, 1703) in favor of the college of physicians and against an apothecary, William Rose, who had been accused of prescribing medicines. However, the House of Lords ordered (Journal of the House for the period March 15, 1703/04) "That the said Judgement given in Queen's Bench . . . against the said William Rose shall be, and is hereby, reversed." From this time on the apothecaries were recognized medico-pharmaceutical practitioners.[16]

The battle on the other front, against their competitors, the chemists and the druggists, was not so favorable for the apothecaries. Here they were on the defensive, and they were forced—willingly or unwillingly—to use in this quarrel the same arguments which the physicians had used against them shortly before.

The apothecaries failed to get powers to search chemist shops and they were likewise unable to persuade parliament to pass a measure to prohibit druggists from practising pharmacy and to make it unlawful for physicians and surgeons to prepare and sell medicines.[17]

Similar attempts were equally unsuccessful until 1815. In that year an Apothecaries' Act forbade "unqualified persons"—and there were no qualified ones besides the physicians, the surgeons and the apothecaries— to judge disease by external indications.

Apothecaries were now practicing throughout England, either belonging to guilds of their own or joined with related occupations (e.g., barber-surgeons). For the first time, the 1815 Act gave the London Society of Apothecaries certain powers over professional standards and medical education throughout England and Wales.[18]

As the apothecaries became more preoccupied with their now accepted role as general medical practitioners, the chemists and the druggists claimed an increasing share of the pharmaceutical work. Through an emergency organization the chemists and druggists bid successfully to amend the Apothecaries Act to preserve as rights the pharmaceutical services that it had now become customary for them to render. They defined these rights as consisting of the buying, the compounding and the dispensing of drugs and medicinal compounds, wholesale and retail. With this definition the chemists and the druggists, excluding all medical ambition, drew the boundary between the medical and the pharmaceutical professions.

Naturally, the more the apothecaries became medical practitioners, the more their original tasks passed into other hands.

By the end of the 18th century the chemists and druggists had absorbed a considerable proportion of the sale of drugs and medicines and after the first few years of the 19th century, had practically monopolized it.[19]

In Scotland and Ireland the pharmacist took a similarly winding historical path, but not quite the same path as his English counterpart.

No guildlike connection with "spicers" and "grocers" has shown up in the antecedents of the Scottish apothecary, and, although he, too, eventually merged into medicine, the amalgamation was mainly with surgery, rather than with internal medicine as in England. To perform surgery, the surgeon-apothecary in Edinburgh had to belong to the surgeons' guild (1575).

However, the boundaries were drawn loosely, and the surgeon-apothecary came into service as the general practitioner for ordinary folk by the 17th century in some parts of Scotland. Pharmacy now was taught with surgery and, despite divisive tendencies, eventually (1721) all apothecaries were permitted to become members of the corporation of surgeons without examination, on payment of 50 pounds each!

As in England, a new class of practitioners of pharmacy now arose. Unlike their English colleagues, they received immediate and full recognition by physicians; what is more, the College of Physicians in Edinburgh prohibited its members from operating pharmacies.[20]

In Ireland, too, the apothecaries were in a guild with the surgeons (1456), but, after a few centuries, the apothecaries of Dublin were granted an independent charter as the Guild of St. Luke (1745). This later amalgamated with the Company of Apothecaries' Hall, whose jurisdiction extended over the whole of Ireland. Like their counterparts elsewhere in the British Isles, Irish apothecaries drifted into the general practice of medicine, and the Medical Act of 1858 included Apothecaries' Hall as one of the licensing bodies for medical practitioners.

Many medical apothecaries eventually refused to operate pharmacies open to the public, which further stimulated a rising class of "druggists." The Irish "druggist," on the other hand, was blocked from taking a place beside the dispensing "chemist" as a fully recognized pharmacy practitioner (Act of 1875), being held in a subordinate class reminiscent of the German "Drogist," but permitted a wider scope of function. He has been continually at odds with Irish "chemists" (pharmacists), frequently trespassing illegally on their services. Finally, an enactment of 1951 discontinued any further registration of new druggists, while permitting those now in practice who could pass a special examination to become pharmaceutical chemists in everything but name.

What became of the apothecary?

Today, in Ireland, as in England and Wales, the Irish apothecary is a medical practitioner and the Licentiate of Apothecaries' Hall (L.A.H.) is a registerable medical qualification . . . The Irish apothecaries, like the English, have passed from pharmacy to medicine, but not so completely. . . . Many own pharmacies as well as medical practices. Some call their pharmacy "Apothecary's Hall" but the term "Medical Hall" is more popular. The latter term is also occasionally used by pharmacists who acquired medical halls from apothecaries. Thus the Irish apothecaries have the best of both worlds, being both physicians and pharmacists; a truly Irish situation.[21]

Although England serves as the main focus of discussion for the present purpose, in the British Isles in general can be discerned the history of the tangled skein that results when closely related occupational functions are exercised in a social atmosphere more heavily charged with the idea of "wait and see how it develops" than with preconceived ideas of discipline and planned development of a health system.

THE PHARMACEUTICAL SOCIETY OF GREAT BRITAIN

In the course of negotiations with the College of Physicians in 1841, the members of the board of examiners of the Society of Apothecaries, declared

. . . that one of the chief evils in the present position of the Apothecary is his name, which has little reference to his actual duties, that he is in fact the Medical Attendant on the larger mass of the community, and should be designated the General Practitioner of Medicine.[22]

In the same year the present Pharmaceutical Society was founded "to benefit the public and elevate the profession of Pharmacy, by furnishing the means of proper instruction."[23] According to Jacob Bell, the low prestige of pharmacy conducted as a trade induced the apothecaries to aspire to medical practice as a profession. Generally, they seemed to be unaware that it was their own fault if pharmacy in England had not attained a professional standard more comparable with that on the Continent. Bell felt that he voiced a central idea for satisfying the ambitions of chemist and druggist when he said in 1842 that pharmacy had become so complicated and had embraced so many sciences "that a complete knowledge of the subject can only be acquired by those who devote their exclusive attention to the pursuit."[24]

The Pharmaceutical Society continued on a road diverging from that of the apothecaries, moving slowly but continuously toward professional status for a new class of practitioners of pharmacy. The Society's charter (1843) empowered it to regulate the education and the admission of members. The objectives specified were (1) advancement of chemistry and pharmacy; (2) promotion of a uniform system of education for practitioners; (3) protection of "those who carry on the business of Chemist and Druggist"; (4) relief of needy members, associates and their widows and orphans.

The first Pharmacy Act in 1852 empowered the Society to conduct examinations by means of two boards (one for England and Wales and another for Scotland) and to grant certificates of qualification for "pharmaceutical chemists," the title being restricted legally to those so registered.[25] Medical men engaged in practice could not be registered as pharmaceutical chemists, although they could dispense (and a majority did so). The most important change in a new Pharmacy Act of 1868 made qualification and registration compulsory for all members of the profession. In addition, the sale of poisons was henceforth permitted only in pharmacies serving the general public.[26]

An amendment passed by Parliament in 1898 extended full membership—reserved hitherto to the Pharmaceutical Chemists (title of all those who had passed the major examination)—to the Chemist and Druggist (title of all those who had passed the minor examination). After another decade the law (1908) brought the calling of pharmacy more fully under the control of the Society and gave the Society the power to institute a compulsory curriculum. However, membership was voluntary, and, despite the Society's examination and registration activities, it remained an auxiliary institution to the official authority. It became such an authority itself in Great Britain in 1933.

The Pharmacy Act of 1933 made membership in the Pharmaceutical Society *compulsory*. Every person registered as a British pharmacist becomes a member of the Society by virtue of his registration. The titles "pharmaceutical chemist," "pharmaceutist," "pharmacist," "chemist and druggist" or "druggist" are protected. The term "chemist" became and remains the most popular designation used by community pharmacists. The statutory committee has the power, subject to appeal to the High Court, to remove names from the register. Each registered pharmacist conducting an establishment for the dispensing of drugs is authorized to dispense poisons also. Inspectors, who must be registered pharmacists, are appointed by the Society.

The Act of 1933 became the Magna Charta of British pharmacy. In an editorial explaining the new Act, the Society's journal proclaimed, "Pharmacy is recognized as a self-governing community, free to conduct its own affairs and subjected to governmental control only in those matters where its activities affect the public."[27] "Self-governing community!" The principle employed by England in relation to her colonies (advancing them to dominions if they have proved to be sufficiently mature for self-government) is here applied in internal affairs.

The Pharmacy and Medicines Act of 1941, among other changes, relaxed distributive controls on certain poisons, abolished the stamp duty on proprietary medicines and differentiated between pharmacists and other persons distributing them

and dealt with the advertising of medicines.[28]

Further legal changes in 1953 allowed everyone on a single register of pharmacists to use the title pharmaceutical chemist (usually shortened to "chemist"), and authorized the Society to register without examination (or with a modified examination) persons granted degrees in pharmacy by universities in the United Kingdom. Additional changes in the operating framework of the Pharmaceutical Society came with a Supplemental Charter granted to it by the government (1954), which included the following amended objectives for the Society: (1) To advance chemistry and pharmacy; (2) to promote pharmaceutical education and the application of pharmaceutical knowledge; (3) to maintain the honour and safeguard and promote the interests of the members in the exercise of the profession of pharmacy; and (4) to provide relief for distressed persons (enlarging the scope of the Society's Benevolent Fund).[29]

Behind the British concept of *laissez faire* stands a belief in natural development and a readiness to acknowledge it. A startling illustration of this concept, described previously, was the circumstance that a nation's apothecaries evolved into recognized medical practitioners. Still another illustrative event occurred in British pharmacy (1878) when a large number of druggists became dentists![30]

PHARMACEUTICAL ASSOCIATIONS AND JOURNALS

As a necessary first goal in its early decades, the Pharmaceutical Society aimed at the gradual formation of a class of uniformly and sufficiently educated pharmaceutical practitioners, on whom could be conferred the legal right to supply the people with drugs and medicines. The Society tried to make pharmaceutical science available to the average chemist and druggist, but it could not promote scientific research to the desired extent, since many pharmaceutical scientists were not members.

For this reason the British Pharmaceutical Conference, "an organization for the encouragement of pharmaceutical research," was founded in 1863. The Conference was not connected officially with the Pharmaceutical Society until 1922, when it became an autonomous part of the Society. Significantly, however, prominent leaders of the Pharmaceutical Society were among the first elected officers of the Conference, and this close connection between the associations has continued even though it is not compulsory for a Conference member to belong to the Society.

According to Gamble,[31] the founders and the foundation of the Conference were influenced by

. . . the good work done . . . by the American Pharmaceutical Association . . . in the field of pharmaceutical science particularly . . .

Reynolds described the American method of allotting subjects for investigation to individuals for report at the annual meeting, and referred to the inclusion in the published "Proceedings" of the American Association of a section which formed a "Year-Book of Pharmacy" both home and foreign.

The present monthly *Journal of Pharmacy and Pharmacology* (which includes the *Transactions* of the British Pharmaceutical Conference as a supplement) traces its lineage back to the beginning of the Conference. At first the *Transactions* (or *Proceedings*) of the Conference appeared in the *Pharmaceutical Journal* (1864) and as a reprinted booklet, later (1870) as part of a *Year-Book of Pharmacy*, which (1928) was divided into a *Quarterly Journal of Pharmacy and Pharmacology*. Expanding its scope, this quarterly became the present monthly *Journal* in 1950.

The Pharmaceutical Society had developed into the administrative and educational body of British pharmacy, with the British Pharmaceutical Conference representing its scientific work, supplemented by the Society's Department of Pharmaceutical Sciences (as such since 1959). There was a need for an institution devoted especially to the commercial interests of the profession. Consequently, in 1921 the Retail Pharmacists' Union (known as the National Phar-

maceutical Union since 1932) was created with the support of the Pharmaceutical Society, since the latter's quite different task was to represent all pharmacists professionally.[31a] The new Union mainly served the interests of pharmacy owners as entrepreneurs and has the important duty of representing pharmacy in all affairs concerning national health insurance. In Scotland, similar functions are shared between the Scottish Pharmaceutical Federation (founded in 1919) and the Pharmaceutical Standing Committee (Scotland).

The representative association of hospital pharmacists, called the Guild of Public Pharmacists, was founded (1923) by amalgamating the Public Pharmacists Association with members of the pharmacists' section of the Hospital Officers' Association. It now includes about 90 per cent of the hospital pharmacists in England, Scotland and Wales and has branches throughout the three countries. Similar organizations exist in Northern Ireland and the Irish Republic. The Guild publishes the *Journal of Hospital Pharmacy* (before 1963 *The Public Pharmacist*; quarterly, 1932 to 1959; bimonthly since 1960).

The weekly *Pharmaceutical Journal* has been the official organ of the Pharmaceutical Society of Great Britain since the beginning in 1841 (although it was founded on the private initiative of Jacob Bell, who presented the copyright to the Society in 1859). Subsequent changes in the title are significant. Until 1895 it was called *The Pharmaceutical Journal and Transactions*, then simply, *The Pharmaceutical Journal*. Coincidental with an official attempt to popularize the designation "pharmacist," the title was changed to *The Pharmaceutical Journal and Pharmacist* (1909). The designation "pharmacist," not having been adopted by the majority of the English dispensing "chemists," was dropped, and the title again reads *The Pharmaceutical Journal*.

The Chemist and Druggist, another important English pharmaceutical journal founded in 1859, has never changed either its name or its objectives. The main idea was to produce for the average practitioner a general and practical journal, "simply use-ful—a trade journal," to borrow a phrase from its editorial on the founders.[32] Another monthly journal is *Pharmacy Digest* (pub-lished from 1920 to 1958 as *The Alchemist*).

Apparently the first English journal con-nected with pharmacy was *The Chemist*, which existed for only 13 months (1824 to 1825). Around the mid-19th century, a number of other journals (now supplanted) helped to convey pharmaceutical informa-tion to the rising new class of practitioners of pharmacy, the "chemists and drug-gists."[33]

INSPECTION OF PHARMACIES

The inspection of the pharmacies reflects the general development of English phar-macy. A royal order of Henry VI first gave the grocers power to examine "anis, worm-seed, rhubarb, scammony, spikenard, senna and all sort of drugs belonging to medicine, so as not, in the buying of these to be hurt in their bodily health" (1447).[34] Later de-crees (1540, 1553) gave the supervision of pharmacies to the medical profession. How-ever, when the Society of Apothecaries was chartered independently (1617), its master and wardens were empowered to inspect any pharmacy and to burn before the of-fender's door all drugs and preparations they deemed corrupt or unwholesome.[35]

In the 18th century, power to examine the shops of apothecaries, chemists and druggists was given to the College of Physi-cians (1723), and cases involving question-able drugs were judged by a court com-posed partly of physicians and partly of apothecaries (1730).[36]

Scotland also placed inspection of the apothecaries' stock in the hands of physi-cians (e.g., the Glasgow Faculty for West-ern Scotland, 1599; the Edinburgh College, 1621, 1684), sometimes with assistance from representatives of the apothecaries them-selves.[37]

The present regulation (stemming from the Pharmacy Act of 1933) makes the pharmacists throughout England, Scotland and Wales definitely self-governing, under the supervision of their own Society.

SOCIAL STANDING

To gain an impression of the social posi-tion held by the members of the pharma-ceutical calling in England, we must choose as representatives, until the end of the 18th century, the apothecaries. From the middle of the 17th century on, we also must con-sider the chemist and, from the beginning of the 19th century, the new professional group resulting from the gradual amalga-mation of chemists and druggists, which constitutes the rank-and-file of modern British pharmacy.

As in all other countries, the social posi-tion of the British apothecary was based, on the one hand, on respect for his profes-sional work and, on the other hand, on the fact that most of the apothecaries were, or at least were considered to be, well-to-do.

Thompson describes two apothecary shops of the 16th century as well equipped with furniture, containers of various kinds and sizes, and weights and balances. The prescriptions of the physicians were copied in a great book which stood on a raised desk or table. As in other countries, the apothe-cary shops in England in this period had "a windowframe over which canvas was stretched, but when this was rolled up they were open to the street."[38]

The equipment of English apothecaries of the 17th and the 18th centuries—unlike that of their counterparts on the Continent, in general—does not seem to have reflected their prosperity and social position. The fact that the apothecary considered himself to be primarily a medical practitioner prob-ably made it seem unnecessary to aspire to a dignified and representative pharmaceu-tical atmosphere.

On the wall hang saws, knives, forceps and other surgical instruments; for the apothecary was ready to perform any operation, from the cutting off of a wen to the amputation of a leg. . . . The walls are lined with shelves bear-ing an array of Delft jars of blue and white for which the Lambeth potters were famous.[39]

Another type of pharmaceutical estab-lishment was represented by the chemist's shops, which are hinted at in 1553 but did not become numerous before the second half of the 17th century. The most famous of these chemists was the German-born Ambrose Hanckwitz (who in England took the name of Godfrey). He was brought to England by no less a person than Robert Boyle, who "conveyed to chemistry that direction of work which it kept up since that time with so much success."[40] Together with Hanckwitz, Boyle found a new method for preparing phosphorus and "for many years the 'English phosphorus' supplied by Hanckwitz from his laboratory ... monopolized the European market."[41] In 1706 Godfrey Hanckwitz built a laboratory and shop that "became a fashionable resort in the afternoon when he performed popular experiments for the amusement of his friends."[42]

Around 1800, such manufacturing chemists parted company with the dispensing chemists, although some of them retained both functions and carried on (or, rather, created) the idea of professional pharmacy and, later, became founders of the Pharmaceutical Society of Great Britain. In general, however, little of the old glory of the art of the apothecaries or of the recent fame of chemistry came down to the new combination of chemists and druggists. They practiced pharmacy, it is true, but primarily as merchants like their predecessors, the druggists. With the number of exceptions to be expected, this background differentiated the character of their shops and their general social position from those of their continental colleagues. In continental Europe the pharmaceutical profession, as a profession, gave and gives to all of its members a certain traditional reputation. In England, Wales and Ireland most of the tradition and the prestige of pharmacy passed with the apothecaries into medicine. However, through the Pharmaceutical Society, during more than 120 years, the modern calling of pharmacy has done much to regain lost ground and create new prestige, even though at times progress has been slow or uneven.

PHARMACEUTICAL EDUCATION

One of the most important means of building up a professional reputation is, naturally, the education of the rising generation. An examination was required by law for the first time in the British Isles in Glasgow, Scotland. On the basis of the charter granted to the Glasgow faculty by James VI in 1599, the faculty "issued a license to practice pharmacy to candidates who passed its examination in pharmacy, and still retains the right to do so, but has not exercised it since the advent of the Pharmacy Act of 1868."[43] In 1657, in Edinburgh, an examination became compulsory for all those who wished to practice pharmacy within the city.[44] In England the first official requirement of a definite time of apprenticeship and an examination of the presumptive apothecaries is contained in the charter of December 6, 1617, which created the Society of Apothecaries of London. It is ordered that:

No Person or Persons whatsoever may have, hold, or keep, an Apothecary's Shop or Warehouse, or . . . may exercise or use the Art or Mystery of Apothecaries, or . . . may sell, set on sale, utter, set forth, or lend any Compound or Composition to any person or persons whatsoever, within the City of London and the Liberties thereof, or within Seven Miles of the said City, unless such person or persons have been brought up, instructed, and taught by the space of Seven Years at the least, as Apprentice or Apprentices, with some Apothecary or Apothecaries exercising the same Art, and being a Freeman of the said Mystery. And after such Seven Years Service or Apprenticeship as is aforesaid, shall be expired and finished, that then every such Apprentice may appear and be presented to the Master and Wardens, . . . calling unto them the President of the College or Commonalty of the Faculty of Physicians of London for the time being, or any Physician or Physicians by the said President to be nominated, and thereunto to be assigned from time to time, if upon warning thereof given, such Physician . . . will be present, and taking advice with the same Physician or Physicians, shall be examined, proved and tried concerning his knowledge and election of Simples, and concerning the preparing, dispensing, handling, commixing and compounding of Medicines, and shall be by them the said Physicians, Masters and Wardens, approved and allowed, before he shall presume to have, keep or furnish an Apothecary's Shop, or to prepare, make, mingle, work, compound, give, apply, minister, utter, put forth, sell or set on sale, any Medicines, or otherwise by any other ways or means exercise the Art of an Apothecary or any part thereof, within the City of London and Liberties and Suburbs of the same, or within Seven Miles of the same city.[45]

The Society of Apothecaries held its first examination two years later, resulting in the refusal of the candidate. Botanic courses were organized (1627), which led to the leasing of land and to the establishment of "a physic garden" at Chelsea (1673). Later, it was presented to the Society of Apothecaries by Sir Hans Sloane, one of the most active and best known medical practitioners of his period.

Apprentices were examined before entering the calling and, on occasion, were rejected "for insufficiency in the Latin tongue." Lectures in materia medica were offered after 1753. When the first regular curriculum of the Society of the Apothecaries was issued (1827), it was mainly medical. It required 5 years of apprenticeship, including attendance at courses in such subjects as anatomy, physiology and the theory and the practice of medicine.[46]

Real pharmaceutical education began in England only after the founding of the Pharmaceutical Society. One of the fundamental demands in the program of the Society was "the development of scientific acquirements . . . to remove our [the English pharmacists'] apparent deficiency as pharmacopolists, when compared with other nations." With the establishment of a laboratory (1844-1845), the society's school of pharmacy became the first institution in London to offer chemical laboratory instruction all day, under proper guidance.[47]

Because of the central importance of education as a tool for shaping a new profession out of the original heterogeneous group of "chemists" and "druggists," the Society consistently has fostered and valued the role of education in the life of British pharmacy. The Society's commendable history in this area, says J. W. Fairbairn, "rises up from the past like a signpost pointing out that the only way to maintain and improve professional status in an increasingly scientific society is by continually increasing academic standards." Fairbairn recalls that the two levels of qualification characteristic of British pharmacy go back as far as the founding generation of the Society:

Originally they envisaged a society of registered pharmaceutical chemists and registered assistants, but by 1869 the Assistants' examination (Chemist and Druggist Diploma) became the basic one for membership while the Pharmaceutical Chemist Examination became a sort of extra qualification which carried with it higher status. Those with the Pharmaceutical Chemist Diploma (Ph.C.) tended to enter the manufacturing, teaching, or hospital branches of pharmacy whereas those with the Chemist and Druggist Diploma remained in retail practice. This two-class system of pharmaceutical education persisted for almost a hundred years, and, although the Pharmaceutical Society in 1954 abolished the old chemist and druggist course, the idea of an ordinary and a more advanced pharmacist still persists.[47a]

To enter pharmacy in Great Britain today, the aspirant must earn either a university degree or the pharmaceutical-chemist diploma of the Pharmaceutical Society of Great Britain.

The level of preprofessional education in either case is the same. In the examination for a General Certificate of Education (given mainly to assess British students' capacity for more advanced studies) a prospective pharmacy student must pass with grades at the ordinary level in the English language, another language and mathematics and in chemistry, physics and biology, botany or zoology at the advanced level. (In Scotland the examinations are slightly different but the subjects and the standard are approximately the same.) Some believe that this standard may be estimated fairly as about equivalent to 1 year or more of preprofessional college study in the United States.

Most of the universities that offer a general degree in pharmacy (Bachelor) include the study of pharmacology and physiology, pharmaceutics, pharmaceutical chemistry, pharmacognosy and forensic pharmacy. Degree courses ordinarily have a curriculum of 3 academic years.

The alternative nondegree course also lasts 3 years and covers the same subjects, but it emphasizes the practical side somewhat more and often is not as concentrated. This course of instruction may be taken at a number of institutions still, but it is losing ground in popularity.

Whichever academic preparation the prospective pharmacist offers, he also must have one year of practical training under a pharmacist.[48]

A substantial minority earn the university degree in pharmacy and may then qualify for registration by passing the examination of the Pharmaceutical Society in forensic pharmacy. The majority complete the alternative course of instruction, and they must pass the comprehensive qualifying (diploma) examination of the Society.

Successful candidates are registered as "pharmaceutical chemists" and become eligible for Membership in the Pharmaceutical Society ("M.P.S.").

Before 1954 the two standards of examinations led to different types of registration—as "Chemist and Druggist" and as "Pharmaceutical Chemist." On amalgamation of the two registers, holders of the higher qualification (Ph. C.) were titled "Fellow of the Pharmaceutical Society" (F.P.S.). Members may now proceed to the Fellowship by means of postgraduate research.

The research degrees of Master of Pharmacy or Science, Doctor of Philosophy (in Medicine, Pharmacy or Science), and the esteemed Doctor of Science are available from several universities and are attracting an increasing number of students.

London's famous old school of pharmacy on Bloomsbury Square was operated by the Pharmaceutical Society of Great Britain from 1842 until 1948, when it became a school of the University of London. The Society is still represented on its governing body.

The Pharmaceutical Society of Northern Ireland offers a Pharmaceutical Chemist Diploma and the University of Belfast offers the degree of Bachelor of Science in Pharmacy. These two different standards are similar to those of Great Britain, and there are reciprocal agreements between the two societies. The Pharmaceutical Society of Ireland also has the Pharmaceutical Chemist Diploma (but it appears that this Society is about to insist on a university degree for qualification). Reciprocity between Ireland and Great Britain probably will be arranged, in view of the increased standard of the Irish qualification.[49]

An examination qualifying for a certificate as "Assistant in Dispensing" has been conducted by the London Society of Apothecaries since 1815. Holders of this certificate acted as drug dispensers in the dispensing practices that the apothecaries continued as they moved from pharmacy into medicine. However, creation of the National Health Service (1948), resulted in the virtual disappearance of the "dispensing doctor." Hence, the training for the dispensing assistant's examination was amended to make successful candidates suitable to serve as technicians under the supervision of pharmacists in community pharmacies as well as in hospital pharmacies.

This development was possible because the modern practice of pharmacy, while it involves a heavy responsibility, involves many routine technical tasks that do not necessarily have to be performed personally by a university graduate in pharmacy. Says a report to the Pharmaceutical Society:

The function of a pharmaceutical assistant is to undertake work of a routine nature in the preparation and/or supply of medicines under the supervision of a pharmacist. The training should produce a person who can act as a general assistant in pharmacy, though in practice he or she may be primarily engaged in one branch of work, e.g., in serving customers or dispensing.[50]

Diplomas in biochemical analysis and in pharmaceutical analysis, offered for some years by the Pharmaceutical Society, now have been discontinued. Postgraduate diplomas in pharmaceutical analysis, clinical chemistry and food and drug analysis are now offered by the Royal Institute of Chemistry. Pharmacists took an active part in the founding of this Institute, and many pharmacists have been Fellows throughout the Institute's existence. Pharmacists also were prominent in the founding of the Chemical Society, the Society for Analytical Chemistry and the British Pharmacological Society.

Even though it may be seen that British pharmacy retains the elements of a double standard of pharmaceutical education, the differences have been narrowed and the requirements advanced. In addition, an increasing number (in 1962 still a minority) of the students choose the regular degree course of the universities. The extent to which the burgeoning of advanced and postgraduate education will bypass community practice or find in it renewed potential is a part of British history that is still unfolding.[51]

PHARMACOPEIAS AND FORMULARIES

There were three official pharmacopeias in the United Kingdom until 1864, published in London, Edinburgh and Dublin, respectively. The first edition of the *Pharmacopoeia Londinensis* had an unusual fate. As a matter of fact, there are two "first" editions of this standard—one issued May 7, 1618, and another December 7 of the same year. The latter replaced the earlier edition and became the basis of the editions that followed.

An epilogue in the later book explains the necessity for withdrawal of the first issue. The printer is blamed by the College of Physicians of London for having "snatched away from our hands this little work not yet finished off . . ." Actually, differences among the members of the College about the scope of this first English pharmacopeia were responsible for the replacement of the earlier book by the later one. In both issues the Galenic-Arabic school, which still dominated the drug therapy of this period, offered the main basis; however, the second issue represented the victory of baroque abundance over renaissance simplicity.[52] The first issue listed 680 simple

and 712 compounded drugs compared with 1,190 simple and 963 compounded drugs in the second. The number of animals used pharmaceutically rose in the second issue from 10 to 31, and the number of parts of animals (among them various excrements and urines) rose from 47 to 162.[53] However, there were some signs indicating the dawn of a new era. Chemical preparations (among them calomel and preparations of iron and antimony for internal use) and those regarded as chemical at this period had been included in both issues of the new pharmacopeia. The French immigrant Theodore de Mayerne (1573-1655) almost certainly was responsible for the introduction of calomel—and probably the other chemicals also.[54]

Eight subsequent editions preserve for us a pharmacopeial picture of the state of pharmaceutical, chemical and medical knowledge and thought of their time.[55]

The first *Edinburgh Pharmacopoeia* appeared in 1699—a distinguished book that lived to see twelve editions (the last published in 1841).[56] The *Dublin Pharmacopoeia*, first published in 1807, lived only until the third edition (1850) and was supplanted by a pharmacopeia for the whole of the British Isles. While the *Dublin Pharmacopoeia* did not gain much attention beyond Ireland, during the 18th century the *Edinburgh Pharmacopoeia* ranked high among the internationally acknowledged pharmaceutical standards.

The first *British Pharmacopoeia*, issued in 1864, replaced the London, the Edinburgh and the Dublin standards, but it disappointed the mass of the medical and the pharmaceutical practitioners because in it many of the preparations that they were in the habit of dispensing were omitted or changed.[57] Consequently, it already was superseded by a second edition in 1867.

After World War II, a long-delayed seventh *British Pharmocopoeia* appeared (1948), and, since then, a new revision has appeared every 5 years (parallel with the American revision schedule), plus an interim addendum.[58]

Until the end of the 18th century, the preparation of the official pharmacopeias in

England was apparently the exclusive business of the medical profession. In 1785 we find the first mention of pharmaceutical cooperation. An entry in the proceedings of the Society of Apothecaries reports an invitation from the College of Physicians to assist the college in revising the *London Pharmacopoeia*, in order that it should be "as correct and free from errors as possible, and that all the formulae should be such as can be easily prepared by the gentlemen of your Society." A smiliar invitation followed in 1806.[59]

The "gentlemen of the society of apothecaries," after having become primarily medical practitioners, no longer could be considered the representatives of pharmaceutical practice. In this situation a new proof was given of the English tendency to take the good wherever it may be found and to confer tasks and responsibilities on those who have shown the necessary ability. The College of Physicians, editing the *London Pharmacopoeia*, had encountered much criticism on the part of the pharmaceutical chemists. The impossibility of editing such a standard treatise exclusively from the medical point of view and knowledge had become evident, and the necessity of pharmaceutical cooperation had become apparent. Neither the old apothecaries nor their successors, the chemists and the druggists, unorganized as the latter were at that time, had as yet produced the experts needed. However, a learned pharmacist, Richard Phillips, had criticized the edition of 1809 and the corrected reprint of 1815 with the utmost acrimony. It was he who was commissioned to translate the *Pharmacopoeia* of 1824 from Latin and to prepare a commentary. "Subsequently he assumed a more responsible position with reference to the work as editor as well as translator and commentator, in which capacities his name is associated with the editions of 1836 and 1851."[60]

These two editions of the *London Pharmacopoeia* are therefore to be considered essentially the work of a pharmacist. On the other hand, the *British Pharmacopoeia* was edited not by the College but by the General Council of Medical Education and Registration. With it the Pharmaceutical Society, which was now the representative of British pharmacy, has long cooperated, and in 1926 a permanent Pharmacopeia Commission was created on which pharmacy and medicine have equal representation.

It is of interest to note that, after the appearance of the first edition (1864), a representative pharmacist, Peter Squire, "brought out a book called 'A Companion to the British Pharmacopoeia' which proved a useful guide to medical practitioners, and acquired a great circulation."[61] In 1952 this book was absorbed into the *Extra Pharmacopoeia*, a comprehensive ready-reference work for practitioners (first edition, 1883). British pharmacists refer to this work informally as "Martindale" (as Americans refer to "Remington"), in remembrance of the original author, William Martindale, who was once chief pharmacist at University College Hospital in London and later founder of wholesale and retail pharmacies.

The Pharmaceutical Society has published at irregular intervals since 1907 the *British Pharmaceutical Codex*. A more comprehensive formulary than the *Pharmacopoeia*, it includes monographs on drug actions and uses and is the legal standard for surgical dressings in Great Britain. The *Codex* now appears every 5 years, with increasing authority (from 1963, simultaneously with new editions of the *Pharmacopoeia*). A *British Veterinary Codex* also is published by the Pharmaceutical Society (first edition, 1953).

A *National Formulary* was first issued for use in the old National Health Insurance plan and has been continued under the title *British National Formulary*, to avoid confusion with the *National Formulary* of the United States. Now used in the universal National Health Service (government-paid services), it has been made a comprehensive book of drug preparations, compiled by a joint committee of the British Medical Association and the Pharmaceutical Society of Great Britain.

PHARMACEUTICAL LITERATURE

Prior to the 19th century, the general conditions in English medicine and pharmacy were not conducive to a large and systematic literature on pharmaceutical subjects. In Britain until the 16th century, the same books of the Galenic-Arabic school that formed the professional library of pharmacists in all European countries were used, such as the *Antidotaria Nicolai,* the *Grabadin* of Mesuë, the *Book of Symon Januensis,* and the others. Later on, the most important French and German pharmaceutical literature was introduced.

Among English books issued in the 16th century, we should mention *The New Herbal* (1551) by William Turner, physician to the court of Edward VI; Robert Recorde's *The Urinal of Physick* (1548) and William Bulleyn's *Bulwarke of Defence* (1562). Bulleyn's *Bulwarke* was quoted frequently because of the 21 rules it contained for the apothecary's guidance. Rule 19, admonishing the apothecary "that he doe remember his office is only to be the physicians coke," has often been quoted by physicians during their disagreements with apothecaries. The popular *Herball* (1597) of John Gerard, a barber-surgeon, was based on a Belgian herbal by Dodoens; it was revised and much improved by the scholarly apothecary Thomas Johnson.

In the 17th century an English translation of *The Charitable Physician* and *The Charitable Apothecary* by the French physician Guibert (see p. 67) was popular.[62] The voluminous herbal *Theatrum botanicum* . . . (1640) was written by John Parkinson of London, one of the last representatives of a herbalist tradition soon to be pushed aside by modern botanists.

In 1688, the apothecary James Shipton published a collection of formulas which he said were prescribed by the physician George Bate, and which he therefore titled *Bate's Dispensatory.* The book (usually known as the *Pharmacopoeia Bateana)* lived to see several editions in Latin and in English and was used as a book of reference until the end of the 18th century.[63]

Quincy's *Pharmacopoeia officinalis & extemporanea: or, A Compleat English Dispensatory* (1718) was so popular that it was issued in ten editions by 1736.[64] There were a few other compilations from Continental works and some commentaries on the London and the Edinburgh pharmacopeias —among them Salmon's *New London Dispensatory,*[65] Lewis' *New Dispensatory,*[66] Duncan's *Edinburgh New Dispensatory* and Thomson's *London Dispensatory*— but no sign of the lively, fruitful and sometimes creative activity so characteristic of the Continental pharmacists—the French and the Germans especially.

Nineteenth-century books by pharmacists included *Practical Pharmacy* by the German Carl F. Mohr and the Briton Theophilus Redwood, *Pharmacographia* by the Swiss F. A. Flückiger and the Briton Daniel Hanbury and *Microscopical Examination of Foods and Drugs* and *Introduction to the Study of Materia Medica* by H. G. Greenish. Meanwhile, various books written by men from the ranks of British pharmacy currently serve aspects of the art, the science and the industry.

Since there was no want of chemical interest or great chemists in England—as is witnessed by the names of Boyle, Mayow, Black, Priestley, Dalton and Davy—a relative deficiency in pharmaco-chemical literature may be explained by the fact that during this period the ambitions of the English apothecaries were directed to the practice of medicine.

Remembering the abundance of pharmaceutical textbooks on the Continent around 1800, particularly in France and Germany, it seems almost incredible that in 1843, when the young Pharmaceutical Society of Great Britain tried to organize a systematic pharmaceutical education, "books and periodic publications, conveying educational knowledge in the department of pharmacy, were . . . wanting."[67]

SCIENTIFIC CONTRIBUTIONS

While a similar limitation affected the contribution that pharmacy could make to British science, it should be noted that the scientific contributions—whether growing from the ranks of apothecaries or chemists-and-druggists—have been by no means fully explored historically. If we include apothecaries in this pharmaceutical contribution (and that involves questions of both dating and definition), significant work already can be identified in the development of botany, chemistry and other sciences.

Apothecaries took part in the founding of the Royal Society; T. D. Whittet has found that at least 30 British apothecaries and 12 pharmacists have been elected Fellows. The apothecaries contributed many papers to the Society's *Philosophical Transactions.*

At one time, botanic science in Great Britain was largely the province of apothecaries such as John Houghton (a pioneer of good agriculture), Samuel Doody, William Hudson, James Sherard, Isaac Rand, Phillip Miller, R. Pulteney and Nathaniel B. Ward, all of whom became Fellows of the Royal Society.

Among those who made important contributions to chemistry and were elected Fellows of the Royal Society were Timothy Lane, who made some of the earliest investigations on rusting of iron; Josiah Colebrook, who investigated paints used by the ancients; Thomas Henry, a founder of the Manchester Philosophical Society and of a chemical manufactory, and William Thomas Brande, a pioneer of organic and clinical chemistry, who also conducted important metallurgic investigations.

Sir William Watson, F. R. S., a versatile scientist and apothecary, made significant contributions to botany, chemistry and physics. At least four of the "chemical operators of the Apothecaries' Hall" became Fellows of the Royal Society (Godfrey-Hanckwitz, Henry Hennell, W. T. Brande and Robert Warington).

Six apothecaries or pharmacists associated with the firm of Allen and Hanbury became Fellows of the Royal Society: Silvanus Bevan, William Allen (distinguished as a chemist), Daniel Hanbury (botanist), Luke Howard (botanist and pioneer meteorologist), Richard Phillips (analytic chemist) and William West (chemist and inventor). Luke Howard's son John Eliot Howard, the quinologist, also was honored as a Fellow of the Royal Society—the highest distinction a scientist can be given.

A. W. Gerrard, while chief pharmacist of University College Hospital in London, was the first to isolate pilocarpine and several other plant principles. He later founded the present firm of Cuxson, Gerrard and Co. at Birmingham.

A chemist-and-druggist in community practice, John Walker, invented the friction match. Sir Joseph Wilson Swan, F. R. S., pioneer of photography and electricity and one of the first to produce artificial silk, remained a practicing pharmacist most of his life, as did H. B. Brady, F. R. S., a great naturalist and George C. Druce, F. R. S., the greatest British field botanist of his time.

Sir Robert Kane, F. R. S., a prominent member of the Dublin Apothecaries' Society, became one of Ireland's greatest chemists and a founder of Ireland's chemical industry. William Higgins, F. R. S., who anticipated some of Dalton's atomic theory, was for a few years operator to the Dublin Apothecaries' Hall. Other important names include those of Thomas Johnson, the previously mentioned apothecary and early botanist (d. 1644), and the 19th-century figures Jonathan Pereira, F. R. S., apothecary-physician-professor, William Tilden, F. R. S., organic chemist, Edward Morell Homes, botanist, John Attfield, pharmacist-professor-author, and Edward Frank Harrison, who contributed to the defense of the allied armies against gas attacks during World War I.[68]

TIES BETWEEN DISPENSING AND PRODUCTION

It is significant that the organizers of the Pharmaceutical Society—William Allen,[69] its first president, and Jacob Bell—were owners not only of pharmacies but also of pharmaceutical manufactories (founded about 1800) that still exist. This union between professional interest and technico-commercial intelligence and activity was not rare in British pharmacy. Of the British pharmaceutical industry in the Manchester area, in Scotland, London and Leeds, a number of the industrial pharmaceutical laboratories, wholesale drug houses and

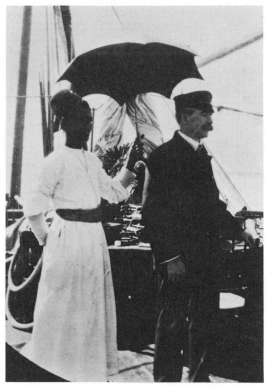

Sir Henry Wellcome, who had emigrated to Britain as a young American pharmacist, is shown aboard his floating research laboratory on the Upper Nile; the laboratory was an auxiliary to the Wellcome Tropical Research Laboratories at Khartoum. Besides his varied enterprises in pharmaceutical manufacturing, research and philanthropy, Sir Henry (1853-1936) personally led an archaeologic expedition in Ethiopia, published a book on Alaskan Indians and collected many of the rare books and objects for the great medico-historical library and museum that he established in London. (Photographed after 1907; from Burroughs Wellcome & Co.)

several nonpharmaceutical establishments[70] originated in the shops of dispensing "chemists" and often can be traced back a century and more. Several of the founders of the Pharmaceutical Society extended their pharmacies to make them industrial or wholesale establishments. To the names of Allen and Bell there should be added those of John May, Thomas Morson and John Savory, all of London, and those of F. B. Benger of Manchester and Richard Raimes of York—founders of firms still serving British medical care. The chemist John Fletcher Macfarlan of Edinburgh was one of the pioneer British manufacturers of alkaloids, at first in the laboratory of his pharmacy and later on in the manufactory that grew out of it. The fact that some of the same people in England who, in the beginning of the 19th century, created anew the profession of pharmacy, simultaneously took an important part in the development of the British pharmaceutical industry is a further proof of the intimate historic ties between dispensing and production in pharmacy, which one finds internationally.

One of the largest pharmaceutical concerns in England, with headquarters in London and with associated houses across the world, was developed by men with American pharmaceutical education. S. M. Burroughs as well as Henry Wellcome, the two late founders of Burroughs Wellcome and Company, were graduates of the Philadelphia College of Pharmacy. Although Henry Wellcome became a naturalized British subject and later on an English knight and Fellow of the Royal Society, he never lost his connections with his native country and, through his life membership in the American Pharmaceutical Association, he maintained his relations with American pharmacy. Perhaps this is symbolic.

Interest in pharmacy's history has increased notably in the British Isles during recent years. The stimulus coming from Committees for the History of Pharmacy formed by the Pharmaceutical Society and by its Scottish Department, and from the Faculty of the History of Medicine and Pharmacy founded by the Society of Apothecaries of London (1959), will yield broader illumination of the rich complex of events that were destined to help shape pharmacy in America.

8:   Some International Trends

Since the Middle Ages, European peoples have been so interrelated that most developments within individual countries can be considered as a national reaction to general European trends. Naturally, special conditions and the character of the people concerned often yield interesting differences. In one sphere we may find national trends predominant (see the chapters on Italy, France, Germany and England), only to find them submerged elsewhere by common ideas and facts that seem to be borne along by a genie of the time that cannot long be barred by boundaries. The powerful thrust of science and its technologic applications are in this category, as are movements originating from the facilitation of trade and commerce and from the rise and the spread of democratic-humanitarian ideas in their wake.

For the purposes of this discussion, such international trends will be considered in three categories: (1) commercial, (2) social and (3) professional-pharmaceutical.

TRENDS OF INTERNATIONAL COMMERCE

The development of manufacturing drugs on a large scale was accompanied and promoted by legislation that created an exclusive right to exploit new products or processes. These patent and trademark laws exerted a great and steadily growing influence on the practice of pharmacy.

Large-scale production, though by hand methods, existed for certain drugs already in the time of Greco-Roman antiquity and in the Middle Ages. For example, the *terra sigillata* tablets consisting of a special clay found on the island of Lemnos (and elsewhere) were sold over the entire known world up to early modern times. There was large-scale manufacture of distilled waters and perfumes in some monasteries of Italy, France and Germany[1] in the 13th century

and later, and of troches of vipers in Venice. However, these early precursors of pharmaceutical mass production were almost exclusively an accident of circumstance—the presence of local raw material granting a practical monopoly to the producers.

In other words, with only a few exceptions (for instance the preparation of corrosive sublimate, cinnabar, sugar of lead, borax, etc., at Venice around the year 1300) quantity manufacture of pharmaceuticals was incidental and conservative. Modern mass production has been systematically planned and progressive.

Drug manufacture in the United States began to convert to mass production technics in this sense after the middle of the 19th century and, within a century, transformed not only the pharmaceutical industry but also the practice of pharmacy. In industries based on science and elaborate technology, the vigorous, steady thrust of this development scarcely could be expected without a two-pronged legal support that society gave to the massive investment ordinarily demanded by mass production. This support consisted of the legal definition and protection of the *patent* and the *trademark*, two quite abstract forms of property that have had far-reaching—and sometimes controversial—effects in the pharmaceutical field.

In general, when a government grants a patent, it intends to protect the rights and the rewards of discovery. If a drug product represents nothing particularly new, or if, for some other reason, it is not patented, the manufacturer then may rely on a trademark to protect rights and rewards accruing from the public's belief in the merits of the manufacturer or his product (merits that may be real or, on occasion, largely imaginary).

Linked to this development in the early modern period were the nostrums, fancifully promoted to physicians and laymen

111

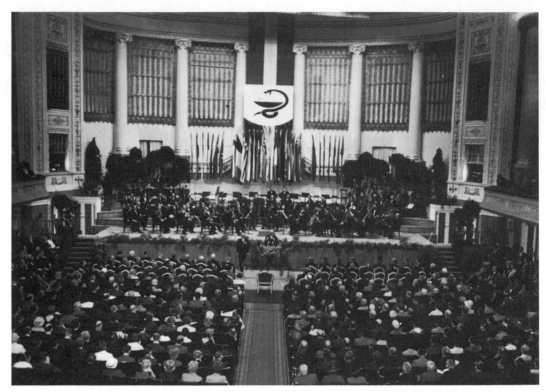

Beneath the symbol of the profession and a panoply of national flags, the opening session of the 19th General Assembly of the International Pharmaceutical Federation, at Vienna, is addressed by the President of the Austrian Republic. (Photograph from the American Pharmaceutical Association and Foto Schikola, 1962)

alike. Lacking legal and scientific means to expose and curb extravagant claims, the responsible drug maker and medical practitioner often were no match for the impostor and charlatan.

Some nostrums prepared in the 17th and the 18th centuries were so highly regarded that rulers bought the formulas from their inventors and published them for the benefit of their people. Here are several famous examples: The formula for a decoction of cinchona bark was sold (1680) by the Englishman Talbor to Louis XIV of France, for an extraordinarily high price.[2] An act of the English parliament (1739) permitted the payment of 5,000 pounds to Joanna Stephens for her remedy for vesical calculus, consisting of alicante soap and burnt eggshells.[3] Frederick the Great of Prussia (1775) gave the inventor of a nostrum against tapeworm (consisting of filix, jalapa and scammonium) not only an annuity but also a title.[4] Similar "bargains" are reported elsewhere.[5]

Cleverly promoted into high esteem, such remedies came to represent large enterprise and high monetary value. Purveyed with an air of mystery, if not actually secret in composition, they were supposed to represent some unique virtue or invention. Through this circumstance such drugs found a role in bringing about legal rights that formed the basis of modern patent legislation.

Patents

Reigning princes, as part of their prerogatives, granted privileges—whether for safe passage, for a trading monopoly, or for exploiting invention—to anyone who had gained their favor or had paid the rather considerable amounts asked for. Here we find the beginning of patent legislation in most countries. Such privileges for the production and the sale of nostrums were granted by the German emperors and princes, as well as by the French kings until the end of the 18th century and by the English kings until the first third of the 17th century.

Many drug preparations that were granted the early and rather arbitrary "letters patent" held too little that was original to be considered for a patent today. Today's so-called "patent medicines" commonly are *not* in fact patented, but rather derive their misnomer by lineal descent from the class of early English nostrums.

It is significant that England was the first country to establish governmental regulation in lieu of princely arbitrariness. Business interests were concerned, and thus the usual *laissez-faire* policy had to cease. A statute of King James I of England (1624) declared all monopolies that were grievous and inconvenient to the subjects of the realm to be void, with the exception of those privileges for the

sole working or making of any manner of new manufacture within the realm to the true and first inventor of such manufacture, which others at the time of making such letters patent or grants should not use, so they be not contrary to law nor mischievous to the state by raising of the prices of commodities at home or hurt of trade or generally inconvenient.[6]

On these words rests the modern legal concept of patents for inventions.

The first real medicinal patent was granted in England in 1698 for Epsom salts (Patent No. 354). Subsequent patents included *Sal oleosum volatile* (1711), Stoughton's elixir (1712) and Turlington's balsam (1744).

Of special interest is the patent granted to the London pharmacist Thomas Wilson for his Patent Ague Drops (1781). These drops were employed with success by a Dr. Thomas Fowler, physician to the general infirmary of the county of Stafford. The drops were analyzed by Mr. Hughes, the apothecary to the infirmary, who found them to be a solution of arsenic. The famous Fowler's solution was the final result of the cooperation of the physician Fowler and the apothecary Hughes.[7]

Thus, patent legislation and its application to the pharmaceutical field, as we know it, was born in England. In the American colonies, the British monarch or his governors granted letters-patent of the old type for exclusive privilege (land, trading companies, manufacture), but this practice never was more than casual. The explanation lies in a combination of circumstances: the colonial preoccupation with agriculture, the restrictive policies of the Crown on the dissemination of industrial information and enterprise in the colonies and the sheer red tape in which patent grants were entangled.

Apparently there was no Colonial concept of patenting inventions on a systematic basis, thereby lagging behind the mother country's marked shift toward emphasizing patents of industrial or inventive purpose. This was rectified rather suddenly after the Revolution, and "between 1790 and 1836, five major statutes were enacted in pursuance of the constitutional provision of the granting of patents."[8]

That this American development was part of an international trend of the 19th century—a concomitant of the rise of large-scale industry—may be seen in the emergence of modern patent laws elsewhere (e.g., France, 1844; England, 1852; Italy, 1864; Germany 1877). In the United States, the modern regulation of patent rights is based on the patent law as revised by an enactment of 1870.

It is noteworthy that the patent law for a federated Germany (supplanting earlier laws for the separate German states) adopted the English concept that only a new method of manufacture—not the product itself—is patentable for medicines, foodstuffs and substances prepared by means of chemical processes. This stand was taken in order to avoid the granting of monopolies on such vital necessities of daily life. The idea—which raises a complicated social issue that meanwhile has been much debated—has not been adopted in the United States, where drugs as well as the processes for making them can be patented.

The development of the patent system provided a legal property of far-reaching importance to pharmaceutical industry (and industry at large). With the signing of an International Patent Convention it was confirmed as an international trend at Paris in 1883, which in its present form is adhered to by nearly all of the principal countries.

The patent laws protecting inventors and their inventions strongly influenced the progress of applied science in all fields, including pharmacy. The extensive development of large pharmaceutical firms, based on research, could not have occurred in the same way without patent laws. The fact that the industry, the ingenuity and the money invested in the discovery of new drugs and processes have been rewarded by a temporary monopoly has helped to stimulate the startling advances since the last quarter of the 19th century.

Trademarks

Because of the limited term of patent protection (17 years in U.S.A.), and the requirement of full disclosure of what is being patented, most pharmaceutical manufacturers have preferred to reinforce the property value of a new product by trademarking. Robert P. Fischelis summarized an important advantage to be gained when he said:

If the individual who registers a trademark for a patented product is careful enough to apply his trademark in such a manner that it will indicate the brand of the patented product rather than the patented product itself, he can acquire unlimited exclusive rights to the brand name and by clever advertising he can continue to enjoy a virtual monopoly on a given product even after his patent rights have expired.[9]

Historically, the "trade mark" has been a mark—such as a sign or a symbol—used to identify the origin or the ownership of the goods to which it is affixed. The mark of ownership (such as a cattle brand) has a history interwoven with the mark of origin (such as the design embossed on a medicinal tablet), which is today the primary function of trademarks. At first such marks generally were not adopted in the makers' own interest

. . . but were imposed upon them in the interest of the public, in order to locate responsibility for short weight, inferior material or poor workmanship. Like the finger prints taken today by the police, they established a liability rather than a right. But since this liability tended to secure honest and efficient workmanship, the trade-mark came to be regarded as an assurance of quality, and the confidence of the public in the quality of wares bearing a trade-mark of good repute became an asset.[10]

The use of trademarks in pharmacy represents no modern innovation, for the mark of origin may be traced back into classical times. For example, when Lemnian clay was processed into pastilles (as early as the 5th century B.C.) each pastille was stamped with a seal to indicate its authentic origin (hence called Sealed Earth). This type of troche still survived in early modern therapy; by then they were made from earths of varied origin, each "sealed" with a distinctive design.[11]

By the 17th century, the use of trademarks had been systematized and regulated to a certain extent by the guilds, such as those that gave pharmacy its first organized and regulated form on European soil. These old guild provisions were transformed into common law and, hence, given their modern meaning as trademarks—a process that involved a particularly tangled legal history. Suffice it to say that adequate legal recognition came, concomitant with the rise of large-scale industry and patent legislation. The two-part modern British legislation was inaugurated in 1862 and 1875.[12] In the United States a statute was enacted in 1870[13] (superseded currently by the Lanham Act of 1946).[14] The fundamental enactments came in France beginning in 1857 and in Germany in 1874. Events in other countries likewise give evidence that this international trend was in floodtide during the late 19th century, culminating in an international trademark agreement of 1883 at Paris, which was signed by 25 countries.

As long as the pharmacist prepared most of his own drugs, guided by a pharmacopeia or a formulary and based on raw materials gathered locally or bought from men whom he knew, the system of trademarking could not have seemed as important to him professionally as it has since the development of remote mass production. Thereafter, his prescription ingredients passed through the hands of many men he would never meet, under conditions he could not know. This half-blind dependence on the identity and the responsibility of the pharmacist's remote suppliers helped to catapult pharmaceutical trademarks into modern importance, especially under American conditions that prevailed between the end of the Civil War and the passage of the first Federal food and drug legislation (1906).

Intensifying the pharmacist's dependence and perplexity was a disturbing circumstance. At the very time when more potent drugs were being marketed—and in more concentrated forms—the changing character of drugs and drug tests made it impracticable for the community pharmacist to verify personally the quality of drugs he dispensed. Therefore, a drug guaranteed by its maker's mark gained an enhanced practical value in the professional practice of both pharmacists and physicians.

Thus, the emphasis on trademarking drugs, which once had served mainly to tout nostrums and quack remedies, in the 20th century came to dominate the field of prescription drugs likewise. This second line of development in pharmaceutical trademarking was encouraged by a growing realization among marketing experts, i.e., that physicians are influenced by advertising technics coupled to easily remembered trademarks (when choosing between drugs of similar quality and effectiveness), even as human beings in general are influenced in other kinds of choices.

As refinements in mass marketing and promotional psychology magnified the commercial effectiveness of trademarks internationally, so the proliferation of improved, privately controlled medications expanded the area of the application of trademarks. In the United States soon after the turn of the present century, programs of industrial research increasingly generated products the distinctiveness of which could be maximized by reliance on trademarks in the form of product names (trade names). In the struggle for markets, less creative manufacturers often used the same trademarking weapon of distinctive trade names to obscure their paucity of distinctive products. The trademark as a manufacturer's house mark signifying quality began to be subordinated to trademarks used as a primary system of drug nomenclature.

Arguments about what seemed to be a "needlessly irrational" system of nomenclature (i.e., fanciful trade names) applied to a professional-scientific area were already old in 1903, when one of the distinguished American pharmacists of his time, M. I. Wilbert, commented:

The nuisance arising from this self-evident right [to trademarks] is that we, particularly in connection with the medical and pharmaceutical professions, are being overwhelmed with a multitude of meaningless and in many cases misleading names. Many of these names are dangerously similar, and are likely to lead to serious misunderstanding and possibly fatal mistakes. The injustice to the public, as well as the pharmacist, is evidenced by the unnecessary duplication of names and titles for substances or mixtures that are not themselves covered by patents.[15]

In America the validity of the trademarking system has never been at stake, but the question of its appropriate limits came back into pharmaceutical focus with Congressional hearings on policies and methods of drug pricing, beginning in the late 1050's. In this context, emphasis has centered on the possible exploitation of the patient that may occur if the value of product trademarks should be unduly inflated. Additionally, the scientifically oriented segment of the medical profession has continued to feel uncomfortable with what one medical editor called

. . . the peculiarity of the present system of drug terminology whereby the number of names that can be given to a product is limited only by the number of manufacturers that are producing it . . . a system that is confusing and irritating and should be to a degree humiliating to the presumably intelligent members of a profession that is forced to conform to it.[16]

Apprehensive that the patent system alone would not assure adequate protection to investments in research and promotion, manufacturers have tended to construe such attacks as attacks on the trademark system itself—perhaps, even on the system of free enterprise—and as fostering a market for substandard drugs. Speaking on behalf of American pharmaceutical manufacturers in the early 1960's, the National Pharmaceutical Council termed the prescribing of drugs by nonproprietary names "second-class medical care" and proposed that "the crux of the controversy is whether all drugs with the same generic name even when they bear U.S.P. on their label are equivalent therapeutically."[17]

In a closely reasoned definition and discussion of a somewhat different view (substantially representative of the "opposition"), George F. Archambault observed:

Unquestionably, this [tradenaming] is a sound and probably the only, sensible approach for true specialties, that is, those medications that contain *several active ingredients and that have no official U.S.P. or N.F. titles.*

However, many in the medical and pharmacy professions believe the drug industry makes a serious mistake in permitting the trade name philosophy to be the advertising and sales promotion technique for pharmaceutical specialties of *single drug entities and official preparations.* They believe the house quality designation to be the better approach. . . . This right of "house designation" is a right we all respect. By the same token, many physicians rely on the professional judgment of the pharmacist in selecting the source or manufacturer of a drug.[18]

As the controversy wore on,[19] arguments pro and con from previous decades were repeated with renewed vigor, though without apparent prospect of altering the massive shift of the past century to a pharmaceutical nomenclature based, in normal practice, on product trademarks.

INTERNATIONAL SOCIAL TRENDS

Modern social legislation, of which health insurance laws are a part, has been one consequence of the change in the structure and the living conditions of human society produced by industrialization and mechanization of life.

A harbinger of later social welfare legislation were the laws (1802-47) by which the English administrative policy of *laissez-faire* received its death sentence. This factory legislation was born out of the necessity of protecting working people, in this case women and children especially, from exploitation by industry.

Compulsory Health Insurance

In ancient Rome, as well as in the Middle Ages, organizations built on compulsory membership were devoted to the care of the sick. This care became the required or the self-imposed duty of almost all guilds. Particularly in mining (the first European large-scale industrial undertaking) there were early institutions of a rather modern character, requiring regular fees and affording medical care. However, the change from private cooperative assistance in cases of sickness to authoritative institutions introduced by law and guaranteed by the government was made for the first time during the middle of the 19th century, in Germany. The laws were perfected by social legislation introduced in 1881 by a special public message of the German Emperor. They were intended to make ineffective the agitation of the German socialists through a well-planned government-fostered social welfare program.[20] A publication of the International Labour Office (1925) stated that

the motive of the reform was a desire to improve the living conditions of the workers in order to reconcile them with the state as an institution defending the capitalistic organization of [paternal] protection, and at the same time to deprive the workers' occupational organizations of the potential weapon they possessed in numerous mutual aid and provident bodies attached to the trade unions.

Disadvantages of the original German system, not only for the physician and the pharmacist but for the insured as well, were that the contracts concerning medical and medicinal care were negotiated, not by a centralized governmental authority, but by individual representatives of local independent health insurance bodies. Frequently, these representatives tried to deprive the physicians of their liberty of action by prescribing detailed rules for the medical treatment of the insured. Moreover, they endeavored to exclude the pharmacist as much as possible—for example, by delivering bandages, and many remedies directly to the insured, and they produced drugs in laboratories conducted by or affiliated with individual health insurance bodies or their central organizations. The final objective was socialization of the healing arts.[21] Restrictions placed on both physician and pharmacist in the providing of medicaments for the insured were numerous.[22] From the beginning, the remuneration of the pharmacist was based on governmental price lists issued annually, less discounts to insurance agencies of 10 to 20 per cent. Austria established (1888) a health insurance plan similar to that of Germany.

A number of social circumstances[23] united to carry the idea of social insurance around the globe and, with it, provision for health insurance, usually under government supervision or sponsorship. Within 70 years after the German innovation, 44 countries had a social security program, all but 5 including health insurance. Most programs with health benefits included a pharmaceutical component. By the early 1960's 59 nations were providing health benefits.[24]

The contributory principle of paying for health insurance was already established in the final form of the German plan. Both worker and employer contributed, but under certain circumstances the government would pay a worker's share. Manual workers were insured no matter what their income; others could participate on a voluntary basis.[25] In most versions of health insurance, the goal of providing primarily for low-income classes has never been far out of sight, although the appeal of health insurance eventually tends to broaden benefits and expand the occupational strata covered. American preoccupation with the social implications of the British experiment in universal compulsory health insurance tends to obscure the fact that it is perhaps

unique in offering comprehensive health insurance to so large a population.

In England, too, the original provision was for lower-income classes. This provision was effective from 1912 until 1948, when parliament placed all citizens under the government health insurance scheme (National Health Service). After one of the most penetrating historic studies made of the British plan, Eckstein concluded—in a statement curiously analogous to the analysis of the German innovation—that "In a very real sense the institution of the [British] Service marks a triumph of nonsocialist over socialist ideas, however much we have become used to calling systems like the National Health Service 'socialized' medicine."[26] Nevertheless, with this popular and far-reaching move, England went far toward realization of the "welfare state" idea.

Although British pharmacists (as in other nonsocialist states) remain private entrepreneurs, most of their prescription practice falls within the National Health Service. As such, it is paid for through government-collected funds. Prescriptions that have been filled are sent periodically to a bureau that prices them according to a negotiated schedule of fees covering ingredients, professional service and other costs. To discourage the careless use of pharmaceutical services that was encountered originally, a token payment from the patient's pocket is now required in England, as in France and some other countries.

A steady rise in the cost of pharmaceutical service has attracted the government's attention repeatedly over the years. The Senior Secretary of the Pharmaceutical Society of Great Britain, Sir Hugh Linstead, interpreted this circumstance (1962) as follows:

The number of prescriptions has remained fairly steady—about 210 million annually for 50 million people. But the cost of each item has steadily risen owing to the increasing use of new and more expensive drugs . . . about three times the cost in 1948 when the service started, and it has only been kept down by the most strenuous efforts with what we call the *British National Formulary*, which gives recipes for non-specialty medicines and advice about equivalent preparations for expensive specialties. . . . In consequence about 60 percent of the medicines prescribed under the National Health Service are for specialties and the remainder are not. On the European continent 90 percent or more prescribed medicines are for specialties, and I suspect that in the United States and Canada the percentage is even higher.[27]

Until the introduction of health insurance, England was the only one of the larger European countries in which the physicians enjoyed full liberty to dispense and deliver medicines. Under the English health insurance plan the physician is forbidden to do so. Dispensing of medicines is restricted to pharmacists.[28]

In France and Germany, where the separation between physician and pharmacist has been compulsory for centuries, such a clause was not necessary. Yet, here another danger existed: the dispensing and the delivery of medicaments and medicinal supplies by the health insurance bodies, and the establishment of special pharmacies for the insured. In both countries clauses within the act itself (in France) or in other laws (in Germany) exclude such possibilities, at least to a great extent. In Poland, where a similar precaution was not taken, the local health insurance bodies established their own pharmacies (numbering 200 in 1925), depriving private pharmacies of a great part of their legitimate field. As a consequence, "many private pharmacies, especially in highly industrialized centers, became completely ruined and had to be closed."[29] Meanwhile, sickness-benefit agencies in at least five other countries have tried to operate some pharmacies of their own.[30]

In most countries pharmaceutical and other health services remain in traditional and private channels. However, the amount of government regulation and compensation for insured services varies.

The circumstance has been quite different in the Soviet Union and in other communist countries, such as Yugoslavia. There, pharmacists and other health practitioners are truly socialized and practice as employees of the state. Under socialistic arrangements the patient may either pay for

pharmaceutical service out of his own pocket or obtain government-paid services, depending on particular regulations.[31]

In America a contest between the contrasting ideas of compulsory government health insurance and a private fee-for-service medical care for the allegiance of the American public has been resolved in a typically American way: lacking zeal for either choice, Americans since World War II have joined voluntary health insurance agencies on a scale unprecedented anywhere in the world. By 1961 three fourths of Americans held voluntary health insurance to some extent and were obtaining in benefits about one fourth of the nation's total personal medical expenditures (predominantly hospitalization and surgery). To see this in perspective, it may be noted that the share of total costs covered in countries with health benefits under social security ranges from about 25 per cent to as high as 95 per cent.[32]

The United States had become fully conscious of the issue just before World War I, when the British parliament and public were considering their first health insurance legislation for the lower-income groups. In following years, when workmen's compensation laws were being passed in state legislatures here as an early social welfare measure, several state health insurance bills were proposed, but none were passed.

By 1920 the American Medical Association awakened to the implications and passed a policy resolution, the fundamentals of which have survived the ensuing decades:

. . . The American Medical Association declares its opposition to the institution of any plan embodying the system of compulsory contributory insurance against illness, or any other plan of compulsory insurance which provides for medical service to be rendered contributors or their dependents, provided, controlled, or regulated by any state or the Federal government.*

During the prosperous years before the Great Depression the principle of insurance

---

* House of Delegates 1920, J. A. M. A. 74:1319, 1920.

applied to medical care persisted mainly as a matter of social study rather than political action. With the depression, problems of medical care became more acute, and a broader segment of the public became acutely aware of the issues of medical economics. As had happened in other countries, experience with an American social security system (adopted in 1935) brought wider interest and support to proposals for broader social-welfare functions. Bills for compulsory health insurance went into the Congressional hopper repeatedly in the ensuing years, the first to make a serious bid being the Wagner bill of 1939.

Even voluntary group insurance had been considered an unacceptable alternative to traditional fee-for-service by many American physicians and other conservatives until a few years after the adoption of the social security system. However, in the other direction stood a threat of government-sponsored health insurance, against which the voluntary insurance movement now was thrust as a counterforce by many who originally opposed or ignored it.

By the late 1940's insurance as such no longer was controversial in America as a device for reducing the economic risks of illness. After another decade the voluntary movement, aided by contributory plans of both employers and unions, which blanketed large groups from all economic classes, was keeping pace with the hopes of its most optimistic advocates.[33] Compared with health insurance plans in some countries, the American voluntary coverage remained somewhat more limited in scope, leaving pharmacy as practiced outside hospital walls largely untouched. However, insured prescription service had come up for local experimentation by the 1950's. In the subsequent decade the only part of proposals for government insurance that seemed to retain major support among the American people was the question of partial health care under social security for aging citizens, the group with the lowest income and the highest risk of medical expenses.

A broader question must wait to be answered definitely: has the freer, "typically American" system of dealing with the exigencies of medical expense been stabilized lastingly, or is voluntary insurance only a prologue—as it has been in certain other countries (such as Norway)—to some form of government participation or control?

Opium Convention—Narcotic Laws

The introduction as well as the scope of health insurance, while an international trend, has remained strictly a separate national decision of the individual country. However, the trade in opiates and other narcotic drugs became a matter of international cooperation and decision. The reason was that no boundaries or informal arrangements could prevent the spreading of drug addiction, with all its demoralizing consequences, from one country into the other. Nevertheless, it was the second half of the 19th century before the great European trading nations and the United States of America became aware of the threat to themselves of what originally was considered to be peculiarly an Eastern vice.[34]

It is not to the credit of the white race that in the early 19th century the English government, in order to retain the profitable trade in opium, overcame by force of arms attempts of the Chinese government to eliminate the import of the drug from English-dominated India. Defeated in two so-called opium wars (1839-1843 and 1856-1860), the Chinese government had to compensate the English traders for their losses and withdraw laws prohibiting the trade in opium. It is an irony of history that the rapidly developing cultivation of the poppy in China itself soon turned the tables, making opium a Chinese export to India.

All over the world, medicine came to place opiates high on the list of the drugs most useful to mankind, because of their unmatched analgesic power. The isolation of narcotic alkaloids and the development of hypodermic injection by the mid-19th century formed a two-edged sword that on one side enhanced medicinal use and, on the other, intensified widespread abuse.

As both the character and the dimensions of the addiction problem were perceived more clearly, West European and American interest in some form of cooperative control came to a focus early in the present century. This culminated in an international convention or treaty agreed on at The Hague in 1912. Eventually, most governments of the world signed the agreement (i.e., one or more of the eight multilateral treaties concluded 1912-1948), which stimulated corresponding legal restrictions in the individual countries.

The United States of America was among the very first to implement her moral and legal obligations, by Congressional enactment of the Harrison Narcotic Act in 1914. Earlier legal concern with the problem could be seen in the prohibition of nonmedicinal imports (1877) and of nonmedicinal use (1908). However, it was the Harrison Narcotic Act that gave American expression and force to the far-reaching control envisioned by The Hague Convention, and still provides today the basic framework within which the narcotic traffic, both licit and illicit, is controlled.

After World War I, supervision of the international agreement was given to the League of Nations, through its Opium Advisory Board. This supervision has continued through a commission of the United Nations' Economic and Social Council since World War II. Thus, an addiction problem that mankind had created and shared in common evoked at least one early demonstration of the possibility of international cooperation for bringing about a common solution to such problems.[35]

It is understood that the narcotic control laws place a great responsibility on international pharmacy, emphasizing its importance from the point of view of public health. It might even be doubted that the satisfactory enforcement of the laws would be possible without the strategically distributed pharmacies, with their professional standing and their fixed place within health administration, all over the civilized world.

INTERNATIONAL PROFESSIONAL TRENDS

In the development of industrial pharmacy, of health insurance under governmental control and of laws controlling narcotics, the pharmacist had to adapt as best he could to a given situation. However, there was a wide field left to the initiative of the members of the profession that could be cultivated fruitfully on an international basis.

It was the old pharmaceutical dream of an international pharmacopeia which may be regarded as the main incentive for the creation of organized international intercourse. The *Allgemeiner deutscher Apothekerverein* (General Association of German Pharmacists) decided (in 1864) to convene an International Congress of Pharmacy to discuss matters of international pharmaceutical interest, primarily to plan an international pharmacopeia and to tackle the problem of the nostrum evil. At this first Congress, convened in Germany in 1865, the planning of international drug standards proved to be too difficult to accomplish. But the usefulness of such conferences was so obvious that the pharmaceutical congresses, once started, became a standing feature of the life of the profession.

Fédération Internationale Pharmaceutique

International Congresses of Pharmacy continued to be held every few years in various countries,[36] but there was no continuity through year-around organization or support of services through regular membership fees. Participation in a Congress was open to everyone interested in the pharmaceutical topics to be discussed, regardless of the type of affiliation with pharmacy or with a national pharmaceutical association. With adjournment of each Congress the international cooperation and communication thus established risked disruption.[37]

These handicaps of the occasional Congresses led the Dutch Pharmaceutical Association to propose (in 1908) that professional pharmaceutical associations in Europe be circularized to interest them in organizing a permanent international association of pharmacy. Two years later at the Tenth International Congress of Pharmacy in Brussels, when the Dutch suggested the

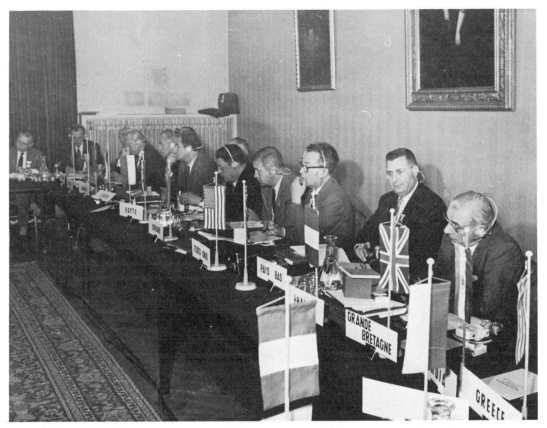

Organizational leaders of pharmacy avoid linguistic barriers by tuning headphones to one of the simultaneous translations into several languages. At this meeting of the council of the International Pharmaceutical Federation, William S. Apple, Executive Director of the American Pharmaceutical Association (2nd from right) represents the United States. (Vienna, 1962; photograph from the American Pharmaceutical Association and Foto Schikola)

founding of such an association, the suggestion won approval. It was decided to place the headquarters and the secretariat at The Hague. During 1911, promises of collaboration were gained from pharmaceutical societies around the world, culminating in an organizational meeting of delegates that summer, at which the first statutes were presented.

The new International Pharmaceutical Federation became a federation of the important national pharmaceutical associations, dedicated to the furtherance of the profession and of pharmaceutical knowledge, and seeking better collaboration and understanding on issues of common concern. The *Bulletin* of the Federation was

established (in 1912), which more recently became the *Journal Mondial de Pharmacie* (1957).

Since the federation of national associations represented a new concept of international cooperation, it was decided to continue the old International Congresses of Pharmacy for all interested pharmacists; however, the staging of the periodic Congress would be kept within the framework of the Federation.

The First General Assembly convened at The Hague in 1912, thus giving new expression to pharmacy as a world-wide brotherhood dedicated to providing the same responsible services wherever civilization thrives. After the Third General Assembly, and before the Federation had matured, World War I and its aftermath reduced activities largely to keeping a foundation intact.

Between the two World Wars, the International Pharmaceutical Federation came of age. Its assemblies were increasingly well-attended and productive. It gave pharmacy an organized link with international bodies of related professions and with intergovernmental agencies. It continued to foster efforts toward unifying drug standards internationally. A Federation commission studied the control of medicaments aboard ships at sea and, in 1934, issued the International Ships' Formulary. A Scientific Section was established (1926), and the later development of other sections permits special-interest meetings and studies that, for Americans, resemble the modern structure of the American Pharmaceutical Association. Pharmacy leaders were gaining new insight into the varied national guises in which common problems could be posed and could be attacked.

Then a harbinger of catastrophe met the Federation in 1939 when the Assembly scheduled for Berlin had to be abandoned. In the following year the Germans overran Holland, and the Federation headquarters had to go underground. With the war's end, the records were pulled back together and the representatives of the Federation were recalled, activities were revived (such as the International Commission on Specialties), and the revival was completed with the staging of the Twelfth General Assembly (Zurich, 1947).

The American Pharmaceutical Association became a member of the Federation in 1925, although the United States had been represented recurrently at the International Congresses since 1867. After sharing with the country at large a period of relative isolationism, American pharmacy entered the present period of active collaboration and support of the International Federation during the early 1950's under the leadership particularly of Don E. Francke of Michigan, a distinguished editor and practitioner in hospital pharmacy. A large group of American pharmacists have linked themselves with other pharmacists internationally through Associate Membership. During the past decade or so, a number of them attend each biennial General Assembly, as do the delegates officially representing the American Pharmaceutical Association. At a recent typical Assembly these pharmacists met their counterparts among more than 2,000 representatives of 35 countries.[38]

As a junior counterpart of the International Federation, the International Pharmaceutical Students' Federation was organized in 1949 by 24 students from 11 countries meeting in London. The national organizations of pharmacy students are federated into the "IPSF" as full members; individual pharmacy students of the world may affiliate as associate members. In 1962 there were 29 member nations, including the United States.

The Students' Federation promotes the interests of pharmacy students, encourages international cooperation among students, holds a study-tour in a different country nearly every year and publishes an *IPSF News Bulletin*. Students convened their eighth study-tour and Congress at Barcelona in 1962. One of the most significant accomplishments of the Students' Federation has been a developing exchange program, which permits selected pharmacy students and young graduates to experience life and pharmaceutical work in another country for a time, at low cost.[39]

The international pharmaceutical congresses, as well as the International Federation, have done remarkable work. Not only have they discussed almost all questions of general pharmaceutical interest but, more important, they have proved the necessity of such an international intercourse. The Federation has organized many inquiries and investigations, and publication of the results in the *Bulletin* of the Federation, has given to pharmacy an invaluable fund of information. By representing and expressing a pharmaceutical world ideology, they have brought the concept of pharmacy as a profession, and the importance to public welfare of its professional status, to the knowledge and the appreciation of all governments of the civilized world.

Unification of Drug Standards

Why the unification of drug standards internationally has persisted so long as a pharmaceutical ambition and effort has been epitomized by the British pharmacopeial expert, C. H. Hampshire:

Differences in national standards for widely used materials are a hindrance to the spread of medical knowledge, an inconvenience to pharmacists who have to dispense prescriptions brought from various countries, a source of trouble and possibly of danger to travellers. . . . An International Pharmacopoeia will help to resolve these difficulties, will tend to economy of production and will facilitate commerce in drugs between the nations.[40]

As we noted, from the beginning of the International Congresses of Pharmacy, there was concern about the international tangle of diverse names for medication of the same specification, and about diverse specifications for medication of the same name. An international pharmacopeia came before the Congress in 1885, but never found acceptance. Henceforth, efforts to achieve effective influence concentrated on the more potent drugs.

At the only international pharmaceutical congress so far held on American soil, at the initiative of the American Pharmaceutical Association and with its active support, practical steps were taken toward making more uniform at least some of the potent drugs listed with different strengths in the various national pharmacopeias.

At the Chicago congress in 1893, the idea of an international code of potent medicaments was supported by the American Pharmaceutical Association, and was backed by its contribution of $1,000 to launch the undertaking. The delegates of 18 countries agreed on the principles of such a code,[41] and in 1906 the first convention concerning the unification of potent medicaments met. The *Protocole International* (also called "P.I." and "International Formulary") was signed. A revision and enlargement of this formulary (by the Federation's committee for pharmaceutical nomenclature) was accepted by the second international conference on the unification of potent medicaments (signed on behalf of 26 countries, including the United States of America) and was completed in 1929. These efforts were hampered by the disruptive effect of two World Wars, and, although the agreements achieved had a constructive influence, they seem not to have been as far-reaching in their influence as sanguine proponents had expected.

The 1929 agreement applied mainly to standards for 27 potent drugs and preparations, methods of preparation, nomenclature and maximum doses. Another important clause of the agreement proposed the continuing of such endeavors through the medium of the League of Nations and the establishment of a permanent secretariat for that purpose within the League's Health Organization. As a consequence, the League of Nations set up in 1937 a Technical Commission of Pharmacopoeial Experts, which held its first meeting the next year.

When World War II struck, it shattered this promising new medium of collaboration, as it did much else in European life. Some technical work for the Commission was kept alive through the war, especially by British and American representatives.[42] Postwar work built on the foundation from previous decades, finding a new home within the World Health Organization that emerged in 1946 as a part of the United Nations. Several previous members of the defunct League's Technical Commission could be called on to help to form the W. H. O. Expert Committee on the Unification of Pharmacopoeias. It first met in 1947 and, "by all odds, has been the most active of all such W. H. O. expert groups ever since." This Committee is aided (since 1950) by an Expert Advisory Panel on the International Pharmacopoeia, comprised of experts on drug standards from all parts of the world, serving on a voluntary basis. Administrative head of this endeavor (since 1948) is the pharmacist and pharmacopeial expert, Paul Blanc, chief of the Pharmaceutical Section

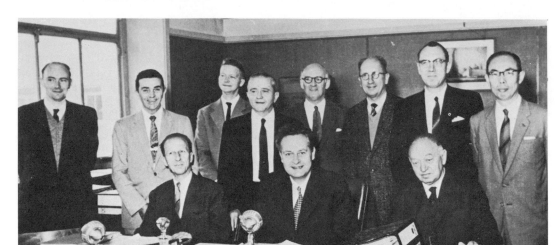

The Expert Committee on the *International Pharmacopoeia* gathers for its 15th session, at the United Nations' facilities in Geneva. (*Left to right, seated*) P. Blanc (chief of W. H. O. Pharmaceutical Section, Geneva); T. Canbäck (Stockholm); H. Baggesgaard-Rasmussen (Copenhagen); (*standing*) G. R. Brown (consultant, London); F. A. Maurina (Detroit); O. Wallén (consultant, Stockholm); J. L. Powers (Washington, D. C.); T. C. Denston (London); H. Flück (Zürich); L. C. Miller (New York); and T. Itai (Tokyo). R. Hazard (Paris) not present. (From Dr. Maurina, Parke, Davis & Co., 1957)

of the World Health Organization in Geneva. The American pharmacist and then U.S.P. chairman, E. Fullerton Cook of Philadelphia, served as a member of the small expert committee that held the main responsibility for pharmacopeial work in the League of Nations and later in the United Nations (W. H. O.). His contribution has been carried forward by other Americans.

As a fruit of this work there appeared the first edition of *Pharmacopoea Internationalis* (published by the World Health Organization, Geneva), Volume I in 1951, Volume II in 1955 and the first supplemental volume in 1959. The W. H. O. edition appeared in English, French and Spanish, and other translations have been published in German and Japanese.

In accord with a resolution of the Third World Health Assembly, the International Pharmacopoeia ("Ph.I.") is presented as "a collection of recommended specifications, which are not intended to have legal status as such in any country, but are offered to serve as references so that national specifications can be established on a similar basis in any country."* Thus, the International Pharmacopoeia is not a pharmacopeia in any legal sense, and for that reason officials of the Pharmacopeia of the United States objected to the title as adopted.[43] It is actually a compendium of suggestions, and the fact that it is the work of representatives of a limited number of countries makes the use of the term *internationalis* the expression of a worthwhile goal rather than the statement of global acceptance.

The World Health Organization also has developed a supplementary project through a Subcommittee (of the Expert Committee) on International Non-Proprietary Names.

* Pharmacopoea Internationalis, Supp., Geneva, 1959, p. xx.

The Subcommittee mainly tries to attain international agreement on common or public names for new drugs (trying to avoid conflict with trademarked names) and to publicize their selections, with the aim of fostering a more standardized and rational pharmaceutical nomenclature. The multiplicity of nonproprietary names for drugs has been, on record, a matter of international concern among pharmacists since 1892. The program is said to have met with "universal approval" except for the United States, where there is an unusually intense fear that scientific names may dilute the benefits of brand-name advertising. Also American legal counsel has considered the program to be "contrary to principles of international law."[44]

International Groups of Specialized Scope

Because fully developed professions and sciences are predominantly international, rather than national, in their knowledge, ethos, technics and services, they have been particularly prone to ignore artificial political boundaries in spheres of specialized interest. Countertendencies are the cultural (including linguistic) differences and the fact that while the "space age" has banished the handicap of time, it has not banished cost in spanning great distances. For such reasons, pharmaceutical workers have established supranational assemblies that are limited to a specific cultural region of the world rather than being global—perhaps encouraged by the circumstance that the International Pharmaceutical Federation itself has tended to be more European in cast than is suggested by its global concept.

Among the periodic regional congresses, nations of the Americas find common pharmaceutical ground in a triennial Pan-American Congress of Pharmacy and Biochemistry. Leadership in organizing the first such Congress in 1948, which was attended in Havana by delegates from most of the countries of both North and South America, including the United States, fell to the energetic Cuban pharmacist, Hector Zayas-Bazán. By 1963 six such Pan-American Congresses of Pharmacy had been held.[45] As Alejandro Orfila of the Pan American Union pointed out on the occasion of the Fourth Congress, at Washington, D. C.:

This Congress—by its very name and composition—is a living example of the broad, all-inclusive scope and influence of the Pan American movement of the 20th century. We can multiply this example many times; for this Congress is only 1 of 12 inter-American conferences that will take place during the present month in 10 different countries of the Western Hemisphere.[46]

Standing regulations and by-laws were adopted (also at the 1957 Congress) for a continuing agency, consisting of national associations in the Americas and functioning as a Pan-American Pharmaceutical and Biochemical Federation between meetings (Congresses). This pattern of inter-American cooperation among pharmacists and pharmaceutical workers now seems to be permanently established and finds its main role in matters of common pharmaceutical concern. The biochemical aspect is to be understood mainly in terms of the clinical chemistry that has been so closely associated in South America with pharmaceutically-trained personnel.

Similar regional congresses have been staged by countries of the Near and the Middle East, for both professional and scientific interchange. The First Middle East Pharmaceutical Conference was held in Lebanon in 1956, with 11 nations represented.[47]

Other international congresses that are part of the organized development of pharmacy have been restricted in scope by the subject rather than by geography. These have included an International Congress of Military Medicine and Pharmacy (first meeting in 1921, at Brussels), an international union of pharmaceutical employees (first meeting in 1925, at Vienna), International Congress for Hospital Pharmacy (first meeting in 1953, at Basel), and international congresses for the history of pharmacy (first meeting in 1934, at Basel, sponsored by the Gesellschaft für Geschichte der Pharmazie). Since 1952, international historical meetings also have been staged by the World Union of Societies for

Pharmaceutical History, in conjunction with F.I.P. General Assemblies.

AWARENESS OF HERITAGE

Because pharmacists are convinced that they have in common the task of serving public health and welfare, their international agreements, congresses and associations of various kinds have by their very nature been based on professional ethics and hence have had a cultural tendency. One trend, particularly, has brought together members of the profession all over the civilized world on exclusively cultural grounds, and has gained recognition as an indisputable basis for a truly professional conscience and atmosphere: the pharmaceutico-historical movement.

Written History

By the 18th century, pharmacy was sufficiently aware of itself, and sufficiently mature, to begin to capture what it had accomplished and experienced as a part of the recorded history of our civilization. One of the early attempts was a local history appearing at Nuremberg.[48] Shortly after 1800 we find essays on pharmacy's history as the introductory part of several textbooks, for example, those of J. C. Wiegleb, J. Fr. Gmelin and J. B. Trommsdorff. J. A. Buchner's textbook (*Vollständiger Inbegriff der Pharmacie*, 1822-1827) contains a more elaborate sketch. In his history of chemistry (1843-1847), H. Kopp pays much attention to pharmacy.

The first comprehensive history of pharmacy was published by the Frenchman Adrian Philippe (1853; with a German version by J. F. H. Ludwig). However, the epoch of historical research and interest really began with the work of three great German pharmaceutical historians: Julius Berendes (1837-1914), Hermann Peters (1847-1920) and especially Hermann Schelenz (1848-1922), whose voluminous history of pharmacy (*Geschichte der Pharmazie*, 1904) presents such an inexhaustible treasure of information that the original edition was reprinted after more than a half century (1961).[49] Since that time a

flood of historical literature, including several national histories quoted in earlier chapters, has appeared. Bibliographies are readily available to guide the interested reader to the rich store of historical literature about the pharmaceutical profession, science and industry that is being built up.[50]

History in Artifacts

Hermann Peters took steps toward the establishment of a pharmaceutical museum within the *Germanisches Museum* in Nuremberg (1883).[51] His example found many successors. Häfliger lists no less than 230 European public and private pharmaceutico-historical collections, including museums or monasteries and hospitals which display rare old pharmaceutical equipment.[52] Through the American Institute of the History of Pharmacy, Griffenhagen has published guides to museum collections in America and, also, to pharmacy museums overseas (see Appendix 5).[53] Three examples of remarkable collections about pharmacy, each quite distinct in character, are at Basel, Switzerland (begun by Häfliger at the University in 1924), at London, England (opened in 1913 by the pharmacist Sir Henry Wellcome as part of the Wellcome Historical Medical Museum) and at Washington, D. C. (developed mainly after 1919 as part of the present Division of Medical Sciences in the Smithsonian Institution).

An international guide for visiting or reading about museum collections dedicated to pharmacy appears as Appendix 5.

Organized Endeavor

The first European society devoted especially to the history of pharmacy was founded in Paris (1913): *La Société d'histoire de la pharmacie*. Since then it has published a remarkable *Bulletin*, appearing since 1930 under the title *Revue d'histoire de la pharmacie*. Thirteen years later (1926) an Austrian, three Germans and an American founded the Germanic *Gesellschaft für Geschichte der Pharmazie* (Society for the History of Pharmacy). This society took up the task of publishing books and pamphlets, setting a high standard that has been maintained to the present day. More or less

dormant between 1939 and 1949, the Gesellschaft resumed with a meeting attended not
only by Germans but also by French, English, Swiss, Dutch and Scandinavian pharmacists, which testifies to the international
recognition of its work and to unifying
tendencies which it expresses and promotes.
On this ground (1949) the *Gesellschaft*
added the significant adjective "international" to its name (*Internationale Gesellschaft für Geschichte der Pharmazie*).

The credit for having been the first country to make the history of pharmacy a
required part of the pharmaceutical curriculum goes to Spain. In 1923, the Austrian
government made the history of pharmacy
an obligatory part of the pharmaceutical
curriculum and appointed lecturers on this
subject at the three universities of the country (Vienna, Graz and Innsbruck). In Germany lectures on the history of pharmacy
were delivered at the University of Berlin
beginning in 1926. Meanwhile, significant
programs in pharmaceutical history have
developed in other German universities
such as Braunschweig, Marburg and Kiel,
and in other countries, such as France,
Holland, Yugoslavia, Czechoslovakia, England, Italy, Argentina, Brazil, Canada and
the United States of America. At least half
the American schools (including Puerto
Rico) offer a course in pharmaceutical history[54] to provide students with an understanding of the development of their profession and the genesis of some of its
achievements and its issues.

There have been other American efforts
in the same direction, led particularly by
the two original authors of the present book.
As early as 1904 Edward Kremers insti-
gated the establishment of a Section on
Historical Pharmacy in the American Pharmaceutical Association, which has meanwhile served as an annual forum for presenting and discussing papers on the
profession's past.[55] At the University of
Wisconsin Kremers was also responsible for
developing a course in the history of pharmacy, for creating a pharmacy museum and
for bringing to Madison George Urdang, a
distinguished pharmacist and historian,
who had fled Nazi Germany in 1938. Here

Urdang helped to found the American Institute of the History of Pharmacy (as he
had the *Gesellschaft* in Germany), and as
the Institute's first Director (1941-1957),
he made this national society and center for
research and publication a humanistic force
in American pharmacy. Impressed by Urdang's erudition and writings, the University of Wisconsin extended to him (1947)
a full professorship and the authority to
train the first American pharmacists to the
Doctor of Philosophy level as pharmaceutical historians.[56]

At the first Pan-American Congress of
Pharmacy, the Institute was recognized as
the "Pan-American research center in the
history of pharmacy." Beyond the Americas,
the Institute's first Director stimulated
ideas and organizations and inspired men
in many lands. By mid-century Urdang and
his counterparts overseas could rightfully
speak of an international movement toward
activities and appreciation for pharmacy in
its historical and cultural relations to civilization. Urdang wrote:

For many years this writer has cherished the
hope that some day there would be national
associations (societies, institutes, etc.) devoted
to the history of pharmacy in a sufficient number of countries to make possible a world
organization, a kind of "entente cordiale" for
the worldwide exchange of ideas, for publication and for world congresses every two or
three years in one of the member countries.
The list of national pharmaceutico-historical
groups seems to be comprehensive enough for
the realization of such a superstructure. Furthermore, the mere existence of a world organization for the history of pharmacy would,
in the long run, be an incentive for the founding of historical associations in countries still
without one. . . .[57]

At that time Urdang was working with
colleagues abroad—particularly two pharmacists and historians of Holland, P. H.
Brans and D. A. Wittop-Koning—to make
this idea a reality, and in May 1952 a World
Union of Societies for Pharmaceutical History was founded by constituent national
societies of France, Spain, the Benelux and
the United States of America. Within 4
years the World Union, as a "roof organiza-

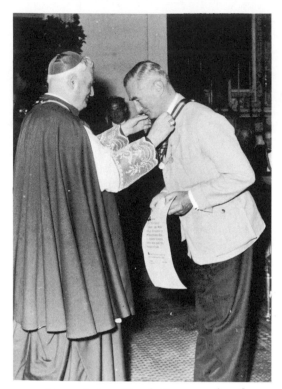

At an International Congress for the History of Pharmacy (Rome, 1954), Bishop Giordani confers the honorary membership of the Nobile Collegio Chimico-Farmaceutico on Sir Hugh Linstead, a British pharmacist. Sir Hugh has served as Senior Secretary of the Pharmaceutical Society of Great Britain (since 1926), President of the International Pharmaceutical Federation (since 1954) and as a member of Parliament (since 1942). (From Federazione Ordini Farmacisti Italiani, and Surlano Studio, Rome)

tion," linked historical societies of 12 countries.

The Union was intended to strengthen organized endeavor among all those interested; the International Academy of the History of Pharmacy was created to honor and bring into closer collaboration those historians judged by their colleagues to be working at a particularly high level of scholarship in their respective countries. Only two persons from each country may hold full membership simultaneously. The idea for this more elite organization has been put forward by G. E. Dann of Germany, president of the *Gesellschaft* and, like Urdang, one of the elder statesmen of this sphere of the world of pharmacy. Again with the assistance of Wittop-Koning and Brans in The Netherlands, where the secretariat of both organizations has been placed, the Academy was founded on the seventieth birthday of George Urdang, who became the Academy's first president and, later, honorary president for life.

Although some pharmaceutical historians have differed from Urdang in their view of the relative roles of the World Union and the Academy, a basic distinction was expressed by P. H. Brans when he said, "On the part of the Academy, one may consider it a horizontal world organization [of elected peers], while there is also a vertical world organization, a Union, which unites all the pharmaceutico-historical societies of the world."[58]

This uniting tendency, leaping national boundaries, reflects a community of tasks that creates professional solidarity among pharmacists in various spheres of their lifework. The basic strivings find roots in a common professional idealism internationally; someday, indeed, looking back on the history of our own decades, it may seem that the values and the issues that make a difference to pharmacy's status in society were more divergent and discordant within than between individual countries of the world of pharmacy.

For a century there have been developing at diverse levels of human thought and activity more threads of international contact and cooperation, despite disruptive wars and conflicting social philosophies. Pharmacy has participated in this development and has been affected by it. In the future, the grave—if not desperate—need to give more substance to the age-old dream of a brotherhood or "one world" of man will probably give still more significance within the pharmaceutical segment of that world to the term "international trends," of which we have mentioned a few examples.

Speaking before the American Pharmaceutical Association as president of the

International Pharmaceutical Federation, Sir Hugh Linstead observed:

In spite of the special example of some of the newly born countries, it is broadly true to say that the 19th century was a century of nationalism while the 20th century is a century of internationalism. We in Europe are moving fairly rapidly towards the integration of that continent just as you in the Americas are groping towards closer unity between the United States and Central and Southern America. Similar tendencies are showing themselves in embryo in Africa and among the Arab States.

Within these large international movements there are moves to secure closer coopera- tion and understanding between professional groups. You have your Pan-American Congress of Pharmacy, we have in Europe a committee representing the pharmaceutical organizations of the six countries of the European Economic Community. I have only this month had the privilege of attending the Eighth Pan-Arabic Congress in Cairo. The oldest organization in this field is of course the International Pharmaceutical Federation . . . ; [and though we have not] yet found the answer to the coordination of professional pharmacy internationally . . . our problems are essentially the same in every country; our ideals are the same; all of us are bound to profit from an increasing interchange of experience and ideas which modern communications make possible.[59]

Part Three

Pharmacy in the United States

SECTION ONE
The Period of Unorganized Development

9: The North American Colonies

THE SPREAD OF EUROPEAN SETTLEMENTS

When the Italian Cristoforo Colombo sighted land in the Bahamas off the coast of Florida, he thought excitedly that he had reached the wealth of the East Indies. In common with other explorers of his day, he had dreamed of precious spices, gold and gems, and he had hoped to bring them back for his employers, the king and queen of Spain. Columbus never knew that he had discovered a new world offering to old Europe more than mercantile goods: new homes for many millions of people and a refuge for the persecuted and oppressed. In America, for the first time in recorded history, it has been proved that with soil and climate favorable a new commonwealth and culture can be developed on the basis of the freedom of the individual.

It required centuries before the ideology associated with "America" became strong and sufficiently significant to form a unifying framework, a specifically American sentiment. During the first century after the discovery of the new continent, a sentiment of this kind could not arise for the simple reason that the endeavors of the European peoples with regard to America were concentrated on the quick, comprehensive and profitable exploitation of the assumed riches of the country. Even the first settlements were not intended to become agricultural colonies. They were established to organize the fur trade and to export ginseng, timber and other valuable goods used in the old countries or to be used in exchange for goods from the Orient. However, in 1608, John Smith wrote from Virginia to the London corporation (which owned the land by Royal charter) to the effect that "here was a land, unlike Mexico and Peru, that would yield only to toil; that held no spoil for the predatory classes of Europe."[1]

With the beginning of the 17th century, North America gradually became a land for colonization, instead of a collection of colonies destined for exploitation by European sovereigns.

Among the European colonizing nations, Spain*, France and England particularly left their early political impress on the civilization that developed within the territory that has become the United States of America. Spanish influence was felt in the area now included in Florida, Louisiana, Texas and the Southwest, and it is still dominant in Puerto Rico. Characteristic of the relatively small attention paid to North America by European governments during the first century after its discovery, there were no settlements in this area until St. Augustine, Florida, was settled by the Spaniards in 1565. It remained the only abode of white men in this vast area until Spaniards from Mexico settled in New Mexico in 1598.[2]

French influence manifested itself north of the St. Lawrence river and along the Great Lakes, penetrated the wilds of Michigan and Wisconsin and the prairies of Illinois, and drifted down the Mississippi to Louisiana, which was originally a French territory, named in honor of Louis XIV. English civilization remained the dominant factor in the thirteen original colonies and throughout the vast domain west of the Alleghenies, and later beyond the Mississippi and the Rockies.

---

* For an excellent summary of the Spanish contribution to the history of pharmacy, of particular interest here because of its influence on Spanish-held territories of America, see Chapter 6 of the Second Edition (p. 97), which may be consulted in most pharmacy libraries. The chapter was prepared by the distinguished pharmacist-historians at the University of Madrid, Professors Guillermo Folch Jou and Rafael Folch Andreu. To restrict the present textbook edition to a scope feasible for the usual instructional program, it has been expedient to omit the chapter.

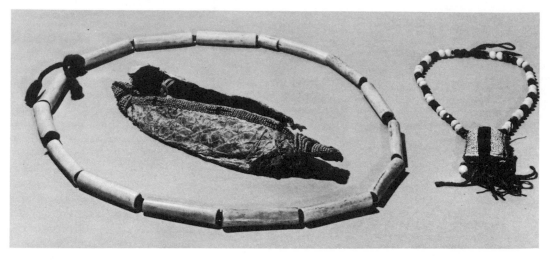

The medicine man of the American Indians relied heavily on his command of the spirit powers—although Europeans on both sides of the Atlantic found therapeutic activity, real or imagined, in various botanic substances which he used. In the photograph, three aspects of Indian medicine are illustrated: (1) The individual bone tubes in the necklace (left) could be used by the medicine man (Chippewa "juggler") to suck disease-causing foreign matter or spirits out of the body. (2) Lying within the necklace is a diuretic device (Menominee) consisting of a wood twig covered with blue cloth, which is encased in a bladder ornamented with beadwork. The patient drinks hot water in which this device has been boiled. (3) The amulet bag on a beaded cord (right) could be worn to fend off or help overcome disease. (From the State Historical Society of Wisconsin; Joan Freeman, Anthropologist)

Dutch influence acquired an early footing in New Amsterdam and continued to play an important part there long after this city had become New York. Although Germany does not figure among the colonizing nations, Germans contributed a considerable number of colonists to Penn's woods (shown, for example, by the name of Germantown, now a part of Philadelphia).[3] To a slight extent, Swedish influence had gained a footing on the Delaware even before the Dutch and William Penn's coreligionists, the so called Quakers, took possession.

DEVELOPMENT OF PHARMACEUTICAL PRACTICE

Drugs in the New World

The early development of pharmacy in the colonies went hand in hand with medical practice. It would be impossible to assign to each nation its quota in the development of this medicopharmaceutical practice. Often it was not even in the hands of medical practitioners. Men of other professions or women, who have played an important part in the primitive and pioneer medical practice of all peoples, served as pharmacists.

Naturally, it is of great pharmaceutical and medical interest to learn which indigenous drugs were known and used by the American aborigines. In South America, under European exploitation, the search for aromatics, spices and medicinal plants started immediately after the discovery of the new continent, but in North America, the land of colonization, this search began almost a century later.

The knowledge of drugs and of their medicinal use varied with the cultural levels of various Indian tribes. Several lists of drugs have been made on the basis of research and inquiry among these tribes[4] (see the tabulation in Appendix 1). The Maya Indians had an extensive botanic knowledge and more than four hundred uses for botanic drugs,[5] and an Aztec,

Martin de la Cruz, compiled a herbal in the 16th century, which another Aztec, Juannes Badianus, translated into Latin (1552). The original "Badianus manuscript" (as it is now called) became one of the treasures of the Vatican Library; a facsimile has been published in an annotated American edition.[6, 7]

The knowledge of drugs used by the Indians of northern America comes from a different kind of source. These drugs and their uses can be gleaned from the accounts of explorers of the new continent, and also from early medical practitioners.[8] No less than 56 Indian drugs were still recognized in 1925 in the *United States Pharmacopoeia* or in the *National Formulary*.

It is of interest that an organized endeavor was made, during the early part of the 18th century, to transplant valuable medicinal herbs from Spanish Central and South America to Georgia. The London Society of Apothecaries, together with the Board of Trustees for the Colony of Georgia, made this attempt on the initiative of the well-known English physician Dr. Hans Sloane. The botanist Robert Miller was commissioned to secure ipecacuanha, jalap, sarsaparilla, contrayerva, cochineal and the trees producing Jesuit bark (cinchona), balsam of copaiba and tolu balsam. However, the Spaniards guarded their monopoly jealously; after 5 years of traveling and intense work Miller died in 1740 without achieving success, and the Society of the Apothecaries withdrew further subscriptions "to promote agriculture in Georgia."[9]

A more literary attempt in the same direction was made in 1769 by John Ellis, a fellow of the Royal Society and the agent for West Florida, when he published a *Catalogue of Plants That May Be Useful in America*, comprised of 82 different medicinal plants.

The list is to be found in William Stork's introduction of the fourth edition of John Bartram's "Journal." In 1770, Ellis published "Directions for bringing over seeds and plants from the East Indies and other distant countries in a state of vegetation; together with a catalogue of foreign plants worthy of being encouraged in our American Colony." This was probably one of the earliest steps taken along the lines of our present seed and plant introduction work of U. S. Department of Agriculture.[10]

Much more significant was the introduction of American drugs into the European materia medica. The first treatises on American drugs were published by Nicolas Monardes, a physician in Seville. The title of the complete work (1574) was *Historia Medicinal de las Cosas que se Traen de Nuestras Indias Occidentales, que Sirven en Medicina*. It is significant of the great interest in the medicinal and the botanic treasures of the New World that new editions soon followed. As early as 1574, Carolus Clusius published a Latin translation in Antwerp, which in turn was translated into other languages.[11] Monardes himself (1493-1578) never had been in South America, but, living in one of the principal ports for imports from the "Occidental Indies," he had opportunity to collect much information about new medicinal plants and to secure samples of the drugs.

Other such works followed. Among them was Francisco Hernandez's *Quatro libros de la naturaleza y virtudes de las plantas y animales que estan recevidos en el uso de medicina en la Nueva Espana . . .* (Mexico, 1615). Guielmo Piso's *De medicina Brasilensi libri 4* appeared in Amsterdam (1648) and William Hughes' *The American Physician, or a treatise of the roots, plants, trees, shrubs, fruit, herbs, etc. growing in the British Plantations in America* was published in London (1672). In Paris appeared a *Traité ou Abrégé des Plantes Usuelles des Domingue,* which included an extensive section called *Pharmacopée Americaine . . .,* by Pouppé Desportes (1770).[12] The German materia medica likewise absorbed strange plants brought from the New World, and, throughout Europe, hope for a new therapeutic resource spawned optimistic reports.[13]

Of these drugs cinchona deserves special mention. However, it should be noted that the use of cinchona by the natives appears to be improbable, since Alexander von Humboldt and other explorers did not find the bark in the medicine bags of Indian medicine men. Credit for discovering the specific value of cinchona in treating malaria, it is now assumed, probably goes to the Jesuits. Introduction of the drug to Europe once was attributed to the supposed cure of the wife of the Spanish viceroy in Lima, Peru (the Count of Chinchon) by cinchona bark given on the advice of native Indians, but this romantic legend has long since been discredited.[14]

New Spain

Columbus and those explorers of the new continent who succeeded him could be expected to pay attention to the medicinal uses of plants, and their special interest in the spice trade is well known.

During his first voyage (1492-1493), Columbus was accompanied by a surgeon, but neither his name nor his journal has been preserved. The admiral himself diligently wrote a journal until the day of his return to Palos, to which Las Casas (1474-1566) still had access when he wrote his history of the Indies.[15] The second expedition of Columbus included a surgeon and Doctor Chanca, a physician. The latter wrote (1493) a letter to the Chapter of Seville containing a few remarks on drugs.[16] He mentions cotton, turpentine, tragacanth, nutmeg, ginger, aloes, cinnamon, mirobalans and mastic.

The works of Badianus, Monardes, Hernandez and others indicate that the Spaniards were interested in pharmaceutical matters throughout the colonial period. However, their greatest impact on the pharmacy of North America came during the 28 years that Spain controlled the vast territory of Louisiana.

On February 12, 1770, Don Alexandre O Reilly, governer of Louisiana, issued an edict regulating the practice of surgery that contains the first legal definition of pharmacy, as a separate branch of medicine, to be issued in North America:

Medicine . . . embraces three parts, namely: medicine proper, which is the science of recognizing diseases and the relation which they have with remedies, and of prescribing the latter together with the diet. The other two parts, which are surgery and pharmacy, are its attendants and have their special field. Surgery includes the use in general of hands and of external remedies. Pharmacy is concerned, generally speaking, with the preparation of remedies.[17]

The Rudolph Matas History of Medicine in Louisiana, under the editorship of John Duffy, reveals that O Reilly's interest in pharmacy was not fortuitous. The Spanish regulated medicine and pharmacy more strictly than did the French who preceded them in Louisiana. Records indicate that the Spanish required that a chief pharmacist be responsible for compounding prescriptions in all colonial hospitals. More important, in 1769 one Jean Peyroux was examined in materia medica by the Royal Physician and was given a certificate to operate a pharmacy. He is the first pharmacist known to have been examined and licensed within the territorial limits of what is now the United States.

Peyroux's certification was based on his acceptance of seven conditions: to maintain what might be called a poison register; to notify the authorities of drugs purchased by him; to dispense them at honest and reasonable fees; to compound prescriptions exactly as written; to submit to the "code of Paris"; to compound medicines on prescription but not prescribe them himself; to agree to inspection of his stock by the Royal Physician. These requirements—so reminiscent of professional oaths often required of European pharmacists—were intended by Don Alexandre to apply to all pharmacists. The names of four additional pharmacists who submitted to examination during the Spanish period are known. In one instance (1792) examination was by a board of two pharmacists, in others, by a board of from one to three pharmacists, together with physicians and surgeons (or at least in their presence). Probably more pharmacists than the five known presently were examined and licensed under the Spanish regulation.

New France

From the time Cartier sailed up the St. Lawrence (1535) until the first family effected permanent settlement (1617), New France was visited by explorers, fur traders and missionaries, seeking glory, wealth and the extension of Christianity. The credit of being the first real French settler in America belongs to a pharmacist, Louis Hébert. For this reason he has been designated (next to the explorer, founder and governor of Canada, Samuel de Champlain) as the "father of New France."

Champlain saw the necessity of establishing homes if the French settlement was to be permanent. He finally induced Hébert, who had been with him on his first trip to New France (1604), to establish his home in the new country. It is indicative of the pioneer character of Hébert that he again and again left security and his regular profession, following the voice of what he considered to be his proper vocation. He had been born in Paris, the son of a well-known pharmacist; he possessed a pharmacy of his own on the banks of the Seine, but he sold it[18] to go to Port Royal (now Annapolis Royal, Nova Scotia) with the expedition of De Monts. Hébert arrived there with 50 other colonists in 1606. When the English destroyed the place and took over the land, Hébert returned to Paris and reopened his shop. However, when his friend Champlain decided to establish a new colony, to be called Quebec, and asked Hébert to accompany him, the courageous pharmacist sold his possessions once more and migrated to Quebec in 1617 with his family, his household goods and a small store of drugs. Hébert well knew from his previous experience that he would have to devote himself to husbandry. We are told of his cattle and his apple trees, "the first to be planted in America."[19] He also made a study of the indigenous grapes, which he cultivated and improved.

On the other hand, the fur company, which had been induced by Champlain to support Hébert and his family for 3 years, had required his bond for free medical attention at all times to the settlers and the clerks employed by the company. Thus, while devoting his time primarily to the cultivation of the soil and to the study of the native plants of his new home, Hébert

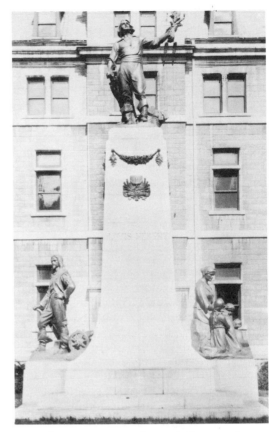

The monument to Louis Hébert in the city of Quebec (between City Hall Garden and Saint Anne Street) shows the French pharmacist holding aloft the first sheaf of wheat harvested from Canadian soil. At the base (right) his wife is also depicted in bronze, teaching the children of the first colonists, while a statue of Hébert's son-in-law stands on the left. The sculptor was Alfred Laliberté.

put to good use his pharmaceutical skill as well as his supply of drugs brought from France. With and without contract obligation, he tried to help in Quebec as he had previously helped in Annapolis (Port) Royal.

Hébert was royal procurator for a time and received, simultaneously with the grant of a large fief, the title of Sieur de L'Espinay. His activity was cut short after 10 years by an accident which caused his death. Canada honored the memory of Hébert, this earliest and eminent pioneer, by erecting a monument to him in Quebec (1917). "His work as the first pharmacist to settle in North America is commemorated by a tablet in the town hall of Annapolis Royal, Nova Scotia."[20] Hébert was succeeded by Giffard, a surgeon, who, following Hébert's example, cultivated the soil.

The activity of the *Soeurs hospitaliers* (Sisters of Charity) and of the Jesuit missionaries was important in developing early medicine and pharmacy in New France. Four of the important documents connected with the early history of pharmacy there are lists of drugs and medicaments, which were sent to Paris by the sisters of the hospital at Quebec (1664 to 1668) with requests for new supplies. These lists reveal a rather extensive materia medica for so early a period in the development of a distant colony.[21] It may be assumed that the colonists also were supplied from any surplus in the medicine chests of vessels from French ports.[22]

Whereas both the pharmacist Hébert and the surgeon Giffard as farmers, and the *Soeurs hospitaliers* of necessity, led a settled life, the Jesuit missionaries often led an itinerant life among the Indians and the trappers; however, some of them occupied semipermanent stations at such outposts as De Pere and Sault Ste. Marie. With the advancement of the colony, some of them occupied permanent positions at colleges and other institutions. Thus the *Catalogue of Persons and Officers in the Society of Jesus for the Province of France at the end of the year 1749* mentions two *pharmacopoles* or apothecary-brethren: Charles Boispineau, of Aquitaine, stationed at the college of Quebec, and Jean François Parisel, whose residence is given as The Isle of Orleans.

The itinerant missionaries made the best use of such medical and pharmaceutical knowledge as they possessed in befriending the Red Man. In the instance of Father Hennepin, who was a member of La Salle's party which explored the Great West in 1680, specific examples of such practice are recorded.[23] In their reports to superiors, these Jesuit missionaries also occasionally mentioned the use of drugs by the Indians. During one expedition south of the Great Lakes, the Father was taken by his Indian guides to a spring that was not only salty but had a film of oil on its surface. The salt water was used by the Indians as a purgative, the oil as a remedy against rheumatism. Another Jesuit, Father Lafitau, discovered ginseng in Canada and wrote a detailed account of this plant and drug.[24]

In French Louisiana a "physic garden," growing imported herbs mainly, was begun as early as 1724 in New Orleans. Its overseer, Sieur Dameron, also had charge of a "laboratory" in which medicines for the garrison and the hospitals were produced. At least two surgeon-apothecaries are known to have been in New Orleans at this time; one of them, Sieur Bernard Alexandre, may have first suggested establishment of the laboratory, which probably was located in the Royal Hospital. In general, hospital pharmacy became the responsibility of the Ursuline Sisters and remained so until after the arrival of the Spanish.[25]

In his Creole stories, G. W. Cable gives an interesting account of social conditions of the former French colony of Louisiana toward the close of the 18th and the beginning of the 19th centuries. An Alsatian pharmacist is one of his heroes.[26]

In 1803, the territory of Louisiana—which included much more territory than the present state of Louisiana—became by purchase a part of the United States of America. Thus ended New France as a political unit, though the romantic history of the French settlers and *coureurs de bois* continued on the St. Lawrence, throughout the Great Lake region and down the Mississippi.

New Sweden and New Netherlands

The political units of New Sweden and New Netherlands were short-lived on the North American continent.

On board a Dutch vessel, Henry Hudson had sailed up the river that now bears his name in the same year (1609) that Champlain penetrated to the lake named after him. It was nearly three decades before the founding of New Sweden.

Dutch settlers followed the early explorers and fur traders and, in 1626, Peter

Minuit transacted the well-known real estate deal in which he bought Manhattan Island from the Indians for about $25. The colony was prosperous and an example of tolerance, permitting the settlement of persons of all nationalities and faiths.

Sweden's colony on the Delaware by 1654 comprised the territory of the present state of Delaware and parts of Pennsylvania, New Jersey and Maryland. The settlers were Finnish rather than Scandinavian.[27] In 1655 New Netherlands captured New Sweden and united it with the Dutch colony. A few years later this greater New Netherlands had to suffer a like fate at the hands of the English. It was captured by an English fleet with the Duke of York on board, and thenceforth the former New Amsterdam was called "New York." "In the further course of time, intermarriage of both Dutch and Swedes with the English settlers blended the three races in a common strain."[28]

One medical person is known to have come over from Sweden to the new colony, the barber-surgeon Hans Jancke.[29]

The first known surgeon in New Netherlands was Herman Meynders van den Boogaerdt (1631).[30] He was appointed commissary of stores at New Amsterdam and later at Fort Orange. It is not reported whether or not he dealt in drugs. Another surgeon, Gysbert van Imbroch (van Emburgh, d. 1665) "kept a shop at New Amsterdam" in 1653 and served as a "shepen" of Wildwyck.

Besides being the local physician and pharmacist, he kept a general store, and the inventory of his estate includes a wide variety of objects, from high priced books down to the commonest necessaries of life.[31]

Was Imbroch's "shop" at New Amsterdam a drugstore? It may have been a surgeon's and barber's shop. However, the "general store," carried on in Wildwyck (since 1669 called Kingston) from 1663 to 1665 may be considered one of the first drugstores in North America.

Another medical person of pharmaceutical interest in New Netherlands was the surgeon Hans Kiersted from Germany, who came to New Amsterdam with Governor Kieff (1638). For a long time he was in the employ of the Dutch West India Company. While nothing is known about a pharmacy kept by him, some of his drug formulas have survived.

Many of his descendants have been identified in the medical profession. His great-great-grandson, the late general Henry T. Kierstedt, of Harlem, at his well known drugstore on Broadway dispensed the "Kierstedt ointment," made from a recipe left by Dr. Hans.[32]

This Henry T. Kierstedt was president of the American Pharmaceutical Association (1860-1862), one of two presidents who have held the office for 2 years.[33]

New England

In North America pharmacy practiced and developed by white settlers began in New England. In 1602, Bartholomew Gosnold and his crew landed in Massachusetts to load the first cargo of New England's exports. "It consisted of the bark and pith of the sassafras tree."[34]

In 1606, King James I granted the London corporation a charter which gave to it the ownership of Virginia, at that time including all the unoccupied country between the settlements of the Spanish in Florida and those of the French in Canada. In 1607 the first English colonists sailed into Hampton Roads, and the very next year two "apothecaries," Thomas Field and John Harford, arrived. There are no records of their fate.[35] Two years later a "Table of such as are required to this Plantation" was sent by the settlers to their "Virginia Company" at London, asking for "foure honest and learned Ministers, two Surgeons, two Druggists." Letters sent to London by the settlers requested "that the Company would send them some Phisitians and Apothycaries of which they stand much need off."[36]

Whether these "Phisitians and Apothycaries" ever arrived, history does not record. However, there is an entry in the Records of the Virginia Company (1621) reading as follows:

It was signified unto the Court that an apothecary offered to transport himself and his

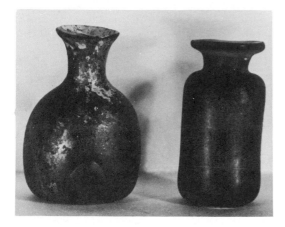

Medicine vials used by the American colonists, as unearthed by the National Park Service. A glass-bottle factory established in the woods near the Jamestown settlement (1607) has been considered to have been the earliest industrial enterprise within present United States territory. (From the National Park Service, Jamestown, Va.)

wife on his own charge to Virginia if the Company would please to give them their transport of two children . . . which offer the Council did very well like of in respect of the great want of men of his profession, and being put to the question did agree thereunto; provided that the Apothecary at his coming over did exercise his skill and practise in that profession.

According to Blanton, "there is no further record of apothecaries living in the colony in this [the 17th] century, the physician being 'for the most part his own apothecary.' "[37]

Apparently changes of occupation for financial reasons were by no means exceptional among the people coming to these shores. There is quite a record of a man by the name of Richard Townshend who, at the age of 15, was apprenticed to a Doctor Pott in Jamestown to learn "the art of an Apothecarye" and, more than 5 years later (1626) sued his master for having neglected his teaching. The court ordered that Doctor Pott "doe henceforth from time to time endeavour to teach & instruct the said Richard Townshend in ye art of an Apothecarye by all convenient wayes & means

. . . " or pay him for his services. Whatever pharmaceutical education Townshend may have received from his medical preceptor, he did not make much use of it. In 1628, 2 years after this judgment had been passed, the young man was a planter and a member of the House of Burgesses. Six years of study under the well-educated Dr. Pott, says his biographer, "set him above his fellows, among whom was little reading and writing. . . . Townshend advanced with phenomenal rapidity to the highest positions in the Colony."[38]

The records as yet unearthed prove only that in the early days of the Virginia Settlement need was felt for the presence of "druggists" and "apothycaries." They do not mention the establishment of pharmacies or of general stores dealing in drugs and performing pharmaceutical activities.

As important as the early Virginia Settlement was, as the first English foothold on the American continent, the decisive dates for English colonization are 1620 and 1628. In 1620 the Pilgrims sailed on board the Mayflower from Plymouth, landing by accident not within the limits of Virginia as they should have done according to their patent, but at a place they called Plymouth in remembrance of their English port of embarkation. In 1628, the Puritans founded Salem; they were followed a year later by 400 additional colonists and, in 1630, by the main group with governor John Winthrop, who founded Boston in the same year. This man and this town became the two most important landmarks of early American cultural life, including medicine and pharmacy.

"Medicine was promulgated, for the first hundred years of colonial America, by three types of individuals: the governors, the churchmen, and the educators."[39] As always in primitive and in pioneer society, it was practiced to a large extent by the housewives. The housewives of the early English emigrants brought their peculiar kind of knowledge and practice over from their native country. Books giving advice for self-treatment, as well as for the cultivation of herbs furnishing the drugs recommended, were much cherished and used by the English emigrants. The most important of these books were Gervase Markham's *The English Housewife* and *The English Husbandman* (1613). Then, too, there was apothecary John Parkinson's *Paradisi in sole* (1629) and *Theatrum botanicum* (1640), and especially the herbal of John Gerarde, in the edition (1636) prepared by Thomas Johnson, a "Citizen and Apothecarye of London."

Nicholas Culpeper's *The English Physician* (1652) was reprinted again and again and used for centuries, in many editions. The book is described on the title page as:

Being an Astrologo-Physical Discourse of the Vulgar Herbs of this Nation: Containing a Compleat Method of Physick. Whereby a man may preserve his body in Health, or Cure himself, being Sick, for three pence Charge with such things only as grow in England, they being most fit for English Bodies.

The American colonists planted these "English things" in their gardens.[40] Apparently the colonists were sure, since both the herbs and the "Bodies" using them had been transplanted from England, that the mysterious mutual reaction would remain in force!

In addition to these European plants, the New England housewives and others practicing medicine within the colonies used a gradually increasing number of native herbs. The kinds of native drugs employed in the first decades of the settlement we learn from William Wood's *New England's Prospect* and John Josselyn's *New England Rarities*. Of the 56 Indian drugs still holding official recognition in 1925, 30 of them had been used by the Indians of New England.[41]

The first governor of Massachusetts Colony, John Winthrop, and his son John Winthrop, Jr., first governor of Connecticut Colony, are the most outstanding examples of North American governors interested in and practicing medicine. They apparently often asked friends in England for advice on medical topics. In 1643 one of them

Pharmacopœia Londinenſis; OR, THE London Diſpenſatory FURTHER Adorned by the *STUDIES* and *Collections* of the *Fellows* now living, of the ſaid *COLLEGE*...

The first full-scale pharmaco-medical book published in British North America was introduced by this title page, dated 1720, Boston. It is an American edition of an English work written by the controversial Nicholas Culpeper, who was introduced to medicine through his apprenticeship to apothecaries. (From the National Library of Medicine)

received from London a list of "Receipts to cure various disorders,"[42] sent by Edward Stafford. These "receipts," mostly of household character, show us something of the pharmaceutical resources used. They had been drawn "from John Gerard's herbal."[43]

The younger Winthrop was a political leader of importance and at the same time an outstanding figure in the history of science in North America during the 17th century.

It is doubtful if there was any doctor of medicine in the American colonies during the 17th century who could equal Winthrop in the extent of his medical practice, in the number of his acquaintances among the leading physicians and chemists of Europe, or in the completeness of his laboratory and library.[44]

The great interest that Winthrop, Jr., took in chemistry makes understandable his use of many medicinal chemicals—such as saltpeter, preparations of antimony and mercury, tartar, copperas, white vitriol, sulphur and iron—in addition to red coral, powdered ivory, rosin, some American and European vegetable drugs and several galenics. He prepared some chemical compounds and galenics himself. Thus, he was one of the first to do real pharmaceutical work in North America.

George Starkey, a Harvard College graduate (1646) was a protégé of Winthrop. He won a great reputation as a chemical practitioner and invented numerous remedies, of which his oil of sulphur was best known. Having built a furnace in Boston, he wrote to Winthrop asking for "a little mercury and antimony." These two substances, of which especially the latter had been the subject of many a quarrel in Europe about this time (see p. 67), became "principal bases of the chemical remedies used in America for the next two centuries."[45]

A year before the death of John Winthrop, Jr., the so-called King Philip's War broke out. The Indians, under their "King" Philip, fought desperately, and there was much need of medicaments among the troops from the Bay Colony. A letter written (1676) by a surgeon who had joined the troops to the secretary of Massachusetts Bay Colony contains a list of medicaments that the writer urgently demanded. It is noteworthy that most of these items were from the London pharmacopoeia of 1650.

In all probability the articles were not compounded in the colonies but imported from England. A list of the ingredients necessary to compound the several galenicals called for reveals clearly that such was in all probability the case, for it could scarcely be expected that the "shop" or office of a colonial physician, no matter how extensive his medical practice or

his drugstore, would contain one-half of the simples necessary.[46]

There were few physicians in the New England colonies until 1700. The first apothecary who entered New England came to die rather than to live there. This Englishman, Giles Firmin of Sudbury, arrived at Boston probably toward the end of 1632 and died in 1634. Nothing is known of Firmin's opening a shop in Boston. Presumably he practiced medicine "as one of Boston's few physicians. His son became a physician as well as an apothecary."[47] It may be recalled that during this period the apothecaries in England became, more and more, general medical practitioners (see p. 97). However, the primary occupation of this first English apothecary on North American soil seems to have been preaching, and that by vocation as well as by necessity. Even the younger Firmin is quoted as having written to Governor Winthrop: "I am strongly set upon to study devinitie, my studies else must be lost, for physic is but a meene helpe."

Indeed, most of the male medical practitioners of the early colonial days seem to have resorted to other callings for a livelihood.

[Among 134 medical practitioners who settled in Massachusetts Colony before 1692] twelve and probably many more, practiced surgery; three were barber-surgeons. . . . Six or seven, probably a larger number, were ministers as well as physicians. . . . One was not only a doctor, but also schoolmaster and poet. One was a butcher, but called himself a surgeon in his will, a union of callings which suggests an obvious pleasantry.[48]

Whatever else the early medical practitioners may have done to earn their livelihood, in one particular they were no doubt alike, with few exceptions they dispensed their own medicines, unless they directed the relatives of the patient to prepare potions from indigenous or cultivated herbs or roots.

The apothecary shop, as it existed at a later period in the larger cities of the American colonies, was usually the dispensary of a more or less progressive or successful medical practitioner who occasionally deigned to enlarge on his otherwise meagre income by the sale of sundry articles like spices or tea, which at that time were counted among the luxuries of the more settled portions of the country.[49]

That the legislators in the early times of American colonization considered the dispensing of drugs by the medical practitioners as obviously necessary may be discerned in various official statements.[50]

The "general store" of the surgeon Gysbert van Imbroch at Wildwyck (Kingston), mentioned above (see p. 139), was doubtless an enlarged dispensary. William Davis (Davice) is usually considered to have been the earliest owner of a pharmacy in North America, an assumption based on an official record of 1646. According to this, the selectmen in Boston ordered for the benefit of the apothecary Davice that a payle or fence be erected before his hall window.

One of the earliest records that gives a detailed picture of the practice of a dispensing "pharmaceutical chemist" has been studied by Griffenhagen in an account book begun in 1698. Most of the income recorded by Bartholomew Browne of Salem was for dispensing medicines, but occasionally he charged for "attendance," suggesting that he was practicing medicine to a very limited extent. As was common then (and long afterward) among practitioners of the health professions, Browne took a considerable amount of produce and merchandise in exchange for his services, spent a great deal of time collecting, and still had time and need to work his own farm.

The remedy most widely used by the 200 or so patrons identified in Browne's accounts was White Samech, the neutral salt of potassium tartrate made by adding potassium carbonate to cream of tartar (335 pots). In addition, 104 pots or vials of other types of Samech, tartar combined with herbs, were dispensed. Second in popularity was an unidentified "Elixir" (326 pots). A cordial powder was dispensed on 145 occasions.

Soon after the period covered by the account book, Browne apparently turned to the practice of medicine. Thus he exemplifies not only the practice of pharmacy in the late 17th century, but also the casual migration from one profession to another and the particular lack of separation or definite standards with regard to the practice of medicine and pharmacy.[51]

EIGHTEENTH CENTURY PHARMACY

The increase in population about 1700 had its effect on the trade in drugs and other articles then sold in drugstores. As early as the first decades of the 18th century, there must have been a considerable number of apothecary shops or drugstores in North America. (There were 14 apothecary shops in Boston in 1721.) Advertisements of the owners of such stores appeared in daily and weekly newspapers. Zabdiel Boylston, reportedly the first medical practitioner in America to inoculate against smallpox and "the most meritorious physician of his day in America,"[52] industriously advertised his drugs. In the *Boston Gazette* (1723-1724), he offered "good cassia fistula, good saffron and good jalap root, juniper berries and other druggs and medicines at reasonable rates."

In 1721, "Robert Gibbs at his apothecary shop in Corn-Hill-Street, Boston," offered English Starch, fresh cinnamon and mace and "all sorts of painters colors." Thomas Aston, "next door to the governor's house, Boston," offered (1732) "all sorts of drugs and medicines" and a list of spices, tea, coffee, etc., calling himself "apothecary and grocer." The same man advertised drugs and apothecary's wares "imported in the last ship from London." Such references to the "fresh" import of drugs from London are met again and again. In 1759 at Boston, B. Church, Jr., "just arrived from London," offered to "town and country physicians etc. . . . the best medicines at the most reasonable rate, also some noted modern authors in physick, surgery and midwifery."

In the Colonies the proprietaries, which started their astounding rise in England early in the 18th century, gained enormous popularity. To the busy settler with little time and small means, these ready-made and not too high-priced remedies seemed to solve at once, conveniently, all the prob-

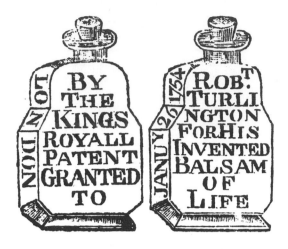

In early America, the need for simple means of therapy, ready at hand, gave English patent medicines (and, later, American imitations) a large place in medical care. Turlington's Balsam of Life was one of the most popular products and "very dear," according to a Colonial apothecary. The distinctive bottle, reproduced here from a Colonial brochure, was designed by Turlington "to prevent the villainy of . . . a vile spurious counterfeit sort." (From the Smithsonian Institution; original at the Pennsylvania Historical Society; see Griffinhagen, G., and Young, J. H.: Old English Patent Medicines in America, U. S. National Museum Bull. 218, Washington, D. C., 1959)

lems of medical and pharmaceutical aid—and even of finance—arising in sickness; the daring advertising appealed to his plain and optimistic turn of thought. Bateman's "Elixir," Godfrey's "British Oyl," Duffie's "Elixir," "Scotch Pills" and others were advertised in Colonial newspapers almost immediately after their appearance on the English market and were sold everywhere.

In these advertisements the shops are mostly referred to as "apothecary shops." Some are designated with special sign names, such as "William Rand, apothecary at the unicorn" (1733) and Ph. Godfrid Kast, "at his shop at the sign of the lyon and mortar, in Salem" (1764).

Most of the drugstores of that time—whether operated by physician-pharmacists, by the few real apothecaries or pharmacists or by the many self-styled ones—did

not restrict themselves to the sale of drugs, but dealt in every possible commodity. The sale of materials needed for the building and the upkeep of houses in rapidly growing communities—such as paints, oils, varnishes, brushes, wallpaper and glass—almost became a specialty of the American colonial drugstore.

In the *Boston Gazette* during the first half of the 18th century the greatest variety of goods advertised in connection with drugs is to be found in the advertisements of Silvester Gardiner, "one of the outstanding New England physicians before the American revolution."[53] Dr. Gardiner offered on several occasions (1748-1750) "all kinds of apothecary and grocery ware by wholesale and retail, dye stuff, painters colours, linseed oyl, etc," and a series of nostrums "by appointment of the patentees." Gardiner's stock of drugs filled over 20 wagons when it was sold at public auction, after Gardiner's escape to England during the Revolutionary War.[54]

In New York newspapers, the advertisements of 18th century apothecaries, insofar as drugs are mentioned by name, show the usual chemicals and galenics used in Europe in this period. However, it scarcely would be possible to offer a greater variety of merchandise, together with drugs and medicines, than was offered in a characteristic advertisement (August 3, 1769, supplement to the *New York Journal or General Advertiser*) as for sale "at the sign of the looking glass & druggist pot."[55]

In Philadelphia the *Pennsylvania Gazette*, founded by Benjamin Franklin in 1729, was a popular means for advertising. About the time of his marriage, Franklin opened a store and offered in his *Gazette* all "commodities varied from needles and pins to horses and slaves." Among these "commodities" we find advertised coffee, tea, chocolate, palm oil, saffron, spermacety, crown soap, powdered mustard, linseed oil, patent medicines and "seneca rattlesnake root, with directions how to use it in pleurisy." Franklin doubtless prescribed over the counter.[56]

For pharmacy this dabbling in drug dispensing by one of the most eminent and influential Americans during the 18th century had its favorable consequences. Franklin retired from business in 1749, but never lost his interest in medicine and pharmacy. It was he who, having dabbled in both professions without being educated in either, was the first to bring about an obvious practical example of the separation of pharmacy and medicine in America. In the Pennsylvania Hospital, founded on his initiative, he appointed an apothecary whose only task was that of preparing medicines.

There are several other proofs of Franklin's interest in pharmacy. From London, he sent his friend John Bartram, the famous American botanist, "some of the true rhubarb seed" (1770). This reportedly was the first attempt on American soil to cultivate Chinese rhubarb, which yields the medicinally used rhizome.[57]

In Philadelphia of the early 18th century, as in other towns of the American colonies, the number of drugstores owned by pharmacists and devoted exclusively to supplying medicines to physicians and household remedies to the public was very small.[58] Evan Jones was located at Philadelphia, in 1730, at the sign of "Paracelsus' Head."[59] Christopher Marshall established himself in Philadelphia in 1729. His biographer calls him "an apothecary, druggist, botanist, and chemist," first in a family line of Philadelphia pharmacists.[60]

Pennsylvania was the first American colony to have a pharmacy conducted according to the German model and designated *Apotheke*. After the foundation of the Moravian sectarian settlement in Bethlehem in 1741 the Brethren operated, among other institutions for mutual assistance, a pharmacy under the direction of the German physician Dr. Friederich Otto and, later, of his brother, Matthes Otto. The pharmacy was in the possession of the Moravian church community until 1796, when it was purchased by Doctor Freytag.[61] Another Germanic pharmacy in Philadelphia (around 1780) supplied the German farmers and settlers in Pennsylvania with all the domestic remedies to which they had been accustomed in the old country.[62]

COLONIAL LEGISLATION RELATED TO PHARMACY

The English colonies, influenced by the initiative of private individuals and not by governmental actions, enacted laws dictated by immediate needs of these individuals. It is but natural that the laws mirror English custom and spirit. Not until 1736 did an English-American colony deal legally with pharmacy. So far as is known, the first North American law concretely mentioning the apothecary and having a direct bearing on pharmacy is the Virginia "act for regulation of the fees and accounts of the practicers in physic," passed in 1736. As David L. Cowen points out, this act has no "direct relation to the pharmacy laws of today," but it reveals much about the pharmaceutical situation in colonial America and deserves to be quoted here:

I. WHEREAS the Practice of Physic, in this Colony, is most commonly taken up and followed, by Surgeons, Apothecaries, or such as have only served Apprenticeships to those Trades, who often prove very unskillful in the Art of a Physician; and yet do demand excessive Fees and exact unreasonable Prices for the Medicines which they administer, and do too often, for the Sake of making up long and expensive Bills, load their Patients with greater Quantities thereof, than are necessary or useful, concealing all their Compositions, as well to prevent the Discovery of their Practice, as of the true Value of what they administer; which is become a Grievance, dangerous and intolerable, as well to the poorer Sort of People, as others, and doth require the most effectual Remedy that the Nature of the Thing will admit:

II. Be It therefore Enacted, by the Lieutenant-Governor, Council, and Burgesses of this present General Assembly, and it is hereby Enacted, by the Authority of the same, That from and after the Passing of this Act, no Practicer in Physic, in any Action or Suit whatsoever, hereafter to be commenced in any Court of Record in this Colony, shall recover, for Visiting any sick Person, more than the Rates hereafter mentioned.[63]

(In the list the "Rates" allowed "those Persons who have studied Physic in any University, and taken any Degree therein" are about twice as high as the fees allowed

"Surgeons, and Apothecaries, who have served an Apprenticeship to those Trades.")

III. AND, to the End the true Value of the Medicines administred by any Practicer in Physic, may be better known, and judged of, Be it further Enacted, by the Authority aforesaid, That whenever any Pills, Bolus, Potion, Draught, Electuary, Decoction or any Medicines, in any Form whatsoever, shall be administred to any sick Person, The Person administring the same shall, at the same Time, deliver in his Bill, expressing every particular Thing made up therein; or if the Medicine administred, be a Simple, or Compound, directed in the Dispensatories, the true Name thereof shall be expressed in the same Bill, together with the Quantities and Prices, in both Cases. And in Failure thereof, such Practicer, or any Apothecary making up the Prescription of another, shall be nonsuited, in any Action or Suit hereafter commenced, which shall be grounded upon such Bill or Bills: Nor shall any Book, or Account, of any Practicer in Physic, or any Apothecary, be permitted to be given in Evidence, before a Court; unless the Articles therein contained, be charged according to the Directions of this Act.

IV. AND be it further Enacted, by the Authority aforesaid, That this Act shall continue and be in Force, for and during Two Years, next after the Passing thereof, and from thence to the End of the next Session of Assembly.

Influenced if not drafted by an academically educated and graduated physician, this act reflects the attitude of London physicians of this period toward the medical ambitions of the apothecaries. On the one hand, it is contemptuous in its judgment of both surgeons and apothecaries who have only served an apprenticeship and is, in a way, an answer to the denial by London apothecaries (1724) of the necessity of academic education for the practice of medicine (see p. 97). On the other hand, the act reluctantly recognizes the apothecary as a medical practitioner. Since only the fees of graduate physicians and those of surgeons and apothecaries who had "served an apprenticeship" were enumerated, the conclusion seems justified that only such skilled apothecaries as were eligible to practice in Virginia could legally

demand remuneration for services mentioned in the act.

Of special importance is Section III of the act. Cowen states that "the bill of particulars took the place of the practitioner's oaths of the earlier laws, and such particularization often became an integral part of later medical legislation throughout the country."

The reference to "dispensatories" is new and perhaps indicates European academic training of the author of the act. According to Cowen, "this is the first legal recognition of such compilations" in the colonies. (The only such work that had been published in British America by that time was a reissue of Culpeper's *Pharmacopoeia Londinensis* of 1653, which apparently attained no professional status.)

Another reference in the act to which attention should be directed refers to "any apothecary, making up the prescription of another." This is the first official statement up to that time that there may have been medical practitioners who, at least at times, wrote prescriptions instead of dispensing their medicines themselves. Hence, it may be assumed that the most significant pharmaceutical task, the dispensing of the prescriptions of medical practitioners, was carried out by apothecaries in North America before 1736.

The first legal mention of the term "druggist," as well as "apothecary," appears in an "Act for the better Ordering and governing Negroes and other Slaves . . .", promulgated in South Carolina (1751), prohibiting "any Physician, Apothecary, or Druggist" from employing any slave "in the Shops or Places where they keep their Medicines or Drugs."[64] The designation "druggist" usually was applied to people who imported drugs and sold them at wholesale, while the term "apothecary" was restricted to the pharmaceutical dispenser and second-class medical practitioner.

ATTEMPTED SEPARATION OF PHARMACY FROM MEDICINE

The above-quoted Virginia act of 1736 contains a general confirmation of the fact that apothecaries in Colonial America sometimes must have had the opportunity to "make up prescriptions" brought or sent to them by medical practitioners. However, a specific record of the appointment of an individual apothecary to fill prescriptions, other than his own or those of his preceptor, is to be found in the *Account of the Pennsylvania Hospital, from Its Rise To the Beginning of the Fifth Month, called May,* 1754, written by Benjamin Franklin, then the clerk or secretary of the board of trustees of this institution. In this interesting account we find the following paragraph:

The practitioners charitably supplied the medicines gratis till December, 1752, when the managers having procured an assortment of drugs from London, opened an apothecary's shop in the hospital; and it being found necessary appointed an apothecary to attend and make up the medicines daily, according to the prescription, with an allowance of fifteen pounds per annum for his care and trouble, he giving bond, with two sufficient sureties, for the faithful performance of his trust.[65]

Jonathan Roberts, who was warmly recommended by Dr. Thomas Bond, was appointed as the first apothecary to the hospital and served the institution faithfully and well until the spring of 1755, when he resigned to accept more remunerative employment. John Morgan, an apprentice of Dr. John Redman, became the second apothecary at the Pennsylvania Hospital (1755-56), resigning after a year to complete a medical education.

A decade later (including 5 years' study and experience in European medical centers) this former hospital pharmacist, John Morgan, was attempting to make the Continental practice of writing prescriptions, "the regular mode of practicing physic" (as he called it in his *Discourse upon the Institution of Medical Schools in America*[66]) a generally recognized American custom. In his *Discourse*, which he wrote during his residence in Paris and in Italy, then gave as an introductory lecture at the inauguration (1765) of a medical school in connection with the College of Philadelphia, he recommended the complete separation of pharmacy and surgery from the practice of

medicine. "We must regret," he said, "that the very different employment of physician, surgeon, and apothecary should be promiscuously followed by any one man: They certainly require different talents." Morgan's prime object in advising the separation of the several branches of medical practice was doubtless to improve the entire profession by having each department cultivated successfully. "The knowledge of medicine will then be daily improved," he pointed out; "and it may be practiced with greater accuracy and skill."

To objections that were raised to this idea, which was strange and, from a business point of view, inconvenient to most American medical practitioners of this time, Morgan made the following reply:

Practitioners in general business never do, or can do, the business of an apothecary in this place themselves. They have apprentices for the purpose. After visiting the sick, do not their apprentices make up their prescriptions? I should ask, is not an apothecary acquainted with the art of compounding and making up medicines as skillful in it as an apprentice? Is not a man educated in the profession to be trusted in preference to one who is only learning the business?

The resolution concerning the separation of pharmacy from medicine adopted by the College of Physicians in Edinburgh (1754) and the beneficial results of this separation that Morgan had observed not only in Edinburgh but also in continental Europe (together with his own experience as "apothecary" in the Pennsylvania Hospital) undoubtedly account for Morgan's advocacy of "the regular [European] mode of practicing physic." Furthermore, there is hardly any doubt that Morgan was familiar with the famous *Elémens de pharmacie théorique et pratique,* by the French pharmacist Antoine Baumé. Hence, it may be supposed that he had read this statement in the introduction:

Those who in the early times devoted themselves to the art of healing, practiced simultaneously medicine, pharmacy, and surgery; but gradually it became obvious that each one of these different branches requires the entire devotion of an individual person.

The time was not yet ripe for effective separation of the professions of medicine and pharmacy in the American colonies. Some physicians here and there unostentatiously adopted Morgan's practice of sending prescriptions to a pharmacy. Others eventually became public advocates on principle—for example, Dr. Abraham Covet, in Philadelphia (1774), and Dr. John Jones, the first professor of surgery in the New York Medical School.[67]

English spirit and English customs, the philosophy of *laissez faire*, dominated pharmacy in Colonial America despite the sometimes large influx of people of other nationalities. This influence was not to be neutralized easily by ideas brought from the European continent or by such men as Morgan, who had been influenced by the progressive Scottish University of Edinburgh.

Like English pharmacy during that period, American pharmacy showed little scientific life of its own. The earliest publications in North America that were devoted substantially to pharmaceutical information were written characteristically as much for physicians and for "home doctoring" as for practitioners of pharmacy—books such as Nicholas Culpeper's "*The English Physician . . . Containing, admirable and approved remedies . . .* (Boston, 1708); *The Husbandman's Guide: In four parts . . . Part second, Choice physical recepts . . .* (Boston, 1710); Culpeper's *Pharmacopoeia Londinensis; or the London dispensatory . . .* (Boston, 1720),[68] and a tract by the Reverend Thomas Harward, *Electuarium novum Alexipharmacum* (Boston, 1732).

The first teacher of pharmacy and pharmaceutical chemistry was the oft-mentioned physician John Morgan, who also taught materia medica and the theory and the practice of medicine in the first medical school in America. The school had been founded at his initiative, as part of the College of Philadelphia (later the University of Pennsylvania).[69] Morgan, like his successor Benjamin Rush, taught pharmacy, pharmaceutical chemistry and materia medica to medical students, as a part of the medical curriculum.

It remained to be proved that pharmaceutical knowledge as a basis for pharmaceutical practice separated from the practice of medicine was important for public welfare. Only then could professional pharmacy be established firmly in America. This proof was supplied during the Revolutionary War.

10:   The Revolutionary War

MEDICAL MEN IN THE AMERICAN REVOLUTION

When the Revolutionary War began, forty years after the rather blunt classification in the Virginia act of 1736 (see p. 145) of medical personnel who lacked academic education, the overwhelming majority of North American medical practitioners still consisted of "surgeons, apothecaries, or such as have only served apprenticeships to those trades."

If there were any notable differences between the kinds of practice carried on by these men, they were a matter of volition or were dictated by general circumstances and not by a special kind of education or examination. It was up to the practitioners themselves to decide whether they preferred to act as physicians, surgeons or apothecaries and to choose their titles accordingly. In their apprenticeship they had learned the practice of all these branches of medicine; for the most part, they tried to make the best of all of them.

Almost all medical practitioners of this period dispensed their prescriptions themselves, and many of them practiced pharmacy in a shop open to the public. Not infrequently, one of the few physicians with academic education and degrees, such as Silvester Gardiner, was especially successful in pharmacy. Another example was the American military hero, Hugh Mercer,[1] a graduate of the Scottish university of Aberdeen. As a medical practitioner, he conducted an open pharmacy in Fredericksburg, Va. (1771 until the beginning of the Revolution). This made him an apothecary as much or as little as Benjamin Franklin became an apothecary by dealing in drugs and patent medicines in his store (see p. 144).

During this period the designation *doctor,* especially for American-born practitioners, rarely meant a university degree. Some practitioners without academic education later on received an honorary doctor's degree (e.g., Samuel Danforth,[2] John Brooks[3] and Isaac Senter[4]). However, for the most part it was a title of courtesy applied to all kinds of medical men, including the apothecaries.

Before the Revolutionary War and for some time thereafter, the drug field belonged to the following three classes:

1. Persons who had served a more or less lengthy apprenticeship with a medical practitioner, whose prescriptions they had learned to compound; not infrequently they seem to have had greater interest in their commercial talents and prospects than in their medical accomplishments;

2. Those who had been trained as apothecaries, chemists, or druggist, and all who had pharmaceutical education, such as the *apothicaires* or *Apotheker* in their native countries. However, most of these preferred medical practice combined with dispensing; and

3. Storekeepers who specialized in drugs to some extent without having any special pharmaceutical training.

MILITARY PHARMACY IN THE REVOLUTION

Pharmaceutical arrangements of the several forces fighting in the Revolution reflected the particular civil pattern of each. For example, the medical service in the British army was in accord with the situation in the mother country, where physicians had to be examined and graduated; and apothecaries, although entitled to attend the sick, considered themselves to be the legitimate representatives of the art of pharmacy.

Hence, only a graduate of one of the great universities or of the College of Physicians of London could become an army physician.[5] The surgeons and the apothe-

149

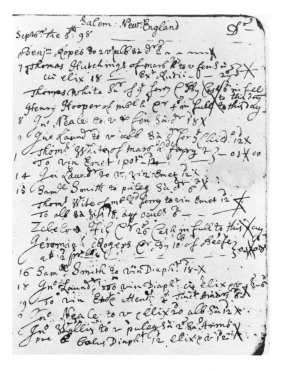

Among financial records of an American pharmacy, one of the very earliest known was kept by a dispensing "pharmaceutical chemist," Bartholomew Browne. The excerpt (above) from his 90-page account book was written September 5, 1698, at Salem, New England. "White Samech" was the drug most frequently dispensed. (Original in the Essex Institute, Salem, Mass.; from Griffenhagen, G.: Essex Institute Historical Collections, pp. 19-30, January, 1961)

caries had to prove that they had a professional education; their service in the army was restricted to their special field. Within the German ("Hessian") corps of the British North American Army, a distinct separation between the different branches of medicine reflected the German authoritarian system.

The medical staff of the British army on American soil consisted of physicians and surgeons with administrative or with practicing medical functions, purveyors, apothecaries and mates. (Among apothecaries whose names survive in military history are Robert Bishopp, George Brown, Michael Croker, Arthur Edwards, Richard Huddleston, John Johnston, Benjamin Mace, Daniel Maudeville, William Payne, Richard Proctor, John Watson, Gregory West. Furthermore, a surgeon, John Rush, was "appointed apothecary to the general hospital.") The medical staff of the German troops in British service included the pharmacists Becker, Keller, Rudolph and Schirmer.[6]

The French auxiliary army fighting on the side of the Americans likewise had its own medical staff consisting of well-educated physicians, surgeons and pharmacists. The *Pharmacien-en-chef*, C. H. Ferrand, after his return to France, received the honorary title "Apothecary Major of the Battlefields and of the Armies of the King," in acknowledgment of his services.[7] (The usual title of the French chief military pharmacist at that time was "apothicaire-major général.")

The French pharmacist-historian, Maurice Bouvet, says:

There were French pharmacists among the civil personnel, the military service, the surgeons of the navy and even among the soldiers. Ten French pharmacists—Augé, Chefdieu, La Chesnaye, La Crampe, Métaver, Rollandeau, Rosancelin, Souchet, Tarrault, Tual—died for the noble cause which they defended.[8]

The American army used the British army as its pattern, naturally enough, including a military medical service imitative of British forms.[9]

For example, the professional education required of the surgeons in the British army found its parallel in an obligatory examination introduced in the Continental Army (as early as May 8, 1775).[10] Duncan states that "although regimental and hospital surgeons were in demand, examinations of a somewhat rigid character were, as a rule, insisted upon as a prerequisite for appointment."[11]

There is no evidence of any examination or proof of skill required of the apothecaries active in the American revolutionary army. Compared with the surgeons, their number was small. Apparently, there was no complaint concerning their activity throughout the war. Moreover, as early as October, 1775, a man whose knowledge and understanding of the special tasks of pharmacy had already stood the test became director general of the military hospitals and chief physician of the army. This man was Dr. John Morgan. Dr. Morgan was the second of the four medical directors of the American revolutionary army—three of whom were academically educated and the fourth a man of approved theoretical knowledge.[12]

The Continental Congress passed a resolution (1775) establishing an army hospital with a staff consisting of a director-general and chief physician, 4 surgeons, 1 apothecary, 20 mates, and others. According to this resolution, it was the duty of the "surgeons, apothecaries and mates to visit and attend the sick, and mates to obey the orders of the physician, surgeons, and the apothecary."[13] The appointment of the apothecary and the surgeons was left to the director-general. The resolution does not show any differentiation of duties performed by the apothecary and the surgeons. It was up to Morgan to point out and to secure this differentiation.

A letter by Morgan to Doctor Potts, who was at that time the director of a department hospital, is characteristic. Morgan writes that he had given "a warrant to Mr. Andrew Craigie, to act as an apothecary" under Potts and expresses the opinion that Potts will find this appointment "particularly useful," because of the necessity of experience in the apothecary business. "Without such a one I know not how you could either procure sufficient medicines for your department or dispense them when got." Morgan admonishes Potts "to make it a part of the duty of the mates to assist the apothecary in making up and dispensing medicine." He states that "the apothecary to all intents is to be looked on in rank as well as pay in the light of a surgeon and respected accordingly and if he is capable he should in return do part of the surgeon's duty."[14]

The "making up and dispensing medicine" was, according to Morgan, the prime task of the apothecary in the army. When Congress passed a resolution effecting the reorganization of the medical department of the army (1777), the plan was prepared by William Shippen and John Cochran. However, it bears some marks of Morgan's mind and experience. Here, for the first time in the history of American pharmacy, the duties of the apothecary were officially stated and restricted exclusively to professional pharmaceutical tasks. The paragraphs concerning pharmacy read:

That there be one apothecary general for each district, whose duty it shall be to receive, prepare, and deliver medicines and other articles of his department to the hospitals and army, as shall be ordered by the director general, or deputy director general respectively.

That the apothecaries [general] be allowed as many mates as the director general, or respective deputy general, shall think necessary.[15]

The country was divided into four districts. However, the Southern department had an administration of its own and did not adopt the title "apothecary general." While there were three bearers of this title at the same time in the army, the Southern department had, simply, an "apothecary" on its medical staff. In addition, the appointment of second apothecaries was authorized. In salary, the apothecaries-general ranked between the senior surgeons and the second surgeons.

A further reorganization of the military medical department (1780) abolished the different departments and concentrated all authority in one medical staff. The title "apothecary general," borne by several persons of the same rank, disappeared. There was now one "apothecary," with five assistants, to be appointed, like the other principal officers, directly by Congress. Andrew Craigie became this "apothecary" and kept the position until the end of the war.[16]

Through a resolution of Congress, a "continental druggist" was "appointed at Philadelphia whose business it shall be to receive and deliver all medicines, instruments, and shop furniture for the benefit of the United States."[17]

APOTHECARY-GENERAL ANDREW CRAIGIE

There is some mystery surrounding Andrew Craigie, the apothecary-general. Noth-

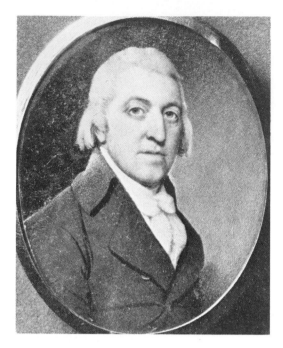

Andrew Craigie, patriotic Whig and prosperous druggist, who became Apothecary General during the Revolution. (Miniature painted about 1791 by Benjamin West; reproduced from Pratt, F. H.: *The Craigies*, Cambridge, 1942)

ing is known of his professional training or of what his proper profession was. On May 14, 1775, "Mr. Andrew Craigie, who had been made commissary of medical stores, was directed to impress beds, bedding, and other necessities for the sick.[18] A few months later the Massachusetts Provincial Congress appointed Craigie, "being informed of his skill in medicine . . . to be medical commissary *and apothecary* to the army raised by this Congress."[19] Although restricted to the Massachusetts troops, this was the first official appointment of an army apothecary in America.

There can be no doubt that Craigie was efficient in fulfilling his duties and, also, had a talent for making friends. His reappointment after the radical reorganization of the military medical department (resolutions of Congress of October 6, 1780) was certainly helped by the mentioning of his name by General Washington in a letter written to an influential member of Congress. In this significant letter, after referring to several physicians and surgeons as having "a just claim to be continued, from their abilities, attention, and other considerations," General Washington wrote the following: "Dr. Craigie, the present Apothecary General, a gentleman not personally known to me, has been reported as very deserving of the appointment." The concluding lines read: "The reason of my mentioning these [gentlemen] particularly proceeds from a hint given me, that the new arrangement might be influenced by a spirit of party out of doors, which would not operate in their favor."[20]

Craigie, more than two years before the reorganization of the military medical department, discussed with Doctor Potts the consequential idea of the establishment of general department laboratories and storehouses to serve the medicinal needs of the army. Craigie wrote to Doctor Potts, that "the department is at present in chaos," and added:

I beg leave to query whether this will not be the plan. To have the principle store at Carlisle, where all the medicines shall be prepared and the chests completed. Under the supposition that the general hospitals will be more collected and the number lessened, I would propose that an apothecary attend each with a complete chest of medicines; that the surgeon and physician general of the army be attended by an apothecary with a good chest. . . . I would have an issuing store at a convenient distance from the army, from which the hospital and regimental chests might occasionally be replenished.[21]

That Craigie's proposal found acceptance and support is confirmed by a later report "that hospital drugs were prepared and compounded mostly in apothecary general Craigie's shop at Carlisle, Pennsylvania."[22]

After the war, Craigie entered the wholesale drug business, based on a wartime fortune said to have been acquired by "buying up government promises and other speculations."[23] The commercial abilities of this first and most prominent American apothecary in military service were at least as great as his pharmaceutical skill.

MILITARY DRUG SUPPLY AND FORMULARIES

Shortages of drug supplies, speculation and uncertain transport were problems that continually plagued the Continental armies. In the attempts to meet these and similar difficulties, Apothecary-General Craigie's business acumen, and his professional skills as well, were of no little value.

At first, the Revolutionary Army drew on the stocks of private pharmacies such as the Greenleaf shop at Boston, where at least five of fifteen medicine chests wanted by the Provincial Congress of Massachusetts (1775) were assembled, and the pharmacy of Christopher Jr. and Charles Marshall at Philadelphia where medicine chests authorized by the Continental Congress (1776) were prepared. The contents of these field chests provide concrete evidence of the drug therapy available to the wounded and the afflicted under the conditions of the revolutionary years. The detailed drug lists may be readily consulted in George Griffenhagen's account of *Drug Supplies in the American Revolution.*[24]

Private drug stocks became totally inadequate for medical needs in the war that ensued. Imports were cut off from England, and channels for medicinal supplies from other countries did not develop effectively until late in the war and afterward. The most immediate relief from drug shortages, Griffenhagen concluded, came from American privateers who preyed on British shipping. "Drug cargoes from British prize ships, many of which were en route to New York, served as a most important source of supply, particularly in 1777 and 1778."

The place of purging and emesis in therapeutics of the late 18th century is reflected in the drugs most in demand, although cinchona headed the pharmaceutical needs of military medicine. In discussing the drugs in most critical supply, Griffenhagen also mentions that prices had skyrocketed:

Jalap, ipecac, and rhubarb were the botanical favorites, while bitter purging salts (Epsom salts) and Glauber's purging salts were the chemical choices for purging. Tartar emetic (antimony and potassium tartrate) was the choice for a vomit, and cantharides (Spanish flies) was the most important ingredient of blistering plasters. Gum opium was administered for its narcotic effects, while gum camphor, nitre (saltpetre or potassium nitrate), and mercury (pure metal as well as certain salts) were employed for a variety of purposes. Lint, a form of absorbent material made by scraping or picking apart old woven material, also often was short in supply.

Equipment shortages included surgical instruments and mortar and pestles for pulverizing the crude drugs. Glass vials for holding compounded medicines were also a supply problem, especially after essential drugs were again available.

Some of the shortages were eased, if not solved, by local manufacture. Lint was produced in large quantities in the Colonies, and glass vials were manufactured in numerous glasshouses. Even local manufacture of the purging salts and nitre aided in eliminating shortages of these essential items, and at the same time initiated the first large-scale pharmaceutical manufacturing in America.[25]

As time went on, both the medical organization of the army and the drug supply situation improved. One facet of this improvement and, at the same time, a basis for its continuance was the publication of a military formulary in 1778, the so-called "Lititz pharmacopoeia." This small booklet, modest in appearance, proved to be a landmark in the history of American pharmacy.

Lititz Pharmacopoeia

The Lititz pharmacopoeia illustrates in a most remarkable way the choice of items suggested by the medical knowledge (particularly English medical knowledge) that was current, the results of the American experience, and, finally, the difficulties arising from the actual situation of a nation at war, which was restricted in its imports. The Lititz pharmacopoeia is so called because the booklet was written, at least in part, in the Moravian village of Lititz (preface dated at Lititz, March 12, 1778). It was first used in the military hospitals of Lititz and Bethlehem, Pennsylvania. The actual title (see p. 154) may be translated, "Formulary of simple and yet efficacious remedies for use of the military hospital, belonging

PHARMACOPOEIA

SIMPLICIORUM

ET

EFFICACIORUM,

IN USUM

NOSOCOMII MILITARIS,

AD EXERCITUM

Fœderatarum *Americæ* Civitatum

PERTINENTIS;

HODIERNÆ NOSTRÆ INOPIÆ RERUMQUE
ANGUSTIIS,

Feroci hostium sævitiæ, belloque crudeli ex inopinatò
patriæ nostræ illato debitis,

MAXIME ACCOMMODATA.

PHILADELPHIÆ:

Ex Officina STYNER & CIST. M DCC LXXVIII.

A modest military formulary was the first publication compiled on American soil to be termed a "pharmacopeia" (original, 4½ by 2½ inches; 32 pages). It is commonly called the Lititz pharmacopeia, after the Pennsylvania town of that name, which was the site of an army hospital for wounded patriots. The reproductions show the title page and sample pages of text. The annotations in this copy by "BR" are those of Benjamin Rush, one of the most competent American physicians of the 18th century. (From the Library Company of Philadelphia)

[22]

61. * PULVIS AROMATICUS.

REC. Canellæ albæ.
      Rad. zingiber. ana P. Æ. M.
      Fiat pulvis.
Dosis a gr. v. ad scrupul. i.

62. * PULVIS ALUMINOSUS.

REC. Alum. crudi.
      Terræ japonicæ, ana P. Æ. M.
Dosis a gr. viii. ad drachm. ss.

63. PULVIS ANTIMONIALIS.

REC. Tartar. emetic. drachm. i.
      Cretæ ppt. unc. i. M.
Dosis a gr. x. ad scrupul. i. pro emetico;
vel a gr. ii. ad gr. viii. 3tia vel 4ta quaque
hora, pro diaphoretico.

64. PULVIS ANTIMONIALIS
NITROSUS.

REC. Tartar. emetic. gr. ii.
      Salis-nitri drachm. iii. M. -
                                    Dosis

[23]

Dosis a gr. xv. ad drachm. ss. 2da vel 3tia
quaque hora.

65. Fit etiam cum OPIO, addendo

      Gum. opii gr. ii.
Eodem modo sumendus.

66. PULVIS CAMPHORATUS,
NITROSUS.

REC. Camphor. drachm. ss.
      Sal. nitri drachm. ii. M.
Dosis a gr. xv. ad drachm. ss. 2da vel 3tia
quaque hora.

67. Fit etiam cum OPIO, addendo

      Gum. opii gr. ii.
Eodem modo sumendus.

68. * PULVIS CORTICIS PERUVIANI.

Dosis a drachm. ss. ad drachm. i. quaque vel
2da quaque hora.

                              69. PUL-

to the army of the Federated States of America. Especially adapted to our present poverty and straitened circumstances, caused by the ferocious inhumanity of the enemy, and the cruel war unexpectedly brought upon our fatherland." The author of this "pharmacopoeia"—or, more truly, emergency military hospital formulary—was, in all probability, Dr. William Brown, an American graduate of the University of Edinburgh.[26] The first edition did not actually carry an author's name (leading to some doubts later on about assignment of credit), but the second edition shows the name of Dr. William Brown on the title page.

About half the formulas listed seem to stem from the experience of the author and his American colleagues. The most important overseas source for this first book of its kind in America was the *Pharmacopoeia Edinburgensis* (1756), which was official when Brown himself was studying at Edinburgh. Other sources of formulas, in order of importance, were the *Pharmacopoeia of the Royal Hospital of Edinburgh*, the *Pharmacopoeia Londinensis* (1746) and the *Pharmacopoeia contracta* of *Beth Holim* (House for the Sick; sometimes called the Portuguese Hospital) in London. Alex Berman suggests that the last perhaps was more influential on the Lititz pharmacopoeia than was previously supposed.[27]

Because of perplexing and unpredictable drug shortages, the Lititz pharmacopoeia followed an old pharmaceutical tradition of permitting official substitution of therapeutically equivalent substances for drugs in uncertain supply. In official European drug books of the 16th and the 17th centuries, when imports were irregular, lists of authorized substitutes were sometimes annexed under the heading *Quid pro quo* or *De succedaniis*. The earliest known list of this kind goes back 1800 years to Galen.[28]

Another feature of the military formulary was indicated in its introduction by the statement:

There are distinguished by an asterisk the formulas of medicaments which must be prepared and compounded in a general laboratory; the others are to be mixed, as needed, in our hospital dispensaries. [Translation by Sister Mary Francis Xavier.][29]

This remark is the first official mention of large-scale manufacture of pharmaceutical products in America. The purpose was to relieve the apothecary in the hospital of the preparation of compounded medicines which could not be made quickly or without special effort and unnecessary waste of time and material. A comparison of the preparations with and without asterisks makes it evident that there was no differentiation as to the professional skill required.

The Lititz pharmacopoeia was published about the same time that Apothecary-General Craigie's proposed establishment of a "principle store at Carlisle" was realized. This "principle store" was, in all probability, the "general laboratory" mentioned in the Lititz pharmacopoeia. Thus, officially recognized American manufacture of pharmaceutical products on a large scale—the first we know of—was established according to the proposal of an apothecary, under his direction and for the public welfare.

Coste's Compendium

Two years after the issuance of this formulary "for the use of the military hospitals belonging to the army of the Federated States of America," there appeared (1780) a "Pharmaceutical Compendium compiled for the French military hospitals in North America" (*Compendium pharmaceuticum militaribus gallorum nosocomiis in orbe novo boreali adscriptum*). It was compiled by Jean-François Coste, Chief Physician to the French army fighting with the American patriots against the British. It is understood that this booklet, limited to the use of the comparatively small French contingent on American soil, did not gain the practical or the historical significance of the Lititz pharmacopoeia.

Necessity had stood godfather to both books. "The incertitudes of war, of the sea and of a long voyage," says Coste in his introductory remarks to his formulary, "called for the employment of a few remedies," i.e., of a selected number. While the Lititz pharmacopoeia is based on Scottish and English sources, Coste's book naturally follows French patterns, especially the *Codex medicamentarius seu pharmacopoea Parisiensis* (1758). A significant difference lies in the fact that the Lititz pharmacopoeia makes use of indigenous North American drugs, such as sassafras and serpentaria, while Coste's formulary does not. It is amusing that the only indigenous North American products admitted to the *Compendium pharmaceuticum* (although merely in a kind of annex headed *Post-scriptum*) is "*cerevisia Newport, abietina dicta*," commonly called Newport or Spruce beer. It was used as a menstruum to macerate freshly grated horseradish (2%). Doctor Coste resided at Newport, and his formulary was printed there.

Both Coste's *Compendium* and the Lititz pharmacopoeia may be readily consulted in modern facsimile editions, with English translations by Sister Mary Francis Xavier and annotations by Edward Kremers.[29]

The meeting of English and foreign pharmacy on American soil, during the War of Independence, was not restricted to such literature. Notwithstanding a sprinkling of immigrants from non-English countries, it was the English "apothecary" (to be more precise, the second-class physician conducting an open store) who had served as a model for American Colonial pharmacy. The American counterpart of this English model now came in touch with representatives of the well-organized pharmaceutical service of two continental European countries in which pharmacy had achieved a high professional as well as social standing. France was represented by the pharmacists in General Rochambeau's army, and Germany by the pharmacists in the German auxiliary contingent fighting on the side of the British. While this did not cause an immediate change in American pharmacy from a state of undisciplined growth to an attempt at stabilization and professionalization of the trade, it did broaden the pharmaceutical outlook.

IMPORTANCE OF THE REVOLUTION FOR PHARMACY

When we try to understand the significance of the Revolutionary War for pharmacy as a profession, the following seem to be especially prominent: (1) Eight years of successful pharmaceutical activity, separate from medicine but equally recognized and given the same official status; (2) the first known American manufacture of pharmaceutical products on a large scale, initiated by an apothecary in order to meet national needs; (3) the first practical attempt at a uniform and obligatory formulary as a basis for satisfactory and reliable pharmaceutical work (in this case, military pharmacy); and (4) the meeting of American pharmacists with European colleagues who were more advanced professionally.

The importance—indeed, the necessity—of professionalized pharmacy for the public welfare had been proved by the tests to which it had been put by the American Revolutionary War.

11: Young Republic and Pioneer Expansion

The Revolutionary War was over. The American people were free. The question then was, free from what and for what? The first part of this question may easily be answered. The American people had severed their connection with Great Britain and, hence, with Europe. They had gained the liberty to work out their own destiny. This destiny was not apparent at the time, although it had found its basic and, perhaps, prophetic expression in that declaration of the inborn and eternal rights of men—the first amendment of the Constitution of the United States.

The United States was the first nation in the world to be founded not on the organization of kindred tribes or on dynastic imperialism, but as the result of the free decision of peoples of varying descent. It had won a victory, but, simultaneously, a task had been assigned to it. This task was to prove that liberty of the individual was within, not beyond, the limits of human nature and political wisdom.

After the war, the first and immediate necessities of the new nation were to find as firm a basis for the life of professions and trades as for the individual, and to derive the greatest possible benefit from the natural resources of the country.

INDIGENOUS MATERIA MEDICA

This War of Independence and the new nation emerging from it not only had a special and alluring ideology but seemed to open up a limitless country to all peoples. It awakened the interest of the whole civilized world. Thousands of former enemies, especially many of the German soldiers in English service, remained in America. Others stayed for a while to explore the country and to study its resources and pos-

sibilities. One of the latter, the physician-botanist Johann Schoepf, traveled through the country for more than a year and published (1787) a book about the indigenous American materia medica, titled *Materia Medica Americana Potissimum Regni Vegetabilis*. Schoepf's journey was only one of the successful botanic and medicobotanical expeditions by foreigners following the Revolutionary War. They were supported and supplemented by intensive research on the part of American botanists.

Botany, and especially medicinal botany, had been cultivated in North America during early Colonial times. Thus there was a fund of experience on which to build.[1] Schoepf's *Materia Medica Americana* is based largely on the observations of the excellent American botanist G. H. E. Muehlenberg and the work of Bartram, Clayton, Colden, Kalm, Catesby and others.[2] To Muehlenberg, Schoepf wrote from Baireuth, Germany:

My lists [describing about 400 North American plants] make it certain that North America owns a rich indigenous materia medica in her plants and can find all she needs, apart from few East Indian spices and plants, on her own soil. . . . I almost may flatter myself in writing this little book to have rendered sufficient services to America to be pardoned for my assistance in combatting her.[3]

Schoepf was not the only one who took advantage of the diligent, comprehensive and unselfish work of Muehlenberg. Numerous European and American botanists, among them Benjamin Smith Barton, author of the *Collections for an Essay Towards a Materia Medica of the United States,*[4] and Manasseh Cutler,[5] author of the first scientific treatise on New England botany, were in close scientific contact with Muehlenberg.

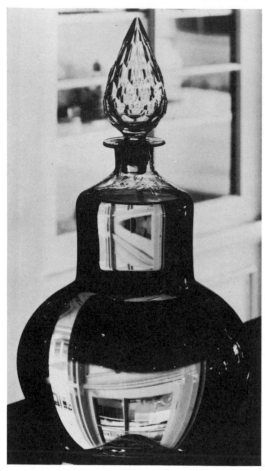

An early type of show bottle (or "show-globe") of the 19th century, brought to America from England, is similar to the carboys that contained stock solutions in a pharmacy. (Specimen in The Upjohn Company's pharmacy restoration at Disneyland, Anaheim, Calif.)

Barton's treatise on American materia medica (two parts, 1798 and 1804) was the first of its kind in English and simultaneously was a critique of the work of Schoepf. Evidence of the inspiration that Barton imparted to research on the medicinal value of American plants can be found in numerous theses of medical graduates of the University of Pennsylvania, where he taught natural history and botany.

Muehlenberg considered the pharmacist an authority to be consulted for information about indigenous *officinalia,* in regard to their strength as well as their common names. Twice in his notebook he mentions the necessity of consulting a pharmacist for this purpose.[6]

All this valuable scientific work, besides enriching American medical and pharmaceutical science and practice, added to the international materia medica. It was supplemented by the observations of unscientific empirics. These observations of laymen formed the basis of sectarian movements and, later on, were subjected to scientific evaluation. Coupled with the results of early research work previously mentioned, they played an influential part in American medicine and pharmacy.

The first gardens in North America devoted largely, if not entirely, to the cultivation and the study of medicinal herbs were established and used by members of religious sects;[7] and medicinal use of plants in America was to be associated again and again with sectarian movements.

THE "THOMSONIANS" AND THE "ECLECTICS"

About 1800, Samuel Thomson entered the scene. His personality and work gained nation-wide recognition in spite of the simplicity and the lack of originality of what he called his "system"—or, perhaps, because of these characteristics. Thomson was an uneducated man, the son of a farmer and originally, a farmer himself. His early desire to become an apprentice to a doctor could not be fulfilled because of his almost complete lack of education. In 19th-century America he rediscovered the fundamentals of the ancient theory of Galen (see p. 16) and used them for his own theory, the "Thomsonian system"! His doctrine reads like a slightly modified abstract from Galen's writings when he states:

I found, after maturely considering the subject, that all animal bodies are formed of the four elements, earth, air, fire and water . . . that a state of perfect health arises from a due balance or temperature of the four elements.[8]

Before Thomson there had been so-called botanic physicians and herb doctors, the latter strengthening their offerings with supposed medicinal "secrets" of the American Indians; but they remained inividualistic practitioners, local or itinerant in their practice. Unlike them, Samuel Thomson systematized his crude teachings, patented his therapeutics, and propagandized his band of rabid followers, who launched a movement accepted by large segments of the American public.

The appeal of these "irregular" practitioners undoubtedly drew strength from therapeutic excesses of regular practitioners, who were still bloodletting with abandon and giving massive doses of cathartic and emetic as veritable cure-alls. Thomsonians played openly on the citizen's fears that the "heroic" treatments might be worse than the disease. They offered to substitute "milder" and "safer" botanic remedies for the "harsh minerals" of the orthodox school. However, their "less lethal remedies" could be characterized as "frequent lobelia emetics, scalding capsicum and herb teas, medicated enemas, and parboiling steam baths —all built around a distinctive monistic pathology."[9]

The founder of the sect divided the main part of his materia medica into six classes, each based on the properties of the drugs. The original Thomsonians usually prepared and dispensed their own medications, based on drugs marketed by special manufacturers through authorized botanic drug depots.

A large botanic medical literature was produced on two levels: a literature for lay consumption and suited to the needs of uneducated practitioners, and a literature largely designed to attract educated readers, serve as a reference for more ambitious students and practitioners, and in general obtain scientific recognition.[10]

Thomson's policies and attitudes eventually generated a disastrous schism in the ranks of the movement (1838), producing the Neo-Thomsonians. After mid-century, the color and the fanaticism of the Thomsonian medical sect had disappeared. Left on the scene were Botanic splinter groups with more scientific pretensions than their predecessors. In evaluating their ambitions, Alex Berman stresses their limitations:

The laudable objective of investigating indigenous plants for curative purposes could not be realized as long as Botanic practitioners were not scientifically trained in this direction. Moreover, mere appropriation and compilation of facts established through investigation by non-Botanics could not be substituted for original research on the plant materia medica. Finally, the Botanic practitioners as a group evinced a marked disinclination and lack of ability to conduct phytochemical work. A noteworthy exception to this was John Uri Lloyd. Despite these faults, a number of plant drugs employed exclusively in Botanic practice eventually entered the general pharmaceutical literature and the official compendia.

. . . Indeed it was in the development of a distinctive pharmacy of indigenous plant remedies that the Eclectics made their most determined bid for scientific recognition. In early Eclectic pharmacy of the "antiphlogistic" period, Eclectic practitioners generally compounded their own medicines for their saddle bags and home stock. Ingredients were obtained through wholesale botanic houses, from the Shakers and their agents, by personally gathering plant medicinals in the field, or through regular drug channels.[11]

The disadvantage of large and unpleasant doses of Eclectic remedies gave way to their concentrated "resinoid" plant medicinals (e.g., resin of podophyllum), which were first introduced by Wm. S. Merrell and Company of Cincinnati (1847), then by other firms. This development stimulated Eclectic optimism that "they could match the alkaloidal pharmacy of the regulars with concentrated medicines of their own."

The name *eclectics* probably was taken by practitioners of the reformed botanico-medical system from a classification of medical practitioners put forward earlier by a prominent botanist, C. S. Rafinesque, in his *Medical Flora; or Manual of Medical Botany of the United States of North America* (1828-1830). Rafinesque intended this book to serve the "daily use of medical students, physicians, druggists, pharmacians [a term revealing the French origin of the author!],

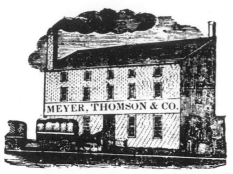

An advertisement of 1835, by one of the special drug depots serving the botanic system (or fad) of therapy. (The

chemists, botanists." He stated that "pharmacy, by the aid of botany and chemistry, has become a science," and that "druggists and chemists" must be able "to distinguish the genuine kinds and detect the frauds of the collectors and herbalists."[12] Rafinesque also laid down rules for the pharmaceutical treatment of plants in order to get efficient medicaments.[13]

The scientist Rafinesque naturally welcomed the scientific turn which the botani-comedical movement was given by Wooster Beach and his followers. "I belong, like yourself," he wrote to Dr. Beach, "to the Reformed Practice of Medicine, and agree with you much better than with the Thomsonian, Homoeopathic, and Botanical Empirics."[14]

Rafinesque's *Medical Flora* had urged American research in plant chemistry comparable with that being conducted in Europe, praising especially the work of the Society of Pharmacists of Paris. Yet, Rafinesque may not have shaped the Eclectic movement as much as might be supposed from his belated recognition as one of its "fathers," possibly in part for "propaganda purposes, to bolster up a declining movement."[15]

Rafinesque had described Eclectics as "those who subject and adopt in practice whatever is found beneficial, and who change their prescriptions according to emergencies, circumstances, and acquired knowledge."

This definition holds true for classical eclectics who did not recognize any dogma. However, the American eclectic medical practitioners clung to one dogma, namely, the rejection of a large number of remedies of mineral origin, particularly all mercury compounds. Nevertheless, compared with the Thomsonians, they were liberal.

The materia medica of the early followers of Samuel Thomson consisted of botanical products and combinations thereof. The aim was to exclude all poisons, in which list lobelia was not by them included. Their remedies, there-

Thomsonian Manual, vol. 1, p. xvi; from Alex Berman)

fore, excluded such energetics as podophyllum, sanguinaria, rhus, etc., which became important agents with Beach and his followers, the Eclectics. Whilst the Thomsonians rejected mineral salts and the inorganics, these substances were conservatively employed in Eclecticism.[16]

The development of the Thomsonian as well as the Eclectic school of medicine is of general interest,[17] partly because this American botanical movement, originating in the period of reconstruction after the Revolutionary War and growing out of its atmosphere, had a greater influence on pharmacy than is generally realized. For example, many plants and plant preparations listed in various editions of the *United States Pharmacopeia*, the *National Formulary*, or other books of reference, were introduced into medical practice by the eclectic school of medicine.[18] One of the outstanding figures in American pharmacy, John Uri Lloyd, devoted the greater part of his life and scientific effort to pharmaceutical work in the service of eclectic medicine.[19]

MEDICAL SECTARIANISM AND PHARMACY

The influence of the botanicomedical movement on the practice of pharmacy goes back to Samuel Thomson, the founder of the new school or sect. He and his cause became a touchstone for the meaning of constitutional "liberty." This question had to be answered: Which was of greater importance and broader general consequence, the recently acquired and legally guaranteed "liberty" of the individual to take up any profession, or the protection of the people from the dangers arising, particularly in the field of medicine, from the unchecked activity of individuals practicing their profession by no other standard than their own belief in their ability and a modicum of empiric experience?

This question always becomes acute and must be decided whenever and wherever "liberty" is introduced as the inborn right of the individual. This happened in France after the great revolution and in Germany (Prussia) with the introduction of the so-

called "liberty of trades." In both countries the idea of protection of the people proved to be stronger than the dogma of liberty. The attempts made in France (1791) to introduce unrestricted liberty to practice pharmacy without educational requirements were short-lived. This was true also in Germany (1810 and 1811). Even the customary English *laissez-faire* attitude, although confirming the right to practice medicine and pharmacy to persons who had previously practiced these callings, did not recognize the liberty of everyone to do so. The American people and their legislators and courts decided otherwise. The meaning of American constitutional liberty proved to be, and probably at this time had to be, dogmatic.

What this meant to the formation and the development of the health professions becomes evident from the fact that for decades the attempts by physicians to regulate the practice of medicine—through educational requirements, examinations and licenses—and to control the professional conduct of practitioners proved to be futile. True, regulations requiring the licensing of medical practitioners had been issued before the Revolutionary War in New York, New Jersey and, soon afterward, Massachusetts and New Hampshire. Other states followed with similar laws.[20]

The passage of laws restricting medical practice reached its highest point in 1825; and thereafter, due to the attacks of the empirics and the realization by the profession of the futility of regulation, practically all laws were repealed.[21]

If such was the situation for medicine, what had pharmacy to hope for in recognition and protection of its professional aims?

The lack of enforceable standards in the health field left the way open for unbridled and profitable promotion of drugs—whether patented medications administered by irregular practitioners such as the Thomsonians, or preparations for self-medication.

In early America even regular medical practitioners made liberal use of the so-called patent medicines. Later, as the growth of newspapers developed a nationwide medium of promotion and as improved

transport could place the promoted remedies in stores available to all and without
legal hindrance, the trade in medicines
flourished in all sorts of unlikely places.
Imitations of English patent medicines, prepared on a large scale by American wholesale druggists, evolved into independent
large-scale enterprises.[22] Thus, the trade in
English and American patent medicines became the backbone of many American
"drugstores" that came to make drugs something of a specialty and often vied successfully with the waning drug shops operated
by physician-apothecaries. In the young republic there were no effective definitions
of a pharmacist or pharmacy to guide the
erratic course of such establishments, in the
majority of which the professional and scientific pharmacy of older European countries was not merely a strange but probably
even an unknown way of life.

*The origin and development of European
pharmacy was, in general, parallel with
professional medicine, as a profession concerned with public health, the nonprofessional aspects being incidental. To a very
great extent, nonprofessional medicine was
responsible for the development of American pharmacy as an independent calling,
the professional aspects being incidental.*
Many of the peculiarities in the evolution
of American pharmacy can be explained by
this fact. Fortunately, however, a group of
individuals who fought for higher aims in
time created professional American pharmacy. These people came, for the most part,
from the wholesale drug field.

BEGINNINGS OF AMERICAN
PROFESSIONAL PHARMACY

As long as the dispensing of medicine was
primarily in the hands of the physician-
apothecary, the only domain of the "chemist
and druggist" proper was the wholesale
distribution of drugs. The wholesale druggists provided the country physicians with
the imported or indigenous drugs and chemicals needed by physicians in their practice,
and they naturally were held responsible
by their clients if the expected effects of
the drugs were not realized. Furthermore,

the Revolutionary War had taught wholesale druggists the advantage of domestic
manufacture of products previously imported. Thus, to be able to detect adulterations and to do their own manufacturing,
they became highly interested in a better
knowledge of drugs and chemicals. The interest in real pharmaceutical activity had
begun.

Advertisements of the period immediately
after the Revolutionary War reveal this
active interest in professional pharmaceutical knowledge. Thus Th. B. Atwood, owner
of "Atwood's medicinal store" in New York,
announced (1784) "the latest arrivals from
Europe" in the *New York Packet* and simultaneously made known that he would like
to engage a partner. "The want of capital,
with good security, will be no objection to
a man of abilities. He must understand
pharmacy thoroughly, and he should be
grounded in chemistry."[23] Effingham Lawrence in New York advertised the receipt
of "a large and general assortment of genuine drugs and medicines from London and
Amsterdam" and asked for "a person well
acquainted with practical chemistry."[24]

During the period of reconstruction,
wholesale druggists began to issue printed
lists enumerating the goods they had in
stock. The title of one of these lists (Boston,
1795) reads: "Catalogue of drugs and medicines, instruments and utensils, dyestuffs,
groceries, and painters' colours, imported,
prepared, and sold by Smith and Bartlett
at their druggists store and apothecaries
shop." This title is the best possible illustration of the combination of importing with
manufacturing, of wholesale business (the
"druggist's store") with dispensing (the
"apothecary's shop"), operated in this period by prominent American "druggists."
A remark at the end of the catalogue of
22 pages states that "physicians' prescriptions will always meet an exact and particular attention."

Some of the wholesale druggists very
early started to manufacture chemicals, thus
establishing a basis for large American
chemical and pharmaceutical industries.[25]
Again the name of Marshall of Philadelphia
appears. The firm of Christopher Marshall,

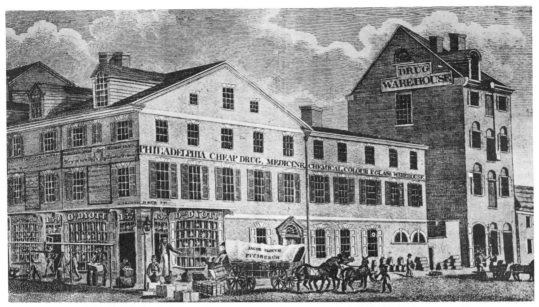

Crates and barrels of drugs are being loaded onto a Conestoga wagon before the door of one of the first American druggists to develop a national wholesale trade. Excessively shrewd and unusually successful financially, Thomas Dyott was operating his "Drug Warehouse" in Philadelphia as early as 1807 and, later, manufactured his own line of household remedies. Such patent-medicine makers have been called by an American historian "the first American business men to exploit goods bearing brand names in a market as large as the nation, the first to pioneer in their advertising a wide variety of psychological lures." (Young, J. H.: J. Am. Pharm. Assoc. n.s. *1*:290, 1961; illustration from Porter, T.: The Picture of Philadelphia, 1831)

Jr., and Charles Marshall (sons of and successors to the druggist Christopher Marshall, Sr., the founder of the venture) "had, as early as 1786, entered quite extensively into the business of making muriate of ammonia and Glauber's salt." The Philadelphia druggist, John Harrison, began (1793) to manufacture various chemicals, notably sulfuric acid. Other druggists took up similar lines of manufacture.

People working as apprentices or clerks in such establishments of necessity acquired pharmaceutical knowledge and skill and, finally, professional pride and aims.[26] The number of apprentices was large. In Marshall's pharmacy it ranged from six to twelve. These men, who were accustomed to real pharmaceutical work, later on became pioneers in the professional practice of pharmacy in the United States and, to some extent, the first teachers of pharmacy for pharmacists.[27]

A parallel with the development in England is evident. There, too, wholesale druggists initiated professional pharmacy during the first half of the 19th century, filling, in this way, the gap left by the transformation of the apothecaries into medical practitioners. The main difference was that the establishment of the Philadelphia College of Apothecaries (1821) represented the first obvious manifestation of a pharmaceutical profession in America, whereas the organization of the Pharmaceutical Society of Great Britain (1841) implied a revival.

"An Act Concerning Physicians, Surgeons and Apothecaries," issued in 1808 by the legislature of the Territory of Orleans (Louisiana), for the first time known of in the United States of America, made a diploma and an examination prerequisites for "practice . . . as . . . apothecary," as well as for practice as a physician or a surgeon. In spite of this Act, no record of such an examination of an "apothecary" has come down to us. When the Act was revised by the legislature of the State of Louisiana (1816) "one apothecary" was added to the four representatives of medicine and of surgery entrusted with the examination of applicants for licensure in one of the health professions.[28]

On the other hand, we are informed by David L. Cowen that, even in the year of issuance of the revised Act, a committee of the Louisiana House of Representatives reported that it preferred not to "insist on the examination of apothecaries which had been urged in the law submitted to us."[29] However, two gentlemen of New Orleans, F. Grandchamp and L. J. Dufilho, must be regarded as the first pharmacists known to have been licensed within the United States.[30, 31]

The State of South Carolina was the first of the former British colonies of which there is undeniable evidence of a pharmaceutical examination (1818) as a prerequisite for a pharmaceutical license. The legislature had passed an act (1817) obliging every apothecary to obtain a license from "the medical society of South Carolina or board of physicians," thus empowering these bodies "to examine any apothecary, who may apply to them for a license." In 1818, a Richard Johnson was granted the license "to pursue the business of druggist," after being examined:

1. on the definition of chemistry and pharmacy, 2. on the preparation of mercury and phosphorus, 3. on the preparation of phosphate of antimony and tartar emetic, 4. on the doses of Laudanum, tartar emetic, ipecac, and Fowler's mineral solution of arsenic, 5. on the mode of making the common plaster and mixing the ol. ricini with water.[32]

Thus, during the period of reconstruction after the Revolutionary War, the groundwork was laid for a large number of commercial drugstores, and, in addition, for a few establishments with professional aims. In place of the six drugstores in Philadelphia about 1750, which were not owned by physicians, there were twenty in 1785.[33] At that time the population numbered 40,000.

Kellocks' *New York Directory* of 1786, when the city had a population of 23,600, mentions six "druggists and apothecaries," besides one "physician and apothecary" and one "surgeon and apothecary."[34] Of interest is the separate listing of the medical men with open shops from the "druggists and apothecaries" proper. In 1821, in Philadelphia and its outlying districts with a population of 137,000, there were about 130 stores "identified with the trade in drugs."[35] In Boston, with a population of 43,000, there were at the same time 7 wholesale and 23 retail establishments,[36] the wholesale druggists also dispensing directly to the public.

The gradual separation of pharmacy from medicine had progressed rapidly since 1783, so far as the drugstores were concerned. The open shops of the physicians, although not disappearing entirely until the end of the 19th century, were definitely on their way out. However, only a few of the medical practitioners surrendered the dispensing of medicines within their practice. As late as 1819, this custom was taken for granted by physicians to such an extent that the president of the New York College of Physicians and Surgeons in "remarks" submitted to the regents of the University of New York, argued that it was unnecessary for the students of medicine to attend a course in materia medica because, according to the rules of admission, before entering the school the candidate must have "studied three years with some regular practitioner." In this time, he claimed, the candidate would learn "better than in any other school, the nature, powers, and doses, of all the remedies in common use, by daily handling and preparing them in putting up the prescriptions of his teacher."[37]

The importance of pharmacy in times of emergency, which had been indicated during the Revolutionary War, was soon to be re-emphasized. In 1793, the first plague—believed to have come to the city with refugees from Haiti—broke out in Philadelphia. (At that time the seat of the national government was located there.) It is said that 5,000 died and 17,000 left the city. "The national government removed its offices; papers stopped publication; business, except dealing in drugs, almost ceased to exist."[38]

It may be assumed that the active part taken by Philadelphia apothecaries in fighting the plague increased the general respect in which they were held and their own professional self-esteem—the two bases on which the first American professional association was later founded. It may here be recalled that a similar event occurred in the history of English pharmacy (see p. 97).

The period of reconstruction after the Revolutionary War was a time of ferment. Some problems were touched on, ways of clarification were attempted, many a beginning was made. While all of this was necessary and not in vain, nothing assumed definite shape. The first attempts at regulation of medical and pharmaceutical practice failed. America was not yet amenable to the firm regulation and limitation of professional activity that are not necessary in more densely populated countries, but impracticable in a continent with vast undeveloped areas.

The rapid conquest of these areas for civilization and their development commensurate with the progress which had been made in the older parts of the United States would not have been possible without giving the pioneers all possible "liberty" to do what the actual circumstances and their personal incentives demanded of them.

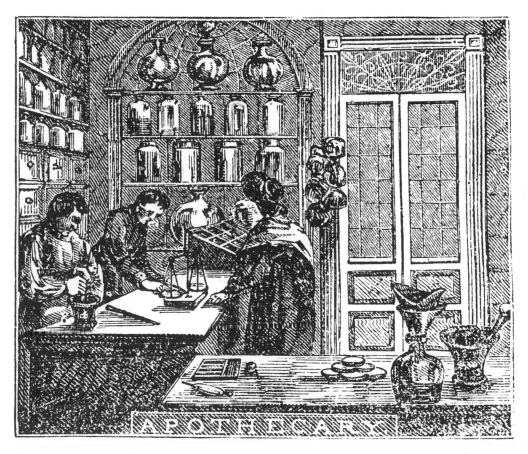

This depiction of the interior of an American pharmacy is one of the earliest known in the literature. It appeared in a vocational guidance book first published in 1836. (Edward Hazen: Popular Technology; or, Professions and Trades, vol. 1, New York, 1841, p. 236; photograph from the University of Wisconsin)

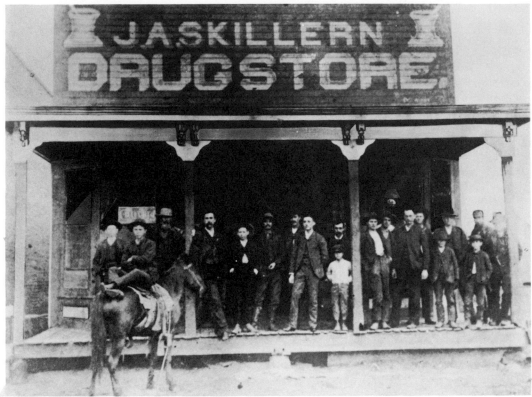

A drugstore in a Texas town of the 1880's reminds us that those practicing pharmacy faced the same rude conditions of life and work as did most people who migrated Westward. Uneven development of the country long hindered attempts to establish national standards for pharmacy and other occupations with professional aspirations. (Photograph of first drugstore in Lewisville, Texas; from Chain Store Age)

Thus, for a long time regulation was left to self-discipline and initiative by the professional groups.

WESTWARD MOVEMENT OF THE FRONTIER

The "westward movement" before the Revolutionary War had been, in large part at least, a movement to the south—down the fertile valley of the Shenandoah, for example. After the Revolution the mountain barriers were overcome, and the movement west of the Alleghenies became one of the dominant factors of American national life. As a result of the Revolutionary War, all the western areas which had been partly ceded to the province of Quebec by England shortly before the war were transferred to the United States. Furthermore, the war necessitated a rapid westward development for both political and financial reasons.

If the soldiers who had fought for American independence could not be paid in full during the time of their service, after the war the government was even less able financially to give them back pay. For this reason Congress sought a way out of the difficulty. "As early as September, 1776, Congress tried to encourage enlistments by offering bounties of land—500 acres to a colonel, 100 acres to a private, and other ranks in proportion."[39]

Saying farewell to his officers after the war, George Washington gave them this admonition: "The extensive and fertile regions of the West will yield a most happy asylum to those fond of domestic enjoyment, and seeking for personal independence."[40] Many people poured across the free land that held promise of this "personal independence." With every wave of this movement, extending westward the boundaries of the United States, pioneer scenes of the Atlantic coast were re-enacted.

In 1800, it was estimated that there were a million people inhabiting the area west of the Alleghenies. Ten years later, the number had risen to two and a half million; by 1830, to three and one-half million.[41] In 1960, in only five states of the old Northwest (Ohio, Indiana, Illinois, Michigan, and Wisconsin) dwelt more than 36 millions of people.

The medicopharmaceutical scenes described by Cooper in *The Pioneers* are redescribed, though in modified form, in Gerstäcker's *Die Regulatoren von Arkansas*,[42] and other writings.[43]

In a Milwaukee journal, advertisements were published similar to those common toward the end of the 18th century in the old 13 states: "Higby and Wardner, dealers in drugs, medicines, paints, oils, dye-woods & stuffs" recommended (1841) an extensive assortment of these goods, listed as "just ar-rived," together with "brushes, perfumery, patent medicines and a general assortment of physician's and chemist's preparations, among them Corrosive Sub, Red Precip, Opium, etc." In another advertisement, Fred Wardner announces a most varied line of goods (steel, stoves, glassware, etc.) as well as drugs and medicines.[44]

It would be a mistake to conclude, from some crudities and turbulent scenes in these new states that the pioneers had only material objectives and ideals. Already in 1787, the charter of the settlements in the old Northwest Territory stated that "religion, morality, and knowledge, being necessary to good government and the happiness of mankind, schools and the means of education shall forever be encouraged."[45] In its contract with Congress the Ohio Company provided, on its own initiative, two entire townships for a university. "Under this provision Ohio university was established at Athens in 1808 as the first state university in the world under democratic government."[46]

In these new states, after the period of infancy, ideas of importance for pharmacy developed, such as state university departments of pharmacy and state organizations.

Part Three

Pharmacy in the United States

SECTION TWO

The Period of Organized Development

12:   The Growth of Associations

LOCAL ORGANIZATIONS

In the preceding chapter it was pointed out how the restrictions and regulations necessary to raise American pharmacy to the status of a profession were, for a long time, left to the initiative of individual pharmacists. This initiative was not always taken spontaneously.

On the one hand, the few people who combined professional vision with pharmaceutical education and skill prospered, requiring no regulations for the proper conduct of their establishments. On the other hand, the uneducated merchants who called themselves druggists did not want them. The merchant class may be divided into two groups. One was worried about its ability to meet regulations requiring even a modicum of knowledge. The other group conducted an unscrupulous business, possible only because there was no regulation and control.

Pressure from outside forced pharmacists and druggists in the United States to form their first associations. This pressure came from the medical profession. During the first half of the 18th century, the situation within the medical profession was not much better than that of pharmacy. However, one center of American cultural and scientific life had the oldest American school of medicine and the greatest number of well-educated physicians. This city was Philadelphia, where a proper separation of pharmacy and medicine already had been undertaken by the founder of its medical school. Hence, it is not surprising that the next step in the direction of professional pharmacy was taken in Philadelphia, originating in the proposal of a Philadelphia professor of medicine. In response to the implied challenge, pharmacists organized the first pharmaceutical association striving to attain professional aims, based on adequate education.

This undertaking was not the first attempt by physicians to secure better regulation of the drug trade. Shortly after the Revolutionary War the Massachusetts Medical Society petitioned the legislature to prohibit the sale of bad or adulterated drugs.[1] Laws in Louisiana (1808 and 1816) and South Carolina (1817) established the principle of examination and licensure as prerequisites for the practice of pharmacy.

A difference between these movements and the one in Philadelphia is noteworthy: In their earlier efforts, the medical societies in Massachusetts and the legislators in Louisiana introduced measures affecting future druggists. In the attempt at Philadelphia (March, 1820), all shopowners in the city who called themselves apothecaries, chemists or druggists were affected directly and immediately. J. Redman Coxe, with the support of the University of Pennsylvania, made a "suggestion" to which 16 prominent Philadelphia druggists affixed their signatures, proposing that an honorary degree be granted to such apothecaries "as have taken every measure to become perfect masters of their profession. . . ." The proposal read as follows:

It is suggested that by a close attention for at least three years in an apothecary's shop to the practical part of their duties and after two courses of lectures on the subject of chemistry, materia medica, and pharmacy, such persons may be subjected to an examination by the professors of those branches in the University, and if found qualified, may receive a degree under some appropriate denomination which, being publicly known, may ensure them a greater chance of popular favor than will probably be granted to those who are neglectful or indifferent to the high responsibility they are invested with.[2]

Druggists not included in the group of 16 offered their vehement opposition to the entire plan. Those not distinguished by the proffered degree of "master of pharmacy" and not able or willing to obtain it by pass-

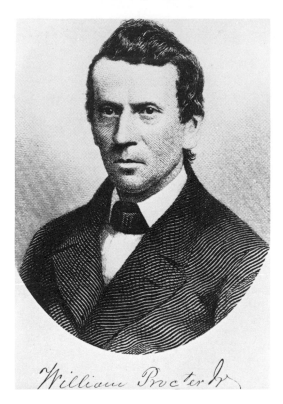

William Procter, Jr. (1817-1874), one of the most admired of all American pharmacists, is depicted in this contemporary engraving as a young and vigorous leader. An unruffled and unpretentious "Quaker" of solid integrity, Procter was astonishingly productive (about 550 articles) and versatile (practitioner, experimenter, editor, association leader, professor). "The favorite child of his genius was the American Pharmaceutical Association," said Albert Ebert, who knew him well. An inspiring tribute to the professional legacy that Procter left is the bronze statue of him in the Association's headquarters building in Washington, D.C. (From A.I.H.P. Archive)

ing the examination apparently were to be branded as "neglectful or indifferent." However, the same statement which caused Philadelphia druggists to resent the action of the medical faculty also suggested the proper way of counteraction. In his final sentence, having referred to the English Society of Apothecaries, Dr. Redman Coxe remarked that the progress (in Philadelphia) which he had in mind could not be achieved in any "other way than by the measure proposed," because "such an incorporated association does not exist here."

Apothecaries and druggists held their first meeting only 4 days after the board of trustees of the University of Pennsylvania published its resolution concerning the examination (February 1821). This was the first united action of members of the calling known in the history of American pharmacy. A committee was appointed to determine whether it might not be "preferable to adopt a plan as a substitute, distinct from the one proposed."[3] This committee consisted of 9 men, among them the most prominent Philadelphia wholesale druggists. Henry Troth[4] was the leader. "It was an enterprise of youth, for the average age of the five whose ages we know was but 28 years at the time of the founding, the oldest being Samuel Jackson, who was 34, and the youngest, Peter Williamson, who was but 24."[5]

The report of the committee, delivered at a second meeting, admits that "medicines of inferior or sophisticated qualities" were "too often introduced into the shops," due to "the want of proper pharmacological information on the part of some druggists and apothecaries who vend" and also "of physicians who buy." One passage frankly states that it was the "happy effect" of the action of the University to rouse the druggists "to a sense of the propriety of placing their business on the respectable footing it ought to possess as a branch of the science of medicine." As the best method "to effectuate the reformation generally desired in the business," the committee recommended "the establishment of a College of Apothecaries, the attention of which will be constantly directed to the qualities of articles brought into the drug market," and furthermore of "a school of pharmacy."

Despite that, the University of Pennsylvania carried through its arrangements, conferred the honorary degree of a Master of Pharmacy on 16 Philadelphia pharmacists, and opened a course in pharmacy. However, "not a single student ever attended the lectures in the Medical Department with the view of securing the degree of Master of Pharmacy."[6]

The "College of Apothecaries,"[7] established after the hearing of the report by those present at the meeting of March 13, 1821, changed its name about a year later. In the charter then issued, it is called by the name "College of Pharmacy," which was to be applied also to other early American pharmaceutical associations but later on became restricted to pharmaceutical schools.

The designation "College" was obviously chosen with the intent of placing the new corporation on the same footing with its well-known medical sister, the Philadelphia College of Physicians. This in turn had followed an old English custom, the English Royal College of Physicians having been founded in 1518. However, the change of wording, from "apothecaries" to "pharmacy," shows an understanding of the situation in the world of pharmacy at this time, perhaps especially by the vice-president of the College, William Lehman, a pharmacist who was representative of that intellectual group of Philadelphians which had made the "city of brotherly love" the intellectual center of the United States.[8]

The English "apothecaries" had become medical practitioners to an increasing extent and could no longer be considered as typical representatives of the profession of pharmacy. Hence, the designation of apothecary was misleading. What designation should be used, both to characterize the calling and to describe its professional aims? The more recent English terms "chemist" and "druggist" did not solve the dilemma, for neither the one nor the other had as yet achieved the recognition and the status of a profession.

France and, to a certain extent, Germany offered the solution to this problem. Almost half a century earlier, the French term *apothicaire* had been replaced by the term *pharmacien*. A *Collège de pharmacie*, an association of Parisian pharmacists, based not on private initiative but on law, had included members of the highest scientific

attainment (1777 1796). This made the word *pharmacie* the recognized European designation for the entirety of professional pharmaceutical activity. Even in Germany, where the pharmaceutical practitioner still called himself by the old term *Apotheker*, the word *pharmacie* had replaced the expression *Apothekerkunst* to designate the profession as a whole. The two pharmaceutical journals which at that time enjoyed international fame and were well known to Lehman, were the French *Bulletin* [later *Journal*] *de pharmacie* and the German Trommsdorff's *Journal der Pharmacie*. Hence, "College of Pharmacy" was the term of choice for an association of practitioners who were eager to conduct their activities on the basis of scientific knowledge and professional ideals. It was Lehman, on his own initiative and without questioning the other members of the board of trustees, who baptized this firstborn child of American pharmaceutical solidarity as the Philadelphia College of Pharmacy.

Still another action of the young College revealed the broad spirit of its members: the appointment of honorary members shortly after the College had begun to function. This has been a custom characteristic of associations with scientific or professional standards. Thus, the Philadelphia College of Pharmacy, from its very beginning, considered itself on a par with other professional societies. Moreover, the names of its honorary members helped to justify this claim.

During this period of glorious rivalry between French and German scientific and professional pharmacy, both countries possessed a considerable number of pharmacists whose achievements received worldwide recognition. France led particularly in developing elegant procedures in the preparation of drug products and elegant appearance of the products themselves. Probably due to the Francophile tradition of Benjamin Franklin the French honorary members —Derosne, Pelletier, Robiquet, Vauquelin and Virey—outnumbered the German members, Brandes, Doebereiner and Trommsdorff. It is indicative of the English situ-

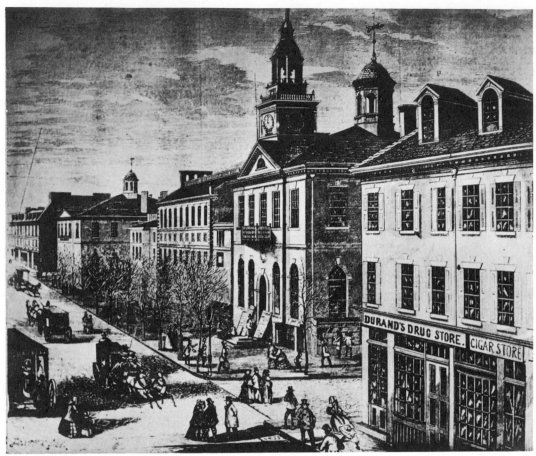

Many contributions to American pharmacy during its formative period stemmed from this corner pharmacy at Chestnut and 6th Streets in Philadelphia, shown as it appeared in the 1850's. It was outfitted in the most elegant French manner by a French immigrant pharmacist, Elias Durand. Durand and his chief staff pharmacist, Augustine J. L. Duhamel, kept American pharmacy in touch with pharmaceutical developments in France, published investigations of their own in American pharmacy's first journal and were active in the first association (Philadelphia). Pharmacist Durand presented a herbarium of 12,000 specimens to the Philadelphia College of Pharmacy, then brought together 100,000 specimens for the Jardin des Plantes at Paris ("Herbia Durand" gallery).

ation of that period that no one in the ranks of English pharmacy seemed to be prominent enough to be added to this list of illustrious French and German pharmacists.

A French pharmacist in Philadelphia, in connection with the Philadelphia College of Pharmacy, immediately exerted a strong foreign influence on American pharmacy. This was the former *pharmacien* of the Grand Army of Napoleon I, Elias Durand, who established a pharmacy in Philadelphia (1825). William Procter, Jr., describes

the activity and the importance of this man as follows:

His [Durand's] store became an important center of pharmaceutical information, which directly and indirectly, had much to do with the introduction of scientific pharmacy into Philadelphia, and through this college, his journal, and graduates, into the United States. Many of the finer medicinal chemicals were made in this country first by Durand.[9]

Augustine J. L. Duhamel, a pupil of Durand, was of French extraction, like his master, although born in Philadelphia. He strengthened the French influence on American scientific pharmacy. By the age of 33, he had published 34 papers in the *American Journal of Pharmacy*, all of them

> eminently practical in their character. . . . Two of his communications relate to Boullay's filter and method of displacement [percolation], and we believe that he was the first on this side of the Atlantic to comment on this valuable improvement in pharmaceutical manipulation. . . . His familiarity with the French language gave him access to the writers of that country, of which he extensively availed himself.[10]

Since the Philadelphia College of Pharmacy had been founded as an association (like the early colleges of physicians and the French *Collège de pharmacie*), its professional activity was by no means restricted to the establishment and the administration of its school. Its constitution provided for "a committee of inspection" for the examination of drugs "brought into the market and submitted to them," and a "committee of equity, to settle any disputes that may arise in the transactions of the members of the college." The constitution stated finally, that members "guilty of adulterating or sophisticating any articles of medicine or drugs or of knowingly vending articles of that character, or of deteriorated qualities may be expelled."[11]

The leaders of the College maintained a balance between the scientific and the commercial interests of the calling which they represented and tried to promote. One of the first steps was the publication (1824) of carefully determined formulas for the imitation of English patent medicines. Such imitations were a general American custom, but it is somewhat peculiar that the first professional pharmaceutical association in America sanctioned them, in effect if not in plain words.[12]

The leaders of the College founded the first American pharmaceutical journal (1825), the *Journal of the Philadelphia College of Pharmacy*, to disseminate current scientific and professional information.[13] The College also issued (1826) *The Druggist's Manual*, "a price current of drugs, medicines, paints, dyestuffs, glass, patent medicines, etc., with Latin and English synonyms, a German, French, and Spanish catalogue of drugs, tables of specific gravities, etc., etc., and a variety of useful matter." In this first American guide for retail pharmacy prices were not supplied by the editor but had to be filled in by the druggist.[14]

Having laid down in its constitution the fundamentals of professional pharmacy and having tried to realize them partially, it is not surprising that the Philadelphia College of Pharmacy became the model and sometimes the advisor of other local American pharmaceutical associations founded between 1821 and the Civil War—that event which so greatly changed the political, economic and spiritual life of the United States. The following list shows the spread of the early pharmaceutical associations:

1821	Philadelphia College of Pharmacy
1823	Massachusetts College of Pharmacy
1829	College of Pharmacy of the City (and County) of New York
1840	Maryland College of Pharmacy
1850	Cincinnati College of Pharmacy
1859	Chicago College of Pharmacy
1864	St. Louis College of Pharmacy (precursors in 1854 and 1857)

As was to be expected, Boston and New York were the first American cities to follow the example of Philadelphia in organizing pharmaceutical associations. These three cities were at that time not only leaders in general cultural standards but also the most important ports for the entrance of drugs. Moreover, they were the homes of the three oldest medical schools of the country. The medical associations of these three cities took the first steps toward the establishment of uniform drug standards, which finally brought about the first *United States Pharmacopoeia* (1820).

Repeating an earlier attempt to bring about a legal regulation of pharmacy, the Massachusetts Medical Society petitioned the legislature (1823) to give the counsellors of the society, "together with an association of apothecaries for all parts of the Commonwealth, if such an association should hereafter be incorporated," the power to appoint "Boards of Examiners," to examine all people "who may hereafter wish to compound or retail medicines in small quanties or to put up the prescriptions of physicians," and to grant licenses. In justifying the interest of the physicians in this regulation, the petition stated that:

physicians are daily discontinuing the practice of compounding or preparing the medicines which they use, and have therefore become in a great measure dependent upon the druggists and other retailers of medicine.[15]

This separation of pharmacy from medicine had been advocated as a desirable goal, and noted as partly achieved in the big cities, in the *Pharmacopoeia* of the Massachusetts Medical Society 15 years earlier (1808).

The attempt of Boston physicians to play a decisive role in pharmaceutical affairs suffered the same fate as that of their Philadelphia colleagues. As a result of the opposition led by several wholesale druggists, it was defeated.[16] However, the pharmaceutical association recommended in the medical petition was founded, on December 26, 1823, in accordance with advice asked of and given by trustees of the Philadelphia College of Pharmacy.[17] The constitution of the new Massachusetts College of Pharmacy emphasized the same points as its Philadelphia model. In the activity of the two first American pharmaceutical colleges the main difference was that in Philadelphia lectures were provided in the year of founding and were continued without interruption and continually improved, whereas in Boston no serious attempt at regular instruction was made until 1867.

"Almost all the business transacted was in reference to prices."[18] In contrast with the Philadelphia manual, the early drug lists published by the Massachusetts College (e.g., 1828) contained prices. They may be considered the first American attempt to fix the prices for drugs and medicines on the basis of associative agreement. The preface of the "Catalogue of the Materia Medica and of the Pharmaceutical Preparations with the Uniform Prices of the Massachusetts College of Pharmacy" gives in classic brevity the motives for the "uniform prices." It states:

a judicious arrangement as to prices is no small means of adding support and dignity to the business. . . . One evil where there is a difference in price is, that the purchaser either thinks that the one who charged high wronged him as to price, or that the one who charged low wronged him as to quality. . . . A competition as to prices must be eventually ruinous to all; but a competition as to the quality of the medicines and attention to business will add to the respectability and standing of the profession.

Significantly, this preface still appears with exactly the same wording in the price list published in 1854.

The list of founders of the College of Pharmacy of the City of New York shows that here, too, the wholesale druggists were instrumental in promoting American professional pharmacy.[19] These proud and self-conscious men, like their colleagues in Boston and Philadelphia, wished to regulate their affairs according to their own ideas and not under the supervision of the medical profession. The College was founded as "an association of pharmacists, druggists, and others interested in the progress of the profession, for purposes of mutual instruction, protection and assistance in all matters pertaining to their professional welfare; the school for undergraduates forming merely the teaching department of the institution."[20]

The Maryland College was founded, not in counteracting some action or demand on the part of physicians, but as a fruit of friendly understanding. The Maryland medical and chirurgical faculty initiated a meeting with representatives of Baltimore pharmacists "with the idea of elevating pharmacy." At this meeting, a committee of five pharmacists was appointed, which undertook all further steps leading to the founding, in 1840, of the Maryland College of Pharmacy. This association was more or less active until 1847, "but thereafter languished until 1856, when . . . it was thoroughly reorganized."[21]

The foundation of the Cincinnati College of Pharmacy was more indirectly influenced by the sister profession of medicine, when

"The meeting of the American Medical Association in Cincinnati in the year of 1850 . . . was so fraught with the high ideals in medicine that the founders of the Cincinnati College of Pharmacy were stimulated to greater effort in the accomplishment of their plans.[22] This influence probably was mediated in part by the leading personality among the quartet of talented men who founded the college, William B. Chapman, who was a graduate of the Philadelphia College of Pharmacy, as well as a graduate of the Ohio Medical College.

The history of the local St. Louis pharmaceutical association goes back to 1854, when the St. Louis Medical Society protested against the "habit of prescribing for and administering medicines" by druggists and the refilling of prescriptions without authorization by the physician, resolving "to withdraw the medical influence from any druggist, who may thus act." The *Journal of the Philadelphia College of Pharmacy* thought this resolution was "too threatening for a Western city, where men of all classes are less controlled by custom and chartered privilege than in the older cities."[23] In self-defense, and encouraged by the attitude of the Philadelphia *Journal*, the pharmacists founded the St. Louis Pharmaceutical Association, "for the purpose of exciting a more generous and brotherly feeling among the members of the profession of pharmacy . . . and [for] the improvement of the educational status of the apothecaries and druggists."[24]

This association was not very active. It was reorganized in 1857[25] but died during the Civil War. It "did not survive the shock of the upturning influences which marked the breaking out of the rebellion."[26] Finally, on November 11, 1864, the St. Louis College of Pharmacy was founded, not in defense against but in close harmony with the medical profession. The meeting at which the College was organized was held in the hall of the St. Louis Medical College, "largely attended by the physicians of the city." Of the 23 members announced as officers or trustees of the new college, not less than 9 had "M.D." attached to their names.[27] Like the older associations, this new St. Louis pharmaceutical organization was influenced by Philadelphia, for example, adopting for its own use the constitution and by-laws of the Philadelphia College."[28]

The foundation of the Chicago College of Pharmacy, in 1859, was influenced by the American Pharmaceutical Association,[29] which had been established in 1852 and gradually became inseparable from each progressive step in American pharmacy. The constitution, the by-laws and the code of ethics of the Chicago College were unmistakable offspring of those of the Philadelphia College and of the American Pharmaceutical Association.

In addition to these organizations, which developed into institutions in which the educational branch (i.e., the school) became dominant, there were other early local pharmaceutical associations.[30]

As demonstrated in the course of this chapter, the rise of early local pharmaceutical associations was due to outer circumstances more than to the professional enthusiasm of member druggists. Even the Philadelphia College of Pharmacy, the early and consistent herald and standard-bearer of American professional pharmacy, experienced times in which indifference among the passive majority of practitioners became threateningly obvious in the decrease of its members.

The general American appetite for independence expressed itself both in the formation of the early American pharmaceutical associations and in their decline when the independence of the drug trade no longer seemed endangered. The average American of this period did not desire any restrictions, whether by a special group thinking itself superior to him (in this special case the medical profession), by his own associations, or even by laws which tried to regulate his conduct. Legislators respected this sentiment. It was this typically American spirit that had defeated early medical endeavor to regulate legislatively the practice of medicine in all its branches, including pharmacy, by forcing it under the control of legally authorized and chartered medical associations.

German Influence

On the other hand, there were pharmacists in America imbued, because of their origin and education, with an appreciation for authority. These individuals were pharmacists of German descent who came to the United States in the turbulent years before the German Revolution (1848) or in consequence thereof. Often ambitious and competent, they gained a steadily growing influence over the development of American pharmacy.

Even in early colonial times there were German pharmacists in North America who enjoyed a high reputation. However, these men were neither numerous nor ambitious enough to exert any lasting influence. Thus the early development of American professional pharmacy found its model more in the French pharmacist, whose native country was America's ally in the struggle for independence. Had the later period between 1830 and 1860 brought as many French pharmacists to the United States as it did of German pharmacists, the development of American pharmacy might have taken other directions. In France, the July Revolution of 1830 (as well as that of 1848) was successful and hence caused no emigration. The German upheaval of 1848 failed, and the stern measures of the German princes against the revolutionaries forced thousands of the best-educated Germans to seek refuge in the United States. This fact doubtless has been of great importance in American cultural life. The fact that German physicians and pharmacists had played an important part in the German political movement of 1848 brought a great number of them to America.[31]

These German pharmacists spread over the country. All of them possessed practical and scientific training and a professional standard which at that time could not be equalled either by the English chemists and druggists or by the few graduates of early American colleges of pharmacy, not to mention the druggists without college education. As a result, their pharmaceutical practice was recognized as exemplary and was imitated. In some cities, such as St. Louis, Cincinnati and Milwaukee, a great number of the genuine pharmacies were for a long time in the hands of such "Forty-eight-ers" or of German immigrant pharmacists following them. Others were owned by American-born citizens trained by German immigrants; occasionally they completed their pharmaceutical education in Germany. These people were inclined to foster professional ideals and to endeavor to promote them by means of associations.[32]

The reputation which these German pharmacists enjoyed and their importance as preceptors is reflected in a biographic sketch of the distinguished John Uri Lloyd. In describing the 2-year apprenticeship of the young boy with an Anglo-American pharmacist, the author writes:

> The large number of Germans living in Cincinnati gave a pronounced Teutonic flavor to the drug business, no clerk being proficient unless drilled in German. In order to learn that phase of the business, it was deemed expedient for John Uri to become apprenticed to a German pharmacist. He found an opening with Mr. George Eger. . . . Mr. Eger, who had been educated as a pharmacist at a German university, gave careful attention to the young apprentice. . . . The lad who finished his apprenticeship under George Eger . . .was everywhere accepted as a competent pharmacist.[33]

A group of such German pharmacists founded (1851) an association named *New Yorker Pharmaceutischer Leseverein* (New York Pharmaceutical Literary Society), the first American pharmaceutical group formed with the purpose of improving the scientific, cultural and professional standards of its members without any regard to business affairs. Furthermore, it was the first to obligate its members to notify the board of the society when taking an apprentice, to fix the period of apprenticeship, and to make the examination of apprentices obligatory. "These apprentices, after the time of their apprenticeship, have to pass a stringent examination before a commission, and on passing the examination receive a certificate."[34]

In the first years of its existence the members of the New York German Pharmaceutical Society sent their apprentices to the New York College of Pharmacy.

In 1857 the society instituted the system of examinations for the apprentices that many members had trained in their establishments, and certificates of proficiency were issued to those who wished them. The College of Pharmacy at that time was in a somnolent condition, no students had graduated in 1857 and only two in 1858 and 1859. The examining board of the German Apothecaries Society filled the gap for a number of years, until the college revived its work, whereupon the apprentices were again sent to that institution.[35]

Another type of local pharmaceutical association originally influenced by the German element is the so-called Veteran Druggists' Association. The first such association was organized in 1898 by the pharmacist Thomas Nevin Jamieson. Since World War I, under the influence of William Bodemann, of Chicago, the idea of associations of "veteran" (older) pharmacists has spread to many of the larger American cities, largely as social groups.

The two German immigrants who exerted the greatest influence on the development of American pharmacy were John M. Maisch, the first general secretary of the American Pharmaceutical Association, and Charles Rice, the creator of the modern American pharmacopeia. They did not come to America as German pharmacists but became pharmacists after their immigration. Perhaps that fact helped them to give more to American pharmacy in general. The danger of isolation because of special professional education and traditions acquired abroad did not exist for them. They thought in terms of American pharmacy and tried to improve it in accord with their general background. A third man who should be named together with these two great American pharmacists of German birth is Frederick Hoffman. He was a German pharmacist, having passed all German pharmaceutical examinations, but, nevertheless, one of the greatest journalists and the most stimulating spirits that American pharmacy has had.

Some of the later local pharmaceutical associations have been branches of national organizations, e.g., the American Pharmaceutical Association branches (after 1905)[36] and the Greek-letter chapters of academic fraternities and sororities in pharmacy.[37] Of a different type are the alumni associations of the colleges (the first, in Philadelphia, 1864).

It required a central, nation-wide organization, which on its part fostered the founding and the existence of state organizations, in order gradually to develop a general professional feeling among pharmacists in America. With this came, as will be shown later, a greater willingness on the part of individual pharmacists to give up part of their independence for the benefit of all, to submit themselves to legal restrictions, and even to ask for them. However, this central organization, the American Pharmaceutical Association, originated not so much in a growing understanding of the necessity of professional solidarity and intercourse among pharmacists as in the same pressure from outside that had brought into existence the early local associations. This pressure arose from bad conditions in the drug trade.

STATE ORGANIZATIONS

Fifteen years after the founding of the American Pharmaceutical Association, the first state association, that of Maine, was founded (1867). It is significant that the establishment of this association coincided with the appointment of a "committee on legislation regulating the practice of pharmacy" by the American Pharmaceutical Association and was heartily welcomed by the *American Journal of Pharmacy*, whose editors were among the most active leaders of the American Pharmaceutical Association.[38] However, the *Journal* apparently did not recognize at this time that the Maine association of pharmacists, representing an entire state, was not merely another local group, but the beginning of something entirely new.

The fate of the Maine Association is somewhat shrouded in mystery. Its activities continued to be reported in the press through the 1870's[39]; then a peculiar change appears in the *Proceedings* of the American Pharmaceutical Association. Instead of the Maine Pharmaceutical Association it lists (beginning 1881) the Maine Insane Asylum.[40] This institution received the proceedings even after the Maine association, "having been dormant for a number of years," was reorganized (1890).[41] Thus there may have been an interested pharmacist in charge of the Maine Insane Asylum, who was a member of the old organization and participated in the founding of the new one.

This story is of general interest because it shows how state organization frequently was brought about. A few persons, sometimes only one, held the organization together. With their death or withdrawal from public life, interest waned, and the association died, to be revived later. Such was the fate of several state pharmaceutical associations. Their necessity had become so obvious that none disappeared permanently, as so many local associations had done. John M. Maisch saw the main task of the state associations as follows:

A few subjects that ought to claim their attention are the enactments of laws for the regulation of pharmacy where none such exist, and the amendment of those now in force where they are inadequate to the public or oppressive to those engaged in the practice of pharmacy. The co-operation of these various societies ought to be secured in an endeavor to modify the laws and rulings of the general government where they oppress the true liberty of those engaged in business.[42]

C. Lewis Diehl called these state pharmaceutical associations "the children of the American Pharmaceutical Association."[43] Indeed, the American Pharmaceutical Association inspired the founding of these organizations wherever and whenever it could. "Thus we often find, that the early officers of the state organizations are also active members of the American association, and that the organization of a state body followed a meeting of the American association near the birth place of the new society."[44]

However, the medical influence, which had been so decisive in the formation of early local pharmaceutical societies, was

sometimes an impelling force also in the establishment of state associations. For instance, it was only after definite steps by the Medical Society of New Jersey to force legislative measures on "all dispensers of medicines" in the state, that the New Jersey Pharmaceutical Association was founded (1870) "to establish the relation between them [the pharmacists] and physicians, and the people at large, upon just principles . . ."[45]

The State Medical Association of Mississippi resolved (1871) "that the druggists, pharmacists, and chemists of the State of Mississippi be requested to call a convention at an early day, and organize a State Pharmaceutical Association, to meet annually at the same time and place that the Medical Association does, and cooperate with it in any and all measures of mutual interest and importance."[46] Only a month later, the Mississippi Pharmaceutical Association was founded. This new organization tried to stabilize the good relations with its older medical sister on the one hand and at the same time to gain recognition and support within the profession of pharmacy. One of the first resolutions of the new association was to the effect that the president was to be an ex-officio delegate to the State Medical Association and that the two organizations should cooperate. At the same time, it adopted the constitution of the American Pharmaceutical Association and urged "all pharmacists in the State to join" the national representative of American professional pharmacy.[47]

Yet, the founding of state pharmaceutical associations soon became a self-propelled and independent movement. At least potentially, these associations gave pharmacists a more effective medium for organized cooperation, but until the present century they usually represented—as did the earlier local associations—only a small ambitious minority of pharmacists. How the organization of pharmacists into state blocs spread through the country may be perceived from the chronologic list of the founding of the state associations (see Appendix 2).[48] That more than half of them were organized in little more than a decade, centering in the 1880's, gives striking evidence that the "time was ripe" for pharmacists to put their group efforts on a wider stage. During this period, also, most of the state pharmacy acts came into existence. Both lines of activity were stimulated by the American Pharmaceutical Association and, more particularly, by its general secretary, John M. Maisch.

The desire to secure a pharmacy law, or amendments to a law considered unsatisfactory, caused most of the revivals of early and inactive state associations.[49-52]

While pharmacists themselves, through their associations, often were responsible for establishing schools and even operating them, by the turn of the century the associations and the schools tended increasingly to go separate ways. The influence of the local associations dwindled as state associations became dominant, and pharmacy schools, following an example set in some of the midwestern state universities, gradually associated themselves with general colleges or universities.

For a long time state pharmaceutical associations strongly reflected the business orientation and the limited education of the average American practitioner. They only slowly gathered support and more adequate staffs (even as late as 1947, of 39 associations reporting, 15 had no full-time executive officer)[53]; and their programs tended to be dominated by commercial concerns. But by midcentury, state associations in general were gaining wider support (partly by giving employee-pharmacists a status more nearly comparable with that of pharmacy owners), enlarging administrative facilities, and sharing more fully in the professional as well as the economic concerns of pharmacy.

Symptomatic of the change was the increasingly widespread debate on how American pharmacy might be organized for more effective action. In 1962, first in Michigan, then in Virginia, Delaware and Wisconsin, the state associations voted to integrate more closely with the American Pharmaceutical Association at the national level and, at the same time, to try to revivify local associations. Whether or not this will become a general trend or represents the

standard pattern of the future, it appears that the incursions of crassly commercial interests after World War II failed to overwhelm the independent pharmacist and, indeed, gave him a new conviction that his professional heritage and prerogatives must be safeguarded cooperatively. In that cause, the American Pharmaceutical Association already had invested more than a century of consistent thought and endeavor. For, paradoxically, the Association was not erected on the foundation of an established professional pharmacy; rather, it had largely created American professional pharmacy.

NATIONAL ORGANIZATIONS

The American Pharmaceutical Association

The American Pharmaceutical Association was the first national pharmaceutical organization, and for a long time the only one. It represented, defended and promoted, during the decades in which the calling gained its distinctive shape, all fields of pharmaceutical enterprise and interest, the scientific and educational as well as the commercial, the ethical and the legal. It always has been the guardian, although not always the initiator, of progressive movements concerning American pharmacy.

Until 1852, the concept of professional pharmacy was only a dream of the few colleges of pharmacy. Even if their influence extended beyond local boundaries, as that of the Philadelphia College of Pharmacy did, no means was available to promote the concept of professional pharmacy on a larger scale, making the presumptive members of the should-be-profession, the general public, and especially the legislators, conscious of this concept. The American Pharmaceutical Association was founded by the early colleges of pharmacy to provide this means.

The immediate incentive for the founding of the American Pharmaceutical Association lay elsewhere, in bad conditions of the drug market, whose dangers were accidentally made evident once again.

In New York, Ewen McIntyre, at that time a pharmacist for George D. Coggeshall, discovered that a portion of supposed calcium carbonate, imported from England, was in fact calcium sulfate. Coggeshall and his friend John Milhau brought the matter before the New York College of Pharmacy. Other preparations were examined and likewise proved to be substituted, adulterated or deficient in strength. Protests made to British manufacturers and exporters brought a significant reply from one Englishman who stated that the products were "as good as the Americans would pay for."[54]

A petition to Congress, signed by pharmacists as well as by physicians all over the country, resulted in the subsequent passage of a law requiring the observance of certain standards, which went into force in 1848. The effect was unsatisfactory. The Medical Association of South Carolina requested the Secretary of the Treasury to appoint a more efficient inspector for the port of Charleston and "in its meeting of 1850 the society was pleased to note that the unsatisfactory inspector had been removed."[55] However, since the occasional change of inspectors did not mean a change of the whole system, it brought little or no improvement.

This failure to secure the desired results was attributed to the lack of fitness on the part of the inspectors installed at the several ports of entry, who were appointed for their political affiliation rather than for their ability, although they were to some extent handicapped by the lack of clearness in the wording of the law in regard to standard books.[56]

At this time, there was still no strict borderline between medicine and pharmacy in the United States. Many men with medical degrees made their living chiefly, if not exclusively, by operating pharmacies. One of these, C. B. Guthrie, a doctor of medicine and a practicing pharmacist in the city of New York, requested (following the advice of the New York College of Pharmacy) that the American Medical Association act against drug adulteration. As a delegate of this pharmaceutical group, he presented a proposal concerning standards to be used by drug inspectors (1851).

The result was illuminating. The physicians attending the meeting were in doubt, apparently, as to whether this proposal of a local group of pharmacists was indeed representative of the opinion of American pharmacy as a whole. As the report in the *American Journal of Pharmacy* puts it, "the sentiment of the [American Medical] Association was evidently in favor of such a tariff of standards, but they wanted it to be more fully matured by a convention of Colleges [local associations] of Pharmacy."[57] Moreover, the action of a delegate of a *pharmaceutical* group at this *medical* forum prompted the offering of a resolution declaring the ineligibility of delegates of colleges of pharmacy and dentistry. This resolution, although not adopted but referred to a committee, was symptomatic.

What a striking demonstration of the necessity for a national pharmaceutical organization which would be representative of American pharmacy and could speak for the whole profession. Four months later (September 9, 1851) the New York College of Pharmacy invited the sister Colleges (associations) in Philadelphia, Baltimore, Boston and Cincinnati to send delegates to a convention to be held in the city of New York on October 15 and 16 of the same year. This convention was called with the restricted purpose of complying with the medical demands made at Charleston for united action of medicine and pharmacy in the question of drug adulteration. As the invitation put it, the convention was convened "for the purpose of considering the propriety and practicability of fixing a set of standard strengths and qualities of drugs and chemicals for the government of the United States Drug Inspectors."[58]

However, there was a strong feeling, at least among the members of one local group (the Philadelphia College of Pharmacy), that the time had come to consider, not one individual problem of American pharmacy, but the all-comprehensive problem of an American profession of pharmacy and its adequate and permanent representation. In the *American Journal of Pharmacy*, William Procter, Jr., then the Editor, gave the following account:

When the invitation . . . was received by the Philadelphia College of Pharmacy, several of the members expressed the opinion that, although the call was for a special object, the Convention might take a wider range in its influence, and form a *point d'appui* from which the pharmaceutical profession of the whole country may be reached, and a course of action instituted, which eventually would revolutionize the condition of Pharmacy in the United States.[59]

Coming to the 1851 New York "Convention of Pharmaceutists and Druggists" with such definite views, the Philadelphia delegation—particularly its most important member, William Procter, Jr.—imbued the minds of the participants from Boston and New York (there were no delegates from Baltimore and Cincinnati) with a broader aim. It exerted a decisive influence on the shaping as well as the unanimous adoption of the memorable resolution recommending

that a Convention be called, consisting of three Delegates each from incorporated and unincorporated Pharmaceutical Societies, to meet at Philadelphia, on the First Wednesday in October 1852, when all the important questions bearing on the Profession may be considered, and *measures adopted for the organization of a National Association,** to meet every year.

The resolution was adopted unanimously. When William Procter, Jr., stated that with the adoption of this resolution "the most sanguine hopes of these members [of the Philadelphia College of Pharmacy] were gratified," he undoubtedly expressed satisfaction with a success which, to a very great extent, was won as a result of his personal insight and endeavor.[60]

When the founding convention met the next year, October 6 to 8, 1852, in the Hall of the Philadelphia College of Pharmacy, probably 20 men from various parts of the country actively participated (including several officially seated although not bearing credentials as delegates of a society).

The venerable Daniel B. Smith, who 31 years earlier had been one of the founders of the Philadelphia College of Pharmacy (and its president from 1829 to 1854) was made the first president of the new national association. William Procter, Jr., of the same

___

* Italics added.

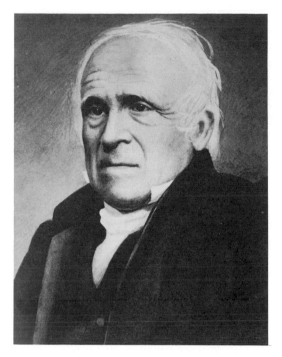

Presiding over the founding meeting of the American Pharmaceutical Association was one of the most respected American pharmacists of his time, Daniel B. Smith, a practicing pharmacist of Philadelphia whose name is associated with diverse civic enterprises. For example, he was one of the organizers of Haverford College as well as the Philadelphia "House of Refuge" and the Apprentice's Library. He was the first President of the American Pharmaceutical Association, the first Secretary of the Philadelphia College of Pharmacy and the first Corresponding Secretary of the Historical Society of Pennsylvania. (From a portrait by John Collins, Philadelphia)

College, was elected corresponding secretary. The other officers were residents of Baltimore, Boston, Cincinnati and New York. The only other states represented at the founding convention were Virginia (Richmond), California (San Francisco) and Connecticut. There is no doubt that the early American Pharmaceutical Association was essentially an Eastern affair. Yet, at this time, so was the whole idea of pharmaceutical education and professionalism.

The *aim* of these pioneers of American

pharmacy was a truly national and all-embracing one. The preamble of the constitution admitted that "a large portion of those in whose hands the practice of pharmacy [in the United States] now exists, are not properly qualified for the responsible offices it involves, chiefly by reason of the many difficulties that impede the acquirement of a correct knowledge of their business."[61] How could this lack of education be remedied if those who needed it most were excluded instead of taken in? Hence the doors were thrown open to "all pharmaceutists and druggists who shall have attained the age of twenty-one years, whose character morally and professionally is fair, and who, after duly considering the obligations of the Constitution and Code of Ethics of this Association, are willing to subscribe to them." [Constitution of 1852, section 11, article I]

Yet, this opening of the doors to "all pharmaceutists and druggists" seems more theoretic than actual so long as the applicants were to subscribe to a "Code of Ethics" advanced far beyond the given realities of common practice. This Code of Ethics, modeled after the one accepted by the Philadelphia College of Pharmacy (1848),[62] asked those who honored it "to discountenance quackery" i.e., to give up the sale of nostrums regarded as "quackery" by official medicine. This obligation, said Edward Parrish, "has never impressed itself as a duty upon many whose aid we desire to invoke in our earliest efforts. It is mainly by the sale of quack medicines that many druggists subsist, who yet desire a reform in their business, and would be glad to cooperate in the laudable objects of the Association . . ."[63] In his opinion, these ethical rules had to be the goal but not the condition for membership, while the new national organization was in its embryonic stage. Assenting to this view (1855), the Association dropped the obligation to subscribe to the Code of Ethics as a prerequisite of membership.

From now on the Code of Ethics disappeared from the literature of the American Pharmaceutical Association, until its modified revival in 1922.[64] At the instigation of Charles La Wall, in that year the Association adopted a new and rather comprehensive code, stating in three chapters the duties of the pharmacist (1) in his services to the public, (2) in his relations to the physician and (3) in his relations to other pharmacists and to the profession of pharmacy at large.[65]

There was still another important compromise between principle and reality which the founders of the American Pharmaceutical Association had to accept. Like the fathers of the American Medical Association, which was founded 5 years earlier, they had adopted the principle of regional representation. The Constitution stated that "the members shall consist of delegates from regularly constituted Colleges of Pharmacy, and Pharmaceutical Societies." It allowed the participation of individual pharmacists, who were not "delegates," only with the consent of "the delegates from the places whence they come," or, if there were no such delegates, "on obtaining the certificates of any three members of the Association. . . ." This statement disappeared in 1855. The revised article was retained unchanged in the reconstruction of the entire constitution in 1856. Thereafter, membership was open to every "pharmaceutist or druggist of good moral and professional standing whether in business on his own account, retired from business or employed by another, who, after duly considering the objects of the association and the obligations of its Constitution is willing to subscribe to them." The power to expel a member "for improper conduct by a vote of two-thirds of the members present at any annual meeting" was retained.

The idea of regional representation was by no means entirely abandoned. It was stated that "every local Pharmaceutical Association shall be entitled to five delegates in the annual meetings, who, if present, become members of the Association, on signing the Constitution, without being balloted for." The idea of adequate representation within the American Pharmaceutical Association of all groups in pharmacy, on both a regional basis and a basis of common special interests, found its most impressive materialization in the "House of Delegates." The idea for such a body came from the creative mind of James H. Beal in 1911 and was adopted that same year by vote of the Council and the Assembly of the Association.[66]

In logical consequence of the abandonment of the code of ethics (1855), the goals of the Association, insofar as they were to be made formal and accepted by the members, had to be included in the Constitution. Therefore, Article I, which originally stated only the name of the organization, read as follows in the form adopted in 1856:

Article I. This association shall be called the American Pharmaceutical Association. Its aim shall be to unite the educated and reputable pharmaceutists and druggists of the United States in the following objects:

1st. To improve and regulate the drug market, by preventing the importation of inferior, adulterated or deteriorated drugs, and by detecting and exposing home adulteration.

2nd. To establish the relations between druggists, pharmaceutists, physicians and the people at large, upon just principles, which shall promote the public welfare and tend to mutual strength and advantage.

3d. To improve the science and the art of pharmacy by diffusing scientific knowledge among apothecaries and druggists, fostering pharmaceutical literature, developing talent, stimulating discovery and invention, and encouraging home production and manufacture in the several departments of the drug business.

4th. To regulate the system of apprenticeship and employment so as to prevent as far as practicable, the evils flowing from deficient training in the responsible duties of preparing, dispensing and selling medicines.

5th. To suppress empiricism [i.e., quackery] and as much as possible to restrict the dispensing and sale of medicines to regularly educated druggists and apothecaries.

An amendment adopted in 1870 implies that it no longer seemed appropriate to concede that "a large portion" of the pharmaceutical practitioners were "not properly qualified." In Section 5 of Article I, the words "as much as possible" were dropped, making it now the unconditional task of the American Pharmaceutical Association "to

suppress empiricism and to restrict the dispensing and sale of medicines to regularly educated druggists and apothecaries." Finally, two new paragraphs were added to Article I:

6th. To uphold standards of authority in the education, theory and practice of pharmacy.

7th. To create and maintain a standard of professional honesty equal to the amount of our professional knowledge, with a view to the highest good and greatest protection to the public.

The wisdom with which these constitutional purposes were originally written (1856) is evidenced by the Association's "Objects" today. For although the phrasing has been modernized extensively (revision of Constitution and By-Laws, 1951), the fundamentals have changed little.[67]

The fact that the early colleges of pharmacy were associations of practicing pharmacists, which maintained educational institutions, was of the highest importance for the development of the new organization. The leaders of the Colleges, who shaped the work of the American Pharmaceutical Association, had experienced in their local districts all the problems faced by pharmacy in this period and therefore were able to deal with them efficiently and realistically within the national organization.

The other great national pharmaceutical associations in the United States, have been, in some sense, specialized outgrowths of the American Pharmaceutical Association. They have rarely lost their connection with the mother organization, since the latter, while delegating certain functions to the younger societies, has maintained its position as the highest court within the profession for all matters pertaining to pharmacy proper.[68]

Wherever continuous systematic work or propagandistic action in a special field was required, specialized organizations have tended to crystallize out. But wherever special interests could be served by an occasional forum and channel for policy formation, these have tended to find expression within the American Pharmaceutical Association itself. Responding to these needs in 1887, the Association established 4 sections

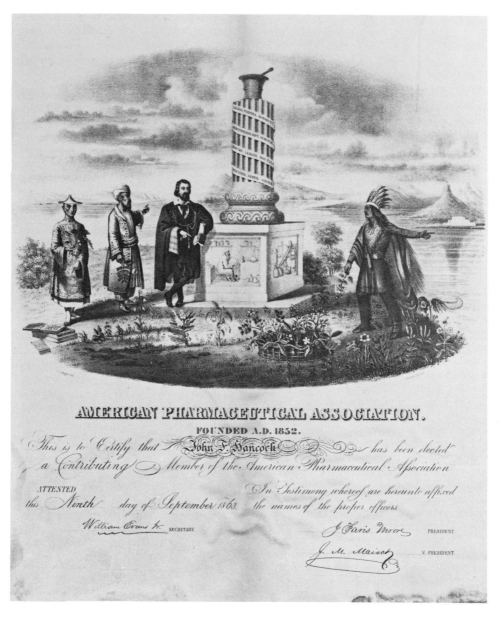

Ornate and symbol-laden, the original membership certificate of the American Pharmaceutical Association was based on the certificate of the Pharmaceutical Society of Great Britain. ". . . Objections were made to the adoption of any part of the English certificate, desiring a picture suggestive only of American ideas, but the Committee very properly pointed to the universality of Pharmaceutic Science . . ." The classic column represents the old and solid foundation of the profession; on it a winding scroll lists some of the great names out of its history; every region contributes to pharmacy and the materia medica (note medicinal plants and books), as suggested by the four figures representing, left to right, the Far East, the Middle East, Europe and the Americas. (See Am. J. Pharm. *27*:483, 485, and *28*:187-188.)

"to expedite and render more efficient the work," apparently using the American Medical Association as a model.

Said Joseph P. Remington, chairman of the Committee on Management, ". . . We believe that a National Association should be so comprehensive in its scope that every important interest should be effectively represented."

Thus arose the "Sections"—annual forums in which specialized pharmaceutical questions could be discussed and whence have come many of the policy proposals debated in the House of Delegates of the American Pharmaceutical Association.[69]

Through the decades the structure of the Sections at annual meetings has changed occasionally as pharmacy or the outlook of the Association has changed, or as a new association made one of the old separate sections less essential. Of the original 4 sections, only the Scientific Section remains unchanged in its scope, reflecting the steadfastness of the Association in trying to represent adequately the scientific basis on which pharmaceutical practice rests. The old Sections on Commercial Interests (called Pharmaceutical Economics after 1937), on Pharmaceutical Education and on Legislation now are merged into a Section on General Practice of Pharmacy. The concerns of these former Sections now have become largely the responsibility of "daughter" associations—respectively, the National Association of Retail Druggists, the American Association of Colleges of Pharmacy, the National Association of Boards of Pharmacy and the American College of Apothecaries.

Besides the Scientific Section and the Section on General Practice of Pharmacy, the annual meetings offer separate sessions and discussion forums through Sections on Pharmaceutical Technology (before 1961, called the Section on Practical Pharmacy), on Industrial Pharmacy (since 1960), on Historical Pharmacy and on Military Pharmacy, and a Student Section (representing the student branches in schools of pharmacy). Other special interests, though distinguishable from the profession as a whole, have not found permanent expression

through a distinct Section or separate affiliate (e.g., the Women's Section, 1914-1923). Conversely, the annual forum of a Section (for papers and discussion) may persist despite the emergence of a specialized organization for year-round work and broader activities (e.g., the Section on Historical Pharmacy [f. 1904] and the American Institute of the History of Pharmacy [f. 1941]).

Some of the specialized organizations that have grown out of activities of the American Pharmaceutical Association, under diverse circumstances and retaining varying degrees of coordination or affiliation with the "mother association," are listed below. (The sequence is according to the founding of the initial organization in a field, even though it died and was later reborn in a new form.)

Conference of Teaching Colleges of Pharmacy[70] (1870-1884), the first organization of school representatives, was succeeded by the present American Association of Colleges of Pharmacy (1900), at first called (before 1925) the Conference of Pharmaceutical Faculties[71] (see p. 222)

National Retail Druggists Association (1883-1887), the first organization devoted mainly to the business and financial interests of the owners of pharmacies or drugstores, was succeeded by the present National Association of Retail Druggists (1898; see below)[72]

Association of Boards of Pharmacy and Secretaries of State Pharmaceutical Associations (1890-?1892),[73] which soon faded away, was succeeded by two separate organizations of today, the National Association of Boards of Pharmacy (1904; see p. 198) and the National Conference of State Pharmaceutical Association Secretaries (1927), at first (before 1949) called the Conference of Pharmaceutical Association Secretaries[74]

Conference of Pharmaceutical Law Enforcement Officials, founded (1929) under the aegis of the A.Ph.A. but since 1944 a component of the National Association of Boards of Pharmacy, has provided a forum on methods and problems[75]

American College of Apothecaries (1939),

the first organization for exclusively professional pharmacies, was called during its first year the Conference of Professional Pharmacists[76]

American Institute of the History of Pharmacy (1941),[77] provides a year-round center for research, information, publication and other sociohistorical activities. (In the same year, a corporation of members of the American Pharmaceutical Association, the Friends of Historical Pharmacy,[78] was formed to maintain the restored colonial apothecary shop of General Hugh Mercer and might similarly take custody of other historic properties.)

American Society of Hospital Pharmacists (1942; see p. 189)

Two of the organizations mentioned that serve practicing pharmacists merit further comment here; the first of these is the large National Association of Retail Druggists, which is to the business sphere of pharmacy what the American Pharmaceutical Association is to the professional and scientific sphere.

National Association of Retail Druggists

In the early 80's of the 19th century, a strong feeling existed among community pharmacists that their business interests could not be taken care of adequately within the frame of the American Pharmaceutical Association. This feeling was strengthened when the Western Wholesale Druggists' Association (founded in 1876) was transformed into a national organization under the name of "National Wholesale Druggists' Association" (1882).

One year later the "National Retail Druggists' Association" was founded. The name itself intimated a close analogy between the two groups. The wholesalers as well as the retailers felt endangered by a growing tendency toward a direct connection between manufacturer and consumer and by rapid expansion of ruinous price cutting. Nevertheless, it soon became obvious that the wholesale druggist could not go the whole way, together with the retail druggist, and that no quick and sweeping results could be expected, especially with regard

to price cutting. Consequently, the National Retail Druggists' Association was dissolved, and the "Section on Commercial Interests" was created within the American Pharmaceutical Association (1887). The last president of the former, A. H. Hollister, served as the first chairman of the latter.

It soon became evident that, while the Section on Commercial Interests, with the moral weight of the American Pharmaceutical Association at its command, could effectively *assist* the endeavor to protect the business interests of pharmacy owners, it was entirely beyond the ability of the Section to watch the situation adequately and to *initiate* and pursue consistently and effectively the actions and the counteractions required.[79]

Again frustrated in dealing with commercial economic forces generated outside their own ranks and not easily controlled, pharmacists decided to begin anew an organization devoted to their business interests. On the initiative of the Chicago Retail Druggists' Association, and with the approval of a committee of the Section on Commercial Interests of the American Pharmaceutical Association, headed by J. P. Remington of the Philadelphia College of Pharmacy, "The National Association of Retail Druggists" was founded at St. Louis, in 1898.

This new organization was there to stay. It had the encouragement of initial success in achieving the abandonment of the war tax imposed on proprietary medicines and toiletries after the Spanish-American war. Moreover, the National Association of Retail Druggists has given the concept and the laws of "fair trade" effective support and skillful defense as the most effective weapon yet devised against ruinous price cutting. After 1911 (Miles case before the Supreme Court), "vertical" agreements for price maintenance (between vendor and distributors) became legally questionable, as "horizontal" agreements (among distributors) had been before. The issues at stake have been, in some form, a matter of legal and legislative controversy ever since. Since attempts to protect the prices of branded products had met with repeated failure into the 1920's, the effective leadership exercised by the Association thereafter in obtaining valid "fair trade" legislation commanded loyal support, especially among the pharmacy owners who constitute its regular membership.

In this and other ways the "N.A.R.D." has demonstrated the compelling need for organized cooperation on questions of business and finance, just as the "A.Ph.A." has done in the professional and scientific sphere. Cooperation between these two great national associations has long been an accepted principle and goal among many American pharmacists. Yet, for periods such as the 1950's this desideratum not only failed to be achieved, but open conflict and cross purposes of the two associations confronted pharmacists with a grave handicap.

Coordination of Organized Endeavor

On the other hand, during the preceding decade, one promising approach toward maintaining effective communication, coordination and division of labor or function between the associations had been demonstrated.[80] Prompted by a request from the Conference of State Pharmaceutical Association Secretaries, negotiations led by the executive secretaries (E. F. Kelly for the A.Ph.A. and John W. Dargavel for the N.A.R.D.) culminated at a combined meeting of their executive boards (1943). They "provided for annual conferences between the executive bodies to be held in the fall of each year," for the purpose of "surveying and studying the resolutions adopted by the A.Ph.A. and the N.A.R.D. and by the state and local associations during the year; and for a competent study of mutual problems of recognized pharmaceutical importance and significance, and for the purpose of each group dealing with these matters as circumstances may indicate."

The following year "plans were made to coordinate future activities of the two organizations in meeting the developing problems of American pharmacy." To further that objective, a continuing joint committee was named to function, between joint conferences, the year round (consisting of the president, the secretary and the board

chairman of both the American Pharmaceutical Association and the National Association of Retail Druggists).[81] Moreover, cross representation was provided on key committees of the two associations.

This productive mechanism disintegrated by the 1950's for a complex of reasons never fully evaluated, including disagreement on legislative issues (Durham-Humphrey bill), overlapping functions, personal incompatibilities and, perhaps not least of all, a question of primacy between professional and commercial values among practitioners. The disharmony that ensued[82] has revived old ambitions and efforts to give the practicing pharmacist a more unified voice and a more effective medium of organized endeavor.

American Society of Hospital Pharmacists

As the National Association of Retail Druggists had drawn strength from the business problems and economic ambitions of pharmacy owners, so the professional ambitions of hospital pharmacists carried them beyond the family circle of the American Pharmaceutical Association into a separate society that developed vigorously.

Until the 1920's American hospital pharmacists had been a subordinate group, in organization as well as in the institutions where they practiced. In a "classic paper" that Alex Berman has called the manifesto of the hospital pharmacy movement, E. C. Austin, Cincinnati hospital pharmacist, spoke of the appalling lack of well-trained hospital pharmacists and of the apathy of the pharmaceutical profession toward its hospital specialty.[83]

Increasingly dissatisfied with the limited status and sphere of activities provided by a Sub-Section on Hospital Pharmacy within the American Pharmaceutical Association, the professionally ambitious hospital pharmacists struck out on their own as the American Society of Hospital Pharmacists during the 1942 meeting of the American Pharmaceutical Association. Like the American College of Apothecaries before them, the hospital pharmacists made membership in the parent Association a prerequisite to membership in their own Society.

The first two chairmen of the Society

were especially influential in maintaining its high level and progressive direction, H. A. K. Whitney particularly in the formative period and, in subsequent years, Don E. Francke, now Scientific Director of the Society and since 1944 editor of the remarkable *American Journal of Hospital Pharmacy*. By the 1950's a hard core of other leaders generated in the ranks of hospital pharmacy a sustained professional enthusiasm and esprit de corps that seemed to contrast with their more affluent but less unified and less optimistic colleagues in community practice. In two decades the membership of the American Society of Hospital Pharmacists had grown from 150 to more than 3,000.

Large-scale hospital construction, mushroom growth of the prepaid medical care, and steadily increasing drug distribution through hospitals all favored the Society's program; yet foresighted planning and energetic work within the Society itself were largely responsible for the first minimum standards for hospital pharmacies, the short postgraduate courses ("institutes") in cooperation with the American and the Catholic Hospital Associations and the American Pharmaceutical Association, the standards for internship in hospital pharmacy, the success of its *Journal* (originally, *The Bulletin*), the *American Hospital Formulary Service*, and the far-reaching Audit of Pharmaceutical Service in Hospitals (jointly sponsored with the American Pharmaceutical Association). An explanation of these achievements, and at the same time itself an achievement, is what Paul Parker as the Society's president termed "the unity of hospital pharmacists throughout America."[84]

Other National Organizations

After the turn of the century the pharmaceutical personnel of America became increasingly segmented under the growing influences of specialization, differences of function and objective and divergent educational backgrounds and socioeconomic circumstances. The deeply probing national "Pharmaceutical Survey" of 1946 to 1949 concluded that

American pharmacy is represented by a wide range of professional and commercial associations and their publications. However, their aims and activities are uncoordinated, ofttimes in conflict, and therefore tend to produce a low rate and quantity of professional accomplishment.[85]

Tangled lines of communication and conflicting representation generated the movement toward better coordination after World War II. At the same time there seemed to be a clearer if tacit recognition that the profession of pharmacy was by no means co-extensive with the pharmaceutical field, a field whose varied, vertically structured components have not favored a stable entente concerning policies and programs.

The tendency toward fragmentation has produced so many temporary organizations during the organized life of American pharmacy that there would be little use in reviewing them all even if space permitted. Some of the organizations encountered repeatedly in pharmaceutical literature (unlike those mentioned previously) did not arise within the circle of the American Pharmaceutical Association; these are listed below:

Owners and Employees of Pharmacies:

National Drug Clerks Association (1910-1934)[86] served employed pharmacists seeking better salary and hours, but also better standards of practice generally and national reciprocity of licenses; before 1912 called the National Association of Pharmacologists

National Association of Chain Drugstores (1933)

National Pharmaceutical Association (1949), for the Negro pharmacist "to improve himself and his economic position"; an outgrowth of two pharmacy seminars for Negroes, 1947 and 1948[87]

National Catholic Pharmacists Guild of the United States (1962), for promoting dedication to Catholic principles and missions, particularly in terms of pharmacy, and for fostering diocesan pharmacists' guilds

Pharmaceutical Manufacturers:

Proprietary Association of America (1881),[88]

PHARMACY ORGANIZATION CHART

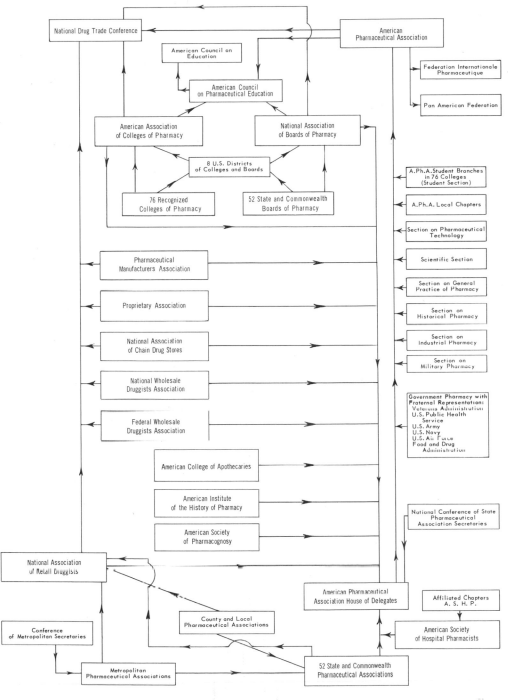

The complexly organized structure that has evolved since the first local association (1821) is shown in its organic relationships. Nonaffiliated organizations are not shown (e.g., American Foundation of Pharmaceutical Education, Druggists Service Council, National Pharmaceutical Council, National Pharmaceutical Assoc., Parenteral Drug Assoc., Pharmaceutical Wholesalers Assoc. and Toilet Goods Assoc.). (Chart from National Pharmaceutical Council, New York, 1963)

for makers of home medications, home medical supplies and cosmetics

American Pharmaceutical Manufacturers Association (1908; known before 1921 as the American Association of Pharmaceutical Chemists) and the American Drug Manufacturers Association (1912; known before 1917 as the National Association of Manufacturers of Medicinal Products) merged in 1958 to form the Pharmaceutical Manufacturers Association, like its predecessors consisting of makers of prescription drugs[89]

Parenteral Drug Association (1946)

Wholesale Druggists:

National Wholesale Druggists Association (1876); before 1882 called Western Wholesale Druggists Association[90] (what would be now known as "Midwestern")

Federal Wholesale Druggists Association (1915),[91] mainly "mutual" or cooperative drug houses in original concept

Pharmaceutical Wholesalers Association, (1957) for houses dealing mainly in prescription products, especially in the western states

The length of such a list could be multiplied in a specialized account of all organizations having pharmaceutical relevance, in the American past and present.[92] This historical circumstance suggests not so much a highly organized profession as it does a profession that has not been as effectively organized and unified as analogous professions such as dentistry, law and medicine have been.

A movement to surmount this handicap by a federation of associations, through the American Pharmaceutical Association, arose in the 1950's following the collapse of hopes that the activities of the pharmacist's professional society (A.Ph.A.) and the pharmacy owners' association (N.A.R.D.) could be coordinated or at least better harmonized. One of the most effective spokesmen for the "federation" movement has been J. Curtis Nottingham of Virginia, although his proposal (1954) at first received scant support.

This movement culminated (1962) in the American Pharmaceutical Association's action to create a new basis for unified professional action among pharmacists. In its fundamentals, the plan permits local, state and national organizations of pharmacists to link themselves together as affiliates of the Association. All who join an "affiliate" must also belong to the American Pharmaceutical Association. An affiliate gains a commanding voice in the policy-making House of Delegates of the Association without yielding its local powers or authority in its specialized field.

In the 1960's it is too early to be certain whether or not this plan will unify pharmacists professionally as they have not been before. Some see the issue as a crucial one. Said the pharmacist and editor Don E. Francke,

Despite the existence of a plan for the federation of American pharmacy with its inherent program for developing a closely knit integrated county-state-national membership structure, the big question remains: Will American pharmacy, and particularly the state associations, become an integral part of it through direct affiliation? We dare not hope otherwise.[93]

13: The Rise of Legislative Standards

Any movement carries within itself the seeds of its own destruction. Reluctantly it nourishes them, tolerates them, helps them to survive. Gradually they grow until the movement itself is overshadowed, until its originators find themselves in the peculiarly uncomfortable position of condoning what they had condemned and of following what they had organized to oppose. Thus it was in pharmacy. Organizations which at first were established to avoid legal restrictions in the practice of pharmacy became the initiators and, subsequently, the guardians of American pharmaceutical legislation.

A number of laws have affected the practice of pharmacy in one way or another. The following explanations are devoted exclusively to legislation that has created the structure of American pharmacy or, at least, has decisively influenced it.

LOCAL LAWS

What we know as "pharmacy laws"—special legislation that covers pharmaceutical activities comprehensively—did not become common in the United States until after 1870. Before that time, American democratic and laissez-faire ideology, frontier conditions, lack of pharmacy schools and like considerations made any systematic attempt at regulating pharmacy the exception rather than the rule.

Pharmacy was, of course, an urban institution, but, even in the cities, few attempts at regulating pharmacy before 1870 are known of. New Orleans (as might be expected) tried briefly (1804) to require dispensers of drugs to register their diplomas or submit to an examination.[1] A statute of the State of New York (1832) required a diploma from a college of pharmacy or an examination before the censors of a county

medical society for the practice of pharmacy in the *city* of New York, but legal difficulties led to revision of the act (1839).[2] Mississippi required for Adams County (Natchez, 1844) that the "apothecary or vender of medicines" obtain a license from the Board of Medical Censors; and gave that Board the power and the duty of inspecting pharmacies.[3] The Charter of the City of Louisville, Kentucky, empowered the General Council (1851) to establish a "Board or Institute of Pharmacy," to require that all apothecaries be examined and licensed by that Board and "to regulate the trade of retail Apothecaries in the business of making up prescriptions, and vending poisonous substances."[4] It was later reported (1868) that the provisions of the Charter were not enforced.[5] A final example is the rather anomalous Pennsylvania statute (1866), which required that only "licensed druggists" could practice in Lycoming County (Williamsport), without establishing either criteria or procedures for licensing.[6]

So far as is known by David Cowen, who is an authority on this branch of pharmacy's history, no other local laws were passed until 1870. As Appendix 3 indicates, laws empowering the licensing of pharmacists were enacted by the respective state legislatures for the cities of Baltimore, San Francisco, Philadelphia, St. Louis, Cincinnati and Milwaukee between 1870 and 1876. In New York an attempt to impose a distasteful law for New York City—the so-called Irving Law (1871)—led to the formation of the New York Apothecaries Union. Under the leadership of Frederick Hoffman, repeal was achieved by joint effort of the Union, the German Apothecaries Society and the College of Pharmacy, thus thwarting an attempt to make pharmacy subservient to

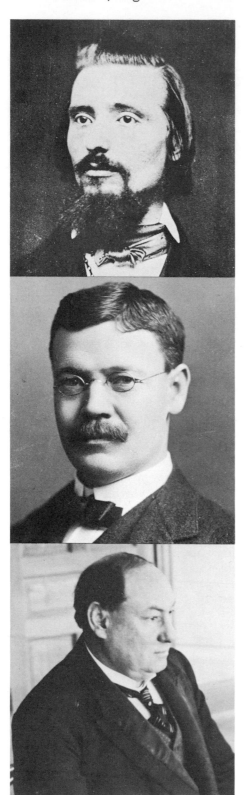

Tammany Hall, and leading to a new pharmacy law for the City of New York (1872)[7] that placed the control of a Board of Pharmacy in the hands of the College of Pharmacy.[8]

The further development of local legislation was made unnecessary by the enactment of state-wide laws after 1870.

STATE PHARMACY LAWS

In the history of American pharmacy, it is interesting that the 4 states that required the licensing of pharmacists before 1870 were all in the South: Louisiana (1808, 1816), South Carolina (1817), Georgia (1825) and Alabama (1851).[9] Louisiana's pioneering efforts are, perhaps, explained by its Franco-Spanish tradition, but legislation in the other states has not yet been satisfactorily explained.

The regulation of pharmacy in each of these states became part of the regulation of the practice of medicine. In 1808 the Territory of Orleans (Louisiana after 1812) not

Three men who were instrumental in laying the foundations of modern legislative standards for pharmacy during the three quarters of a century following the American Civil War: (*top*) John M. Maisch of Philadelphia; (*center*) James H. Beal of Ohio and (*bottom*) Harvey W. Wiley of Indiana. Pharmacist Maisch (1831-1893), as the first permanent Secretary of the American Pharmaceutical Association, assessed the state of pharmaceutical regulation (Report–1868) and led the drafting of the first model pharmacy act for use by the states. Pharmacist-lawyer Beal (1861-1945), a resourceful and influential association leader, was largely responsible three decades later for the issuance of a second model state pharmacy act, as he was also for model state statutes on narcotic and poison controls. While Beal was influential in the national debate on initiating Federal legislation, the physician-chemist Wiley (1844-1930) was the key figure in providing both scientific and polemic underpinning for passage of the first Federal Food and Drug Act. He is shown in his office as Chief of the Bureau of Chemistry, U.S. Department of Agriculture, during the years of legislative controversy.

only required apothecaries to exhibit proof of qualification and to be examined by a board of physicians, but also prohibited the sale of deteriorated drugs and restricted the sale of poisons. In 1816 Louisiana became the first state to pass a law regulating pharmacy. By this statute an apothecary was added to the examining board (a second was added in 1840), and thus there was created not only the first board of pharmacy but, also, the first such board in the United States which had a pharmacist as a permanent member. In 1838 the apothecary A. Delpeuch was secretary of the Eastern Medical Board of Louisiana, and he is, so far, the first pharmacist who is known to have served in such a capacity. The Louisiana statute existed until 1852 (although amended 5 times), when due to a resurgent spirit of laissez-faire coupled with the purported persuasiveness of quacks, all medical legislation was repealed![10]

The South Carolina statute of 1817 provided for examination and licensing of apothecaries either by the Medical Society at Charleston (later by the Medical College there) or by a group of physicians at Columbia who were named in the statute. This act remained on the books until it was replaced by a "modern" statute (1876); however, the act had been emasculated (1838) by repeal of its penalty provisions.[11] The Georgia statute of 1825 repeated almost word for word the first statute for South Carolina, and, although the penalty provisions were removed (1836 to 1839), the act remained in force until it, too, was replaced by a "modern" statute (1881).[12] In Alabama, the licensing of pharmacists found its way into the Code of 1852, and, here, too, the statute remained in effect until it was replaced by a "modern" one (1887).[13]

For some time these statutes were not the "dead letters" which they later became. In Louisiana, records indicate that licensing began as early as 1816 and that, between that year and 1847, no fewer than 124 apothecaries received licenses.[14] The pharmaceutical museum now sponsored by the Loyola College of Pharmacy is located at the site of the shop of L. J. Dufilho[15] (licensed in 1816). (See page 164.) In South Carolina, too, there are indications of the enforcement

of the law.[16] (See p. 164.) The license of Abraham A. Solomons "to carry on the Business of Apothecary and Druggist" in South Carolina (dated December 15, 1835) is the oldest such license known to be extant. In Georgia among those practicing pharmacy in 1868 only 5 were known to be formally licensed. In Alabama there is only presumptive evidence that the law there was ever enforced.[17]

When John M. Maisch presented his report on legislation to the American Pharmaceutical Association in 1868, he believed that only Georgia had a statewide statute. South Carolina did not respond to his inquiry; and the Secretary of the Governor of Alabama reported that the laws of the state were completely silent on pharmacy. Obviously, under the double impact of the growth of medical laissez-faire and of the Civil War, the laws—to use the phrase applied to the New York City statute—had become "dead letter[s] upon the statute books."[18]

But despite prevailing concepts of laissez-faire in the first seven decades of the 19th century, laws regulating pharmacy were not uncommon where public safety or questions of ethical practice appeared to be at stake. Before 1870 at least 25 states or territories had some statutory provisions regarding adulteration, and a few more had some statute concerning poisons.[19] These statutes affected the pharmacist directly. Typically, the sale of "pernicious and adulterated . . . drugs and medicines" was forbidden on the penalty of fine or imprisonment. Poison legislation requiring labeling, frequently enumerated a poison schedule, detailed special care to be taken in dispensing poisons, and, toward the end of the period, required a poison register to be kept (e.g., Pennsylvania, 1860; Wisconsin, 1862).[20] In addition, David Cowen has found that over 25 states had laws on abortion, some specifically prohibiting the advertising and the sale of abortifacients by pharmacists (e.g., Indiana, 1859). At least 15 states had liquor laws that affected the pharmacist, usually by exempting him from the prohibition or from the liquor licensing requirements (e.g., Vermont, 1802).

All this legal activity did not yet add up

to much effective support for the development of professional standards in American pharmacy in general. In particular, the pharmacy practice acts—following some initial enthusiasm—commonly offered only weak penalties and equally weak budgets to apply them. After the Civil War it became evident that the key to effective legislation lay in pharmaceutical organization. The experience of the New York Apothecaries Union (1871-72) was a case in point. Thus it is not surprising that state pharmaceutical laws and state pharmaceutical associations are closely related. Indeed, most of them were organized primarily to bring about state pharmaceutical legislation. Once an association had succeeded, there often has been a consistent fatherly interest in helping to assure proper administration of the pharmacy act.

As shown previously, the American Pharmaceutical Association fostered the organization of state pharmaceutical associations. Naturally, the mother organization did not send her children into battle without providing them with a weapon. This weapon was the so-called model law or "draft of a proposed law to regulate the practice of pharmacy and the sale of poisons and to prevent the adulteration of drugs and medicines."[21] The draft was prepared by a special committee (more particularly by John M. Maisch) and presented at the Chicago meeting of the American Pharmaceutical Association in 1869. The history of this model law shows the transitional character of this period. "The draft was liberally discussed and finally ordered to be printed in the proceedings but without the formal endorsement of the association, as many of the members doubted the advisability of encouraging pharmaceutical legislation."[22]

This inner resistance against legislative restriction, by some of the best men in American pharmacy of that time, had its origin partly in the circumstances described by John M. Maisch 3 years later when he said:

We must remember that in thinly settled districts, where frequently for many miles no drugstore can be found, physicians are compelled to dispense medicines and carry them in suitable forms in their saddle bags, while the sale of popular remedies is usually in the hands of country storekeepers who make no pretensions as to any acquaintance with drugs and their preparations. Hence the necessity which exists in the larger cities to confine the practice of pharmacy to pharmacists alone is not felt there, and the opposition to general laws came, in most cases, only from the representatives of such districts.[23]

However, an additional reason lay in the deep mistrust for the state administrations. "If we propose a law," said Dr. Squibb during the discussion of the draft, "that makes a whole train of offices and office holders, we are simply establishing another political engine in each state that will soon become corrupted to political ends." Only 2 years later the so-called Irving pharmacy law for the city of New York, mentioned previously, proved that the point of view taken by Dr. Squibb was by no means unfounded. At any rate, the knowledge that some states were about to adopt pharmacy laws without guidance, and thus might produce quite undesirable regulations, made the draft the lesser evil. Therefore, a pamphlet was printed, containing the model law and the somewhat lukewarm resolutions and conditional recommendations of the American Pharmaceutical Association. Ten copies were sent to the governors and to the speakers of the legislatures of each state in the Union.

The results confirmed the need for a model law. It became the basis of a majority of the early laws. The way in which some bills were rushed through legislative committees of the state associations and through the legislatures becomes apparent from a comparison of some of the laws with their drafts. In one instance at least, the draft consisted of nothing more nor less than a printed copy of the law of a neighboring state, with the name of the enacting state substituted in red ink.[24] The first success was registered in Rhode Island, where a statute quite close to the model law was passed (1870). But in at least 7 other states proposed laws failed to pass (by 1871).[25] Still the young state pharmaceutical associations persisted in their efforts. In 8 other states and the District of Columbia statewide statutes had been adopted by 1870;

24 more states and territories added laws in the 1880's, 13 more in the 1890's. (Appendix 3 tabulates the passage of these pharmacy laws chronologically.)

In 1900 another model law, of which James H. Beal was the spiritual father, was adopted by the American Pharmaceutical Association, this time unanimously, without long debate and without any reservations.[26] Like its older brother, this model law was sent to the various state governments.

These laws legally defined the difference between a pharmacist and a mere merchant; they established professional pharmacy as a distinct entity, existing for the public good.[27] The first model law suggested that . . .

the incorporated Colleges of Pharmacy and Pharmaceutical Societies of this State shall submit to the Governor the names of twenty pharmacists or professors in Colleges of Pharmacy, out of which number the Governor shall appoint seven persons who shall constitute the Pharmaceutical Board of the State of . . . , who shall hold office for the term of three years and until their successors shall have been appointed. . . .

This part of the model law has been

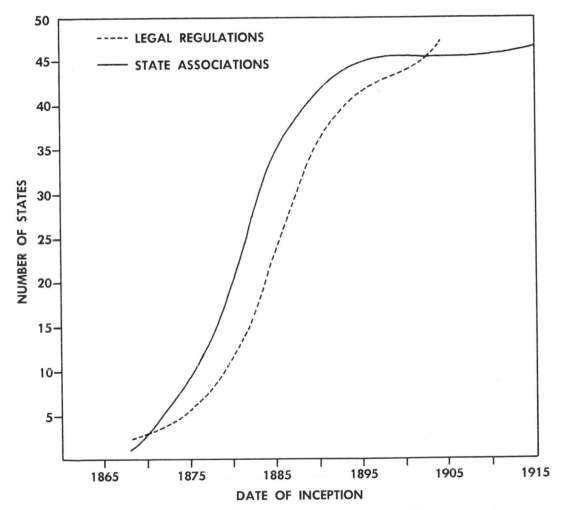

During the last third of the 19th century, state pharmacy acts of the type now known followed in the wake of the founding of state pharmaceutical associations. The influence of the state associations, armed with the American Pharmaceutical Association's model statute, is suggested by these curves plotted from dates of the beginning of state associations and state-wide laws. (Based on Appendices 2 and 3)

adopted and retained (with changes as to the number of the names submitted, the ineligibility of professors and the term of office of the State Board members) in most pharmacy acts since enacted. Thus a pharmaceutical law enforcement agency was created, the duties of which were described in the model law as follows:

The duties of the Pharmaceutical Board shall be to examine all candidates presenting themselves; to direct the registration . . . of all persons properly qualified or entitled under this Act; to cause the prosecution of all persons violating its provisions.

The expansion of state as well as federal legislation pertaining to drugs, within and without the field of pharmacy, has considerably expanded the general law-enforcing duties of the State Boards of Pharmacy. Still, the main task of the Boards consists in the examining, the licensing and the registering of pharmacists: *the guardianship of the identity and the integrity of a well-defined profession of pharmacy*. Without a legally recognized and effective pharmaceutical profession, two important national laws, the Federal Food, Drug and Cosmetic Act and the Harrison Narcotics Act, would have lacked the substratum on which the respective Federal agencies engaged in enforcing them were to rest. The above laws, while not dealing exclusively with pharmacy, still very substantially affected it.

Boards Organize

The new state boards of pharmacy often were not well equipped, by experience, knowledge or budget, to meet the heavy responsibilities thrust upon them. Legal provisions varied widely enough across the country to make reciprocity of state licenses more a wish than a goal. By the late 19th century these conditions made clear the place and the purpose of cooperation among the state boards of pharmacy.

At meetings of the American Pharmaceutical Association after 1887 the Section on Education and Legislation helped to pull together and guide the efforts of board members. From the beginning, it was understood that state board affairs and legislation would be perennial topics in the Section. In the Section, board members found a meeting ground, one that nourished understanding and cooperation, but this annual open forum soon proved to be too cramped as an effective medium for dealing with such specialized problems—especially with the impasse on interchange of pharmacists' licenses between states ("reciprocity").

In the same year that a rather ineffectual National Confederation of State Medical Boards came into existence (1890), there was born a short-lived joint organization between state boards of pharmacy and state association secretaries. However, the principle and the need that gave birth to this ill-fated association did not die with it.

Speaking before the American Conference of Pharmaceutical Faculties (1903), Edward Kremers of the University of Wisconsin suggested that it would be desirable for members of the faculties and the boards to meet together. His Conference colleagues agreed and invited the Boards to a joint conference proposed as part of the next annual meeting (held, by tradition, in association with the meeting of the American Pharmaceutical Association). Six days later, the Association's Section on Education and Legislation heard Henry Whelpley of St. Louis refer to the invitation from the Conference of Pharmaceutical Faculties and again propose, as he had in 1901, that the boards of pharmacy organize.

At the next annual meeting (1904), in the Section on Education and Legislation, Dr. Murray Galt Motter, one of the key figures, announced that representatives of 16 boards had just participated in an organizational conference for a "National Association of Boards of Pharmacy."

Then as now, the autonomy of individual states and their constituent agencies in the control of professions barred any national compulsory standards or uniform patterns of administration, from whatever quarter this might be attempted. Yet, there has been a wide area where interchange of views and agreement on *recommended* practices and minimum standards can be largely effected through the informal federation of state board members represented by the "N.A.B.P."

A common desire for reciprocity strongly motivated the founding; and this keystone of the Association's program long remained a persistent problem. Some boards stood defiantly on "state's rights." Others insisted that their own, and naturally "best" methods be adopted by other boards wanting to reciprocate.

It is to the credit of the National Association of Boards of Pharmacy that, despite these circumstances, a functioning system of reciprocity was evolved that commands the allegiance of all but a few states. Corollary activities have been the encouraging of more valid and uniform state board examinations, the setting up of principles and the improvement of standards for the pharmaceutical internship. After the 1940's, the Association also encouraged the constituent boards to overcome the deficiencies that were rather bluntly pointed out by The Pharmaceutical Survey.

An annual *Proceedings* volume (since 1906) supplemented by the *N.A.B.P. Bulletin* (since 1935) provides a means of communication among board members and between them and the profession.

Effective communication with the schools has been especially important, since legal authority over the qualifications of a pharmacist rests with the boards, but the educational authority rests with the schools. To improve both the communication and the cooperation that such a relationship demands, joint conferences between respective associations of boards and schools have been traditional.

Misunderstandings and dissension limited the effectiveness of this relationship until about the time of the first World War. Across the country in 1921 boards of pharmacy convened in 9 district meetings for the first time, supplementing the annual national meeting; and within a few years these meetings were functioning effectively as joint sessions of the boards and the faculties serving each group of states. Thus a new channel for regional cooperation emerged that still retains a significant place in American pharmacy.

The concern of the National Association of Boards of Pharmacy for the welfare of the American Council on Pharmaceutical Education finds a fundamental basis in the tenet that "all member Boards recognize only such colleges and schools of pharmacy which are on the accredited list of the American Council on Pharmaceutical Education."[27a] (Concerning the Council, see p. 223.)

FOOD AND DRUG LAW

The Constitution of the United States and court decisions have left police power largely with the individual states. However, there are activities for which uniform national regulation is necessary or at least highly desirable. One of these activities is that of supplying the people with good, genuine and unadulterated foods and drugs.

After enacting a drug import control in 1848, which placed inspectors in the principal ports of entry, Congress left the field largely to control by the individual states. The uneven social development among the states, unwillingness to place Federal power against abuses in the domestic drug market, and inadequate recognition of the states' limitations in such a complex field all combined to put federal legislation out of range until the present century. A model food and drug statute issued by the National Board of Trade (U.S.A.) influenced a number of states to try to deal with the problem of substandard and misrepresented foods and drugs.

Meanwhile, experience both abroad and in individual states of this country fostered eventual passage of a Federal law. England had attracted attention with its first broad enactment covering both foods and drugs (1875). And on returning from Germany, Harvey W. Wiley, who was to be enormously influential, said his experience with the German Imperial Board of Health made him enthusiastic about the possibility of enforcing standards of purity in foods and drugs.[28] He gave this enthusiasm scientific backing and, after 1883, political leverage from his vantage point in the Bureau of Chemistry of the U. S. Department of Agriculture. Wiley's work helped to stimulate the enactment of food and drug provisions in state laws, as it later did the national legislation.

Crude controls aimed at fraudulent or willful adulteration often entered state statutes through the first modern pharmacy practice acts, discussed previously. The results were disappointing to the American Pharmaceutical Association, which editorialized that "One reason for this is undoubtedly the fact that to carry on such work systematically and continuously requires such expenditures as have never been granted to any state pharmacy board."[29] It was symptomatic of a new line of development when the section on adulteration was omitted from the second model state pharmacy act drafted by the American Pharmaceutical Association.

More carefully drawn separate statutes also did not prove to be adequate to the task, and frustration became apparent among those who wanted specific drug standards. In 1895 the journal *Pharmaceutical Era* concluded that "state regulation has been fairly tried, and the discovery made that State lines have little force in maintaining standards for food and drugs. . . ."[30]

Meanwhile, Harvey Wiley was demonstrating the effectiveness of scientific technics for both the exposure and the control of abuses; hardy "muckraking" journalists were building up public awareness and concern; and the Progressives were creating a political fervor pointing toward American "social welfare" legislation, of which the Federal Food and Drug Act of 1906 was a pioneer example.

Although exposure of unsavory practices in the food industry had aroused public concern, later revelations about patent medicines gave public opinion an added force that Congress could no longer ignore. Exploitation of the public in the field of health, with an unscrupulous segment of the proprietary manufacturers seemingly uninterested in either adequate self-control or legal control of abuses, helped to unify support for reform.[31]

To the extent that drugs (as well as foods) could be considered *inter*state commerce, the Food and Drug Law that was finally passed in 1906 could exact penalties for certain types of misbranding and adulteration. Despite loopholes in the statute, and consequent problems of administration, it had far-reaching influences that in retrospect have been considered beneficial to the pharmaceutical field as well as to the public. To make state legislation mesh with Federal requirements and reach violators engaging only in *intra*state transactions (hence beyond Federal reach), at least two thirds of the states revamped their food and drug statutes in the years immediately following passage of the Federal law.[32]

While professionally conscious pharmacists welcomed new statutes as desirable improvements,[33] the new style of control ended administration of this segment of pharmaceutical law by boards of pharmacy. Earlier laws were occasionally administered by a dairy and food commission or by a board of health, but by 1912 the new union of food control and drug control left only 7 boards of pharmacy still retaining primary jurisdiction in this field.[34]

In making food and drug control hinge primarily on Federal enforcement, Congress took a historic step in using its power to regulate interstate commerce as a weapon in the direct furtherance of public health and safety for the first time.[35]

Legal loopholes, weak penalties and changing conditions built up pressure for markedly strengthening food and drug legislation by the 1930's, and this was reinforced by wider governmental concern for social welfare during the administration of President Franklin Roosevelt. The need for such control was dramatized and previously effective opposition overcome by a tragic wave of at least 73 deaths in the country (fall of 1937) caused by a toxic "Elixir Sulfanilamide."[36]

This tragedy shocked the country and gave impetus to the passage of the Food, Drug and Cosmetic Act of 1938. Significantly, a new and demanding section on marketing "new drugs" was added to the proposed bill, a section designed to prevent another pharmaceutical catastrophe analogous to the "Elixir Sulfanilamide" case. The drastically revised law also gave the Federal government jurisdiction over medical devices (e.g., instruments, apparatus, sickroom accessories) and cosmetics for the first time; and the requirements and the penalties for violation were broadened in many respects. To provide more effective control over false advertising of foods, drugs and cosmetics, and over deceptive or unfair practices, the same 75th Congress passed separate legislation (called the Wheeler-Lea bill) which amended the Federal Trade Commission Act.

Although pharmaceutical opinion once again had been divided, on principle and on details, the American Pharmaceutical Association expressed "its conviction that further delay was against the public interest, and has done what it could toward the successful outcome."[37]

In 1944 the "biologics law" was likewise renovated (Public Law 410–78th Congress). Responsibility in this field always has been vested in the U. S. Public Health Service. The first such law was passed in 1902 because of special control problems arising from immunologic agents then available for the first time (initially, the diphtheria antitoxin developed in Germany). Trivalent organic arsenicals used as injectable drugs were brought under the same law when World War I cut off imports of early chemotherapeutic drugs from Germany (notably Ehrlich's arsphenamine compounds), thus making home production imperative. The biologics law helps to assure reliable potency and safety of products in its special field through a system of product licensure and inspection of producers.[38]

A particularly important, and debatable, pharmaceutical amendment to the Federal Food, Drug, and Cosmetic Act (Section 503b; effective 1952) holds particular import for practicing pharmacists with respect to dividing drugs more definitely into prescription-only drugs and those that must be labeled with adequate directions, the handling of oral prescriptions, and the requiring of authorization by the physician for prescription refills.[39]

More far-reaching, although not so directly involving the community practice of pharmacy, were the Drug Amendments of 1962 (Public Law 87-781). These resulted from nearly 3 years of Congressional investigation and hearings, during which a sense of persecution pervaded the pharmaceutical industry because of what most industrial leaders considered to be unfair methods and unwarranted sensationalism on the part of the investigating subcommittee in seeking public attention and support for tighter legislative control.[40]

The complexity of the issues and the circumstances surrounding the proposed major amendments left the outcome deeply in doubt until there appeared in Europe a pharmacomedical tragedy even more devastating than the poisonous "Elixir Sulfanilamide" of 1937, which had generated the emotional drive behind revision of the Federal law at that time. Now it was discovered that several thousand infants had congenital malformations resulting from the use of a new sedative by the mothers during early pregnancy. Meanwhile, the offending drug (thalidomide) was undergoing widespread and not too tightly controlled clinical trials in the United States. Although the tragic aftermath experienced in Europe was averted here, press photographs of the grotesque limbs and afflicted infants brought home to Americans once again that many drugs are a two-edged sword and reminded them of the extent of their reliance on the competence and the dependability of the pharmaceutical industry.

Spurred by public apprehension, Congress adopted more stringent drug legislation designed to provide added safeguards of quality, safety and effectiveness of the drugs themselves and of procedures of drug marketing.[41]

CONTROL OF ADDICTIVE DRUGS

The unsupervised illegitimate use of narcotics has such grave consequences and is so difficult to control that early in this century separate and special legislation came to be a common goal among both professional and lay groups, only the approach and the details remaining at issue. Not until the 1870's was the distinctive character of addiction to narcotics made clear by scientific medicine, and even then attempts at control were hampered by the widespread idea that the use of narcotics was largely a private moral concern and, as a social problem, more threatening to the Eastern than to the Western world.[42]

Opiates were dispensed freely and legally without a prescription order; and, perhaps worse still, home remedies of secret composition and high-pressure promotion sometimes contained an opium derivative.

By the early years of this century, what had been of concern among the best informed became alarming to a larger segment of the population. When a committee of the American Pharmaceutical Association looked into the extent of the problem and the demand in pharmacies for addiction-producing drugs (1901), it brought back data termed "appalling."[43] Tradition, the Association's experience (state pharmacy acts) and the members' preference undoubtedly explain the decision for the development and the promotion of a model state narcotic bill rather than an appeal for Federal control.

Although state laws were passed, regulation by individual states alone soon became notorious for inadequate enforcement. An earlier Federal act prohibiting the import of nonmedicinal opium (1877; broadened in 1908) likewise had proved to be quite inadequate. Meanwhile, the Federal government had been an active participant and signatory to the Hague treaty, an international agreement to bring the opium traffic and the addiction problem under control. The United States became one of the first nations to attack the problem forthrightly, within the international framework, when Congress adopted the Harrison Narcotic Act in 1914. To circumvent a constitutional issue, the Act was drafted as a Federal tax measure, which accounts for the traditional association of the Bureau of Narcotics with the Treasury Department. The Harrison Narcotic Act continues in force today, although amended and added to several times. Analogous state legislation still serves in a useful but now supplemental role.[44]

Legislation dealing with addiction to narcotics and for controlling and channeling medicinal use undoubtedly will continue to evolve, for the scientific, moral, legal and social issues are still too complex and intertwined to permit final and uncontroversial answers. Further research progress toward nonaddictive analgesics offers one hope for greatly simplifying this area of drug control.

Pharmacists have been proud of their record in preventing diversion of narcotics from normal channels of medicinal use; and the retired U. S. Commissioner of Narcotics, Harry J. Anslinger, expressed the belief that no evidence exists implicating "pharmacists as being in any way responsible for one case among the 46,000 non-medical addicts known to the authorities." Moreover, he said, "pharmacists accounted for uncovering more forged prescriptions than Federal, state and city authorities combined."[45]

Thus pharmacy as a profession has been gradually recognized by law, and it has been called on to perform special duties for the benefit of the public. This recognition, as well as the fulfillment of the duties imposed on the calling, would not be possible without professional education.

14: The Development of Education

PRIVATE SCHOOLS

The establishment of European civilization in the New World was not to be achieved simply by transferring the European cultural achievements of the late 18th and the early 19th century to the virgin soil of America. Conditions were too different. The exigencies of conquest and settlement, for centuries past only a matter of history in Europe, determined the actual life of people in the United States, up to the time of the Civil War. Thus the young republic had to experience the processes of evolution which had characterized the earlier European development—ultimately arriving at a specifically American culture pattern. Professional education was not a matter of tradition and still less an endeavor to obtain general and comprehensive knowledge. Rather, it centered around the kind of people wanting an education and the kind of actual, practical work for which they were to be educated. For some decades, most of the professions that are now replenished by academic graduates depended largely on preceptors who passed their knowledge on to apprentices, academic study being minimal or entirely optional.

Already in 1789 the College of Philadelphia included pharmacy in the title of one of the professors in its medical school (Samuel P. Griffits, professor of materia medica and pharmacy),[1] and the same was true at some other early medical schools. But this was pharmacy taught by and for physicians. Chemistry also was taught in connection with medicine. At the University of Pennsylvania (about 1810) it was stated that the professorship of chemistry is "almost exclusively" supported by students of medicine, who "are induced to do so in con-

sequence of its application to pharmacy and the different branches of medicine."[2]

Prior to the founding of the Philadelphia College of Pharmacy in 1821, only a few ineffectual attempts to provide instruction in pharmacy for pharmacists are known to have been made.

As early as 1769, a physician (Lewis Mottet) suggested that the colonial commonwealth of South Carolina establish a "botanic garden" and "a chymical Laboratory." He offered himself "for the Direction of the Laboratory, chymical and galenical; and when erected, to collect, analyse and read the General System of Materia Medica." Dr. Mottet was even willing to undertake the venture on his own account, "if the Public will favour him with the Loan of Six Thousand Pounds Currency." As was to be expected, the proposal was " 'found by the learned Committee, appointed by the Honourable House of Assembly, to be too premature' and the public did not favor Dr. Mottet with six thousand pounds, so the project died aborning."[3] Since he was a native of France, it is not surprising that Mottet's suggestion (of a combination botanic garden and chemical laboratory for the teaching of pharmacy) closely followed the example of the *Jardin du roi* in Paris.

An attempt made more than 40 years later was more consequential. James Cutbush, a versatile Philadelphia chemist and apothecary published many valuable articles on chemical subjects, and in 1812 he advertised "a series of Lectures on the Theory and Practice of Pharmacy, accompanied with the necessary chemical elucidations."[4] He was, in America, the first known scientific writer on pharmacy, of some importance, and the first teacher of pharmacy from the point of view of professional phar-

203

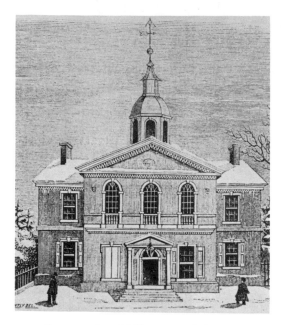

Carpenter's Hall in Philadelphia (woodcut, about 1825), as it looked when the Philadelphia College of Pharmacy was founded there. Erected by a guild of master carpenters (1770), the building has served as the cradle for various national institutions and is still preserved today as a historic landmark in Independence National Historical Park. The Philadelphia College of Pharmacy operated the first and the most influential of the association schools serving 19th-century American pharmacy.

macy. For some decades, he was the only one. The other early attempt at theoretic instruction of pharmacists in the sciences of their profession was made in 1816, by a Philadelphia physician, James Mease. Both attempts evidently were unsuccessful and did not receive much attention, "for no further mention was ever made of them."[5]

At that time pharmacy in America was considered, by most of those active in this field and by the majority of physicians, as an art which did not require theoretic knowledge; it could best be learned by practice, "by daily handling and preparing the remedies in common use." Had it not been necessary to discourage imminent steps by physicians to bring the dispensing of drugs under medical control, educational phar-

maceutical institutions in this country would have remained for a long time only the dream of a few far-seeing pharmacists. Even after their founding, the schools of the early colleges by no means enjoyed continuous prosperity. Thus the Massachusetts College of Pharmacy, founded in 1823, arranged to present occasional lectures but did not provide regular instruction until 1867.

Some of the institutions, while anxious to educate better the rising generation of pharmacists, found that they were in advance of the time. Even the large cities in which these colleges were situated did not provide a sufficient number of students to pay the professors a moderate lecture fee. Thus after several attempts in New York, Dr. Squibb offered his services free and even dragged his lecture equipment from his Brooklyn factory to the lecture room in New York City. In St. Louis the preceptors appear to have been interested more than were their apprentices. Students were few and in order to have any graduates whatever, the St. Louis College offered honorary degrees to its own members.[6]

The New York College of Pharmacy (founded in 1829) was "in a somnolent condition" between 1857 and 1859. The Maryland College (founded in 1841) "languished from 1847-1856." The course given by the Chicago College of Pharmacy (organized in 1859) was suspended on the outbreak of the Civil War, and the school was not reopened until September, 1870. It was destroyed by the great Chicago fire only 1 year later, then re-established with the aid of organized support by pharmacists of all parts of the civilized world. Even the Philadelphia College of Pharmacy graduated only a few in some years (e.g., 3 in 1839, 4 in 1840 and 2 in 1841).[7]

The number of pharmacists attending lectures in the few American colleges of pharmacy before the Civil War was small, and the number who graduated naturally was still smaller. The whole situation cannot be characterized better than it was in the "address to the pharmacists of the United States," which was composed by a commission under the leadership of Wm. Procter, Jr., and Edward Parrish (accepted by the American Pharmaceutical Association in 1854 and printed "for general distribution").[8] The address complained that there was at that time usually neither a legally indentured apprenticeship nor an honor-bound obligation and therefore, that:

Our country has been deluged with incompetent drug clerks, whose claim to the important position they hold or apply for is based on a year or two's service in the shop, perhaps under circumstances illy calculated to increase their knowledge. These clerks in turn become principals, and have the direction of others—alas! for the progeny that some of them bring forth, as ignorance multiplied by ignorance will produce neither knowledge nor skill. . . . It has been found that there are three classes of individuals engaged in pharmaceutical pursuits . . . to whom particularly this address is directed: First, those who are imperfectly acquainted with pharmacy and are in business for themselves; secondly, those who have been but half educated as apprentices and who are now assistants receiving salaries, having the responsibility of business entrusted to them; and thirdly, those who are now apprentices or beginners under circumstances and with ideas unfavorable to the acquirement of the thorough knowledge of the drug and apothecary business.

It is significant that the Association did not expect the people to whom it appealed, even the beginners, to study at one of the pharmacy schools. It merely admonished all of these groups to read pharmaceutical literature "regularly and understandingly" and to "assist the reading when necessary by experiment and observation." The graduates of the schools of pharmacy were given the admonition to "act as examples to their less favored brethren." The address states that the American Pharmaceutical Association, recognizing the "vast importance of good schools of pharmacy, where the sciences are regularly taught," will "freely extend its countenance and encouragement to those already existing and to all new efforts."

A few years before, another important step had been taken: the establishment of a professorship of pharmacy not connected with materia medica, and held not by a physician but by a pharmacist, for the sole purpose of teaching prospective pharmacists. Just 25 years after the founding of the Philadelphia College of Pharmacy (1846) the trustees thus divided the chair of materia medica and pharmacy and unanimously elected to the new chair William Procter, Jr., the senior author of the address just quoted and later called "the father of American pharmacy." In the "report of the committee of nine appointed to consider the propriety of creating a Professorship of Pharmacy," unanimously adopted, the following statements were made:

In organizing the school of pharmacy, it was found necessary to seek professors in the ranks of the medical profession—few, if any, of the apothecaries had so accustomed themselves to the systematic study of the several branches connected with the practice of our profession, as to be prepared to assume the office of teachers. Hence it is not surprising that the theory and practice of pharmacy, although held to be of the highest importance to the student, was not allotted to a professor as a separate branch of instruction, but was appended secondarily to the branches of materia medica and chemistry. The question now arises whether, by the lectures in our school, and by other means tending to create a greater taste for scientific attainment among those who practice our profession, so much advancement has been made, as to warrant the appointment of a practical apothecary to teach in a scientific manner, *what has hitherto, in America and England, been the confused and unsystematized art of Pharmacy.* . . . The professor of Pharmacy, if one should be elected, must enter a field of labor scarcely less extensive than that of either of his colleagues in the school, and one which he will have to traverse in the double capacity of teacher and learner. *We look in vain amongst the medical literature of the English language for a single work devoted exclusively and systematically to this branch of knowledge.* To French and German Pharmaciens and books we are indebted for most that is interesting, instructive and original in regard to Pharmacy. The latter are only available to a limited extent in this country, and are not well adapted to our different circumstances. . . . We would suggest, that as Philadelphia was the first city in the Union to organize a College of Pharmacy, and has continued to be regarded as the metropolis of Pharmaceutical as well as Medical Science in America, it is peculiarly appropriate that this measure, *so imperatively demanded by our present circumstances, and so necessary to an* *advancement of our profession,* corresponding with the progress of science and general intelligence in our country, should be consummated here.[9]*

These two documents (the "address" of 1854 and the "report" of 1846) supplement each other. One pictures the general situation among members of the calling who needed to become educated; the other shows the difficulties the educators had to face in the fulfillment of their task. Conditions in the drug trade for decades afterward made a scientific basis for the whole of American pharmacy a remote objective. The lack of suitable English literature made each American teacher in pharmacy a pioneer in his field. The ostensible motherland of the American people, England, had neglected pharmacy and could offer neither a pattern to be followed nor the means to be used to build up American professional pharmacy. The standard of the French and the German models and achievements was too high, and their spirit was too different. America could not simply copy them. The trustees of the Philadelphia College of Pharmacy were taking a step that, as the report shows, was all the more courageous in that its initiators were painfully aware of the difficulties involved. How great a need was being filled by them, and how highly esteemed this instruction in pharmacy proper was, is illustrated by the following: "There had been an average number [of Philadelphia graduates] annually for the nineteen years preceding the election of Procter to the new chair of pharmacy in 1846 of only 5½, while in the 19 years which followed the average number receiving the diploma annually was 21."[10]

The establishment of the professorship of pharmacy at the Philadelphia College of Pharmacy had a remarkable prelude. William Procter, Jr., the first man to occupy this chair, as well as Edward Parrish, the secretary of the college, were both graduates of the college. Both had experienced the inadequacy of pharmacy "for physicians taught by physicians" as the basis for professional practice of pharmacy. However,

Parrish had gone a step further. If pharmacy was indeed a special branch of medicine, it must receive acknowledgment of its independence. As a separate art, it had the right to declare its own standards and to insist on its own curriculum. Only those who had mastered its scientific foundations and could demonstrate a complete knowledge of all departments, including its practical applications, could qualify as teachers. Pharmacists, physicians or other persons who wished to practice pharmacy were to be taught by these learned pharmacists. Physicians had lost their foothold in the teaching of pharmacy, in the opinion of Parrish; in fact, if they were to practice pharmacy, they should now be taught by pharmacists. Thus Parrish turned the tables on the medical profession. J. W. England says:

In 1843 he [E. Parrish] purchased the drugstore . . . adjoining the building of the University of Pennsylvania, which brought him in contact with medical students and their wants. He believed that those who should return to their homes, often in isolated communities, would be without the information that would enable them to compound and dispense medicines for their patients, and that pharmaceutical knowledge was necessary to them, since they would be far removed from prescription drugstores, *still to be found only in the largest towns and cities.** He therefore started a School of Practical Pharmacy in the rear of his building . . . and gave courses of instruction to those who wished to avail themselves of them. Later (1850) . . . the school was removed to a place, where better accommodations were had and instruction was given to both pharmaceutical and medical students.[11]

When appointed (1859) "superintendent of the practical department of Parrish's" the master pharmacist John M. Maisch offered "all manipulations required in a pharmaceutical establishment" and made known the opening of "a laboratory for practical & analytical chemistry, designed in particular for the wants of pharmaceutists." "For students, sufficiently advanced" Maisch even held out the prospect of "a practical course of toxicological analysis."[12]

---

* Italics added.

* Italics added.

This School of Practical Pharmacy existed side by side with the new chair of pharmacy of the college. The school can be considered a parallel of the pioneer instruction in pharmaceutical and chemical laboratory work, given by German pharmacists about 1800, in their capacity as university professors of pharmacy and materia medica, or of pharmaceutical chemistry. The instruction was given in the rear of their pharmacies, to students of medicine and of pharmacy.

The separate professorship of theory and practice of pharmacy at the Philadelphia College of Pharmacy was not without an American predecessor. The Maryland College of Pharmacy had established such a chair 2 years earlier, in addition to one for chemistry and a third for materia medica. One difference was that the man appointed, David Stewart, was a physician as well as a pharmacist and opened his lectures to students of medicine as well as of pharmacy. A more significant difference was Proctor's long service and far-reaching influence, while Dr. Stewart taught pharmacy only 2 years (1844-46) and thereafter did not long remain prominently active in the profession.[13]

Until well after the Civil War, physician-teachers were more the rule than the exception. To Edward Parrish it was a point of self-respect to "cut loose from that vassalage to physicians . . ."[14] Yet, American pharmacy—underdeveloped and perhaps partly underambitious—did not itself quickly yield men qualified to staff the schools. Teachers holding the "M.D." were first displaced in pharmaceutical chemistry, and by the end of the 19th century were disappearing from all departments.[15]

The courses and the students during the first period of the Chicago School of Pharmacy (1850-60) have been described as follows:

The course continued for twenty weeks. Lectures were given upon three evenings each week, two hours each evening. . . . The students were earnest young fellows, employed in drugstores during the day, and though the course was necessarily presented in the briefest manner, they were encouraged to read, study, and experiment, utilizing the opportunities afforded in the shops. . . . The teachers possessed the equipment necessary for demonstration of the lectures but there were no laboratories.[16]

At Philadelphia in 1868:

The courses of instruction were still given only in the evening—on Monday, Wednesday and Friday evenings, from about October, until the end of February. The school, as from the first day, was set to answer the needs of apothecaries' apprentices. . . . Diplomas were given only to persons of good moral character of the age of at least 21 years. They must have attended two courses of each of the lectures delivered in the college, or one course in the college and one course in some other reputable college of pharmacy *or medical school* in which the same branches might be taught. They also must have served out at least four years with a person or persons qualified to conduct the drug or apothecary business.[17]

These quotations give a true picture of the scope and the quality of professional education enjoyed by that small minority of American pharmacists who attended one of the pharmacy schools before 1870. Materia medica was one of the most prominent subjects taught in this period. Physics, if treated at all, was presented as an introduction to chemistry. Botany was occasionally treated in like manner, as an introduction to materia medica. The instruction was almost exclusively through lectures. Unsatisfactory financial conditions were largely responsible for the lack of laboratory instruction. The fees did not provide a living for the teachers, whose main activities consequently lay outside the college. The colleges, which were without endowment, were not prepared to equip laboratories and to maintain them. Even when the Philadelphia College of Pharmacy erected (1868) a new building, which was remarkable for that period, it did not equip a laboratory immediately. However, by means of funds collected from alumni, "a pharmaceutical and chemical laboratory for individual instruction" was opened in 1870.[18] It was put under the direction of John M. Maisch, the same man who had conducted the first individual laboratory instruction for pharmacists and

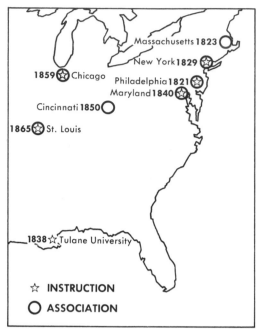

Massachusetts 1823
New York 1829
1859 Chicago
Philadelphia 1821
Maryland 1840
Cincinnati 1850
1865 St. Louis
1838 Tulane University

☆ INSTRUCTION
○ ASSOCIATION

The map illustrates that nearly all organized endeavor and instruction in pharmacy was in the northeastern quarter of the present United States until after the Civil War. An exception was the pharmacy course, in conjunction with medicine, offered in New Orleans. A regular course of instruction was offered by 5 of the 7 local associations of pharmacy founded by 1865. Dates on the map are those of the founding of the associations.

physicians, about 10 years before, in Parrish's School of Practical Pharmacy.

The era of pioneer pharmacy schools, established by the early pharmaceutical associations called colleges of pharmacy (see p. 173), ended with the Civil War. Until 1865, when the St. Louis College of Pharmacy opened, there existed, besides 5 such association schools, only one other pharmaceutical educational institution, the Course in Pharmacy of the Medical Department of Tulane University, New Orleans (founded in 1838). From that time on, pharmacy schools were founded as private schools (by groups of pharmacists organized only for that purpose), as part of private or denominational universities and colleges, or as divisions of medical colleges.

At that time numerous medical colleges

operated not so much to promote medical knowledge as to further the business interests of the people creating them. Henry B. Shafer writes: "A group of physicians who wished to start a medical school approached a college and asked permission to grant degrees under its charter. Since the medical faculty would not be an expense and might even be financially useful and since the charters of most colleges allowed them unlimited powers, it was usually easy to obtain this permission. The faculty in these cases considered the school a business."[19]

Whenever these colleges offered courses in pharmacy, as a rapidly increasing number of them did, it was at least questionable whether their departments of pharmacy were created for bona fide pharmaceutical instruction or whether they were really "feeders" for the medical courses. However, the opposition of the men representing professional pharmacy was not directed primarily against inadequacies within these schools; it was based on principle. These men had created and fostered the old colleges of pharmacy to make American pharmacy an independent profession and to secure a special education for the pharmacist in the United States. While they were ready to recognize a period of study at a medical college as an equivalent of study at a college of pharmacy, they could not sanction any step that might surrender pharmaceutical education to medical domination and thus lead the profession back to the situation from which it had scarcely escaped. On the occasion of the conferring of pharmaceutical degrees by the Medical Department of Georgetown College in Washington (1872) John M. Maisch wrote:

We recognize the correlation of medicine and pharmacy, and that the latter, as a separate art and science, is the offspring of the former; but we do not acknowledge their identity, and look upon the conferring of pharmaceutical degrees by strictly medical educational institutions, which, by such a precedent, might be inaugurated, with the same favor with which we should regard the attempt of a college of pharmacy to confer the degree of Doctor of Medicine, honoris causa or otherwise.[20]. . .

We are earnestly advocating the proper education of the pharmacist, and are in favor of the multiplication of colleges of pharmacy, but not to an indefinite number, which would be fraught with results similar to those which the medical profession throughout the country is endeavoring to correct.[21]

It is understood that the private schools, depending partly on the approval of the practicing pharmacists who functioned as their trustees and financial supporters, and depending always on the fees of their students, developed pharmaceutical education along the same lines as did the old-line colleges (associations). Serviceable in its time, this mold for pharmaceutical education became increasingly cramped and limiting. It was to be broken by a strikingly different educational program, thrusting out of a different environment, the state university.

STATE UNIVERSITIES

As early as 1847, William Procter, Jr., stressed the necessity of state-controlled practice of medicine and pharmacy:

It is a characteristic of our national and state governments to interfere as little as possible with the working of private interests, and competition is left unimpeded to control the business affairs of society. This liberty of action, so advantageous in the common intercourse of men, is unfortunate in reference to medicine, which, as no guarantee of qualification is required by law of its practitioners, is thrown open to any individual who chooses to adopt the title of doctor or apothecary, be he ever so ignorant.[22]

Yet, Procter, and also Maisch, the influential proponent of state pharmacy laws (see p. 196), opposed the advancement of pharmaceutical education through an agency of the state. This seems scarcely comprehensible unless we understand their commitment to an educational ideology of the old-line colleges that was based on an apprenticeship system. Formal study rounded off a prolonged apprenticeship that was prerequisite to graduation.

When pharmacy made connections with general institutions of higher learning, through state universities, old ways and traditions of creating new generations of pharmacists were challenged. Moreover, leaders such as Procter and Maisch knew well the sacrifice and the effort that many had invested in developing pharmaceutical education independent from the medical profession; hence their reluctance to accord the state university the privilege of intrusion in a field that pharmacy had claimed for its own and developed largely on its own is understandable.

At the first state-supported institution to produce graduates in pharmacy (1867), the Medical College of South Carolina, pharmacy instruction had a precarious existence until almost the end of the century.[23]

However, the transformation of pharmaceutical education was to draw its power and pattern from another quarter, the midwestern state universities, first and notably exemplified by the pharmacy curriculum approved at the University of Michigan in 1868. Unlike some states in subsequent years, Michigan embarked on a vigorous and full program of instruction without either the suggestive influence of pharmacy legislation or the support of the profession itself. Instead, the course grew out of pharmacy's earlier connection with medical instruction, through the intermediary of an outstanding chemical laboratory, backed by an administration noted for its pioneering.

In a bold innovation the University of Michigan introduced extensive laboratory instruction coupled with basic science, made the academic study of pharmacy practically a full-time occupation and refused to accept responsibility for apprenticeship as a prerequisite to graduation.

A key figure in this development was the physician-chemist placed in charge of the new pharmacy curriculum, Albert B. Prescott, "Professor of Organic Chemistry and Pharmacy." In pharmaceutical circles Dr. Prescott gained widespread respect for himself but unpopularity for his pharmacy program. Therefore, it was before a rather unwilling audience that Prescott presented his classic address on "Pharmaceutical Education" at the 1871 meeting of the American Pharmaceutical Association.[24]

With brevity and clarity, Prescott explained the advantages of a real scientific

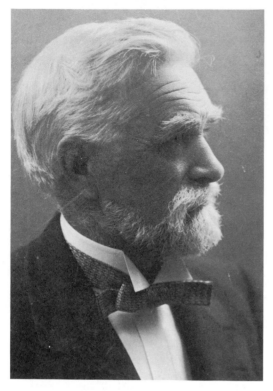

One of the most influential men in the molding of modern pharmaceutical education in America, Albert B. Prescott (1832-1905)· was a physician-chemist at the University of Michigan. There he established a school of pharmacy in a pattern radically different from that of schools elsewhere.

education and gave his reasons for believing a preliminary apprenticeship, before graduation, unnecessary. These reasons are met again and again, in the frequent discussions of the same question in almost all European countries within the past century—a fact which confirms their basic logic and value.

The different nations found different answers. Italy demands a half year practice, permitting part of it during academic study. France requires 1 year of apprenticeship with an authorized pharmacist before study Germany requires 2 years' apprenticeship, with an authorized pharmacist, before study and a year of probation after it. In England the aspirant has to serve an apprenticeship of 2 years if taken between the required preliminary scientific courses, and before

the professional instruction. If taken after academic study, then a single year of practical experience is required.

Because it is contended that the apprenticeship cannot be utilized intelligently without scientific knowledge and that practical experience is advantageous before the professional courses, the 3½ years of study in Switzerland have been divided into 1½ years of general science and 2 years of professional scientific instruction. Between these two phases of academic study, an obligatory apprenticeship of 1½ years is required. This system has served as a model for some other countries; but, in general, diversity rather than uniformity marks the internship of modern history—variety in the length of experience and in its relation to formal study, and in the types of establishments authorized to give practical training to pharmaceutical interns.[25] Yet, in spite of this variation, few instances can be found where full responsibilities of a license have been granted without requiring some supervised practice in a pharmacy, despite the growing importance of academic education (as in all intellectual fields during the past century) and despite difficulties in maintaining meaningful standards of internship.

In this light, apprehension about the University of Michigan's rejection of the responsibility for the apprenticeship can be understood when we recall that in the 1870's few states had a pharmacy law or an administrative board to which that responsibility could be shifted. The idea that the neophyte needs to learn to apply academic knowledge to pharmaceutical practice has been honored by long tradition, both before and since Professor Prescott addressed the meeting of the American Pharmaceutical Association. Thus, the Association's Secretary, John Maisch, could have been writing on similar occasions in other times or countries when he argued:

We grant that as much knowledge in physical and chemical science, and natural history generally, as a young man may possibly acquire before he enters a drugstore, is extremely desirable; but we believe that with all his knowledge of chemistry, natural history, and natural sciences generally, he will not be a pharmacist until he has gone through a regular system of [practical] training, and that is exactly where the colleges of pharmacy throughout the country differ from the University of Michigan. . . . *The colleges are not discouraging preliminary education before the apprentice enters the apothecary business; but what we insist upon is that it is wrong to give a pharmaceutical degree before the graduate has had pharmaceutical experience.*[26]

The break with tradition was sharp and the results uncertain, and within the old framework one could say that the American Pharmaceutical Association only did its duty when it did not recognize the School of Pharmacy of the University of Michigan as a "college of pharmacy within the proper meaning" of the constitution and by-laws of the American Pharmaceutical Association, "it being neither an organization controlled by pharmacists nor an institution of learning which, by its rules and requirements, insures to its graduates the proper practical training to place them on a par with the graduates of the several colleges of pharmacy represented in this association."[27]

The report on the first graduates of the University of Michigan School of Pharmacy shows that non-pharmacists indeed availed themselves of the opportunity to enter the course without practical pharmaceutical experience: "Of the 23 who graduated in the literary department as Pharmaceutical Chemists 13 were medical students, of which 12 graduated as M.D.'s. The pharmacy work was not taken preliminary to the medical work *but along with it*. . . . Of the 23 graduates of 1869 seven were in the practice of medicine and the majority of the remainder in the practice of pharmacy after graduation."[28]

The second state university school of pharmacy, founded 15 years later (1883), although following and even competing with Michigan in its scientific emphasis, remained within the old lines in its relationship to the practice of pharmacy. The reason lies in the different circumstances under which the first two American state university schools of pharmacy were founded. The design of the older one was a bold revolutionary attempt at the beginning of the re-construction after the Civil War, while the younger one was a product of evolution within this period.

The Michigan school was the outgrowth of a course of pharmacy, which "when first established was by no means mainly designed for students looking forward to the practice of pharmacy. . . . In 1860 the design was more for students of medicine, to give them help in handling medicines when they should come into practice, but it was quite as much intended as general practical training in applied science."[29] The school was started without the cooperation of the pharmaceutical practitioners, who in fact were opposed to the idea. This took place 6 years before the founding of a state pharmaceutical association in Michigan and 17 years before a Michigan pharmacy act was enacted.

The Department of Pharmacy at the University of Wisconsin, on the contrary, was established by legislative act on special request of the pharmacists of the state, assembled in an annual meeting of their state association, 3 years after the founding of this association and 1 year after the enactment of a Wisconsin pharmacy law. As a result, Dr. Frederick B. Power, the first leader of the University of Wisconsin School of Pharmacy, had to take into consideration the established pharmaceutical forces and follow the evolution to which his school owed its existence. Unlike Professor Prescott of Michigan (a physician), Professor Power himself came from the ranks of practical pharmacy and was a graduate of the Philadelphia College of Pharmacy. He recognized the desire of pharmacists not to risk losing the identity of the concept of "pharmacy" with that of "drugstore," by awarding a pharmaceutical degree to persons without practical experience. He made this experience a requirement for a diploma, although not necessarily a prerequisite for admission to the course.

The problem of dealing in a balanced way with the science and the practice of pharmacy was solved through the development of the state board examinations. By this means the pharmaceutical practitioners took on themselves the responsibility for

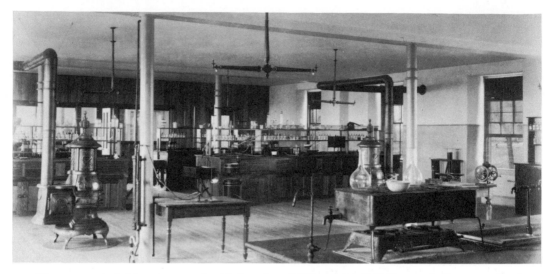

Pharmaceutical laboratory at the University of Wisconsin (1890), just before its school of pharmacy became the first in the country to offer a standard baccalaureate program of four years. Michigan and Wisconsin, like other state schools that followed their pattern, gave a wholly new emphasis to the sciences underlying pharmacy and to laboratory instruction in particular. (Photograph from the Univ. of Wisconsin)

appraising the practical experience and the knowledge of the candidate. The requirement that a candidate for a license have experience before taking the state board examinations made it unnecessary for the schools to require this experience for graduation.

With the raising of academic instruction in pharmacy to a systematic approach to the sciences concerned, corresponding to the needs of practical pharmacy but not dependent on them, the University of Michigan took the first step in the direction of a new educational policy by substituting full-time day instruction for the old time evening courses besides making intensive laboratory work obligatory. Gradually, other schools followed suit. Yet the state university continued to lead in reforms. It was the first, for example, to establish even modest entrance requirements. The announcement of the new School of Pharmacy at Michigan said that the course was to be comprised of "lectures in inorganic and organic chemistry, materia medica and principles of pharmacy; with laboratory courses in qualitative analysis, toxicology, analysis of urine, volumetric analysis, and a somewhat extended course in pharmaceutical

operations. Also class exercise in botany."[30] Quantitative analysis, organic analysis, botany and microscopic botany were optional at first but within a few years were required. This was a comprehensive program and for that time an exemplary one. The course was covered in 2 years, each consisting of 2 terms of 3 months each, which were soon extended to 2 full semesters of about 4½ months each.

Wisconsin started with a similar program. Then, in 1892, the University of Wisconsin School of Pharmacy made a bold innovation. In addition to the 2-year minimum course, its new head, Dr. Edward Kremers, offered the first 4-year course in pharmacy in America, thus placing pharmaceutical instruction on a par with other academic courses. This innovation was not achieved without opposition. Like all ideas that are ahead of the times, its worth was not immediately apparent. It had to run the gauntlet of ridicule before recognition could come. Reluctantly, here and there, it was imitated; finally, it was generally adopted.

The first school to respond enthusiastically was Ohio State University, where the freshman class entering in 1925 faced 4 years of study, before they could receive their pharmacy degrees. Only the Universities of Georgia, Nebraska and Minnesota had the courage to follow Ohio State's bold lead in requiring a 4-year curriculum before it was made a uniform requirement for all accredited schools.[31]

All schools in good standing with what is now the American Association of Colleges of Pharmacy had adopted a 2-year curriculum (at least 50 weeks) as the minimum requirement in 1907, then a 3-year course in 1925, and a 4-year course in 1932.[32]

Every forward step in the pharmaceutical curriculum had been a controversial issue in the profession and would be again when the Pharmaceutical Survey (1946-49) completed its analysis and faced the question of an appropriate length of curriculum for midcentury. The deep division of opinion is partially reflected in the Survey's recommendation that the existing 4-year curriculum be continued and improved but that schools "adequately staffed and financed" develop a 6-year curriculum leading to the professional degree of Doctor of Pharmacy.[33]

The alternatives thus presented did not provide a happy answer to the question, the one choice being considered too conservative by some, the alternative, too progressive by others. However, even before the Survey's *General Report* was off the press, Ohio State University again put forward a "heresy," under the leadership of Dean B. V. Christensen, by requiring a 5-year pharmacy curriculum, beginning with students entering in the fall of 1948. Eventually this "compromise" position, between the status quo and the proposed 6-year professional doctorate, was adopted as the minimum requirement in accredited schools, for students entering college after the spring of 1960.

The University of Southern California, with the entering class of 1950, became the first American school to require a 6-year program (including 2 university years of pre-pharmacy) for a Doctor of Pharmacy degree.[34] By the 1960's a few other schools were offering the same type of program, designed as advanced preparation for professional practice. Education for research careers in pharmacy, with its challenging demand for a high degree of specialization in knowledge and research technics, has developed on the quite different ground tilled by graduate schools, which were getting a foothold in American universities during the last third of the 19th century.

Research Degrees in Pharmacy

If pharmacy students were to be adequately prepared for graduate study and standard research degrees, the standard baccalaureate degree would be necessary as a foundation for such advanced study. Edward Kremers was aware of this when he introduced the 4-year course at the University of Wisconsin. Imbued as he was with scientific standards for pharmacy and a spirit for research brought back from Ph.D. studies in Germany,[35] Kremers superimposed on this foundation the first Doctor of Philosophy programs in pharmaceutical specialties to be based on the regular postgraduate requirements of a recognized American university. The first such Ph.D. was awarded at Wisconsin in 1902.

To give scope to this pioneering program and to reinforce its then meager resources, the University of Wisconsin established the first "Pharmaceutical Experiment Station" in the United States (1913). No person or firm had a claim on the Station's research findings, for in cooperation with the Federal government (Bureau of Plant Industry) it stood under statutory obligation to serve the public. This first American institution of its particular type found endorsement and promotion through the Wisconsin legislature; but the great depression finally choked off its legislative appropriation (1933), and this unique research venture by a school of pharmacy had to be discontinued.

Wisconsin's graduate department was gradually emulated in other strong schools, although at midcentury still only 19 schools offered both master's and doctor's degrees in pharmaceutical research fields. Graduate pharmaceutical students of all types then totalled 357 in American schools, representing a 4-fold increase during the preceding 17 years. After World War II, schools in general were strengthened, and research funds became more readily available, thus bringing a more vigorous response in American pharmaceutical education to the demand for research personnel in pharmaceutical science. By 1955, for example, 612 graduate students could be counted in 49 colleges that were offering graduate work to some extent.[36] Changes in the structure and the dynamics of the pharmaceutical field itself have accelerated a trend toward making such advanced work an increasingly important segment of pharmaceutical education.

Consolidation of the School System

New concepts of American pharmaceutical education, both graduate and undergraduate, flourished in the environment of state universities and land-grant colleges. Unlike the old-line universities on the Eastern seaboard, they did not hesitate to harness intellect for a wide spectrum of the world's work, helping to staff an expanding group of university-educated professions and avidly cultivating applied science. Unlike many of the private and association schools in pharmacy, they had the resources to place the student's instruction in pharmacy on a foundation of basic laboratory sciences and to widen his educational horizons beyond purely vocational limits.

In the end, only the strongest of the old independent schools could compete effectively for students without soiling academic robes with the appeal of cheaper degrees and lower standards. Many did not survive; many others affiliated and merged with general institutions of higher learning. In less than a half century United States pharmacy moved from a handful of hard-pressed night schools in rented rooms to a plethora of schools of disparate standards and types by the turn of the century, and then, after the first World War, into a period of consolidation and strengthening.

In the chronologic table prepared as Appendix 4 can be seen the spread of different types of schools across the country. It will be noted that four of the five schools regularly teaching before the Civil War were operated by local associations of pharmacists, the fifth by a medical college. The

Civil War dealt the adolescent educational system a heavy blow; but after the war each passing decade put formal education within easier reach of prospective students. While each of the four preceding decades had seen one school or at most two begin pharmaceutical instruction, there were ten new schools in each of two postwar decades, a figure doubled in the 1880's and tripled in the 1890's. From the 1880's onward a majority of the new schools were associated with general institutions of higher education; few any longer were born under association auspices. Proprietary schools, which often smacked of being business ventures, helped to swell the total late in the century, although pharmacy was not plagued with them as medicine was.[37]

Shortly after the turn of the century, however, there apparently were more pharmacy schools than there have been at any time since. All evidence suggests there were too many schools, pressed too hard for sufficient students to remain solvent, to permit steady or uniform progress. Among 80 schools teaching pharmacy (surveyed in 1905), 32 were affiliated with a university or a general college, where there were none a half century earlier. A half century later the comparative figure had changed further, strikingly, when 68 of the 74 schools of pharmacy were associated with some broader institution of higher learning. Meanwhile, the distribution of the schools geographically has improved somewhat, with at least one in all but 7 of the states.[38]

What should these schools teach the students who come to them? Before the present century there had been no detailed agreement, either among schools or between the schools and the boards of pharmacy. The question of what qualifications a pharmacist ideally should have came into sharper focus as states began to require a college diploma as a prerequisite to licensure.

When the first state to require a diploma (New York) tried to decide what training the diploma should represent, the problem proved to be of national scope; efforts to solve it led to the formation of a National Syllabus Committee (1906). In its publication, *The Pharmaceutical Syllabus* (1910,

146 pp.) the Committee outlined a curriculum and recommended the proportion and the character of constituent subjects. To continue such work permanently, the Committee was organized formally to represent jointly the American Conference of Pharmaceutical Faculties, the National Association of Boards of Pharmacy and the American Pharmaceutical Association.

In successive editions, the compilers of *The Pharmaceutical Syllabus* endeavored to leave the schools freedom in their methods and curricular decisions and yet provide "suggestions and outlines that may serve as a rational basis for instruction and that will afford scientific tests to determine the fitness of applicants seeking license as pharmacists." However, apprehension about possible regimentation grew, and disagreements became intensified in the 1940's about the direction and the influence of the work of the joint Syllabus Committee. This culminated in the dissolution of the Committee (1946), and a 5th edition of the *Syllabus* never got beyond a tentative mimeographed version.

After the American Council on Pharmaceutical Education became active (1932) as the agency to maintain standards in pharmaceutical education, it emphasized more general requirements for admission and graduation (e.g., years, clock hours of instruction, proportion of laboratory work), while the detailed curricular guides that the Syllabus Committee had provided gradually dropped out of sight. In an advisory capacity, the Curriculum Committee of the American Association of Colleges of Pharmacy has continued to analyze specific issues and segments of the instructional programs.[39]

SPECIAL EDUCATIONAL FACILITIES

Before the passage of pharmacy laws requiring an examination for a pharmacy license, the student's belief in the value of systematic instruction under the guidance of qualified teachers no doubt was the decisive factor inducing college attendance. With attendance hinging on such a farsighted view and so few schools operating, we find that scarcely more than 500 pharmacists had earned an American diploma before the Civil War. The new laws required that all pharmacists have some knowledge but did not state how and where this knowledge was to be obtained. This requirement and the opening of new schools help to account for a sharp increase in the number of graduates by the 1870's, a decade that marked a kind of turning point in education as it did in other areas of pharmaceutical activity. Still, near the end of the century, only about 12 per cent of the pharmacists in American practice apparently had any technical education aside from apprenticeship.[40] If the passing of the state board examination was all that the applicant wanted, there was another and easier way than the toilsome one offered by the colleges of pharmacy.

The new pharmacy laws were not retroactive. They recognized and registered the pharmacists in practice at that time, without an examination, just as the boards of medical examiners had recognized the old medical practitioners as physicians. Consequences sometimes ensuing from this practice are illustrated by the following report concerning such a recognized physician and druggist as late as 1896:

In Bay City, Michigan, there has flourished for some years a practicing physician by the name of O. Barber, who is also a retail druggist. Recently, Dr. Barber had a case of diphtheria which he failed to report. For this oversight he was overhauled by the Health Board and the matter brought into court. To the amazement of that body and probably to the horror of his patients he gave testimony that he could neither read nor write.[41]

Obviously, this was an extreme case. Nevertheless, well-educated pharmacists were rare, and at times it was difficult to find competent examiners within the ranks. For example, when the first West Virginia Pharmacy Act was passed (1881), the legislators did not dare to require a college education even of the examiners. "Five years experience in a drugstore was the only requirement." Of 326 pharmacists registered during 2 years after passage of the act mentioned, only 2 were college graduates.[42]

To pass an examination under such conditions did not require lengthy study. As a matter of fact, another kind of preparation, restricted to a knowledge of questions commonly asked in the state board examinations, promised better success. Therefore, it is not surprising that different ways of preparing for these examinations were offered to all who wanted them, instruction (1) by correspondence courses, (2) by home study of books especially written for this purpose, and (3) by so-called "cramming schools."

Instruction by Correspondence

In view of the widespread lack of even minimal technical education and of the modest legal demands in 19th-century American pharmacy, even home study, at its best, seemed to be a constructive effort to which some pharmaceutical journals and educators offered collaboration. This is reflected in the two best-known attempts of education in pharmacy by correspondence.

The first was operated in Chicago as the "National Institute of Pharmacy"; its commercial management was in the hands of the publisher of the *Western Druggist*. In a series of 24 "lectures," covering a period of 1 year, a complete course in pharmacy, chemistry and materia medica was given. The main purpose, as explained in the announcement, was to enable clerks, assistants and druggists engaged in business and contemplating a removal "to another state having a pharmacy law . . . to cover the most ground in the least possible time (an important advantage when preparing for a Board of Pharmacy examination)." An examination consisting of answering a series of questions sent to the student brought him "a certificate of graduation in the institute." The announcement denied any intention of giving this certificate "any legal force whatever under pharmacy laws, the great advantage in this respect to be derived from the lectures being to qualify members for passing Board of Pharmacy examinations."

The other venture of importance in pharmaceutical instruction by correspondence was launched (1897) by the journal *Pharmaceutical Era*. This course mirrors the progress made during the decade that had passed since the first announcement of a correspondence course by the National Institute of Pharmacy in Chicago. The course was to cover "a period of two years, to be known respectively as junior and senior. Both years will include two series of lectures of twenty weeks length each." For a number of years, the lectures were printed in the regular weekly editions of the journal, while the quizzes and examinations were conducted by mail with individual students.[43] The director of this "Course of Home Study in Pharmacy" was no less a person than J. H. Beal; among the contributors were men of similar standing in American pharmacy (for instance, Virgil Coblentz, Henry Kraemer, Edward Kremers, John Uri Lloyd and Oscar Oldberg). Hence it is not amazing that this course was subscribed to by literally thousands of students.

Of course there were other less ambitious correspondence schools. J. H. Beal probably expressed the opinion of most representatives of scientific and professional American pharmacy when he said,

In so far as these agencies have honestly striven to raise the standard of education among drugclerks and to promote habits of study and selfhelp, they should have our commendation; but any proposition or suggestion to the effect that any course of instruction by mail, is or can be made to be the equivalent of a residence course of instruction at a respectable college of pharmacy is false absolutely, and stamps those who make such claims as guilty of misrepresentation and attempted fraud.[44]

More than a few schools were not above using "bait advertising." For example, a Chicago enterprise, named not so modestly the "Lincoln-Jefferson University," offered "ten large lessons forwarded by mail," for $65 "cash in advance" (marked down from $100). Prospective students were told glowingly that "the diplomas are large and beautiful, bearing no statement that the work was done by correspondence."

This course was not discontinued until 1926, and others survived still longer in states lacking legal restrictions.[45] The deathknell for correspondence courses as a substitute for academic education sounded when one state followed another, led by New York (1905), in requiring graduation from a recognized school as a prerequisite to licensure.

Books Especially Written for Home-Study

A demand for cheap and painless learning spawned a modified form of correspondence work, the home-study books. The best known representative of this type of literature was Oscar Oldberg's *A Course of Home Study for Pharmacists* (1891). It is significant that this method of preparation to meet the state board of pharmacy requirements originated at the same place as the National Institute of Pharmacy, Chicago. Oldberg, a teacher at the Chicago College of Pharmacy, left with a group of dissenting members to organize the Illinois College of Pharmacy, of which he became the dean. This school was affiliated with Northwestern University. Oldberg worded his preface carefully. He emphasized that "no course of study at home takes the place of a good college with its experienced teachers and its invaluable laboratory practice." At the same time he pointed out that of 75,000 persons employed in the drugstores of the United States "only a few thousand have enjoyed the advantages of a college of pharmacy education." He therefore recommended "home study" as being "of the highest importance to those who are prevented by circumstances from entering college. . . . The pharmacy laws, too, oblige many thousands to study at least enough to pass the State Board examinations." In the same year in which the first edition of this *Course of Home Study* was published, the Department of Pharmacy of Northwestern University took up "the work of applying the principles of University Extension by conducting an elementary or preparatory course of home reading in physics, chemistry, materia medica, and pharmacy"[46] or, in other words, instruction by correspondence.

Cramming Schools

If the prime intention of the correspondence courses and of the home study books

and similar attempts was narrowly aimed at preparing for the state board examination, some of them (especially the above-mentioned National Institute of Pharmacy and *Pharmaceutical Era* courses) also endeavored to impart a better understanding of the subject matter. However, this can scarcely be claimed for any of the so-called cramming schools. Their objective was the preparation of their students for state board examinations by cramming their brains in the least possible time with answers to commonly asked questions. As late as 1947, an establishment with the high-sounding name "Bay State Institute of Pharmacy, Inc.," located at Boston, sent out circulars "to the unregistered drug clerks of U. S. A." offering "preparation for the Board of Pharmacy license in the states of Massachusetts, Nevada and Vermont," where graduation from a school of pharmacy still was not a legal requirement for the board examination. The fee for a "Six-Week Resident Course in Pharmacy" or a "Fifteen-Week Correspondence Course in Pharmacy" was $300. Said the circular, "This is the last chance offered to drug clerks. . . ."

However, a few cramming schools survived even the prerequisite laws, which required college graduation. They were given a new lease on life because of the continuation of examinations for a kind of second-class licentiate, legally classed as assistants, "licensed druggists" (as in New York) or otherwise. A strong movement to abolish these second-class certificates entirely arose from abuses and arguments concerning the pharmacy assistant's proper role in a pharmacy. Efforts to solve the problem by abolishing legal provision for licensing any new "assistants" had succeeded by 1947 in all but 8 states. To hasten this solution, a number of states permitted experienced pharmacy assistants of limited education to attempt an examination, during a limited period, to qualify fully as pharmacists. In this situation the surviving "cram" schools found a further market for their brand of instruction.[47]

In-Service Educational Programs

The development of "extension work" in

higher education—beginning in the 1890's, apparently under British influence—offered some encouragement or at least surface justification to home-study endeavors which coincided with a particular need and stage in the development of American pharmacy.[48] However, the most that can be said for home-study endeavors, is that they simplified and systematized the self-education of perhaps thousands of youths in pharmacy who never would enter the doors of a school of pharmacy. In contrast, extension work characteristic of the present century has been primarily to simplify and systematize a continuing education for practitioners who already have a sound academic education.

Although sporadic experiments with pharmacy extension work had gained attention after World War I, it was found after World War II that 43 of 50 schools reporting to the Pharmaceutical Survey still had no "in-service" or "off-campus" training program for practicing pharmacists.[49] Pointing to the importance of pharmacists' keeping up to date with mushrooming pharmaceutical advances, the Survey urged that each school "recognize and assume responsibility for providing organized programs of in-service professional instruction." Such programs should include "refresher courses conducted at the institution, programs of reading, correspondence study courses, and the systematic visitation and personal counseling of pharmacists."[50] Meanwhile, the potential value of such programs to the profession has motivated sufficient cooperation between organized practitioners and the schools to give a national trend to this educational movement. In some areas, however, limited success with the "Council of Pharmaceutical Extension" that had been proposed for each state, a lack of predominantly professional or postgraduate character in the instruction, and emphasis on brief "refresher" courses that reach relatively few practitioners left room for further improvement and expansion of such programs.

While modern extension programs have built upon the pharmacist's college education, nonprofessional personnel involved in operating a pharmacy also can benefit by in-service training of a different kind and on a different level. To the extent that the attainment of this goal has been sought through state-wide training programs, stimulus has been drawn especially from the provision of Federal funds (George-Deen Act of 1937) to states "for training in distributive occupational subjects." With the cooperation of pharmaceutical associations, the U. S. Office of Education issued (1941-43) study outlines and teachers' outlines on distributive skills needed in the average pharmacy. Eight of 38 states reporting in 1946 had instructional programs in this field (5 for nonprofessional employees, 3 for pharmacists themselves).[51]

Preliminary Education

In a first and ill-fated associational effort among schools of pharmacy (1870) the hope was expressed that pharmacists would insist on better educational background in selecting apprentices for their shops. Here was where the screening took place, it was traditionally assumed, and the schools had not ventured to interpose any actual requirement themselves, however modest, in regard to preliminary education.

If a youth of the 1870's had asked how much "book learning" he needed to enter pharmacy, Pharmacist A would have replied, ". . . Any boy of 12 to 15 years, who can read, write or cypher a little, is well enough educated to be placed in any store." If the boy turned to Pharmacist B, he would have been told that to be a real pharmacist he first needed the education "which the common schools supply, supplemented by systematic instruction in natural and physical science where attainable, and by the elements of Latin and Greek, and one or more of the modern languages of Europe."[52] If pressed, this pharmacist might have conceded: "At least that's what we hope to find in coming generations of American pharmacy; but we need sincere lads like you. If you know your arithmetic, grammar and can write a good hand, I'll take you on at my shop."

Whether a preceptor even that demanding of preliminary education was the exception or the rule is no longer easy to discern. It does seem clear that the schools generally found it expedient to accept the apprentices sent to them by members of their association-sponsor, rather than see such youths proceed headlong into the practice of pharmacy without any formal pharmaceutical education at all.

The first serious attempt to require of matriculants some definite preparation arose in the state schools of pharmacy. In this the schools were encouraged by the public support that largely freed them from worrisome dependence on student fees to remain solvent, and by the strong though sometimes hidden forces that hold individual departments to some semblance of a general university standard.

State universities in the old Northwest (i.e., Middle West) were better able to withstand pressure against admission standards. Their requirements around 1885 varied from a common school education as at Purdue, to high school graduation (or, alternatively, scores on an admission examination that probably lay between common-school and high-school attainment) as at Michigan and Wisconsin.[53] Yet, in the country as a whole at this time, Professor E. S. Bastin maintained, "it is the rarest occurrence that an applicant is rejected on the ground of lack of preliminary education."[54]

By the turn of the century, pharmacy seems to have been pretty well abreast of medicine and law in the proportion of schools requiring the equivalent of a high-school education for entrance. Below this top layer in pharmacy—mostly state university schools—requirements fell off sharply, in comparison with medicine and law.[55]

Agitators for better preliminary preparation of students met a sluggish, apathetic response in the profession. A Section of the American Pharmaceutical Association, considering the ignorance of matriculants a pressing problem, attempted for a second time (1898) to sound out opinion among the state boards and state associations. James H. Beal, who conducted the survey, reported back that "Only two state associations seem to have given the matter any consideration . . . No report was received from any Board of Pharmacy."[56]

An organized stand by the schools themselves became possible after they joined together in what is now called the American Association of Colleges of Pharmacy. In a move made effective for the school year 1908-09 "satisfactory completion of at least one year of work in an accredited high school or its equivalent" became an obligatory minimum for member schools (excepting, for a few years, matriculants from 13 Western states and Indian Territory).[57] This standard was soon advanced to a prerequisite of 2 years of high school or the equivalent (effective 1917-18). Finally, in the fall of 1923 a 4-year high school requirement became binding on the 42 schools in the association (of which more than half already were meeting such a standard voluntarily).

The hesitant advance of the schools was conditioned at least partially by a still greater reluctance on the part of the members of the state organizations that supported the schools. The lack of professional recognition (hinging on inadequate educational standards) in the armed forces during World War I led to an awareness, as Blauch and Webster phrase it, "that the profession had suffered from a too-conservative educational philosophy."[58]

Yet in a little more than one decade, between 1920 and 1932, American pharmacy finally caught up with European standards attained about a century before. Within this short time, the united endeavor of the American Pharmaceutical Association, the American Association of Colleges of Pharmacy and the National Association of Boards of Pharmacy placed American pharmacy, so far as education is concerned, on a recognized academic basis and has made it equal to the best contemporary European patterns. However, before this progress could become effective for the whole of American pharmacy, this college standard had to be made a prerequisite of state board examinations and licensing. It is only through this legal requirement that better and more uniformly educated pharmacists can be guaranteed.

New York was the first state (1905) to require college graduation in pharmacy of all candidates appearing before the State Board of Pharmacy[59] and was followed the next year by Pennsylvania. After another decade 17 other states had passed similar laws.[60] By 1949 only Vermont and the Territory of Alaska held out against a mandatory college diploma.

Which Degree?

The question of what degree, if any, should be awarded to graduates of schools of pharmacy has revealed many divergences of opinion. The Philadelphia College of Pharmacy, having started its career by protesting against the Master of Pharmacy offered by the University of Pennsylvania, was at first somewhat shy of titles. At that time the self-styled "doctors" swarmed beyond the doors of the educational institutions of the country and the English "apothecary" had become a misleading designation (see p. 97). Said the president of the College, Daniel B. Smith (1829),

Our diploma bestows no title, for it was the design of the college to avoid any name, which may hereafter acquire a peculiar meaning and become the designation of a new class analogous to the English apothecary. In attempting to avoid this danger, it has committed what may be considered a blunder by establishing a distinction without giving it a specific name.[61]

Thus the diplomas of the college (first issued in 1826) declared the successful student "to be a Graduate in the Philadelphia College of Pharmacy." This simple confirmation of graduation did not prove to be "a blunder." For more than a century the "Graduate in Pharmacy" was the modest but significant title of most graduates of American colleges of pharmacy. True, several other degrees were bestowed on graduates from time to time, but none of them was generally accepted. Not infrequently, colleges offered higher degrees to their regular graduates because of competition. Thus the doctor's degree was offered as a "drawing card" by some colleges. The confused situation about the year 1900 becomes evident from Scoville's survey (1905) which showed the degree of Graduate in Pharmacy was given "by one school for 3 months course, 7 schools for 1 year course, 41

schools for 2 years course, 1 school for 3 years course"; the degree of Doctor of Pharmacy, "by 6 schools for 2 years course, 9 schools for 3 years course, 1 school for 4 years course"; the degree of Pharmaceutical Chemist "by 1 school for 1 year course, 16 schools for 2 years course, 8 schools for 3 years course, 1 school for 4 years course, 1 school for 5 years course"; the degree of Master of Pharmacy, "by 1 school for 1 year course, 2 schools for 2 years course, 6 schools for 3 years course, 1 school for 4 years course"; the degree of Bachelor of Pharmacy "by 4 schools for 2 years course, 1 school for 3 years course"; the degree of Bachelor of Science, "by 1 school for 1 year course, 13 schools for 4 years course"; the degree of Master of Science "by 4 schools for 5 years course each."[62]

Such confusion was certain to attract strong bids for reform. Within a few years (1913) the first official statement of the American Conference of Pharmaceutical Faculties as to degrees was adopted, requiring "for the degree of Graduate in Pharmacy a minimum course of 1200 hours." This was followed (1914) by a recommended standard that the degree of Pharmaceutical Chemist (Ph.C.) be a 3-year course in pharmacy, based on 4 years of high school. The by-laws refer to the Doctor in Pharmacy for the first time (1924) by asking for "at least a four-year college of pharmacy course" as "the minimum requirement." In 1937, the Graduate in Pharmacy diploma disappeared from the by-laws of the American Association of Colleges of Pharmacy, and in 1938 also the degree of Doctor of Pharmacy. The accredited colleges of pharmacy thereafter uniformly awarded the following degrees: Bachelor of Science (B.S.) or Bachelor of Science in Pharmacy (B.S. in Pharm.), for the completion of the 4-year course and later the 5-year course. Although some wanted a more distinguishing degree, to acknowledge the longer curriculum, no accepted designation was at hand. However, as a few schools changed to a 6-year course (first at the University of Southern California in 1950), the awarding of a professional doctorate was approved, thus resurrecting with a quite new significance the old "Doctor of Pharmacy." The degrees of Master of Science (M.S.), Master of Science in Pharmacy (M.S. in Pharm.), Doctor of Philosophy (Ph.D.) or Doctor of Science (D.Sc.) have been awarded in accordance with the general requirements of standard postgraduate schools.

ASSOCIATION OF SCHOOLS AND BOARDS OF PHARMACY

The Conference of Teaching Colleges

Following an invitation of the Maryland College of Pharmacy, delegates from 5 "Teaching Colleges of Pharmacy"—Chicago, Maryland, Massachusetts, New York and Philadelphia—and from the New Jersey Pharmaceutical Association met in 1870 (at the A.Ph.A. meeting).

This led to the first organization for pharmaceutical education, the Conference of the Schools of Pharmacy. By constitutional definition, the Conference consisted of schools requiring apprenticeship before graduation. This explicit exclusion of the University of Michigan confirms other evidence that the threat of change and challenge represented by the state university helped to spark the impulse to form a special organization. In addition, the first association of medical colleges, formed just 4 years earlier, set an example that scarcely could have passed unnoticed among pharmaceutical educators.

Both the nature and the fate of this earliest associative attempt of the medical colleges found a remarkable parallel in the procrastination and the ineffectual short life of the Conference of the Schools of Pharmacy. The Conference was ineffectual largely because, among other reasons, the delegates were without real policy-making powers; they "recommended to the Colleges," which in turn might "urge their members" (practitioners) to take action. For example, recognizing a key limitation in the lack of a uniform requirement of preliminary education, the Conference considered the question at four annual meetings—and four times did nothing—recogniz-

ing that in fact the selection of future students rested with the preceptors who selected youths for the preliminary apprenticeship. The effects of this basic idea can be found in all aspects of the association schools during the 19th century.

One case in which there was action as well as theoretical agreement can be found in the refusal by the Conference (1874 and 1875) to recognize the "Doctor of Pharmacy" degrees offered by two recently established schools (National College of Pharmacy at Washington, D. C., and Tennessee College of Pharmacy, Nashville, Tenn.) for ordinary course work, and partly even to students who did not attend the courses but merely took the examination and paid the fees. Apart from such common defense against unfair competition, there could hardly be any united action of the American schools of pharmacy at this time. There were still no definite educational requirements asked for by the licensing boards (and often no such boards!), such as would make systematic schooling a prerequisite for the pharmacist-to-be. For most of the schools, the necessity of using all possible means to attract students to keep up the mere existence of the school was stronger than the desire of some professors to elevate the educational standards.

After 13 frustrating years the Conference of Schools of Pharmacy was dissolved. The last yellowed page of the minute book reports in the scrawl of an acting secretary that in 1884 only 3 college representatives carried credentials as delegates; no meeting could be held for lack of quorum.

Bitter disappointment with lack of results may have colored the judgment of the Secretary of the American Pharmaceutical Association, John Maisch, when he wryly reflected that "there was very little talked about that can be considered of any importance for pharmaceutical education." Actually much of importance was discussed; delegates saw the problems, grappled with them and failed to solve them. Yet it is difficult to believe that pharmaceutical education did not benefit eventually by the exchange of views and experiences during the years of the Conference.[63]

The American Association of Colleges of Pharmacy

Shortly after the dissolution of the ill-fated Conference, a section on Education and Legislation was established (1887) in the American Pharmaceutical Association, which provided a forum *pro tem* for educational affairs. But when a new Association of American Medical Colleges was founded (1890), Professor William Simon of Baltimore told the Section, "this is what we have to do, and what we ought to have done long ago."[64] Another decade passed before a new association was founded, but this time it would be successful.

James H. Beal, a man who consistently helped to usher in modern American pharmacy, describes in his memoirs the founding of the new college association:

I conceived the idea that if representatives of the various colleges could be brought together where they could speak face to face, their jealousies would subside, and prior to one of the American Pharmaceutical Association meetings I sent a circular letter to the various colleges suggesting that we have a meeting to see if some of these conflicting views could not be harmonized. Only two [individuals] responded favorably, Dr. [William] Simon of the Maryland College of Pharmacy and Henry P. Hynson of Hynson, Westcott and Dunning of Baltimore [likewise professor at the Maryland College of Pharmacy]. When the association [A.Ph.A.] met at Richmond, Virginia (1900), I made the motion to call for a meeting of Pharmaceutical Faculties. A committee was appointed to consider the question, of which Professor Remington of the Philadelphia College of Pharmacy was made Chairman. Remington was very skeptical of the idea but turned it over to me to work out a report, and knowing of the magic in the word "conference," I used it in recommending a meeting. Since there seemed nothing dangerous in the coming together in the same room, the other members of the Committee agreed to the report. When the members found that no compulsion was intended, they discovered they could discuss these questions in good temper and this was the origin of what was known for many years as the American Conference of Pharmaceutical Faculties but is now known [since 1925] as the American Association of Colleges of Pharmacy.[65]

This new organization, founded by the representatives of 21 American pharmacy schools, originated under circumstances quite different from those of the period from 1870 to 1885. In the meantime, the idea of education as a duty of organized society (i.e., of the state) had finally been given recognition by the people of these United States, and farseeing men in American pharmacy, educators and practitioners as well, had taken advantage of this fact. A large proportion of the pharmacy schools founded in this country between 1883 and 1900 were an integral part of the educational systems of individual states, as departments of state universities or of state colleges. In this general and officially approved trend toward higher education, the educational reformers in American pharmacy were given their opportunity.

True, private schools with no university affiliation were still in the majority. A representative of the then still private Maryland College of Pharmacy, Professor Henry P. Hynson, was the temporary President of the meeting to organize "The American Conference of Pharmaceutical Faculties." The dean of the time-honored Philadelphia College of Pharmacy, Joseph P. Remington, acted as the chairman of the Committee on Organization. However, the man who was elected the first president of the Conference was Albert B. Prescott, dean of the first university pharmacy school in the United States, that of Michigan. There could not be any more convincing proof of the change of mind in the field of pharmaceutical education than the selection of this man who 30 years before had been condemned and ostracized by his fellow teachers for introducing and advocating academic pharmaceutical instruction based on scientific considerations only, instead of instruction intended merely as a supplement to the knowledge acquired in "the store."

It is of interest that Joseph P. Remington, president of the Conference in 1902, although emphasizing in his presidential address that drugstore experience should go hand in hand with college work to achieve the best results, did not hesitate to say,[66]

A student who carefully follows the instruction will certainly acquire more sound knowledge of the essential facts which lie at the foundation of pharmacy, in three years at college, than one who has spent his time exclusively in the store for twenty years, gathering knowledge on the installment plan.

Moreover, what had once seemed remote, now became a common goal—hence brought within reach—as this distinguished spokesman of the old-line schools emphasized the necessity "to secure from the legislature of our various states the recognition of the possession of the college diploma before a candidate is permitted to take the state examination."

Whether in private or in university schools, a cornerstone of adequate professional standards thus was recognized, never to be lost sight of again. Besides its successful endeavor in placing pharmaceutical education in this country on a full academic basis, in improving curricula and faculties, and in promoting research, the American Association of Colleges of Pharmacy has created a spirit of collegiate solidarity and friendly emulation among the schools and the teachers of pharmacy which guarantees further progress and finds remarkable expression (since 1937) in its official publication, *The American Journal of Pharmaceutical Education.*

AMERICAN COUNCIL ON PHARMACEUTICAL EDUCATION

When the American Association of Colleges of Pharmacy set up gradually increasing educational standards, their acceptance served as criteria for admission to the Association and for maintenance of a school's membership. In effect, this provided a kind of accreditation system for the American schools until the American Council on Pharmaceutical Education was established (1932).

Through the Council, the Pharmaceutical Survey observed, "the upgrading and the systematization of the training institutions were promoted and the reciprocal recognition of licenses among the several states greatly extended."

The Council originated under stimulus from the National Association of Boards of Pharmacy, which continues as a co-sponsor together with the American Pharmaceutical Association and the American Association of Colleges of Pharmacy (each with 3 representatives on the Council) and the American Council on Education (1 representative). The Council is responsible for drafting standards and periodically sends inspection teams for a searching examination of each school—its staff, program, standards, facilities, administration and finances.

Through its reports to the respective universities and schools, its counsel, and its published list of accredited schools, the Council has had a unifying and elevating influence, has provided one basis for helping prospective students to select schools, enhanced interschool relationships and helped schools to recognize more clearly their potentialities and deficiencies.

The Pharmaceutical Survey gave strong support to the functioning of the Council and proposed the setting up of a central office with a full-time administrative head (subsequently established at Chicago, headed by a Director of Educational Relations, in association with the National Association of Boards of Pharmacy.)[67] The Council's services, like much else of educational value, would have been greatly hampered without the help of the American Foundation for Pharmaceutical Education.

THE AMERICAN FOUNDATION FOR PHARMACEUTICAL EDUCATION

A report of the Committee on Endowments of the National Drug Trade Conference, presented by Chairman Ernest Little of Rutgers University, strongly urged the securing of endowments for the colleges of pharmacy. Although members of the Conference were favorably disposed toward helping American pharmaceutical institutions of learning, a man of rather unusual insight, energy and authority was required to get things done. This man was Dr. E. L.

Newcomb, executive vice-president of the National Wholesale Druggists' Association. Taking independent initiative, the Association (through Newcomb) invited 50 leading pharmaceutical and chemical manufacturers and chain-store executives to attend a meeting for discussion of "facts relative to the future functioning and financial status of colleges of pharmacy, particularly those which did not receive state aid." This conference directed "the group which called the meeting to organize an all-industry committee" for assembling information.[68] Subsequently the National Drug Trade Conference resolved "to advocate the formation of an *American Foundation for Pharmaceutical Education*." As a result of efforts by Dr. E. L. Newcomb and George V. Doerr of McKesson & Robbins, 1 year later, in 1942, the Foundation was organized and incorporated as a permanent institution. It was sponsored by all national pharmaceutical organizations holding membership in the National Drug Trade Conference. This meant sponsorship by organized pharmacy as a whole, manufacturers and wholesalers as well as practicing pharmacists and educators. Among its stated purposes, the Foundation endeavors—

• To uphold and improve pharmaceutical education by aiding . . . colleges of pharmacy and students therein;
• To aid in the creation of sources of unbiased and authoritative investigation and experimentation on pharmaceutical problems;
• To assist in the selection of important research problems and to provide that the investigations be adequately financed, and to insure as far as possible that they be carried out by competent investigators under the supervision of recognized scientific authorities.

The American Foundation for Pharmaceutical Education was especially valuable through its financial help to needy schools during World War II, and, since the war, through a steadily growing number of fellowships and scholarships. Examples of other projects, wholly or partly underwritten by the Foundation, are the American Council on Pharmaceutical Education, the *American Journal of Pharmaceutical Educa-*

tion, the "Pharmaceutical Survey" in the 1940's, and the summer seminars for teachers of pharmacy. (Grants from 1943 to 1955 totalled $1,978,730.) Over two decades (1942 through 1962) the Foundation aided 2,332 undergraduates and 562 graduate students. Of the latter, 219 became teachers, 182 accepted research positions with 74 manufacturing laboratories, and 26 were appointed to posts in governmental or professional organizations.[69]

There scarcely could be a better demonstration of the willingness of the pharmaceutical industry to accept a full share of responsibility to society in matters pertaining to pharmacy.

PHARMACEUTICAL SURVEYS

Because education is basic to renewal and progress in any profession, periodic inquiries into the status of American pharmacy often have been focused sharply on its educational facilities.

Perhaps the first pharmaceutical "survey" was that launched by the American Pharmaceutical Association soon after its founding, to secure statistical data about pharmacy throughout the country (see p. 263). However, not until the 1920's was an attempt made to obtain a comprehensive picture offering, in addition to statistical data, the basis for evaluating the degree to which the needs of present-day society are served by contemporary pharmacy.

There appeared as the result of studies "made possible by a subvention granted by the Commonwealth Fund . . . and by the co-operation of the American Association of Colleges of Pharmacy . . . the National Association of Retail Druggists, and the National Association of Boards of Pharmacy,"[70] a book entitled *Basic Material for a Pharmaceutical Curriculum* (1927). It was prepared by the director of the investigations, Dr. W. W. Charters, then professor at the University of Pittsburgh, and professors A. B. Lemon and Leon M. Monell of the University of Buffalo School of Pharmacy, with collaboration by Dr. Robert P. Fischelis.[71]

The reception of this report was enthusiastic and of great consequence. "A careful study of the Dr. Charters report," said Dean D. B. R. Johnson of the University of Oklahoma, in his address as President of the American Association of Colleges of Pharmacy in 1927, ". . . has convinced me that we must sooner or later come to a four-year course for a degree in pharmacy. I therefore recommend that, as soon as possible, the four-year course be adopted."[72] In the same year, Dr. H. C. Christensen, Secretary of the National Association of Boards of Pharmacy, called the book "a classic . . . so far-reaching in its possibilities for pharmacy . . ." that everyone, in whatever branch of the profession, should read it. He also put a significant question: "Why not have a survey made every ten years . . . ?" In conclusion, Christensen stated: "We now need a survey to show the requirements of the commercial and administrative side of pharmacy. Well, we have opened up a big field."[73]

Immediately after the Charters study was concluded, the National Association of Boards of Pharmacy took steps to initiate a survey on a broader scale. It was joined by the American Association of Colleges of Pharmacy and by the American Pharmaceutical Association. The American Council on Education promised sponsorship provided sufficient financial support could be procured. Just at this time the United States was going through one of its severest economic crises. Support could not be obtained; the project had to be dropped in 1932.

The idea remained alive. Its first fruit was the so-called Bernays Drug and Pharmaceutical Survey, paid for by "a group from the pharmaceutical profession and the drug trades" and conducted by a public relations agency. This study was concerned mainly with "a better relationship between the drug trades and the pharmaceutical profession, and the public." The conglomerate of data collected and the conclusions drawn, covering 1,200 typewritten pages, have remained unpublished. A report, presented to the American Pharmaceutical Associa-

tion (1943)[74] by Edward L. Bernays, the head of the public relations agency conducting the survey, did not find the favorable reception given to the Charters survey.[75]

On the same day, the American Association of Colleges of Pharmacy adopted a resolution recommending a study of "the possibility of supplementing the Charters, Lemon, and Monell Study." An urgent request was submitted to the American Foundation for Pharmaceutical Education, in accord with an agreement by the Executive Committee of the American Association of Colleges of Pharmacy, the Council of the American Pharmaceutical Association, the American Council on Education and the American Council on Pharmaceutical Education, that the Foundation "endorse and underwrite a comprehensive study of pharmacy, pharmaceutical practices, and new areas of pharmaceutical specialization . . ."

The American Foundation reacted favorably, and the study called The Pharmaceutical Survey was inaugurated (April 15, 1946), to be conducted by the American Council on Education and directed by Dr. Edward C. Elliott, a nationally known educator who was a nonpharmacist and a most remarkable man. There were 3 Assistant Directors: Dr. Lloyd E. Blauch (Curriculum Studies), Mr. Solon Mordell, author of *The Prescription Study* (of the Survey) and Dr. H. H. Remmers (Student Personnel). "A committee of fifteen . . . was selected from various branches of pharmacy and from the lay world to act as the advisory group for the Survey. Dr. W. W. Charters was appointed Chairman of this Committee."[76]

This survey produced the evaluation of pharmaceutical education in relation to American pharmacy in general that was expected of it. To whatever extent its diverse recommendations may be realized, The Pharmaceutical Survey represents something unique in the history of world pharmacy. Still today *The General Report of the Pharmaceutical Survey 1946-1949* and its supplemental monographs repay careful study.

While such surveys assumed that new

analysis and insight were to be a prelude to progress, by no means everyone welcomed the change and the uncertainty and even the sacrifice that this might imply. In education for pharmacy, as in many other fields, advances in requirements often have been a response, not to the active demand of a majority, but to that of a minority who aspired to leave their profession a step beyond where they found it. Rufus A. Lyman of Nebraska, a former editor of the *American Journal of Pharmaceutical Education,* looked back on efforts to advance pharmaceutical education as he experienced them over four decades, and concluded:

Some were violently opposed, the majority were indifferent. Support did come from a few farseeing laymen who recognized the importance of the pharmacist and the drugstore in the public health service. It also came from a handful of practicing druggists who were readers of pharmacy history and who had learned the part the pharmacist has played in the past in science, in industry, in research, in education, and in the art of living, and who had a vision of greater things for the future.[77]

15: The Establishment of
a Literature

BOOKS IMPORTED FROM EUROPE

Before America had a pharmaceutical literature of its own, practitioners of medicine and pharmacy generally used the European books with which they felt most at home, whether by tradition or language or training. Most American-born physicians who had an academic education in this early period received their training at medical schools in Edinburgh or London. Naturally, on returning to their native country they used and taught to their students or apprentices the medicine taught in the British Isles and the literature used there.

The literature that seemed important on American soil early in the 19th century may be inferred from resolutions on a proposed American pharmacopeia (New York State Medical Society, 1818) which point out that various pharmacopeias then were used "in the different sections and States of the Union such as: the Edinburgh Dispensatory, the London Dispensatory, the London Pharmacopoeia, the Dublin Pharmacopoeia, the Parisian Pharmacopoeia,"[1] and also mention the few formularies issued in America between 1806 and 1818. This list makes no pretense at completeness, and the omission of the *Edinburgh Pharmacopoeia* was surely not deliberate. However, the fact that the *Edinburgh Dispensatory* was mentioned, and not the pharmacopeia on which the dispensatory was based, tends to confirm that in America the dispensatories (which combined the pharmacopeial text, explanatory comments and additional material) were much more in practical use than the pharmacopeias themselves.

That the *Paris Pharmacopoeia* should be mentioned by the New York State Medical Society as one of the European books used in certain sections of the United States illustrates the French influence. In addition, pharmacopeias and dispensatories of German origin, as well as Italian, Dutch and Swedish pharmaceutical standards, were used by practitioners who had immigrated from these various countries to the United States. This diverse pharmacopeial literature added to the already confusing number of formularies, but it did not negate the dominance of English pharmacopeial literature.

ATTEMPTS TO ESTABLISH AN AMERICAN PHARMACOPEIA

Philadelphia

The first known step toward an American pharmacopeia was taken by John Morgan. He had already distinguished himself in the medical field by establishing the first medical school. American pharmacy was indebted to him for his efforts in the movement to separate pharmacy and medicine in this country. Dr. Morgan now (1787) "proposed to the College of Physicians of Philadelphia the compilation and publication of a pharmacopeia for Pennsylvania."[2] Since the Federal Constitution had not yet been ratified by all of the 13 states, a general standard apparently was not considered. When only 1 year later the United States of America had become a reality, the plan of the College of Physicians of Philadelphia was expanded.

A circular (ordered 1789) was sent to 100 "proper persons." It stated that "one of the objects of the college has been that of forming a pharmacopoeia adapted to the present state of medicine in America; for which purpose a committee of their members has been some time since appointed, who have made some progress in their work." Furthermore, the circular pointed

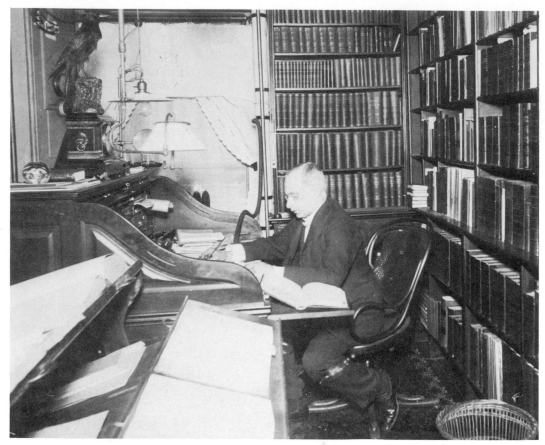

Charles Rice (1841-1901) was one of the most remarkable men to practice pharmacy in America. He was the key figure in giving the U. S. Pharmacopeia (1882) its modern outlook and format; he was chairman of the committee to develop the first National Formulary and he contributed brilliantly to other pharmaceutical publications. Rice did most of his work at his desk in Bellevue Hospital (above), where he served as superintendent of the General Drug Department. Part of his revolving dictionary rack, which he used in reading 18 languages of East and West, can be seen at the lower left.

out "the absolute necessity of some standard amongst ourselves to prevent that uncertainty and irregularity which in our present situation must infallibly attend on the compositions of the apothecary and the prescription of the physician." It asked that the addressee "particularly inform us what native American remedies have been discovered amongst you."[3]

The response to this call was not encouraging. The *Transactions* of the Philadelphia College of Physicians reports 2 replies: one from the president of the Medical Society of the State of Delaware, and the other from the Medical Society of New Haven,

both expressing appreciation of the idea conveyed by the circular.

The College named a committee on pharmacopeia to compile material on pharmaceutical substances and processes, but apparently a completed study was never presented. A new appreciation of native resources and pride in young nationhood after the Revolution reinforced interest in indigenous drugs and in an American pharmacopeia. For example, one member of the Philadelphia committee, the botanist Benjamin Smith Barton, stressed (1798) the desirability of giving American drugs "a place in the Pharmacopoeia of this country," that is, "when such a desideratum shall be supplied."[4]

South Carolina

The idea of "the establishment of an independent American Materia Medica" was mentioned also in a letter published by the Medical Society of South Carolina (1798). In all probability the movement was started by a physician and wholesale druggist (Dr. Johnson) who had graduated from the Philadelphia medical school. Hence, it might be considered to be a continuation of the Philadelphia endeavor. Later on, the society touched on the problem again in a letter (1808) to the Massachusetts Medical Society, refusing to adopt the *Massachusetts Pharmacopoeia.*

Connecticut

The Connecticut Medical Society had voted "that the professors of the Medical College be requested to communicate to the next convention the best mode of producing a general and uniform pharmacopoeia."[5] At the next year's convention, 1816, it was voted "to accept the report of the committee . . . to compile a pharmacopoeia and to submit it to the next convention."[6] Whether the committee appointed for that purpose did any preparatory work is unknown. When the Connecticut Medical Society received the history-making invitation of the New York Medical Society to take part in forming a "National Pharmacopoeia," it appointed as delegates two of the men who had constituted its own pharmacopeial committee, Eli Ives and William Tully.[7]

THE MASSACHUSETTS PRECURSOR

The plans of the physicians in Philadelphia, South Carolina and Connecticut were fully realized by their Massachusetts colleagues. The Massachusetts Medical Society had shown its concern for genuine and adequate medicines as early as 1786, when it petitioned the legislature to prevent the sale of bad or adulterated drugs. The compilation and the publication of a "pharma-copocia" was only another step in the same direction.

At different periods, the Society has expended no small amount of labor to secure a uniform mode of compounding medicines, and to protect the community against the dangers incurred by the use of such as are spurious. At a meeting of the Counsellors, October 3, 1805, a committee was appointed to draw up and lay before them a pharmacopoeia or formulary, for the preparation of compound medicines, with names affixed to the same, to be called the Massachusetts Pharmacopoeia.[8]

In 1807 "the committee . . . presented the manuscript of a pharmacopoeia" at a meeting of the Counsellors of the Society, and it was voted "that the said pharmacopoeia be printed for the use of the Society."[9] The book, a volume of 272 pages listing 536 drugs and preparations, appeared early in 1808. An illuminating preface revealed that the Society

resolved to adopt the pharmacopoeia of the Edinburgh College as the basis of their own; but to permit such omissions, alterations, and additions as, upon minute examination, should be found necessary. It was not desirable however, to give to this the appearance of originality; on the contrary, trifling considerations have not induced any variation from that excellent work.

These words illustrate the honesty of the compilers as well as their modesty.

The most important of the additions mentioned were indigenous American drugs not included in the *Edinburgh Pharmacopoeia.* "The learned physicians of Massachusetts," said a reviewer in the *Medical Repository* (editor Dr. S. L. Mitchill), "have neither neglected the native productions of this country, nor hazarded the introduction of them into their catalogue of materia medica."[10]

The authors of the *Massachusetts Pharmacopoeia* were in advance of their time in another innovation. Their model, the *Edinburgh Pharmacopoeia,* like most similar books of that period, was written in Latin. The text of the Massachusetts book is in English, except for drug titles in Latin as well as English. The preface justified the bold innovation with the statement that a Latin book "is not adapted in this country, where the apothecaries are not necessarily instructed in that language." The same statement naturally held true for most of the American physicians of those days.

The apothecaries are mentioned several times in the preface, such as in the statement that "it is the business of the physician to prescribe, and of the apothecary to prepare medicines."[11] This unreserved recognition of the separation of medicine and pharmacy, as early as 1808, implied an advanced position. It was the first known official declaration of this kind to be made, not by an individual physician like John Morgan (see p. 147), but by an organized group of American medical practitioners. However, the following sentences of the preface imply the recognition that this desirable separation was of necessity restricted to the larger cities:

In them, the professions of physician and apothecary are most distinct; and between those, whose relation to each other is so important, a perfect understanding should exist. As this cannot be established between them as individuals, it is necessary that there should be uniformity, both in the pharmaceutical preparations and language.

The authors chose an excellent way to induce pharmacists to adopt their work. They appealed to self-interest and professional responsibility. "The Medical Society indeed is not empowered to require of apothecaries a compliance with the directions of this pharmacopoeia; nor does such power seem requisite. It has a sufficient substitute in the apothecary's regard to his own interest, and to his duty to the public."[12] This appeal found the expected response within the state of Massachusetts.

Was this local success all the authors of the *Massachusetts Pharmacopoeia* had hoped for? The sentences with which they closed the preface of their work reveal a higher and more comprehensive aim. The authors

cannot hesitate to solicit the aid of all scientific men in effecting a revolution, so very desirable for the correct practice of medicine; a revolu-

tion, which concerns the reputation and success of every medical practitioner, and the health and safety of every individual.

"Revolution" is too strong a word to have been used by men so deliberate as Jackson and Warren with reference only to Massachusetts. They must have had in mind all of the United States. Indeed, attempts were made to secure general recognition for the book. Copies and a circular letter, emphasizing the advantages of "a pharmacopoeia calculated for the practice of the United States"[13] were sent to the medical societies of other states. The New Hampshire Medical Society was the only one to adopt the book.[14] One other response, the letter from the Medical Society of South Carolina mentioned previously, expressed the opinion that "a perfect pharmacopoeia" can be obtained only by "the concurrence of different States," by requesting "the different Medical Societies, at a future date . . . to refer such a compilation to someone of the learned Medical Association."[15]

It was exactly this idea, the recognition of all medical organizations in the compilation of such a standard, that Lyman Spalding of New York made the basis of his attempt at a national pharmacopeia. The Massachusetts Medical Society appointed a committee to revise its pharmacopeia, but after the receipt of the request of the New York State Medical Society for cooperation in preparing a national pharmacopeia according to the plan of Spalding, the Massachusetts Society concurred (1818). Through this collaboration "more than ninety per cent of the articles in the Massachusetts book were included in the later publication."[16] It is one of the ironies of history that in this way the book which had been refused general recognition was destined to constitute, 12 years later, the greatest part of the first generally recognized standard pharmaceutical formulary in the United States of America.

EARLY HOSPITAL "PHARMACOPOEIA"

The *Pharmacopoeia Nosocomii Neo-Eboracensis,* sub-titled in English, *Pharma-*

copoeia of the New York Hospital, was published in 1816 "under the authority of the physicians of that institution" and is usually mentioned as one of the precursors of the *United States Pharmacopeia;* that is true of its earlier appearance but not of its contents or even the ambitions of its authors.

These ambitions are made plain in the remarks introducing the book. A special formulary for the hospital had its beginning with "the adoption, by common consent and common usage, of a few formulae of prescriptions, thrown together upon a single sheet of paper . . . and kept in the apothecary's apartment for his special guidance."[17] A more comprehensive formulary had been begun by Dr. Elihu H. Smith, "for his own individual accommodation, in his practice."[18] The death of Dr. Smith put an end to this attempt, and the manuscript, not considered important by anyone, was lost. It seems doubtful whether a formulary of the New York Hospital ever would have been printed had there not been another incentive: the desire for a convenient means of instruction in the art of prescribing.

The New York Hospital had developed into "a most valuable practical school for the improvement of youth to the exercise of healing art."[19] Instruction could be facilitated by a book containing all necessary information about Latin terms, weights, drug names and synonyms, doses, the diet employed in the hospital, etc., as well as a catalogue of the simple drugs and a list of "preparations and compositions, including the more general prescriptions employed in the practice of the hospital."[20] Besides, there was some hope that such a book could become a good seller. It recommended itself in the preface not only to the students studying medicine in the hospital, but also as "a manual of prescription and selection of official preparations" to those "apothecaries, who reside in parts of the United States where no regular pharmacopoeia has been established." This sentence undoubtedly refers to the *Massachusetts Pharmacopoeia,* the only "regular" pharmacopeia established in the United

States at that time; and it shows furthermore that the authors did not regard their book to be of the same kind. In addition to "private extemporaneous prescriptions as the physicians and surgeons of the establishment have individually suggested,"[21] the preface of the *New York Hospital Pharmacopoeia* mentions as its principal sources the pharmacopeias of London, Edinburgh and Dublin.[22] It does not mention the *Massachusetts Pharmacopoeia,* probably because this book was its only significant competitor. In using English instead of Latin it followed the Massachusetts example.

The New York Hospital book was a good and useful compilation, but it was no state pharmacopeia; neither was it a precursor to the *United States Pharmacopeia* in any proper sense. It was an early American representative of the innumerable printed or unprinted hospital formularies, designed for local use and instruction, which have always been written and still continue to be written.

It is not known who first suggested the issuance of the *New York Hospital Pharmacopoeia.* At a meeting of the physicians and the surgeons of the hospital (April 4, 1815) Samuel L. Mitchill and Valentine Seaman "were appointed to prepare a pharmacopoeia for this institution." Later that same year, they presented a manuscript, previously "admitted to the examination of the members individually, for criticism and amendment." After further amendments, this manuscript was adopted.[23]

Of the two authors, Valentine Seaman, teacher of clinical surgery in the hospital, had earlier (1811) "drawn up a small work for the students attending his lectures, which was printed at their request and for their particular convenience."[24] This *Pharmacopoeia chirurgica in usum Nosocomii Novi Eboracensis* met with acrimonious criticism.[25] The good reception which the new book found was doubtless due to the fact that Dr. Mitchill was its main author. He played an important part in the movement that only a few years later led to the issuance of the first Pharmacopeia of the United States.

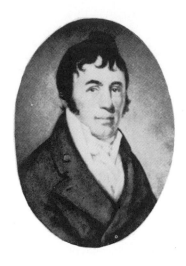

The physician Lyman Spalding (above), more than anyone else, was responsible for the successful planning and work that produced the first Pharmacopeia of the United States. It is said that he was urging the idea of a national pharmacopeia on his friends as early as 1815. At the height of his career, about the time when the first U.S.P. was coming off the press, Spalding was struck down by a box of rubbish falling from an upstairs window. He died less than a year later (1821) at the age of only 47.

THE U. S. PHARMACOPEIA

There has been some discussion as to whether Lyman Spalding is to be regarded as the "father of the United States Pharmacopeia," as stated by historians for more than a century, or whether this proud title should be given to another man, Samuel Latham Mitchill.[26]

In comparison with Spalding, Mitchill was unquestionably the greater and more brilliant personality. A graduate of the University of Edinburgh, Mitchill was older and much more versatile and experienced; his reputation as a physician was of the best. He was one of the founders (1797), and for 16 years the principal editor, of the earliest medical journal in the United States. He had served as teacher and chemist. Once he had been a senator and twice

a representative. Yet, all of this could not guarantee success in a venture which in the previous decades had several times been tried in vain.

The statement, coined by Barton in 1798, that a national pharmacopeia was a "desideratum" of American medicine and pharmacy had been quoted in the medical literature again and again. No one in the country knew this better than Mitchill. He was exactly informed in regard to the different attempts to create such a book. He knew why they had failed. To have tried under the circumstances would have been hazardous for him. True, all scientific and practical sources and resources were at his command; nevertheless, instead of issuing the first *United States Pharmacopeia*, the cautious Mitchill launched a hospital formulary.

To make the dream of an American pharmacopeia a reality required a man who had less to lose and more to gain; a man willing to devote himself entirely to the difficult task. This man was Lyman Spalding. Although Mitchill was not willing to take the risk, he still wished to manage the undertaking. Spalding had gained his friendship through correspondence and Mitchill helped the young doctor to settle in New York. Later he encouraged Spalding in the plan of initiating a *United States Pharmacopeia*, to be prepared as a cooperative task by the medical associations of the entire country. Although Mitchill gave sanction to this plan and assisted in its execution, he left both the responsibility and the glory to Spalding.

The real start of the new and finally successful enterprise was made by Dr. Lyman Spalding on January 6, 1817, when he submitted

to the New York County Medical Society, a project for the formation of a National Pharmacopoeia, by the authority of all the medical societies and medical schools in the United States. The plan proposed was, (1) That a convention should be called in each of the four grand divisions of the United States, to be composed from all the medical societies and schools; (2) That each district convention should form a pharmacopoeia, and elect delegates to meet

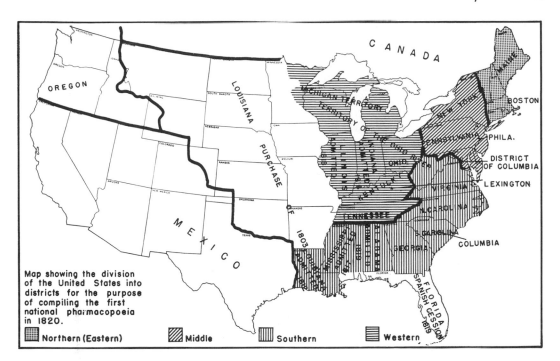

Map showing the division of the United States into districts for the purpose of compiling the first national pharmacopoeia in 1820.

▦ Northern (Eastern)   ▨ Middle   ⫴ Southern   ⊟ Western

in general convention in the city of Washington, on the first of January, 1820: (3) That the general convention should, from the district pharmacopoeia, form the national work.[27]

If at this time there was any possibility of bringing to pass such a work in the United States, Spalding's plan promised success. True, the earlier plans also had included cooperation by the several medical associations and by the practitioners interested in the subject. However, this cooperation consisted of merely adding to a work undertaken by the medical group that had initiated it. Such a group, naturally, claimed the credit. The earlier method had failed in part because it did not satisfy personal ambitions. Spalding's suggestions solved the psychological and the personal difficulties.

The development of the project now proceeded rapidly. Only one month after Spalding submitted his project to the New York County Medical Society, the New York State Medical Society, at the suggestion of Mitchill, approved "the formation of an American Pharmacopoeia of delegates from the several State Medical Societies."[28] A committee with Lyman Spalding as secretary was appointed to "correspond with all the incorporated state medical societies, etc., in the Union and such influential medical men as they may deem proper." On March 4, 1818, the committee issued the first circular. The response received made it clear "that the design of forming a National Pharmacopoeia had met the approbation of a majority of the medical associations in the U. S." A second circular invited "the said associations to designate a time and a place for the meeting of each of the district conventions: and in conformity therewith the following places were designated, viz., Boston, Philadelphia, Columbia, South Carolina, and Lexington, Kentucky."[29]

This division of the country into 4 districts for the purpose of better communication was no invention of Spalding but an early measure (1785) of the Massachusetts Medical Society, which "divided the Commonwealth into four districts, the Eastern, Western, Southern, and the Middle, to encourage the reporting of medical cases."[30]

Most of the work was accomplished within the Northern (Eastern) and the Middle districts, more particularly by the delegates of Massachusetts, New York and Pennsylvania. "There were no conventions held in the Southern and Western districts, but measures were taken by those concerned, to secure a representation of the Southern district in the General Convention at Washington."[31]

Only a scattering of men took seats when the General Convention convened on the first day of January, 1820, in the Senate Chamber of the Capitol in Washington, D. C. They had no power to legislate or even to make the proposed pharmacopeia "official." Yet they formally represented their constituencies and would bring into being the first Pharmacopeia of the United States in a typically American way.

On that first day, we are told, only a half dozen delegates participated; on the second day 5 more delegates appeared. All were physicians, the majority coming from the pharmacopeial Middle District lying just North of the Capital. At that time no society or school of pharmacy existed in the United States, to offer the possibility of organized pharmaceutical representation. (By the time of the second revision of the U.S.P., representatives of American pharmacy assumed a working partnership and in subsequent revisions were officially recognized and increasingly important.)

It was a relatively young group that assembled at the founding Convention, 9 of the 11 being under 48 years of age. Their professional stature varied considerably. The dominance of the College of Philadelphia (later called the University of Pennsylvania) in early medical education shows up in the background of at least half the delegates, who either graduated from its medical department or at least studied there. Two others had studied medicine at the University of Edinburgh, whose famous medical department has been the model for American beginnings at the College of Philadelphia. This educational background suggests an informed awareness of European pharmacopeial experience among the delegates and helps to explain the influence of the respected Edinburgh Pharmacopeia on American developments.[32]

When the first *U. S. Pharmacopeia* was published, the preface mentioned the "Pharmacopoeia of the Massachusetts Medical Society" and the "Pharmacopoeia of the

New York Hospital" in a footnote as two examples of local measures taken "in several of the States . . . by the faculty to regulate the preparation of medicines." Since no other local measures of this kind that resulted in printed books prior to 1820 are known, and since the *New York Hospital Pharmacopoeia*, in contrast with the Massachusetts book, was nothing but a local formulary with some instructive additions, the intention of minimizing the importance of the *Massachusetts Pharmacopoeia* seems evident.

Additional proof will be found in the manner in which the results of the convention for the Northern District are reported in the historical introduction of the first Pharmacopeia. This report says, "A plan for a pharmacopoeia submitted by the delegates from Massachusetts, was taken up, and after being duly revised and amended, was adopted by this convention as their pharmacopoeia." Was indeed only "a plan for a pharmacopoeia . . . taken up" and "adopted" in Boston? The *Transactions* of the College of Physicians of Philadelphia reports the following interesting details:

A convention of delegates from societies and institutions of the Eastern (Northern) district of the United States met in Boston, June 1, 1819. . . . The delegates from Massachusetts submitted a plan of pharmacopoeia, which was referred to Drs. Mussey, Goram, Torrey, Ingalls, and Ives for examination and amendment. On their motion *the Pharmacopoeia of the Massachusetts Medical Society*, as now revised, was adopted by the convention to be presented to the General Convention at Washington, D. C., Jan. 1, 1820.[33]

It was the contents of this revised *Massachusetts Pharmacopoeia* and of "the prospectus agreed upon in the convention of the Middle district[34] which

were duly examined and compared in detail and . . . with such additions as were thought necessary, consolidated into one work, which after full revision, was adopted by the General Convention as the American Pharmacopoeia and ordered to be published by a committee appointed for that purpose.[35]

The report of the Philadelphia delegate states that "in the arrangement of the materia medica the plan proposed in the Middle district [virtually, New York and Philadelphia] has been departed from," but "the list of preparations and compounds is pretty nearly what was agreed on in the convention of the Middle district."[36] Since "more than 90 p.c. of the articles in the Massachusetts Pharmacopoeia were included" in the Pharmacopoeia either the draft of the Middle District was itself based on the Massachusetts book or its authors came independently to similar conclusions.

The entire editorial work naturally had to be done by the committee of publication. Under the active chairmanship of Lyman Spalding, the committee worked diligently, Spalding bearing the responsibility. How thoroughly the original draft was revised and corrected becomes apparent from a printed copy of items of the materia medica as well as of the *medicamenta praeparata* that the chairman sent to his committee members.[37] Finally, the book was printed in Boston and appeared on December 15, 1820, bearing the title *The Pharmacopoeia of the United States of America*, published "By the Authority of the Medical Societies and Colleges."

The national successor to the *Massachusetts Pharmacopoeia* differed most strikingly in that it did not confine itself to the use of the English language. The book placed the text on facing pages in Latin and in English. In contrast with the authors of the *Massachusetts Pharmacopoeia* the majority of the delegates responsible for the national standard was of the opinion that "no well-educated physician or apothecary is unacquainted" with Latin. They believed that the Latin text would render the book "more intelligible to foreigners, and more useful in those districts of the United States where the French and German languages continue to be spoken."[38] Another significant remark in the preface represents one of the earliest official American statements concerning pharmaceutical manufacturing on a large scale. It reads, "Those compound substances which are prepared in the large way at manufactories, and which are to be kept by the apothecary, *though*

*not necessarily prepared by him,** are inserted on the materia medica list. Those which are to be made by the apothecary alone, are placed among the preparations and compositions."[39]

The uncertainty of the authors in selecting drugs is illustrated by the fact that they divided the materia medica list into two parts, one containing "articles of decided reputation or general use" and another containing "those the claims of which are of a more uncertain kind." This dual list was continued until radical changes were effected in 1882 (6th revision).

This procedure had a European pattern. However, there is one difference. In European countries the discrimination had a very practical meaning. There the articles of the first list (*series medicaminum*) had to be kept in stock in even the smallest pharmacy. Thus the availability of these drugs to prescribing physicians was guaranteed.

In general, the new book met with a kind reception, although there were some disapproving voices. In a Philadelphia medical journal, an anonymous reviewer, after a long and detailed criticism, concluded that the work "will probably require immediate revision."[40] The senior surgeon of the Navy, Dr. Edward Cutbush, stated to the Secretary of the Navy that he was not able to give his "unqualified approbation of the work for the use of our naval surgeons."[41] The members of the medical and pharmaceutical professions accepted the book, so far as they were interested, and in 1828 a somewhat modified second issue of the first U.S.P. appeared.[41a]

The importance of first publications such as this lies not so much in their perfection and immediate results as in the simple fact that a beginning has been made. At the close of a 12-page review, the *Medical Repository* stated:

This work forms an era in the history of the profession. It is the first one ever compiled by the authority of the profession throughout a nation. Collections of this sort have been made in other countries, but none, so far, under the

---

* Italics added.

impressive sanction which distinguishes this. Many of the authorities of the Past compiled similar works, later still, the Colleges of Great Britain have followed their examples. France by command of her Monarch has furnished her "Codex," but it has remained for American Physicians to frame a work which emanates from the profession itself, and is founded on the principles of Representation. It embodies a Codex Medicum of the free and independent United States.[42]

REVISING THE PHARMACOPEIA

While the first revision was underway a dangerous schism developed among those most interested in developing effective drug standards for America through the new *Pharmacopeia*. Misunderstandings arose largely because of crude procedures for administering the U.S.P., intensified by an old rivalry between New York and Philadelphia factions. Under the leadership of the eminent New York physician Samuel L. Mitchill, then U.S.P. president, a second General Convention was held in New York, and a FIRST REVISION was published on schedule, at New York in 1830.

A bizarre sequel was the appearance of another and different First Revision, imprinted Philadelphia, 1831![43] This edition gained more recognition than did the competing New York pharmacopeia. And the New York book had no successors. Before the time for a third General Convention, two key figures in the founding period of the *Pharmacopeia*, the New Yorkers Mitchill and Spalding both had died. No one comparable came forward in the New York area to do the work and to fight for it.

However, in the Philadelphia contingent were two physicians whose competent work and influential personalities would be decisive for the future of the *Pharmacopeia of the United States:* George B. Wood and Franklin Bache. Among medical practitioners in general, now that the *Pharmacopeia* seemed to be well established, interest in it waned. So much so that it is doubtful that pharmacopeial work would have persisted except for the sustaining prosperity of the *United States Dispensatory* prepared by Wood and Bache (see p. 246), who were now the key figures in carrying forward the further revision of the *Pharmacopeia*.

These physicians were both on the faculty of the Philadelphia College of Pharmacy, and thus arose a collaboration on the *Pharmacopeia* between physicians and pharmacists of scientific attainment that had been lacking heretofore.

To conduct experiments for use by the Committee on the Pharmacopeia, an eminent Philadelphia pharmacist, Daniel B. Smith, was employed. When the Philadelphia edition (1831) appeared, the preface alluded to this work, to improvements due to the "zeal of pharmacists as well in this country as in Europe," and to the entire *Pharmacopeia* having "passed the examination of pharmacists of acknowledged eminence in their profession."[44]

The pharmacopeial revision work now developed into a definite routine, which persisted through the Fifth Revision (6th edition, 1873). The decennial revisions were carried out by a Committee of Revision authorized and appointed by each subsequent Washington Convention. George B. Wood and Franklin Bache of Philadelphia continued to be the most active members of the Committee.

In the First Revision cooperating pharmacists included only members of the Philadelphia College of Pharmacy. The SECOND REVISION (published 1842) took advantage of the advice of still other pharmacy colleges then operating. Helpful response came from both Boston and New York, but the most important pharmaceutical collaboration again came from Philadelphia, consisting of "amendment of the whole Pharmacopoeia, by a special committee. . . ."[45] Among the collaborators was that remarkable pharmacist, William Procter, Jr.

This Second Revision appeared only in English. A notable technical innovation was the approval of percolation as an optional method of extraction, a progressive step taken earlier only by the French and the Scottish (Edinburgh) pharmacopeias. Brief notes on purity tests for some U.S.P. drugs were introduced, following the example of the London and the Edinburgh pharmacopeias.

Participation of pharmacists in this 1842 edition was more extensive but still only semi-official. With the THIRD REVISION (1851 edition) pharmacy was accorded official representation in the General Convention. A new period dawned. The period of the pharmacopeial convention as a purely medical organization had come to an end.

By including pharmacy, the representatives of medicine publicly recognized two factors: (1) the existence of American professional pharmacy and its representation by the colleges (i.e., local associations), and (2) the necessity of having pharmacy share not only the work but also the responsibility.

At the 1850 Convention 2 of the 5 pharmacists participating were made members of the Committee of Revision: William Procter, Jr., of Philadelphia, and John Milhau of New York City.

When the 1851 edition appeared, fluid extracts were a notable innovation among the dosage forms.

At the U.S.P. General Convention of 1860, 11 pharmacists participated (from 4 colleges along the Eastern seaboard); pharmacists comprised half the new Committee of Revision; and the American Pharmaceutical Association (founded just 8 years before) transmitted new technical material, as published in its *Proceedings*, for use in the work of revision. This convention also was noteworthy for a contribution from the New York medical profession, read by Dr. E. R. Squibb, which was the first proferred from New York in the three decades since the severe schism of 1830.

This FOURTH REVISION appeared as the 5th edition in 1863 (reprinted 1864, 1866, 1868). Its lateness probably can be attributed partly to the numerous changes (requiring some 119 meetings and 138 written reports of subcommittees), partly to a wish to take into account innovations in a forthcoming edition of the *British Pharmacopoeia*, with which there was growing American cooperation. One significant change was the grading of powder fineness according to 5 different sieve meshes. The use of apothecaries' weights was de-emphasized.

Work on the *Pharmacopeia* now had en-

tered a period of transition. When the FIFTH REVISION of the *Pharmacopeia* appeared (1873), Franklin Bache had died and George B. Wood was diligent but old. His energy and authority, after four decades of Pharmacopeial work, were strong enough to hold the new edition within old lines; but there were new men among the 60 delegates at the General Convention (1870), men with new ideas, and their presence implied change.

The old guard, as symbolized by Wood, must have realized that they were on the defensive, since they emphasized (Preface, 1873) the "conservative character necessarily pertaining to a National Pharmacopoeia" and rejected any thought of a "mission to lead in the paths of discovery." They spoke disdainfully of "pandering to fashion or to doubtful novelties in Pharmaceutical Science," and complained of the "meagreness of details" in reports submitted for use by the Committee of Revision.[46]

Although the medical colleges represented at the Convention of 1870 had still outnumbered pharmacy colleges 3 to 1, 4 of the 6 technical contributions presented to the Convention for the next revision came from pharmacists. Without doubt, pharmaceutical interest in the *Pharmacopeia* had increased gradually, while that of the medical profession had decreased.

Dr. E. R. Squibb was among those who felt that the pharmacopeial work had not kept pace with the times; and he was dissatisfied with the dependence of the *Pharmacopeia* on the private success of Dr. Wood's *Dispensatory of the United States*. Some of the proposals Squibb now put forward were a paid full-time director of revision, revision every 5 years (instead of 10), a pharmacopeia embracing so much commentary that it need not be supplemented by a dispensatory, plus publication of an inexpensive annual that would provide a semi-official progress report on innovations in drugs, processes and equipment.[47] Dr. Squibb thought that such a program should be administered by cooperative action of the American Medical Association and the American Pharmaceutical Association, medicine taking the lead and the responsibilities, with pharmacy assisting, as a special branch of medicine.

In pharmaceutical circles this plan was treated with reserve, for rather obvious reasons. At the American Pharmaceutical Association it was clearly recognized that physicians "certainly have a right to direct what substances shall enter into the Pharmacopoeia, their general character, and the preparations, but the details of the work devolve certainly upon pharmacists and pharmaceutical chemists. . . ." The pharmacists' Association seemed ready to cooperate with the American Medical Association—but on a basis of equality.[48]

In medical circles the plan perhaps met more indifference than active opposition. The American Medical Association not only failed to adopt the proposal but called any arrangement for pharmaceutical responsibility "inappropriate" to the Association.[49]

This circumstance created an opportune hour for American pharmacy. Fortunately, members of the American Pharmaceutical Association had the ability and the farsightedness to comprehend the great task confronting them and to grapple with it. At the 1877 meeting, high level discussions were held, with initiative particularly in the hands of Frederick Hoffmann of New York. In a resolution adopted by the assembly, he pointed to the necessity for a more frequent, comprehensive and generally satisfactory revision on a new basis, and placed that task in the hands of the American Pharmaceutical Association.[50]

In place of its old Committee on the Pharmacopeia, which had no authoritative influence, the American Pharmaceutical Association named a new 15-man committee with a great task: not only to draft a new edition of the *Pharmacopeia of the United States*, but actually a new type of pharmacopeia.[51]

There remained a question: What trouble might ensue with distinguished oldsters still in pharmacopeial positions, who felt themselves challenged and their prerogatives put in question? To forestall dissension, the old Convention was left externally untouched. The presidency was filled by a physician,

as from the beginning in 1820. Yet, the internal workings definitely changed.

Previously, the Committee of Revision had played the role of an executive body, largely through the authoritarian dominance of one man, George B. Wood. The Committee was now made the official executive, with the backing of the American Pharmaceutical Association. It was given authority to "report a complete plan for the revision of the Pharmacopoeia at the next Decennial Convention," instead of the traditional procedure of revising and amalgamating various drafts and contributions first brought before the Convention by constituent groups.

Pharmacists now held a majority in the Committee of Revision (14 of 25). At its head was the learned and versatile hospital pharmacist, Charles Rice of New York, who was also chairman of the American Pharmaceutical Association's committee, which presented a remarkable and comprehensive report at the 1878 meeting. When the Association placed the Committee's proposals on the Pharmacopeia before the General Convention, they became the foundation for the renowned Sixth Revision, the 1882 edition.

Any pharmacist who holds this book in his hands and compares it with its predecessor will recognize the advent of the modern *Pharmacopeia of the United States* and will appreciate why this edition signaled a fundamental advance in drug standards for the American health professions and the public.

The new *Pharmacopeia* turned more sharply away from the outworn concept of the community pharmacy as the place of manufacture of most of the pharmaceutical preparations. Instead it tried to establish in the pharmacy another kind of responsibility: examination of medicinal substances by the pharmacist as a check on quality. Casual mention of a few tests was replaced with detailed tests for identifying and determining the purity of many of the drugs. Detailed processes for assaying the alkaloids appeared for the first time. Drugs from the vegetable and the mineral kingdoms were more meaningfully described as to physical characteristics and, where possible, chemical properties. Symbolic formulas and molecular weights were introduced.

The old division of the *Pharmacopeia* into primary and secondary lists of basic drugs and a section of preparations was abandoned. A single alphabetic arrangement of all drugs in the new edition was similar to that in the *British Pharmacopoeia*.[52]

The fullness of description and explanation in the Sixth Revision especially impressed the pharmaceutical and medical world. Two classes of preparations appeared for the first time: abstracts (dilutions of powdered extracts) and elixirs. Still other innovations reinforce the special place that the 1882 edition holds in the history of the *United States Pharmacopeia*.

With authority for drafting subsequent editions now centering in a single executive body, the preparatory work went forward in a more systematic way. One offshoot of work on the SEVENTH REVISION was the serial *Digest of Comments* on the *United States Pharmacopeia*, which would find a useful place in pharmaceutical literature for several decades (after 1905 appearing as *Bulletins* of the Hygienic Laboratory of the U. S. Public Health Service; from 1926 to 1948 as part of the *Abstracts* of the American Pharmaceutical Association).

With the Seventh Revision (8th edition) there was established the present policy that requires announcement of "a definite date, reasonably distant from the actual date of publication, when the new Pharmacopoeia is intended to go into effect and to supersede the preceding one." Thus the new book was made effective on January 1, 1894 (although it had been published in September, 1893). Such evidences of increasing formality in procedure and precision in content reflected increasing legal implications, for although the Federal Food and Drug Act had not yet been passed, the *Pharmacopeia* had already been made "official" under a number of state laws, a fact recognized by the change in this edition from the old term "officinal" to "official."[53]

The *Pharmacopeia* effective from 1894

contained other evidences of a new time. Assays for active principles of both drugs and preparations were added wherever possible. Standards of purity were made "as high as practicable for legal enforcement, but not beyond a point reasonably attainable by the manufacturer." Chemical formulas were modernized. Use of the metric system was encouraged, "solids to be weighed and liquids to be measured." Substances were excluded that could be produced only by a patented process or that were otherwise protected by proprietary rights.

The General Convention of 1900 remains memorable particularly because it took action to incorporate as "The United States Pharmacopoeial Convention" (June 11, 1900), with the purpose of "establishing one uniform standard and guide for the use of those engaged in the practice of medicine and pharmacy in the United States, whereby the identity, strength and purity of all medicines and drugs may be accurately determined and for other like and similar purposes."[54] Some of the organizational changes introduced at this time remain functional today. A Board of Trustees was established to handle business affairs. Additional delegates to the Convention were authorized, including representatives from the American Chemical Society and branches of the United States government (such as the Army, the Navy and the U. S. Marine Hospital Service). With the establishment of this newly chartered organization, the American Pharmaceutical Association had fulfilled its diplomatically pursued goal of giving the *Pharmacopeia* and its revisions a solid and lasting foundation.

Shortly after his re-election as chairman of the Committee of Revision, Charles Rice died (1901). From among the 18 pharmacists and 7 physicians on the Committee there was chosen as Rice's successor Joseph P. Remington of Philadelphia, one of the master pharmacists of his generation.

While the collaboration of physicians was eagerly sought, the preponderance of pharmacists on the Committee of Revision reflects the fact that the entire painstaking and detailed technical work was pharmaceutical in nature and hence devolved on pharmacists, "while the field of the physician in connection with the revision of the Pharmacopoeia is restricted mainly to deciding upon the admission or exclusion of articles."[55]

The General Convention of 1900, faced with the economic realities of modern research and development, modified its policy that had excluded indiscriminately the patented and other proprietary drugs. The Committee of Revision was now permitted to consider any "product of definite composition which is in common use by the medical profession, the identity, purity or strength of which can be determined. No compound or mixture shall be introduced if the composition or mode of manufacture thereof be kept secret, or if it be controlled by unlimited proprietary or patent rights."[56] The Committee also was instructed to introduce average approximate doses (but not to give a minimum or maximum). The general advice that as many assays and tests of identity and purity as possible should be introduced led to a remarkable increase of U.S.P. assays.[57] A purity rubric was to be given for each chemical substance "used solely for medicinal purposes. . . ." With the prospect of Federally enforced drug standards pending, these changes involved new considerations and import.

Under the new chairman, Joseph Remington, revision was carried forward with great care. The United States honored the recommendations of the International Conference on the Unification of Potent Medicaments (1902) in this edition, with one or two exceptions. For example, a strength of about 10 per cent for potent tinctures became a uniform rule. Inauguration of a new class of drugs, the biologicals, was signaled by admission of antidiphtheria serum to the *Pharmacopoeia.*

With this EIGHTH REVISION, which did not appear until 1905, began the practice of dating the *Pharmacopoeia* according to the year when each edition took effect (rather than emphasizing the year of the respective General Convention). The U.S.P. VIII* was the first edition to have full legal recognition of the United States government, which was granted by the first Food and Drug Act (1906). Both this enactment and its successor, the Food, Drug and Cosmetic Act of 1938, made official the *National Formulary* published by the American Pharmaceutical Association (see p. 250), as well as the *Pharmacopeia* published by the independent and newly incorporated United States Pharmacopeial Convention. These books now spoke with the force of law; all they said and did not say took on additional meaning and ramifications. Hence it is not surprising that interim "additions and corrections" became necessary on passage of the Act.[58]

Henceforth the *Pharmacopeia* became nearly indispensable for the entire American trade in drugs, not in pharmacies alone; yet, it is noteworthy that the book could not become "official" in the strict sense of the term "pharmacopeia" traditional elsewhere. That is, under the United States Constitution, the national law could not require possession of a copy nor make observance of the rules and the standards of the *United States Pharmacopeia* compulsory for every licensed pharmacist or pharmacy. Such requirements had to be made effective through laws of the individual states.

When the General Convention (1910) called the general principles that it adopted "recommendations" instead of "instructions," it undoubtedly signaled a trend toward greater authority for the Committee of Revision, with the Convention and its Board of Trustees restricting themselves more to administration and broad policy. With this NINTH REVISION the Committee of Revision was increased to 50 members, plus the president of the Convention ex officio. Fifteen subcommittees were appointed, "of which the chairman, elected by the members of the respective subcommittees, constituted an executive committee. . . ."[59]

The subject areas dealt with by these

---

* Pharmacopeial numbering is according to the *Revision*—not the edition.

subcommittees may be taken as evidence of the need for a pharmaceutical majority in the practical work of pharmacopeial revision.[60] Only 3 subcommittees were devoted to medical subjects, namely those on the scope of the *Pharmacopeia*; on therapeutics, pharmacodynamics and posology; and on biologic products and diagnostic tests. The other 12 subcommittees dealt exclusively with pharmaceutical, pharmacognostic and pharmacochemical problems and hence consisted of pharmacists and other pharmaceutical specialists.

It recognized technical advance in a difficult field when this edition admitted "biological tests or assays" as a matter of principle, whereas in the preceding edition they had been expressly barred.

Indicative of the Convention's reaction to a pharmaceutical trend in formulation and marketing was a paragraph discouraging the introduction of new compound preparations, "as far as possible."

The ninth decennial revision, published in 1916, was translated not only into Spanish, as were predecessors, but also into Chinese.

Remington died 2 years before the Pharmacopeial Convention of 1920,[61] which elected as his successor another pharmacist, E. Fullerton Cook of Philadelphia. Like Remington, he was associated with the Philadelphia College of Pharmacy.

Reflecting the difficulty of the task assigned to the medical subcommittee on scope, a further "Referee Committee on Scope" was now established, consisting of 21 physicians of the General Committee, to take the responsibility of deciding disputed questions concerning the admission and the deletion of therapeutic substances.[62]

No matter how wisely such decisions were made, it became increasingly difficult to keep the *Pharmacopeia* abreast of scientific and therapeutic developments; hence interim supplements became more common. A corollary need was for greater specialization and more participating experts. This was reflected in the number of auxiliary advisors who worked on the TENTH REVISION, which appeared in 1926, including the gov-

ernment "Bureaus and Departments responsible for enforcing drug standards, the various medical associations, numerous national pharmaceutical bodies and hundreds of individuals, all working with the appropriate organized subcommittee."[63]

The demands of pharmacopeial work found formal expression when the Convention revised its Constitution and By-laws (1930). The circle of groups entitled to representation in the Pharmacopeial Convention was enlarged greatly, and the number of individuals participating in revision work greatly increased.

The ELEVENTH REVISION (published 1936) would have been financially prohibitive, it was reported, except for the collaboration without charge by many of these specialized agencies and individuals, including "colleges, universities, industrial organizations, private laboratories and the Government," and "voluntary service . . . by outstanding physicians, pharmacists, and other scientists of this country."[64] Sources of some of the important contributions were acknowledged when the new edition stated,

Portions of monographs, prepared by the American Medical Association and published in "New and Non-official Remedies" have been used to form the basis of a number of new tests. Extensive data published by the American Chemical Society have been utilized in preparing the new reagent standards. The joint "Contact Committee" of the American Drug Manufacturers' Association and the American Pharmaceutical Manufacturers' Association has assisted in developing biological and vitamin assays and in many other problems of the revision.[65]

This Eleventh Revision introduced reference standards for certain drugs and provided for their distribution. It also marked still closer cooperation with the British Pharmacopoeia Convention and, beyond that, increasing adoption of international standards.[66] In this supranational endeavor, which was to culminate in the *Pharmacopoeia Internationalis*, the American U.S.P. chairman, E. Fullerton Cook, played a prominent role.

The TWELFTH REVISION (13th edition,

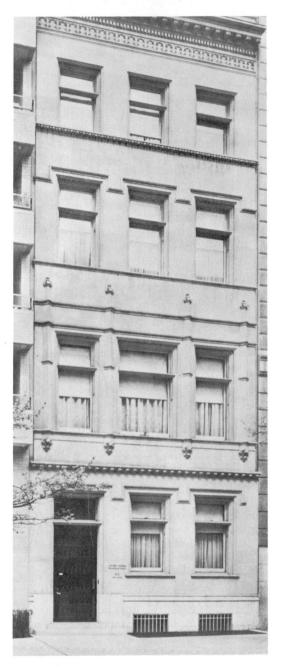

The U. S. Pharmacopeia building in New York City includes administrative and editorial offices, library and archival records, reception room and meeting facilities and the like. The interior arrangement and decor still reflect its former use as an elegant town house. (See Am. Prof. Pharm. *15*:435, 1949)

1942) marked the start of a full-scale program of "continuous revision," under which a new *Pharmacopeia* appears "every five years, a bound 'Supplement' halfway between, and, to meet the frequently occurring situations which require immediate attention, 'Interim Revision Announcements' or sheet 'Supplements' whenever these are required."[67]

This far-reaching decision influenced, and, indeed, even necessitated, another decision that made the chairman of the General Committee of Revision a full-time permanent "Director of Pharmacopoeial Revision" with broad administrative powers. This position is filled through election by each outgoing Board of Trustees.[68]

To house the Director and the Pharmacopeial staff and facilities, a permanent headquarters was purchased at 46 Park Avenue, New York City.[69] This was dedicated in 1950.

The twin innovation of permanent Director and permanent headquarters constitutes one of the most important steps to assure the continuity and the fruitfulness of revision work since the establishment of the United States Pharmacopeial Convention in its modern form (1900). To a large extent this step fulfilled efforts of the pharmacist E. Fullerton Cook, who had been connected with the revision work for about four decades.

His tasks were taken over in 1950 by the first Director of Pharmacopeial Revision elected by the Board of Trustees, Lloyd C. Miller. His selection may be construed to symbolize a transformation that had been taking place in the character of the men and the work of pharmacopeial revision, a shift in emphasis from the high art of professional practice to highly specialized scientific research. Before 1880 the pharmacopeial revision work had been headed by physicians; since then it had been headed by pharmacists; and now (after 1950) by neither a pharmacist nor a physician, but by a pharmacomedical scientist. A biochemist and pharmacologist by education, Dr. Miller brought to his work on the *Pharmacopeia* broad experience in research, industry and the Food and Drug Administration.

In overhauling its Constitution and By-Laws in the 1940's the Convention made other important changes. Formally adopted was the custom of having the General Committee of Revision consist of 60 persons, one third qualified in medical sciences and two thirds in pharmaceutical and allied sciences (plus the President of the Convention and the Director of Revision ex officio). At the same time the composition of the Board of Trustees was defined to consist of 9 persons, including the President of the Convention ex officio. Six are elected from the accredited delegates to the Convention: of these, 2 are from the pharmaceutical colleges and organizations represented and 2 from the medical colleges and organizations; the other 2 are the Treasurer and the Director of Revision ex officio. The last two have no voting privileges.

At this time the number of agencies entitled to representation in the Pharmacopeial Convention was expanded considerably in recognition of the fact that the work must be increasingly a collaboration among the professions, the pure and the applied sciences, the governmental branches, and the trade organizations—all directly involved and particularly knowledgeable in the complex ramifications of drug standards and standardization. One stimulus toward maintaining this work at a uniformly high level of expertness stems from the Federal Food, Drug, and Cosmetic Act, which obligates the Food and Drug Administration to draft standards of its own in the event that standards set by legally designated compendia are deemed inadequate. "Thus far," says the U.S.P. Director, Dr. Miller, "this has not proved necessary and it is our aim to be alert to the point that recourse to such action will never be necessary."[70]

Although the "continuous revision" concept had led to the scheduling of a completely new edition approximately every 5 years, the General Convention continued on the basis of the decennial meeting traditional since the founding.

The THIRTEENTH REVISION became effective (April 1947) less than 5 years after the Twelfth Revision was published. The most striking innovation of this edition placed English drug names ahead of Latin names for the first time, the latter being only vestiges of earlier centuries when Latin had been in common use by physicians and pharmacists.[71]

With English names in first place, the alphabetic arrangement of the Pharmacopeia henceforth gave a quite different sequence to the monographs covering the individual drugs. Moreover, immediately following the material on each basic drug appeared the monographs for its various dosage forms, which heretofore had been grouped by classes (all fluid extracts together, etc.).

After the fundamental changes in the administration, the content and the style of the Pharmacopeia during the 1940's, it is not surprising that the FOURTEENTH REVISION showed little change beyond the routine admissions and deletions of drugs. Becoming effective in 1950, the book invalidated its predecessor after the unprecedentedly brief period of 3 years.

To illustrate a twin function of the *National Formulary*, which has been a companion book of comparable officiality since 1906, it may be mentioned that about 90 per cent of the drugs deleted by the U.S.P. continued to have standards in legal force by transfer into the N.F. Conversely, almost 18 per cent of the drugs newly admitted to the U.S.P. were taken over from the N.F. This edition inaugurated the useful practice of designating with an asterisk each drug known to be protected by a patent.

In preparing the FIFTEENTH REVISION (effective 1955), it was necessary to deal with an unusual number of new drugs vying for admission (the result of the postwar boom in research) and with advances in analytical procedures affecting assays. Administratively, the Revision Committee had been enlarged and diversified, while the subcommittee structure had been pared down by a third and given more autonomy. The revamped working plan respected tradition in that "scope and posology remained the concern of the physicians on the Committee, whereas the pharmaceutical aspects of revision fell to those trained in pharmacy, chemistry, bacteriology, etc."[72]

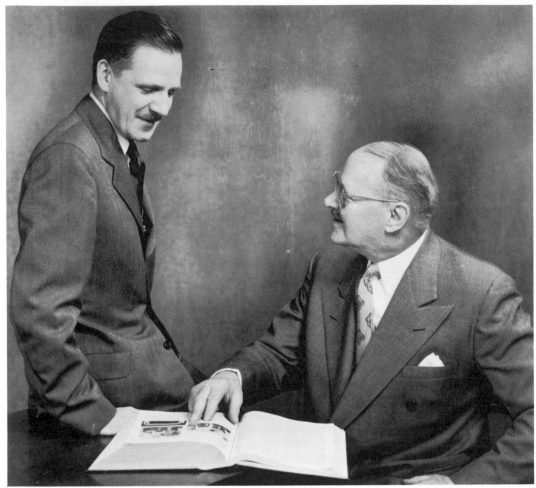

Pharmacist E. Fullerton Cook (right) served as chairman of the Committee of Revision of the U. S. Pharmacopeia for three decades (1920-1950) and became the first American to make a major contribution to the development of international drug standards. A former assistant to Joseph Remington in Philadelphia, Dr. Cook subsequently edited more editions of *Remington's Practice of Pharmacy* than any other single editor since the first edition of this work in 1885. With him is Dr. Eric Martin, co-editor of *Remington*. . . . (Photograph from American Journal of Hospital Pharmacy)

Making the U.S.P. a therapeutic guide to the drugs of medical choice at the time of revision remained a central concept. Already in the first *Pharmacopeia* the scope had hinged on the idea of admitting drugs "the utility of which is most fully established and best understood."

With this edition, Latin names—which had been dropped from primary to secondary position in U.S.P. XII—were now "dropped practically entirely, both because of disuse and because they generally differ so little from the English titles." In instances where the Latin stem did differ markedly, the Latin name was placed among the synonyms. Here, too, began the practice of stating the general therapeutic or pharmaceutic "category" of the substance covered in each monograph. The demise of apothecary weights and measures was either hastened or confirmed by their banishment from statements of dosage and sizes available.

The Sixteenth Revision (effective 1960) stated,

The feature that distinguishes this revision most from all of its recent predecessors is the progress made in adopting new analytical techniques. Thus either much more extensively, or for the first time, use has been made of nonaqueous titrimetry, complexometry, ultraviolet and infrared spectrophotometry, column and paper chromatography, and (in one instance) a phase solubility determination for assay purposes.

Indeed, in the decade that the appearance of U.S.P. XVI brought to a close

the technology of drug standardization underwent a remarkable transition. . . . Chemical analysis attained a new plane in respect to precision and sensitivity, albeit at a decided loss of simplicity. Thus vastly improved techniques of isolation, coupled with refinements in quantitative instrumental measurement provided means of analyzing drug principles for the first time or served to replace more costly and time-consuming biologic assays. During this decade [1950's], the need first arose for standardizing radioactive drugs, and the use of radioactived tracers was introduced into drug analysis.[73]

A continuing trend toward more and longer monographs now called forth a number of editorial stratagems to keep the *Pharmacopeia* within a manageable size. For example, a single monograph sometimes covered two or more closely related substances, which in the traditional style of previous editions would each be covered in a separate monograph. For the first time the *Pharmacopeia* published a list of the articles that had been approved for admission but for which satisfactory monographs could not yet be completed (81 such titles, as compared with 908 titles for which monographs were actually published in U.S.P. XVI).

As the *Pharmacopeia of the United States* approaches its 150th anniversary, it remains the only pharmacopeial standard effective for a large political unit that was originally prepared, and has since been revised, by a

Pharmacopeial Convention of delegates, men sent by interested organizations from various parts of the country. This Convention's only firm bond of unity has been the conviction of the delegates of the necessity of their work. Referring to the unique position of our *Pharmacopeia*, Dr. Albert H. Holland, Jr., of the Federal Food and Drug Administration, stated,

It is recognized by the Federal law as an official standard, yet it is prepared by a private and independent organization and corporation. Fortunately, we do enjoy a friendly and productive working relationship which, I have no doubt, will continue for the long foreseeable future.[74]

Under the responsible leadership of American pharmacy the *Pharmacopeia* thus has become the legally recognized standard of a number of sciences and industries, guaranteeing honesty and security in the trade in drugs, supporting as well as supported by research work in the most widely different fields. At present the *United States Pharmacopeia* is generally recognized to be one of the best and most progressive books of its kind.

COMMENTARIES OR DISPENSATORIES

In the 16th century, when the word *dispensatorium* came into general use as a book title, its meaning did not differ from that of "pharmacopeia." It was in England that "dispensatory" became the designation for a kind of commentary which embraced the text of the pharmacopeia or pharmacopeias. During the 18th and the 19th centuries such dispensatories became an English specialty.

Coxe's American Dispensatory

There were some English dispensatories in common use in America before the creation of an American pharmacopeia because the pharmacopeias on which they were based were recognized in America almost as much as they were in England. However, it may seem strange that America had a dispensatory of its own before it had its own pharmacopeia.

The physician John Redman Coxe, the same man who later on indirectly caused the organization of the first American college of pharmacy (see p. 171), edited the first edition of his *American Dispensatory* in 1806. He used Duncan's *Edinburgh New Dispensatory* to such an extent that it came near being a reprint and was considered as such by Duncan. The book was so successful that it went through 9 editions.[75] Coxe took the good wherever he could find it. When in 1810 the first edition of Thacher's *New Dispensatory* appeared, Coxe did not scruple to profit from the work of his competitor. In the preface to his 3rd edition he stated that "he has not failed to introduce a considerable addition to the materia medica, for which he is chiefly indebted to Dr. Thacher's very excellent dispensatory."

In the preface to his last edition Thacher pointed out that Coxe had transferred "literally from the two last editions" of Thacher's dispensatory more than 40 pages into the 4th edition of his own book. He then adds that these transfers "are not designated by the customary marks of quotation."

After publication of the *United States Pharmacopeia* (1820) the volume by Coxe of necessity became, with some reservations, a commentary on this work. In the quarrel over the two second editions of the *Pharmacopeia* Coxe sided with the New York faction and received a sharp rebuke from George B. Wood in Philadelphia.[76] In the edition of his dispensatory that followed the appearance of these rival pharmacopeias, he nevertheless introduced "all that was essential" from both of them.

Thacher's American New Dispensatory

The fundamental difference between the dispensatory of John Redman Coxe and that of James Thacher was that Coxe based his work for the most part on an English book; moreover, it was written in the English spirit. Thacher, a Boston physician, associated his treatise with the first attempt at an American pharmacopeia and tried to imbue it with the American spirit. The *Pharmacopoeia of the Massachusetts Medical Society* (1808; see p. 229), served as the basis for Thacher's *Dispensatory*. "This Pharmacopoeia," he wrote in the preface of his book, "is not inferior in point of merit to any other and its nomenclature and order of arrangement are strictly followed throughout." Thacher's cooperation with the authors of the *Massachusetts Pharmacopoeia* went so far that he submitted his manuscript to the Massachusetts Medical Society for criticism. "After having been revised by a committee of the counsellors," the *Dispensatory* was published in 1810 and in 3 further editions.[77] Its principal merit was that it paid "proper attention to several indigenous substances, not to be found in any other Dispensatory." As his sources Thacher quoted the publications of Barton and Cutler (see p. 158) and "that excellent publication, the Domestic Encyclopedia, edited by Dr. Mease." Thus Thacher's *Dispensatory* was the first distinctly American publication of its kind.

The United States Dispensatory

Significantly, neither Coxe's nor Thacher's book survived the appearance in 1833 of the *United States Dispensatory*, edited by George B. Wood and Franklin Bache. The name of this commentary on the *United States Pharmacopeia* proved to be of symbolic value. For several decades the only book of its kind in America, the *United States Dispensatory* indeed has been a pharmaceutical book of reference used all over the world. At times it has even put its mother, the *Pharmacopeia*, in the shade; nevertheless, it always has accompanied it with merit and dignity.

The secret of its initial success lay in the personalities of its authors, especially George B. Wood. Both men were principal authors of the *Pharmacopeia* (Philadelphia, 1831), and participated decisively in revising all later editions during their lifetimes. Naturally, they thus gained intimate knowledge of what required exposition. In addition, they were men especially well qualified for their work. While both of them were physicians, they were also professors. For several years, Wood had been a professor of materia medica, and Bache had been a professor of chemistry, at the Philadelphia College of Pharmacy. The fact that

Wood, in his preparation of the *Pharmacopeia* of 1831, insisted on avoiding any explanatory notes "as wholly out of place in a Pharmacopoeia," makes it likely that he was already thinking of issuing some kind of commentary. Doubtless, it was because of the commercial success of the *Dispensatory* that the *Pharmacopeia* could be kept alive. Moreover, the fact that both books were issued by the same publisher made possible the requisite financial balancing. Not until after the death of Wood (1879) were the two books produced and published separately.

In the preface to the first edition of the *Dispensatory*, the authors stated that the *Pharmacopeia* "requires an explanatory commentary," and that "such a work should be in good faith an American work, newly prepared in all its parts, and not a mere edition of one of the European Dispensatories, with here and there additions and alterations." This was doubtless an attack upon the book of Coxe. That of Thacher had not been re-edited since 1821. Wood made this even clearer by stating that the field in America "has not been so fully occupied as to exclude all competition." In the book of Wood and Bache, the English pharmacopeias were considered to the same extent at least as in the earlier American dispensatories, but the "almost untouched . . . pharmacy of continental Europe" was also considered and special attention was paid to the "treatises and dissertations . . . on pharmacy . . . of the French writers, who stand at present at the head of this department of medical science."

All possible literary sources were utilized, and the mass of information was well arranged and presented in a clear style. It seems almost incredible that for more than 30 years the two authors alone did most of the comprehensive and responsible work. During this period they directed no fewer than 11 editions.[78] In the preface to the first edition, the authors thanked "Mr. Daniel B. Smith, president of the Philadelphia College of Pharmacy," for "much important information in relation to the various branches of the apothecary's business," for some "prefatory remarks on pharmacy" and

for "several articles." It was not until after the death of Bache (1864) that, in the preface of the 12th edition, such assistance from outside was again acknowledged. This time it was Wood's "friends, Mr. William Procter, Jr., Prof. of Pharmacy in the Philadelphia College of Pharmacy, and Dr. Robert Bridges, Prof. of Chemistry in the same institution."

The 14th edition was again begun by Wood (with the assistance of Bridges) but completed by his nephew and successor in the chair of materia medica at the University of Pennsylvania, Horatio C. Wood. After George Wood died (1879) his nephew invited Joseph P. Remington, at that time a well-known pharmacist of Philadelphia, and Samuel P. Sadtler, Professor of Chemistry at the Philadelphia College of Pharmacy, to share with him the editorial responsibility of the 15th edition.[79]

This 15th edition (1883) may, as the authors stated in the preface "very justly be looked upon as a new book," though based on the old *Dispensatory*. How much the age and the obstinacy of the late George B. Wood had retarded the adoption of scientific progress in the preceding 20 years becomes evident from the statement that, after the death of Bache (1864) the chemical parts of the work had "had no proper revision and adaptation to the needs of the day." The next four editions appeared under the same editorship (H. C. Wood, J. P. Remington and S. P. Sadtler). By the time the 19th edition appeared, H. C. Wood, Jr., had taken the place of his father. On the next edition he was aided mainly by Remington, who died while the book was on press. H. C. Wood, Jr., held the editor's chair for three more editions, first with Charles LaWall as chief co-editor (21st, 1926, and 22nd, 1937, eds.), then by Arthur Osol (23rd ed., 1943). For the next revision (1947) Osol succeeded Wood, and George E. Farrar became chief co-editor. They have successfully continued the massive *U. S. Dispensatory* as the oldest book of its kind in continuous publication, a book originated in Philadelphia, and edited and published there throughout its long history.[80]

The National Dispensatory

Because of obvious deficiencies of the *United States Dispensatory* from the 12th to the reorganized 15th edition, the monopoly of this book was destroyed at least temporarily. In 1879, Alfred Stillé and John Maisch published the *National Dispensatory*. That the book filled a gap at the time becomes evident from the fact that the 1st edition was sold out in a few months, and that in the same year, a 2nd edition "thoroughly revised, with numerous additions," was issued and had to be reprinted in the following year (1880).[81]

Because of the special inclinations of their authors, two differences in tendency should be noted between the *National Dispensatory* and its older rival, the *United States Dispensatory*. Alfred Stillé as a teacher of clinical medicine at a time when the physiologic action of medicines was to become the subject of exact experimentation, included "for the first time in a Dispensatory, a succinct account" of the results of those experiments, "moreover occasionally in the theoretical language of the day." He added "another feature, novel in a Dispensatory": a therapeutic index. "Such an Index," the authors stated in the preface to the first edition, "becomes to some extent a therapeutical classification of medicines, and it is believed must greatly enhance by its suggestiveness the working value of the book to the practitioner."

The "practitioner" here referred to was naturally the medical practitioner. The *National Dispensatory* appealed much more to the special interests of the physician than did the *United States Dispensatory*. "Of the two works," a reviewer wrote: "the 'United States Dispensatory' seems to find greatest favor with pharmacists."[82] Another difference resulted from the predilection of the German-born second author, John M. Maisch, for the German Pharmacopoeia. In the 2nd edition of the book he included "nearly the entire German Pharmacopoeia."

The National Standard Dispensatory

When John M. Maisch died (1893), the 5th and last edition of the *National Dispensatory* was edited by Stillé, with the cooperation of Maisch's son, Henry C. Maisch, and Charles Caspari, Jr. Caspari participated in a continuation of the Stillé-Maisch book, which first appeared in 1905 (with two further editions in 1908 and 1916) under the title *The National Standard Dispensatory*. It was edited by three men: H. A. Hare, of the Jefferson Medical College, Philadelphia; Charles Caspari, Jr., Maryland College of Pharmacy, Baltimore; and Henry H. Rusby, College of Pharmacy of the City of New York. The *National Standard Dispensatory* was a completely rewritten book, explaining and commenting not only on the individual drugs and chemicals, but also on the groups to which they belong, thus combining a reference book and a textbook.

Although the sections on physiologic action and the therapeutic index (introduced by Stillé) were retained, the medical tendency was not so predominant as it had been in the older work.

Other Volumes of Commentary

Books of similar character, but of less lasting influence than those previously discussed, in their time played a part in the evolving picture of American medical care. Failing to adjust to needs of new times, these publications have long since been discontinued.

The earliest volume of this kind was an American edition of Nicholas Culpeper's *Pharmacopoeia Londinensis or the London Dispensatory* (Boston, 1720).[83] It was well adapted to self-medication in a country where trained medical assistance was usually remote. More widely circulated and of greater professional influence were at least 5 different American versions of the *Edinburgh New Dispensatory* that appeared here between 1791 and 1818,[84] a work we noted had also formed the basis for Coxe's first *American Dispensatory* (1806). A more modest venture in the same direction was an American printing of Robert Graves' *Pocket Conspectus of the London and Edinburgh Pharmacopoeias* (Philadelphia, 1803). Another British book (Squire's *Companion to the British Pharmacopoeia*) quite possibly suggested a similar work to the Americans Oscar Oldberg and Otto Wall when the radically changed sixth revision of the *U. S. Pharmacopeia* appeared. The result was a *Companion to the United States Pharmacopoeia* (1884). Unlike its perennial British counterpart, this *Companion* went into only one more edition (1887).

These dispensatories and related commentaries all served the regular ranks of medicine and pharmacy. One of the more significant books that expressed the pharmaceutical views of a large clan of irregulars was the *American Dispensatory* (1852) edited by two physicians, John King and Robert S. Newton. They represented the "Eclectic" school of medical thought, a more modern and less dogmatic descendant of the American botanicomedical movement of the first half of the 19th century (see p. 160). King's *American Dispensatory* was, more precisely, a specialized formulary and commentary on eclectic drugs (not based on any pharmacopeia), but showed the character typical of the English and the American dispensatories. The book underwent 4 revisions, the rest of the 19 editions up to 1909 being mainly reprints. The demise of King's *American Dispensatory* reflected the decline of "eclecticism" as a self-conscious, separate segment of American medicine.[85]

Some 19th century dispensatories were edited with the needs of physicians primarily in view. Illustrative of this class of dispensatories are a *Treatise on the Materia Medica* (1822; by Jacob Bigelow, author of the botanic part of the then new *U. S. Pharmacopeia*); *Dispensatory and Therapeutical Remembrancer* (1848, American version of the 2nd English edition, by John Mayne); *Dispensatory* (1848), American edition by R. Eglesfield Griffith of the English *Dispensatory* of Robert Christison, based on Duncan); and *The Dispensatory and Pharmacopoeia of North America and Great Britain* (1878; by John Buchanan and John F. Suggins).

HOMEOPATHIC PHARMACOPEIA

To the American pharmacist today, the *Homeopathic Pharmacopoeia of the United States* seems a curious rather than a practical book. Yet, the book retains some current as well as historical interest because its drug standards are "official" under the Federal Food, Drug and Cosmetic Act in the same sense as are the *U. S. Pharmacopeia* and the *National Formulary*.

The strange medical doctrines on which homeopathic drug therapy rests have a small and dwindling place in American medicine. Introduced by Samuel Hahnemann, a German, at the end of the 18th century, homeopathy at first was one of a number of medical systems vying with one another. Eventually discredited and disowned by regular medicine, it has survived in some countries as a small medical sect largely dependent on its appeal to a lay following. (See p. 49.)

The special way of preparing homeopathic remedies[86] makes Hahnemann's system interesting pharmaceutically. Homeopathic pharmacy in the United States, unlike that in some other countries, has never become a special branch of study and practice for the average pharmacist. Hence the *Homeopathic Pharmacopoeia* has found its main use among those practicing homeopathic medicine and among governmental agencies that are responsible for assuring the proper quality and labeling of drugs, whatever the therapeutic theory that calls for them.

Seven editions of the *Homeopathic Pharmacopoeia* have appeared, the last in 1964.

LOCAL FORMULARIES

The first local pharmaceutical formulary to be printed in the United States of America was the *Formulary for the Preparation of Eight Patent Medicines Adopted by the Philadelphia College of Pharmacy*, published in 1824. "When, in 1829, a college of pharmacy was formed in New York City, it adopted the Philadelphia College of Pharmacy formulae . . . , simply adding one for balsam of honey."[87]

While the first formulary had been motivated by a desire to give correct formulas for imitating some of the popular "patent medicines," when the young American Pharmaceutical Association set about to "collect and arrange . . . local unofficial formulae" (1857-59), it denied "any desire to collect the formulae for nostrums or proprietary medicines." The collection of the "unofficial formulae," published in the proceedings of the American Pharmaceutical Association,[88] was restricted to those "recognized by the medical profession." Nevertheless, the Association did not feel well satisfied in promoting such a collection.

The chairman of the committee congratulated his fellow members not so much on their endeavor to collect formulas, but "upon the limited number of such formulas which, however necessary, tend to complicate the labors of the pharmaceutist."[89] The report in the *Proceedings* of the American Pharmaceutical Association laconically states that "the committee was discontinued." Nor did another attempt, made about a decade later, lead to anything of lasting importance. There could be little doubt that most of the leading men in American pharmacy during the 1860's and the 1870's still were not convinced of the advisability of giving the approval of the American Pharmaceutical Association to "unofficial formulae."

In 1886 the *American Druggist* commented on local formularies: The New York and Brooklyn Formulary had the largest circulation of any local work. Other local formularies, prepared for similar purposes, were published by the Kentucky and the Pennsylvania Pharmaceutical Associations. Another was published by a joint committee of physicians and pharmacists in Washington, and still others elsewhere. In addition, there were the formularies published by individual authors.[90] Since Charles Rice, then the recognized authority in the field, was associate editor of the *American Druggist* at this time, his authority appeared behind the journal's implication that such formularies, as well as their unification, were necessary.

THE NATIONAL FORMULARY

When the idea of a semiofficial formulary was revived (1885) conditions were more favorable to such an undertaking than they had been about 1860. Under the influence

of pharmacists, the *Pharmacopeia* (1883) had been radically purified, so far as "obsolete and unused drugs" were concerned.[91] No fewer than 121 preparations had been deleted. No doubt among them were some which conservative physicians in various parts of the country were in the habit of prescribing. Furthermore, preparations representative of so-called "elegant" pharmacy were now being mass-produced under "brands," and prescribed as such by physicians, even though the formulas could be prepared readily in the prescription room of any pharmacy. Practicing pharmacists naturally viewed with concern the growing loss of one of their principal professional functions.

As a counter-measure, support crystallized around the idea of promoting to physicians a variety of formulas improving on or widening the range of drugs recognized by the *Pharmacopeia* and stressing a flexible custom service to fit the needs of the individual patient. It is significant that the father of the modern *Pharmacopoeia* of 1882, Charles Rice, was chairman of the American Pharmaceutical Association committee on unofficial formulas and their ardent advocate. In his report in 1886, Rice explained the origin and the purpose of a proposed formulary to serve this end:

Acting on the suggestion of Mr. S. J. Bendiner of New York, the College of Pharmacy of the City of New York, the German Apothecaries Society of New York and the Kings County Pharmaceutical Society, about two years ago, appointed a joint committee to prepare a Formulary of unofficial preparations which was to be brought to the notice of the medical profession, with the request to accept the formulae therein contained—after examination and approval—and thereafter to abstain from specifying on their prescriptions the products of special manufacturers, whenever ordering any preparation for which a formula was given in the book.[92]

The book on elixirs published by John Uri Lloyd (1883) as well as the *New York and Brooklyn Formulary* (1884) "acted as a decided stimulus" in giving a national scope and reality to the ambitions of pharmacists that here and there had found expression through local formularies. The state pharmaceutical associations participated in the Committee's work; and in 1888 a manuscript was presented to the American Pharmaceutical Association and was published in the same year both as an appendix to the *Proceedings* and as a separate book "by authority of the American Pharmaceutical Association."

Taking the title of the *National Formulary of Unofficinal Preparations* at face value, framers of early food and drug bills did not propose to make the American Pharmaceutical Association's book "official" as they did the *U. S. Pharmacopeia.* However, the 1906 Federal law elevated the *National Formulary* to the same legal standing as the *Pharmacopeia.*[93]

At the first opportunity (4th ed., 1916)* the now incongruous part of the title, ". . . of Unofficinal Preparations," was dropped. Moreover, the *National Formulary* developed its monographs on drug standards in a way analogous with the development of monographs in the *Pharmacopeia*; and since 1938 the American Pharmaceutical Association has maintained a laboratory devoted primarily to determining drug standards. The "N.F." indicates standards for numerous drugs and drug preparations that are used by physicians or laymen but do not qualify for inclusion in the "U.S.P." as the current drugs of choice in their therapeutic class.

A new epoch in the development of the *National Formulary* was initiated in 1938 with a plan for more frequent revisions, approximately every 5 years; and in 1939 the by-laws of the Association were changed to provide for a "Committee on National Formulary" consisting of 10 instead of 15 members and a full-time chairman. A man of proved capacity thus was given enhanced range of action: Justin L. Powers, Director of the Laboratory of the American Pharmaceutical Association, who continued to head the National Formulary until his retirement

---

* The roman numbering of the *National Formulary* refers to the successive *editions* (in contrast with the U.S.P. numbering of revisions).

(1960). Powers' successor, the chemist Edward G. Feldman, serves as Director of Revision of the N.F. as a major part of his responsibility as Director of the Scientific Division of the American Pharmaceutical Association.

When the 7th edition of the book appeared (1942) it showed remarkable changes, testifying to the fact that the men responsible for the *National Formulary* no longer regarded their book as merely a stepping-stone from and to the *United States Pharmacopeia,* supplementary to the latter, but as of comparable character, differing mainly in point of view as to the kind and the scope of material to be admitted.[94]

In an 8th edition (effective on April 1, 1947, in accord with the U.S.P. XIII) "Latin titles are continued but preceded by English titles. Monographs are arranged in alphabetic sequence but in different order than heretofore so that a monograph on a basic drug is followed by monographs on its official [National Formulary] preparations." An 11th edition of the *National Formulary* appeared in 1960.[95] Like the *United States Pharmacopeia,* the *National Formulary* is revised continuously.

The content of legally binding books of standards thereby keeps more nearly abreast of the rapidly changing status of drugs. Exemplifying the transformation wrought by research is the fact that within three decades (1916-1946) the percentage of basically botanical official drugs was cut in half.[96] Other drastic changes in methods of manufacture and testing place an increasing majority of procedures beyond the range of all but the largest and best-equipped pharmacies. Yet, adequate drug standards remain essential for safe practice in a community pharmacy. Even though the American pharmacist increasingly uses the *National Formulary* only as a source of reference information (as he does the *Pharmacopeia* also), he may take pride in the fact that his personal support and his professional society's work together have produced one of the two books of American drug standards and have played a major role in giving the other a consistent and progressive vigor.

THE PHARMACEUTICAL RECIPE BOOK

As the *National Formulary* became more self-consciously "official" and scientific, more removed from the homely appeal of the old "unofficinal preparations," the gap that the original *National Formulary* had tried to fill seemed to reappear. As early as 1912 a committee of the American Pharmaceutical Association published a report on 114 such formulas, under the chairmanship of Otto Raubenheimer. This led to a standing Committee on Recipe Book (under his chairmanship) which published groups of formulas serially in the Association's *Journal* over the next 5 years.

Then a new committee headed by the eminent New York pharmacist J. Leon Lascoff presented the Association with an unedited collection of 1,500 formulas. The accumulation was pruned, edited, and brought between book covers in 1929 under the editorial direction of Ivor Griffith of Philadelphia. The *Pharmaceutical Recipe Book*, as the title implies, included "only preparations that can be compounded by the pharmacist" and abjured ambitions to set drug standards.

Here the pharmacist found compound formulas not only for unofficial drugs but also for materials for diverse technical uses —household compounds, cosmetics, photographic materials, flavorings, reagents, and so on.

Such a book appealed to pharmacists' pride of craftsmanship and met a need as well. It went through a second (1936) and then a third (1942) edition. The fact that no further editions were considered worthwhile is one more indication of the changes taking place in pharmacy.[97]

NEW AND NONOFFICIAL DRUGS

The American Medical Association established the Council on Drugs (called the Council on Pharmacy and Chemistry until 1958) primarily as a medical rather than a pharmaceutical institution. This Council was organized (1905) "primarily for the purpose of gathering and disseminating such information as would protect the medical profession in the prescribing of proprietary medicinal articles."[98] These articles, their advertising, labeling and naming, and even the general policies of the firms manufacturing them, had to comply "with definite rules" and must "present some real advantage," to be admitted, i.e., to be described as to their essential features, "in the annual publication of the Council, the 'N.N.R.' [*New and Nonofficial Remedies*; from 1958 ed. on, called *New and Nonofficial Drugs*]. This description is based in part on investigations made by or under the direction of the Council, but in part also on evidence or information supplied by the manufacturer. . . ."

The Council explicitly stated from the beginning that "the admission of an article does not imply a recommendation. It means only that no conflict with the rules has been found by the Council."[99]

Among the early members of the Council were many pharmacists or persons with pharmaceutical as well as medical education (such as C. S. N. Hallberg of Chicago, R. A. Hatcher of New York, L. F. Kebler of Washington, J. O. Schlotterbeck of Ann Arbor, M. I. Wilbert of Washington and, finally, W. A. Puckner, Ph.G., secretary of the Council and chief of the chemical laboratory of the American Medical Association).[100] At the present the Council consists mainly of representatives of the various branches of medicine (teachers, for the most part).

There is no pharmacist among the Council members, but the pharmacist Joseph B. Jerome, Ph.D., is Assistant to the Secretary of the Council and, since 1960, has been Assistant Director of the A.M.A. Department of Drugs. Although no longer maintaining its own laboratory, the American Medical Association shares with the U.S.P. and the A.Ph.A., the support of the Drug Standards Laboratory at the American Pharmaceutical Association, directed by the pharmacist Jerome I. Bodin, Ph.D.

The importance of *New and Nonofficial*

Drugs cannot be overestimated. For many products, inclusion in the volume represents the preliminary stage before their introduction into one of the "official" books. For other products, inclusion implies admission to the recognized materia medica of the American medical practitioner, even though the Council, as a matter of principle, does not give approval or endorsement to the drugs it "examines and evaluates." Although pharmacy no longer has a large part in preparing these annual volumes, their pharmaceutical importance is second only to that of the legally recognized pharmaceutical publications, the *United States Pharmacopeia* and the *National Formulary*.

TEXT AND REFERENCE BOOKS

When the Philadelphia College of Pharmacy created a professorship of pharmacy and bestowed on William Procter, Jr., the honor and the responsibility of this new charge (1846), the professor looked "in vain amongst the medical literature of the English language for a single work devoted exclusively and systematically to this branch of knowledge." What was the explanation of this? True, English pharmacy at that time was in a period of transition and reconstruction (see p. 99), and an English textbook of pharmacy, written by an English pharmacist, could scarcely be expected.

On the other hand, there was then an abundance of French and German textbooks. England had never—in literature as elsewhere—hesitated to take the good where she found it, and translations of French and German books into English were not uncommon. The reason for the English reserve in taking over one of the continental European textbooks on pharmacy was due to the fact that these books were of little use to the average English "chemist and druggist" of that period. The scientific standards and objectives of these treatises were too high, and the need for elementary instruction in practical pharmaceutical technic could not be filled by them.

As a matter of fact, in continental Europe itself there was an obvious need for a book

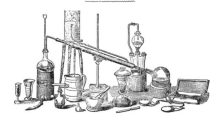

PRACTICAL PHARMACY:

THE ARRANGEMENTS,

APPARATUS, AND MANIPULATIONS,

OF THE

PHARMACEUTICAL SHOP AND LABORATORY.

BY

FRANCIS MOHR, Ph. D.,

ASSESSOR PHARMACIÆ OF THE ROYAL PRUSSIAN COLLEGE OF MEDICINE, COBLENTZ;

AND

THEOPHILUS REDWOOD,

PROFESSOR OF CHEMISTRY AND PHARMACY TO THE PHARMACEUTICAL SOCIETY
OF GREAT BRITAIN.

EDITED, WITH EXTENSIVE ADDITIONS,

BY

WILLIAM PROCTER, Jr.,

PROFESSOR OF PHARMACY IN THE PHILADELPHIA COLLEGE OF PHARMACY.

ILLUSTRATED BY FIVE HUNDRED ENGRAVINGS ON WOOD.

PHILADELPHIA:
LEA AND BLANCHARD.
1849.

The title page of the first pharmaceutical textbook that was adapted to the needs of American students. Significantly, it was based on a British version of a German work by Carl Friedrich Mohr. (Curiously, the first name of the original author is given here erroneously as "Francis.")

describing and explaining in detail all the instruments, apparatus and technical contrivances invented since the rise of modern chemistry and employed by pharmaceutical scientists, manufacturers and practitioners. In the 16th century the German physician Andreas Libavius (Libau) had given such a comprehensive description in an annex to his book *Alchimia*. The Italian pharmacist Antonio de Sgobbis described the pharmaceutical technic and apparatus of his time (1002) in his *Nuovo et Universale Theatro*

Farmaceutico. The book of the French pharmacist Antoine Baumé, *Elémens de pharmacie théorique et pratique* (1762) met the needs of that generation. Now, in the middle of the 19th century, another man was required to fulfill the same task for his time. This man was the German pharmacist Carl Friedrich Mohr,[101] who not only described the modern pharmaceutical contrivances and apparatus but also invented many of them himself. With his *Lehrbuch der pharmaceutischen Technik*, Mohr gave German and Anglo-Saxon pharmacy what it needed. On the continent it was a very useful and much used book. For England and for America it was to become, for the time being, *the* pharmaceutical textbook.

The first German edition of Mohr's book (1847) was scarcely off the press when the English pharmacist and professor at the school of the Pharmaceutical Society of Great Britain, Theophilus Redwood, translated the book and published it under the title *Practical Pharmacy founded on Mohr's Manual* (preface dated December, 1848).

As early as March, 1849, William Procter, Jr., edited an American issue of Redwood's enlarged translation "with extensive additions" under the title *"Practical Pharmacy,* with the subtitle *The Arrangements, Apparatus, and Manipulations of the Pharmaceutical Shop and Laboratory.* The earliest reference to the book in the *American Journal of Pharmacy* begins with the significant remark, "The want of a treatise on practical pharmacy, devoted to apparatus and manipulations, has long been a desideratum both in England and the United States."[102] As stated in a later review, the book comprised "the whole of Mohr and Redwood's book, as published in London, rearranged and classified by the American editor, who has added much valuable new matter, which has increased the size of the book more than one-fourth. . . ."[103]

The book of Mohr-Redwood-Procter "did not go through a second edition by reason of the cost of proper illustrations, which the publishers refused to incur,"[104] and without which Procter apparently did not want a new publication. Thus the way was free for another book of a similar kind. The *Intro-*

duction to Practical Pharmacy, published by Edward Parrish in 1856, is considered the first truly American textbook on pharmacy. This being granted, the question may well arise whether it was a textbook for pharmacists, designed primarily to meet their needs. A review of the first edition, published in the *American Journal of Pharmacy*, gives the answer. Parrish's book "is not based on the superstructure of any foreign publication, as has usually been the case with books, on similar subjects, issued from the American press, but is original in conception with its author, who, from his experience both as a pharmaceutist and as a lecturer and teacher of practical pharmacy to *medical** students, has become aware of the want of a textbook in this department, which he has thus endeavored to supply."[105] This corresponds with a statement made by Parrish himself in the preface of his book as well as with its subtitle: "A textbook for the student and a guide to the Physician and Pharmaceutist." The physician came first.

At the time he wrote his textbook, Parrish conducted a private school of practical pharmacy for *students of medicine* (see p. 206). The *American Journal of Pharmacy* stated, "The book . . . was commenced with a view to satisfy this want [of a book for medical students], but in its progress the author determined to enlarge on his original plan, so as, without claiming for it the fullness of a handbook of Pharmacy, to render it very useful to the strictly pharmaceutical students . . . as well as to pharmacists in general. . . ."[106] It is likely that Parrish decided "to enlarge on his original plan" after having learned that no new edition of the book of Mohr-Redwood-Procter was to be expected. Thus the first textbook on pharmacy that could be considered typically American (written by an American pharmacist) was designed primarily to aid physicians in practicing pharmacy and only secondarily to instruct pharmacists. Although the book retained the traditional subtitle, placing the physician as the primary customer, rather than the pharmacist,

---

* Italics added.

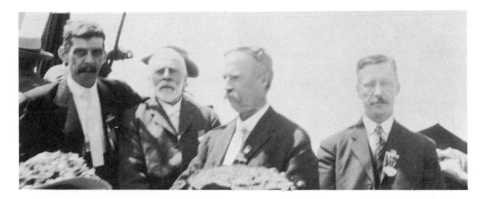

Four pharmacists whose contributions to the pharmaceutical literature had lasting significance for American pharmacy: (l. to r.) Martin I. Wilbert, a Philadelphia hospital pharmacist, later in the U. S. Public Health Service. He coedited the serial *Digest of Comments on the Pharmacopeia of the United States* and was one of the best pharmaco-historical writers of his time. Charles J. Caspari, Jr., Baltimore educator and General Secretary of the American Pharmaceutical Association (1894-1911), who wrote the popular *Treatise on Pharmacy* and was pharmaceutical editor of the *National Standard Dispensary*. Joseph P. Remington, Philadelphia educator and U.S.P. chairman for three decades; he published extensively but is remembered best for *Remington's Practice of Pharmacy*. Joseph W. England, Philadelphia hospital pharmacist and, later, industrial pharmacist; he wrote several hundred articles, helped to found the *Journal of the American Pharmaceutical Association* and edited the comprehensive *First Century of the Philadelphia College*, the first American volume of its kind. All of these pharmacist-authors except England died during the first World War. (The "flying saucers" in the foreground of the photograph (1909) are women's hats.)

it became with each new edition more and more a treatise on pharmacy for pharmacists.[107]

Joseph P. Remington published the first edition of his *Practice of Pharmacy* (1885) as "a treatise on the modes of making and dispensing official, unofficial, and extemporaneous preparations, with descriptions of medical substances, their properties, uses and doses intended as a handbook for pharmacists and physicians and a textbook for students." The analogy to the title of Parrish's *Introduction to Practical Pharmacy* is evident; but here the pharmacist came first, and the limitation to "practice" was, at least in the early editions, still more definite than in the editions of Parrish's *Introduction* issued between 1864 and 1884, which became increasingly scientific and theoretical. With the book of Remington the era of the modern American pharmaceutical textbook started. As Remington himself said, he tried "to frame a system which should embody their [Procter's and Parrish's] valuable fea-

tures, embrace new subjects, and still retain that harmony of plan and proper sequence which are absolutely essential to the success of any system." The book became very popular.

If Remington's *Practice of Pharmacy* today holds a somewhat different place in the literature, it retains its vitality and remains one of the most encyclopedic, voluminous and profusely illustrated of pharmaceutical books for reference and instructional use.[108]

Life implies constant change. The development from the introductory treatises on practical pharmacy to voluminous tomes covering the whole of pharmacy created a renewed demand for smaller and more compendious guides. Reinhold Rother published (1887) the first edition of a book of this kind under the significant title *The Beginnings in Pharmacy*, "an introductory treatise on the practical manipulation of drugs and the various processes employed in the preparation of medicines." The book meant an entirely new type of handbook for America, and was an attempt to provide a real apprenticeship by presenting information perfectly adapted to the material and the implements of the ordinary pharmacy.[109] One reviewer called the book an "eminently useful one, not only to beginners in pharmacy but to pharmacists in general. . . . By its original and masterly treatment and by the elegance of language, this book ranks far above the kindred and more voluminous works."[110] A year later the author died, and his book was not continued.

The idea of a concise treatise on pharmacy also found a realization in the *Handbook of Pharmacy* published by Virgil Coblentz (1894). This book was not restricted to an introduction to practical pharmacy, also embracing "the theory and practice of pharmacy and the art of dispensing." It began a succession of American textbooks on pharmacy that have tried "to supply to the student of pharmacy a compendious and yet sufficiently detailed textbook for systematic study, and to those exercising the art a trustworthy guide to be consulted in daily practice" (preface to the first edition). Among the 25 books mentioned by Coblentz as sources for the illustrations in his treatise, 19 were German and 2 were Anglo-American adaptations of German books.[111] That the book did not live beyond a second edition was most likely due to the appearance of another book, similar in kind, the *Treatise on Pharmacy for Students and Pharmacists*, by Charles Caspari, Jr. (1895).

Caspari's motive for writing a book was much the same as that of Coblentz. Moreover, he expressed it in almost the same words, adding, however, a direct "dig" at Remington's voluminous book. His treatise, he said in the preface, "should be devoid of all unnecessary material, such as official and unofficial formulas, etc., readily accessible in the Pharmacopoeia and such books of reference as are usually found in drug stores." Caspari's book became popular, and went through 8 editions (until 1939).[112]

Of the 3 American textbooks on pharmacy that were begun in the 19th or the early 20th century, the Remington-Cook-LaWall represents the encyclopedic type, the Caspari-Kelly the systematic-informative type, and the youngest, Arny's *Principles of Pharmacy*, the common textbook type. In the preface to the 1st edition of his book (1909), Arny stated that its "frank intention . . . is to explain the Pharmacopoeia from its pharmaceutical standpoint."[113]

Still another type of textbook, the concise informative treatise on practical pharmacy, was represented by Edsel A. Ruddiman's *Pharmacy, Theoretical and Practical* (1917). A newer book with similar intentions, *Fundamental Principles and Processes of Pharmacy* (1944), by Henry M. Burlage and co-authors, has evolved into the present *Orientation in Pharmacy* (1959).

While the textbooks mentioned thus far attempted to cover more or less fully the entire field of pharmacy, another type specialized in the art of compounding and dispensing medicines or, in other words, the theory and the practice of filling prescriptions. One of the earliest and best-known examples of this kind is Wilbur L. Scoville's *The Art of Compounding* (1st edition, 1895), which has been revised by a series of distinguished editors up to the present time.[114] With the book of William J. Husa entitled *Pharmaceutical Dispensing* (1937) the elementary treatment of the subject matter, traditional from an earlier period of pharmaceutical education, was replaced by a systematic scientific treatment.

In a series of pharmaceutical textbooks called *American Pharmacy*, authors belonging for the most part to the younger generation express a new idea. Instead of trying to compile all that the pharmacist should know between two covers, each volume of the series presents one phase of the science and the art of pharmacy within the framework of the respective scientific theories and generalizations and according to a coordinating plan. There have appeared (since 1945): (1) *Pharmaceutical Principles, Processes and Preparations*; (2) *Advanced Pharmacy; Medical, Surgical and Dental Supplies; Animal Health Pharmacy* and (3) *Pharmaceutical Compounding and Dispensing*.

By no means do the books mentioned constitute a complete list of textbooks on the technology and the professional services of pharmacy published in America. However, they are representative of different types of these books and illustrate the development in the demand for professional pharmaceutical information.

Pharmaceutical Sciences

American pharmaceutical education, about 60 years after its first beginnings, had matured sufficiently to begin to provide its own specialized textbooks in the pharmaceutical sciences underlying the development of drugs and the dispensing of them with assurance of proper quality and professional judgment. Until the last quarter of the 19th century, besides the subject of pharmacy, American schools ordinarily required scientific instruction only in materia medica and in pharmaceutical chemistry. Hence it is in these fields that we find the first scientific texts emerging.

A Conspectus of Organic Materia Medica and Pharmaceutical Botany was published (1879) by Lucius E. Sayre, a pharmacist then teaching in Kansas. This was followed (1882) by the more popular *Manual of Organic Materia Medica* by the Philadelphia pharmacist and teacher, John M. Maisch. Other textbooks, often still more specialized, soon followed in biologic areas of pharmaceutical work.[115]

Textbooks on pharmaceutical chemistry written by American pharmacists also were comparatively late. For some decades, *Chemistry, Medical and Pharmaceutical,* written by John Attfield, professor of practical chemistry to the Pharmaceutical Society of Great Britain, was the main textbook on chemistry used by American students of pharmacy, as "revised by the author for the followers of medicine and pharmacy in America, the chemistry of the preparations and materia medica of the United States Pharmacopoeia being introduced" (preface). The practical usefulness of Attfield's book carried it through 19 editions (by 1906). By that time a number of competing American textbooks had appeared; the earliest by pharmacists were written by

Frederick Hoffmann of New York (1873) and by John Uri Lloyd of Cincinnati (1881).[116]

Meanwhile, a wide range of textbooks in the pharmaceutical sciences have appeared, adapting themselves to the changing needs of pharmacy but, more important, helping to determine the character and the depth of American pharmaceutical practice. In them we find the cumulated evidence of the scientific progress of pharmacy. The materials for tomorrow's textbooks are found in a different class of literature, the journals of pharmacy.

JOURNALS

Books represent the static aspect and journals the dynamic aspect of pharmaceutical literature. A remarkable number of American journals have appeared, both national and local, covering widely diverse subject matter. However, they have in common the task of conveying information on all phases of pharmaceutical practice. In addition, they help to mold opinions and to gain support for new enterprises. Hence, the character of the journals, and of the men who determine their content, has an unusual historic interest and influence.

Journals may be classified according to the purpose they try to serve. These purposes may be information or entertainment. Consequently, the highest aim of the ambitious and honest journalist is to achieve educational objectives in the most appealing way. Journals designed for a definite group of readers naturally have to serve the special needs and demands of these people. The needs and demands are by no means always identical. To ascertain the real needs of people and to educate them to the point where they recognize them is one of the primary tasks of a journal. Such efforts are characteristic of journals with higher ambitions. The following or even the creating of trivial or incidental demands, without educational aims, characterize the others.

Accordingly, journals sprang up to serve the two-sided character of pharmacy. One group of publications catered to pharmacy's function in providing professional service to the public based on scientific knowledge. Another group catered to pharmacy as a trade, based on principles and necessities of commercial operation. Hence, some are scientific-professional, and others are commercial. Still others are of a dual nature. Not only the scientific-professional pharmaceutical journals, which of necessity served educational ideals, but also the majority of the more-or-less commercial periodicals, have endeavored to foster professional responsibility.

Association Publications

Scientific-Professional Journals

Significantly, the first American pharmaceutical journal, which at the same time was the first journal of its kind in the English language, was the child of an association. Its European model was the French *Bulletin* [Journal] *de Pharmacie*, initiated by members of the Société de Pharmacie de Paris. But what a difference in the circumstances creating these publications! In France, pharmacy was an old, dignified and widely recognized profession, whose members had prominently, if not decisively, contributed to the various literatures. Evidence in point is that French natural scientists resented the new journal, fearing that the much appreciated pharmaceutical contributions would be diverted from the general scientific periodicals.

When the Philadelphia College of Pharmacy published the first issue of its journal in 1825, no recognized professional pharmacy existed in the United States of America; and only a few people were able and willing to devote themselves to scientific pharmaceutical work. The French journal was nourished by professional wealth and came as a crowning achievement of pharmaceutical progress; the American journal was a child of need and came at the beginning.

As far as ideologic objectives were concerned, the American journal was amazingly successful. The *Journal of the Philadelphia College of Pharmacy*, as it was called by its founders, soon received na-

tionwide and even international attention. In recognition of this fact the title of the publication was changed (1835). The local designation had to give way to a national one. As the *American Journal of Pharmacy*, this oldest American pharmaceutical periodical has served the profession at home and abroad for nearly a century and a half. However, in spite of its national baptism and international reputation, it remained the journal of the Philadelphia College of Pharmacy, and all of its editors have been affiliated with the college.

In the early years the *Journal* could be kept alive only by sacrifices on the part of the Publication Committee. "Let it not be said," wrote Griffith (1832), "that the pharmacists of this country felt too great an apathy and so little zeal in their profession as to permit the only journal devoted to the subjects of their pursuits to languish and die."[117]

The *American Journal of Pharmacy* was indeed the only one of the scientific periodicals, issued by colleges of pharmacy in their capacity as combinations of associations and schools, which survived.[118] Distinctively college organs, such as alumni reports, extension bulletins and student journals, represent a later development, with the main objective of serving as a means of internal communication among members of their restricted groups.

The *Journal of the American Pharmaceutical Association*, published since 1912, was born out of a situation quite different from that faced by the *Journal* of the Philadelphia College of Pharmacy. Mainly through the efforts of Philadelphia men, and later through the American Pharmaceutical Association, a recognized pharmaceutical profession, interested in pharmaceutical activity of a scientific nature, had been created. Like the *Bulletin de Pharmacie* in France more than a century earlier, the *Journal of the American Pharmaceutical Association* was the crowning of a development. The publication of a monthly journal instead of the annual *Proceedings* was discussed many years before it materialized. There was a widespread aversion to involving the American Pharmaceutical Association in any kind of business or competition.[119] The *Journal* replaced both the annual *Proceedings*, published since the founding (except 1861), and the *Bulletin*, an earlier journal issued since 1906. The new journal did not include the comprehensive annual report on the Progress of Pharmacy, which had formed an essential part of the *Proceedings* volumes, but the new *Yearbook of the American Pharmaceutical Association* offered a place for this feature, which evolved into *Pharmaceutical Abstracts* (1935-1948).

True to one of its constitutional purposes, "diffusing scientific knowledge among Apothecaries and Druggists, [and] fostering pharmaceutical literature," the Association has produced a remarkable serial literature through these and other publications which are outlined chronologically in Appendix 6.

Always a means for nurturing American pharmaceutical science, the Association's *Journal* was an indication of a new maturity and stage of specialization when it yielded a separate research journal as an offshoot (Scientific Edition, 1940-1961), which is now called the *Journal of Pharmaceutical Sciences*.

One of the most vigorous and purposeful of the professional journals has been the *American Journal of Hospital Pharmacy*, growing out of modest mimeographed sheets launched (1943-44) as the *Bulletin of the American Society of Hospital Pharmacists*.[120]

Another pharmaceutical group of high importance, the American Association of Colleges of Pharmacy, journalized its proceedings, thus bringing its work to the knowledge of the American profession of pharmacy whose interest and cooperation is asked for. The close relations between the Association of Colleges of Pharmacy and the National Association of Boards of Pharmacy makes the *American Journal of Pharmaceutical Education* the field of discussion for all problems of pharmaceutical education, the theoretical-scientific as well as the professional-practical. It was the first pharmaceutical periodical of its kind (f.

1937). The National Association of Boards of Pharmacy publishes a *Bulletin*.

Commercial-Professional Journals

Having secured the passage of the requisite legislation, the main task of the local and the state associations has been to see to the proper enforcement of the laws concerning pharmacy and to take care of both the professional and the commercial interests of their members. In the course of years, the commercial interests have dominated more and more. As a result, associations have served mainly to promote and defend these commercial interests, a situation reflected in the state association proceedings and in the journals which succeeded them. After World War II at least some state associations seemed to bring professional and commercial concerns more nearly into balance; and the greater dignity and professional substance in some state journals may indicate a reversal of a trend.

The first state association to journalize its proceedings (the original California Pharmaceutical Society having become inactive after 1895) was the California Pharmaceutical Association. From its beginning (1907) the *Pacific Pharmacist* was its official publication. Other state associations followed California's lead, especially after World War I. The highly personal interchange possible through local-association journals found early expression and still survives particularly in urban areas.[121]

The most important association journal stressing the business and management of a pharmacy has been the *N.A.R.D. Journal* (from the beginning in 1902 until 1913 called *N.A.R.D. Notes*), issued by the National Association of Retail Druggists. For its members, the National Association of Chain Drug Stores issues *Chain Drug Store News*.

These owner-oriented journals had a counterpart for employed pharmacists in the *National Drug Clerk* (f. 1913); this ceased publication with the dissolution of the National Association of Drug Clerks and had no successors.

Wide areas of the professional, scientific,

and commercial fields covered by these association-sponsored journals are likewise covered by private publishing enterprises.

Private Enterprises

A number of private pharmaceutical journals have been permitted to designate themselves as the official organs of associations. Bound to serve or at least to respect the special interests of the respective organizations, they form a link between the association periodicals proper and the independent journals.[122]

The first strictly independent trade journal of national circulation was *The American Druggist's Circular and Chemical Gazette* (after 1906, *The Druggist's Circular*), the first number appearing in January, 1857. This journal was followed by a considerable number of independent journals published in various parts of the United States, particularly in drug centers such as New York, Boston, Philadelphia, Baltimore, Detroit, Chicago and Cincinnati.[123] Among such journals that cover a bloc of states and are still published, the oldest are *Western Pharmacy, The Apothecary* and the *Rocky Mountain Druggist* (all f. 1888). Nine independent regional journals now serve the entire United States.[124]

The position of *The Druggist's Circular* (1857-1940) in American pharmacy (at least until the death of its second proprietor and publisher, Dr. Vandeveer Newton, in 1880) cannot be indicated better than by the fact that Frederick Hoffmann rated it on the same level with the *American Journal of Pharmacy*. He stated that *The Druggist's Circular* differed from the *American Journal of Pharmacy*, which was specializing in professional and scientific pharmacy, in devoting "in its larger space an equal consideration to the trade and commercial affairs." He concludes that among the earlier American pharmaceutical periodicals these two "will ever prominently stand forth as models of their kind at their time."[125] A journal of the same type and of like merits was the *Pharmaceutical Era* (1887-1933).

One of the most characteristic features of the American pharmaceutical press is the incessant sequence of consolidations, of mergers and of changes in title, purpose and outer appearance. In the peculiar development of independent American pharmaceutical journalism, why was the dissemination of scientific-professional information left almost entirely to a few association journals and to one or two house organs published by pharmaceutical manufacturers? This cannot be explained entirely in terms of the general trend toward commercializing the entire field of human activity. More probably the stress on dollar appeal and entertainment value could be explained only by a more careful study of the tangled growth of independent journals and their influence. However, among influences that were at work, we can infer the effects of a further commercialization of thought and activities among the readers themselves; more publishers competing to attract reader attention, and hence advertising dollars, by whatever means; and editors who often were more at home dealing with the world of business than that of pharmacy.

A striking example of this development is *The American Druggist*. The first number of a publication then called *New Remedies, a Quarterly Retrospect of Therapeutics, Pharmacy and Allied Subjects* appeared (1871) under the editorship of the physician Horatio C. Wood, who was succeeded (1873) by another physician, Frederick A. Castle. The subtitle of *New Remedies* was changed (1876) to *A Monthly Trade Journal of Materia Medica, Pharmacy and Therapeutics,* and a pharmacist, Charles Rice, to whom American pharmacy is indebted for its first modern pharmacopeia (see p. 238), became associate editor. The transformation from a predominantly medical journal to a pharmaceutical journal found expression (1884) in a further change of title. It now became the *American Druggist, an Illustrated Monthly Journal of Pharmacy, Chemistry, and Materia Medica* (the word "Trade" disappearing). Pharmacy now took the first place, with the intention of making the magazine representative of American pharmacy as a whole, including the allied sciences, and of putting it on a strictly professional footing.[126] After Rice died (1891) another pharmacist, Caswell A. Mayo, was made editor-in-chief. Mayo had been assistant editor of *The Druggist's Circular*, drug editor of the *Oil, Paint & Drug Reporter*, and editor of *Merck's Market Report*. He changed the title to *American Druggist, a Journal of Practical Pharmacy*, thus restricting the scope of the paper as well as expressing the intent to cultivate more the "practical" than the theoretical side of the calling. The *American Druggist* and the *Pharmaceutical Record* then consolidated (1893) under the title *American Druggist and Pharmaceutical Record*, the subtitle remaining unchanged. In 1923 the reference to the *Pharmaceutical Record* was dropped. Under a new proprietorship and editorship, the subtitle was changed (1927) to *The Pharmaceutical Business Paper* ("*Paper*" was replaced by "*Magazine*," 1931, and 2 years later the subtitle disappeared entirely). By this time the paper had in fact become a typical magazine, a clever blend of features on business, professional and cultural aspects of pharmacy, plus some frankly for entertainment. This format of a popular magazine was carried through the 1940's under a succession of editors, mostly nonpharmacists. With Volume 125 (1952), *American Druggist* abandoned its staple, the popularized feature-length article, to become a news magazine for the drug field.

Was the publisher's decision the reflection of an assumption that working Americans no longer can take time for substantial reading? At least partly it was rather a reflection of the forte of a new editor with a record of strength and success on trade newspapers. *American Druggist* now became directly competitive with the independent tabloid, *Drug Topics* (which began, 1884, as a house organ of McKesson & Robbins). The place accorded *Drug Topics* among independent pharmacists, which had been enhanced by its late chief editor, Robert L. Swain (1939-1960), attracted further competition with the founding (1961) of *Drug News Weekly*, a tabloid giving more particular emphasis to chainstore technics and developments.

Insofar as most such journals dealt with scientific progress in pharmacy and allied callings, these reports during recent decades tended, on the average, to be somewhat dilettante. In mid-century an increased emphasis on reporting scientific news can be discerned, in contrast with evaluative, documented discussions of drugs and dosage forms. The case history of *American Druggist*, outlined above, illustrates this change, but it is even more striking in the history of the *American Professional Pharmacist*. Founded (1934) as an exponent of the movement of a segment of American pharmacies toward more strictly professional activity, this professional independent journal heavily stressed documented review articles on drugs and classes of drugs. Then, especially after a change of editors (1961), the *American Professional Pharmacist* turned sharply in the direction of capsule commentaries and concise digests.

This exemplified a seemingly anomalous circumstance of the 1960's: With an entire profession educated as specialists in the field of drugs, there was no longer a specialized journal, widely circulated among community pharmacists, that devoted itself mainly to professional and impartial discussion of drugs.

However, in the burgeoning field of pharmaceutical research, an independent publisher launched (1959) the *Journal of Medicinal and Pharmaceutical Chemistry* (deleting "Pharmaceutical" from the title in 1963). Also, the "journal of biological sciences" called *Lloydia* (f. 1938) could justify a change of subtitle (1961) to "a quarterly journal of pharmacognosy and allied biological sciences."

But none of these journals dealt with the application of science and technology at the operational level of the health professions as well as did, in an earlier period, an American review journal in the scientific-professional sphere called *Pharmazeutische Rundschau*, a journal that testified both to the professional level and the number of pharmacists who were from German immigrant families (founded by Frederick Hoffmann, 1882; in German until 1896; then in English as the *Pharmaceutical Review*).[127]

While the *Pharmazeutische Rundschau*

was notable for its content, it was only one of various foreign-language journals published here,[128] one pharmaceutical reflection of the American "melting pot," especially before World War I.

The fact that many practitioners provided both medical and pharmaceutical services created a market for journals covering both fields. Perhaps the earliest was the *American Lancet*, which began its life as the *Detroit Review of Medicine and Pharmacy* (1866-1876). As the health field in America matured and medicine and pharmacy more clearly separated, these journals also changed.[129]

A similar development may be observed in publications devoted to the wholesale trade in drugs, which sometimes were transformed into journals for practicing pharmacists, as a national network of pharmacies appeared and dispensing associated with wholesale houses disappeared. Consolidations also took place between journals of both types. The history of the *Oil, Paint and Drug Reporter*, once called by H. C. Kassner the "leading journal for manufacturers of drugs and pharmaceuticals and for wholesale distributors," is instructive in this respect. The paper (founded 1871) absorbed (1883) the *Oil, Paint & Drug Review* and (1885) the *Weekly Drug News* (which in turn had consolidated [1883] with the *American Pharmacist* [f. 1882]. Since then it has absorbed the journals *Drug, Paint and Oil Trade, New York Drug Bulletin, New York Druggist's Price Current, Soap Maker's Journal* and *International Petroleum Reporter*.[130]

In the field of pharmaceutical manufacturing, importance has been gained by *Drug and Cosmetic Industry*, started (1914) under the title *Weekly Drug Markets* (changed to *Drug and Chemicals Market* in 1916). After the journal was split into two separate periodicals (1926), *Chemical Markets* and *Drug Markets*, the latter was converted into the elegant and substantial *Drug and Cosmetic Industry* (1932). *Drug Trade News* (founded 1925), a trade newspaper, gained much the same position in the manufacturing field that its sister publication, *Drug Topics*, gained in the retail field.[131]

The general trend of independent pharmaceutical journalism in the United States has manifested itself in the "trade" papers, resembling magazines or newspapers not only in their formats but also in their endeavor to devote themselves to the presumptive surface interests of their readers, stressing breadth of coverage rather than depth.

Striking features of American pharmaceutical journalism are the almost confusing abundance of the journals—of which only a few illustrative examples have been mentioned here—and the incessant changes they have undergone. The list of American pharmaceutical journals compiled by Minnie Marie Meyer (1933) includes some 350 titles, and even this list is not complete.[132] The ups and downs, the unbalanced mass production, the courage to venture and to experiment have not been restricted to the pharmaceutical periodical literature; they have been characteristic of American life and are striking evidence of the youth of this country. Now a trend toward a better regulation and balance apparently has begun.

16: Economic and Structural Development

RETAIL PHARMACY

The community pharmacy has a recognized place in public welfare. This is reflected in legal and educational requirements peculiar to pharmacy's professional functions. Other functions of a pharmacist's establishment are largely commercial and hence are subject to the general laws and rules affecting commercial ventures.

The situation of the "drugstore"* in colonial times and during the first decades of the young republic has been described in previous chapters. The majority of the few educated pharmacists who then practiced their calling in this country were to be found in Boston, Philadelphia and New York. For the most part they were wholesalers as well as retailers; the first pharmaceutical associations and schools were created through the initiative of these men.[1] These wholesale druggists and the dispensing pharmacists filled the prescriptions sent to them by the few physicians who did not dispense their own medicines. However, their main professional activity was to provide the country physicians with drugs, both imported and indigenous, and with compounded medicines that they often produced in their own laboratories.

Before the Civil War

Until the Civil War, and even later, the

* The term *pharmacy* is considered preferable, though interchangeable, in relation to the term *drugstore* (modern U. S. A.). Although in this chapter *drugstore* has been used at times to help imply a pre-professional period (or, for more recent times, an average American pharmacist's establishment) the usage here carries no fixed degree of distinction. There is merit in the idea that in referring to a variety store or supermarket that includes a pharmacist's practice, only a legally defined pharmacy component should be designated by use of the term *pharmacy* (or *drugstore*).

number of such real pharmacists was comparatively small. The general store, with drugs as a sideline, and the physician who kept a public store, left little opportunity for the pharmacist as such. A true American pharmaceutical profession did not exist before the American Pharmaceutical Association created and developed it. One of the first actions of the Association was to secure reliable statistical information about the condition of pharmacy throughout the country (1851 and 1852). The situation cannot be characterized better than by quoting from some of the reports.[2]

The State of Maryland contained in the year 1851 about 139 apothecary shops of all grades, about 100 of them in the city of Baltimore, but only 12 were estimated as being owned by real apothecaries.

In the States of Maine, New Hampshire, Rhode Island and Connecticut the number of drugstores kept by physicians surpassed those kept by apothecaries and the stores of general dealers trading also in drugs and medicines far surpassed the number of legitimate drugstores.

The situation in Philadelphia was typical of the few large American cities of that period. The sale of medicines by general stores was common and extensive. Fifty-seven of the drugstores in Philadelphia were kept by physicians, who left them in the hands of medical apprentices or hired assistants. "The competition among pharmacists in Philadelphia is so excessive," the report goes on to say, "as to be a chief obstacle to the attainment of a higher standard of knowledge and skill among them. There are retail stores in which the whole year's sales do not reach $1,000—and in most of them the annual receipts range from $1,500 to $2,500."

Of California it was reported (1852) that "two-thirds of all the drug stores . . . are

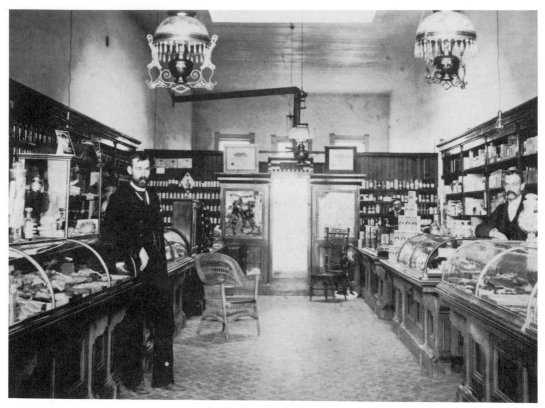

American pharmacies commonly looked like this one in the late 19th century, and many remained basically unchanged until well into the present century. A typical prescription case can be seen in the rear. Fixtures frequently were made of black walnut. Most stock is behind glass or in wall cabinets. Shelves at left hold typical sets of matched salt-mouth and tincture bottles. Handsome cut-glass urns of various shapes, atop display cases, often held toiletries or confections. (Photograph from The White Drug Store, Pullman, Wash.)

kept by physicians." In North Carolina, "throughout the State the dispensing and sale of medicines, including nostrums, was in the hands of the physicians." The report from Georgia states that "pharmacy was yet in its infancy, and pharmacists and physicians equally ignorant about materia medica in general. The use of nostrums was extensive." The conditions just mentioned held true for the early phases of cultural development in most of the southern and western states.

Professional oases could be found where a distinct influence of European continental pharmacy was felt, as in some parts of Pennsylvania and above all in New Orleans, St. Louis and New York. However, even in these places, "many physicians dispensed and dealt in medicines and kept clerks" (New Orleans); "nostrums are kept and are in general and increasing demand throughout the State" (St. Louis); and in one state (New York) an early "enactment to regulate the preparation and dispensing of medicines . . . had proved unavailing."

However, in these parts of the country there was a distinct pharmaceutical calling with professional ambitions, pride and objectives. It was French pharmacy which dominated in New Orleans and tended to make the 12 pharmacies and 4 wholesale druggists professional. Of the 47 pharmacies and the 10 wholesale establishments in St. Louis (1852), 24 of the former and 2 of the latter were kept by Germans. New York City had 273 pharmacies and 51 wholesale drug houses. The part played by Germans at that time is not known exactly, but it was large. When New York first attempted to test the professional and scientific knowledge of the proprietors of drugstores and their clerks (1872), there were 270 candidates of German descent, and 207 of them proved to be scientifically educated people. What that meant becomes obvious from the fact that of the 276 American-born applicants subjected to the same test only 76 had some kind of scientific education. Here, as in Cincinnati, Wisconsin, Indiana and parts of Texas, the German influence on pharmacy was obvious until about 1900. Of Indiana it is said that in 1885 prescriptions were still sometimes written in German, a carry-over from "the early days when a large portion of the doctors and druggists of the community were of German birth."[3]

In 1900 the number of foreign-born persons applying for licensure in the state of New York still almost equaled that of people of American birth. Of 876 candidates for the New York State Board of Pharmacy examination, not less than 409 were immigrants, coming from Russia (226), Germany (59), Great Britain (47), Italy (29), Austria (28), Sweden (5), Denmark (5), France (4), Rumania (3) and Palestine (3).[4] The great number of Russian (mostly Jewish) immigrants was largely a result of the persecution of Jews by governmental restrictions and by governmentally favored mob upheavals (pogroms). The Germans remained the largest group among the non-Russian immigrants, especially if one considers the fact that in regard to language, ethnology and general culture the Austrians are closely related to the Germans.

Published reminiscences of old pharmacists, going back as far as the 40's of the 19th century show 3 basic facts: first, that pharmacy was then considered a simple trade, for the most part, to be changed for another if the expected profit did not materialize; second, that a business frequently had been founded by a physician who later sold it to his clerk; and, third, that because of circumstances the drugstore sometimes became a general store and often a wholesale business, even if it had not been so intended originally.

J. F. Hancock tells the story of a pharmacy opened in Baltimore (1849) by a physician, "who had but recently graduated in medicine" and had "in his younger days learned the trade of house carpenter." After a few years as physician and pharmacist, this man left his calling and sold his drugstore to another doctor of the same type, who made a partner of the young apprentice whom he found in the drugstore. Shortly afterward, this physician likewise discontinued the drugstore and his practice, to become a lawyer. The young apprentice, who had had only 2 years of meager experience, became the sole owner.

Concerning Delaware, Frederick W. Fenn reported that "except in a few instances there were no regular pharmacies outside of Wilmington in 1857. The town drugstores were usually combined with hardware, and additional sidelines were stationery and books, wall-paper, paints, and oils. Some druggists sent out wagons filled with all sorts of domestic medicines to supply country general stores."[5]

Two early representatives of Wilmington pharmacy who grew into general as well as pharmaceutical importance were Joseph Bringhurst, Sr., and Joseph Bringhurst, Jr.[6] The former (1767-1834) was born at Philadelphia and obtained his degree of Doctor of Medicine at the University there. He came to Delaware (1793) where he established a drugstore in connection with his medical practice. He was intimately acquainted with political and industrial figures in England as well as in the United States and was a partner in the first cotton factory erected in Delaware. An ardent Quaker, he wrote a letter expressing his moral views to the then famous poet, William Cowper, which was printed in England under the title "Copy of a Letter from a Young Man, a Quaker, in Pennsylvania [Delaware?], to the Late William Cowper, Poet." Joseph Bringhurst, Jr. (1807-1880), succeeded to his father's pharmacy, from which he retired (1852) to become one of the Delaware pioneers in a number of social and financial ventures.[7]

These pioneers had to be men of courage and industry in the first place. It was with the usual pioneer discomforts that early pharmacists were obliged to study and practice their calling. They did as well as could be expected under the circumstances. By way of illustration, it was not easy to conduct a business in the town of Helena, Mont., where for 3 months of the year supplies could be brought only by way of the Missouri River and for the remaining months had to be carried overland a distance of 1,500 miles, subject to the constant danger of robbery. "During the winter of 1863 and 1864 a vigilance committee was organized which hung all the 'roadagents' who did not escape, and restored law and order." On the other hand, business was profitable, as the following account of a druggist in Helena testifies: "With a capital of $3,500 we sold $99,600 worth of goods the first 15 months we were in business and made a profit of over $18,000."[8]

Chicago's first druggist, Philo Carpenter, wanted to run an exclusively professional pharmacy but was unable to do so, for "owing to the scarcity of currency a large part of the business done was by a system of barter, called 'store pay.' Farmers and others who needed goods took what they had to sell and traded it at the stores for what they needed. The storekeeper then had to dispose of the goods so left in whatever way might be most advantageous."[9] In Detroit the hunters brought buck, beaver and fox skins in exchange for the goods they needed. Such conditions paved the way to the combination drugstore, general store and wholesale establishment. A large portion of the drugstore business in the country consisted of all kinds of dyestuffs and oils and paints, for houses were built which had to be painted, and homespun textiles were made which had to be dyed. The need for these articles was greater than for medicines and drugs, and the latter very often became a sideline, at least in terms of the volume of business transacted.

After the Civil War

All this changed with the Civil War, the decisive turning point in the development of the North American continent. Pioneer society had been self-sufficient as well as primitive. It was scarcely touched, and by no means penetrated, by the intellectual spirit that radiated from individuals and the few centers of learning and culture along the eastern seaboard. At this time society was confronted with a rapidly developing industry that demanded the highest technical achievements. The drugstore business in dyestuffs and similar goods vanished with the rise of the American textile industry, which became one of the largest in the world. A similar dismemberment occurred when the growth of the building industry took away the drugstore's paint and oil business. With these changes, American pharmacy had its great opportunity to develop its professional character. Had full advantage been taken of this, the "pharmacy" might have replaced the "drugstore" permanently.

In some districts, real pharmacy was achieved but could not sustain itself and never became general in scope. The rise of a large and powerful pharmaceutical industry partly accounted for this, taking over the manufacturing previously carried on, to a large extent, in the drugstore laboratories. Another reason for the curtailment of pharmacy as a full-time occupation was the fact that, on the one hand, there were too many drugstores in proportion to the demand for pharmaceutical service; and, on the other hand, the number of educated pharmacists available was comparatively small.

Comparison With Europe

A comparison with the development in Europe helps to support this statement. There also, the rise of a powerful pharmaceutical industry during the second half of the 19th century diminished the manufacturing previously carried on within the pharmacies. However, only the face and not the character of continental European pharmaceutical practice changed. It was controlled by high educational requirements limiting the number of those entitled to ownership of a pharmacy.[10] In addition, the number of pharmacies often was restricted to the proportion needed to handle the demand for pharmaceutical service.

The scientific training and the economic security of the pharmacists enabled them to concentrate profitably on their function as the responsible distributors of medicinal products. The standardization of pharmaceutical products in regard to strength, which began in the late 70's of the 19th century, was no challenge to them; and the manufacture of galenics in the laboratories of the pharmacies was already inspired by professional ambition.

As previously shown, in America the development of pharmaceutical industry encountered conditions very different from those in continental Europe. On the one hand, the dispensing of proprietary medicines directly to the public was of great importance to the American pharmacist at a time when it meant little to European continental pharmacy. On the other hand, the increasing medical tendency to prescribe proprietaries instead of writing individualized prescriptions, which was so dangerous to the continental European pharmacist accustomed to extensive compounding in a large prescription practice, seemed much less important to the average American pharmacist. Since most American physicians dispensed their own medicines, even if they did not have public drugstores, the average American pharmacist had never enjoyed a large prescription practice. The situation is illustrated by the fact that when a law in Missouri excluded the registration of physicians as pharmacists until they had passed the pharmaceutical examination, a privilege previously granted to them, "2,242 physicians registered before the new law went into effect."[11] As late as 1904, an inquiry answered by 41 Illinois pharmacists showed that "in 7 cases the physicians write prescriptions, in sixteen they dispense their own medicines, and in eighteen they do both."[12] Hence, in this respect the situation could scarcely be made worse for the Amer-

ican pharmacist by the influence of industry. At any time, it could only become better by a "tendency for a greater amount of prescribing and a lesser amount of dispensing from the doctor's office."[13]

Another quite different factor, rising out of sharp competition between the too-numerous drugstores, had a remarkable influence on the pharmacist's establishment and on the economic structure of the entire calling. Periodically it has affected even the professional part of his operation. This factor was price cutting.

Chronic Price Cutting

Competition in prices is an integral part of trade and as old as commerce itself. Its advantage to society has its limitations at that point where it becomes profitable only for a certain group of individuals and threatens the actual general economic order on which society is built. It is from this concept that the terms "fair" and "unfair" trade practices are derived.

As early as the first decades of the 19th century, price cutting was a striking feature of American pharmacy. For a long period after the founding of the Massachusetts College of Pharmacy (1823), "almost all the business [it] transacted was in reference to prices." T. W. Dyott, who is considered to have been America's first price-cutter, not only sold drugs and proprietaries more cheaply than his competitors—principally brands of supposedly uniform price—but the example of his own success helped to establish price-cutting and its continuous advertising as a deliberate practice. He came to Philadelphia (1806) from England and opened a patent medicine warehouse.[14] Until its demise during a financial crisis (1837) this venture enjoyed many years of success. The pharmacist-founder of the George A. Kelly Company of Pittsburgh practiced price-cutting, and his methods are considered to be a forerunner of the chain-store system. Under the firm name of Beckham and Kelly, his 4 drugstores in Pittsburgh (around 1860) bore signs that read: "Cut-rate Drugstore."

The demoralizing expansion of price-cutting followed the expansion of the American pharmaceutical industry, which glutted the market with proprietaries. This was caused partly by the fact that proprietaries could be bought in department stores which advertised them at a price lower than that marked by the manufacturer on the package. It was also caused in part by the business methods of the manufacturers and the wholesalers. To induce pharmacists to purchase large amounts of their products, the manufacturers as well as the wholesalers rewarded such purchases with special discounts and bonuses, thus enabling pharmacists to sell the products under the usual resale price.

"It was in the early eighties that the pioneer price-cutting of the 'big four'—Evans of Philadelphia, Robinson of Memphis, Dow of Cincinnati, and Jacobs of Atlanta—aroused national attention. . . . Price cutting became, in a few years, practically universal. . . . The first cut-rate drugstore in New York City was established by George Ramsay, of the Hegeman Company."[15]

Significantly, some of the most successful cut-rate drugstores were established not by educated pharmacists but by enterprising businessmen. Impressed by the success of Hegeman in New York, one man founded the "Economical Drug Store" in Chicago with borrowed money (1892), after he had made and lost a "fortune in the show business."[16] The man who established (1900) in the same city "The Public Drug Company . . . a large drugstore organized and conducted on the Department Store Plan" is described as "not being a pharmacist by training or education, but on the contrary a shrewd and resourceful commercial man."[17]

Co-op and Chain: Two Sides of a Coin

The unification of as many drugstores as possible in one organization had to be resorted to, both in the exploitation of all the possibilities of price cutting as a specific system of business and in the fight against it. This led to the cooperative movement among owners of individual pharmacies on the one hand and to the chain-store movement on the other.

The simpler method of defense against the damage caused by price cutters, and hence the one tried first, was the attempt of the other pharmacists to replace nationally promoted proprietaries with their own preparations or with products made for them by some manufacturer. The next step was cooperative manufacturing by independent pharmacists, exemplified by the formation (1895) of the Minnesota Pharmaceutical Manufacturing Company. In 1896 "companies were formed in almost every section of the United States."[18] Noteworthy were the Empire State Drug Company at Buffalo and the Wisconsin Pharmacal Company. In the same year the United States Pharmacal Company of Chicago was founded, the first attempt to put this cooperative manufacturing on a nationwide basis.

The next cooperative pharmaceutical manufacturer to become a national undertaking was the United Drug Company of Boston. This was not so much a defense measure of small pharmacies against the aggressive "cutters" as it was an attempt to enter pharmaceutical manufacturing on a cooperative basis; but pharmacists were allowed to join under certain conditions.[19] The inaugurator and first general manager of the United Drug Company was L. K. Liggett. When the United Drug Company became (1933) "a subsidiary of Drug Incorporated, a large organization which also manufactures proprietary remedies and conducts an extensive chain-store system," it produced the "Rexall" pharmaceuticals and toiletries for about 10,000 franchised "Rexall" drugstores (1930; 10,500 in 1961). These are financially independent drugstores, found "in every inhabited county of the nation," which "agree to purchase at least minimum amounts of Rexall products in exchange for discounts, local and national advertising advantages, and a distinctive window sign."[20]

After the dissolution of Drug Incorporated, a new Rexall Drug and Chemical Company also developed diversified operations of international scope, including the largest drugstore chain in the world (e.g., 553 units in 1947). Through a planned program the company then contracted the number of its drugstores (e.g., 158 operating in 1961), and expanded many that remained into self-service, large-volume supermarkets that include a pharmacy component. Pharmacy became only one part of the diversified retailing operations of the corporation; and these in turn were joined to diversified manufacturing operations, which in a decade (1953-1962) more than doubled both assets and earnings and increased the annual net sales of Rexall Drug and Chemical from $189,244,000 to $280,850,000.[21]

A nation-wide cooperative manufacturing corporation also founded under the auspices of prominent price-cutting druggists was the American Druggists' Syndicate (established 1905).[22] "There were, in 1930, about 20,000 retail stores purchasing from the syndicate, which in 1926 had been taken over by the D. A. Schulte interests, operators of a large retail chain-store system."[23]

Thus a movement initiated to defend the independent small pharmacies to a large extent turned into a link between independent and chain drugstores, assisting also the latter by strengthening their manufacturing and buying power.

Members of the Independent Druggists' Alliance (founded 1930) were "alleged to reap all the administrative advantages and economies of chain store organization, but to retain independent financial status."[24]

The cooperative manufacturing companies also did some cooperative buying. However, the mainstream of cooperative buying arose as a separate movement. It represented not so much a special means of defense against price-cutting as an attempt to economize by taking advantage of all the allowances, bonuses, etc., granted by manufacturers and wholesalers to big buyers. "The growth of this movement has been rapid, and its history is filled with fewer fruitless attempts and failures than that of co-operative manufacturing."[25] From 1886 to 1907, one buying club after the other was founded.[25a] "These 'co-operative' or 'mutual' wholesale drug companies usually specialize in the distribution of well advertised products and limit their stocks to certain specified items and brands. Some

'mutuals' have grown to tremendous size."[26]

The first attempt at a national buying club association seems to have been made with the establishment of the Associated Drug Companies of America (1906) in New York. It was superseded (1916) by the present Federal Wholesale Druggist's Association.[27] In 1930 this national organization consisted of about 25 members.[28] In 1950 the membership had grown to 66, among them 31 "outright retailer wholesale houses" and 27 associate members consisting of "standard type drug service wholesalers."

"Not to be outdone by a chain composed of former 'old line' jobbers, a group of mutual or cooperative drug companies in 1929 organized a chain system" under the name "Mutual Drug Company." Pharmacists could become shareholders or profit by special discounts, according to the amount of their purchases. Remaining independent, they could gain certain chain-store advantages by joining the company and by identifying their establishments by the name "Ure Druggist, Inc."[29]

The wholesale "chain composed of former 'old line' jobbers" that the Mutual Drug Company desired to counteract, was the combination brought into existence (1928) by McKesson and Robbins, Inc., which was founded (1833) as a small drug wholesaler. The new consolidation embraced (1930) 67 wholesale houses. At this time, about 17,000 independent retail dealers had signed contracts to feature McKesson and Robbins products,[30] a system discontinued by McKesson in 1932. In 1949 each of the firm's 72 wholesale drug divisions represented "a decentralized unit responsible for its own buying, warehousing and sales" but operating "under general policies formulated by the Home Office in New York." The company stated that "more than 38,000 of the country's 49,400 independent drugstores are customers of McKesson Divisions." McKesson extended its wholesaling operations until sales totaled (1958) about $600 millions (almost a third in liquor), a 30-fold increase in less than 4 decades.[31]

The cooperative movement in American pharmacy did not lead to the establishment of a large national manufacturing and wholesale institution like the French *Pharmacie Centrale*, representing both the scientific and the commercial potentialities of the profession. The inner reason was that American pharmacy, although including a highly professional group, lacked the uniformity of education, interests and objectives necessary for establishing or maintaining such an institution. Furthermore, the majority of pharmacists always needed the support of the pharmaceutical manufacturers and the regular wholesale druggists. Official representatives of American practicing pharmacists therefore could not sanction, or at least could not support, a movement that eventually would place them in competition and opposition with these two groups. "The members of the buying clubs are all or nearly all, strong National Association of Retail Druggists (N.A.R.D.) men, although, paradoxically, the National Association of Retail Druggists is theoretically opposed to the buying club idea," wrote the *Druggist's Circular* in 1906.[32]

The Fight for "Fair Trade"

The N.A.R.D. itself (like its forerunner, the N.R.D.A. of 1883-1887) was and remained committed to a cooperative program with established manufacturers and wholesalers to mitigate the recurrent price cutting.

First came the so-called Campion plan, which provided a rebate system applying only to pharmacists selling at regular prices. Concerns which did not employ the rebate system were supposed to be under obligation not to sell to "cutters" at all.[33] The plan proved to be a failure. Other plans were discussed rather than put into force.

When the National Association of Retail Druggists came into existence (1898), it started a successful drive "to relieve the retail trade of the burden of taxation resulting from the imposition of the Spanish-American war tax on proprietary medicines and toilet articles.[34] After this, several plans to curb price cutting were tried with more or less success, until finally the so-called

"tripartite plan" came into being. It derived its name from the fact that it was the result of an agreement between three parties, the National Association of Retail Druggists, the National Wholesale Druggists' Association and the Proprietary Association of America. This agreement, limiting the sale and the distribution of many preparations to dealers who maintained established resale prices, was nullified by legal counteraction by the United States Department of Justice.[35] The three associations were enjoined "from combining and conspiring to restrain trade, from fixing prices by agreement and blacklisting retailers, and from continuing in force the direct contract-serial numbering plan as heretofore enforced."[36] Other decisions seemed to abolish every possibility even for the individual manufacturer to maintain resale prices for his products.

Inasmuch as legislation had enabled the price-cutters to defeat their adversaries, the National Association of Retail Druggists "promptly entered the legislative field."[37] Until 1930 there was not much success. Then, in the throes of the great depression, small business men became more unified in their desire for resale price maintenance. The first "fair trade" law was passed in California (1931), and 45 other states followed suit by 1949. These laws have been fortified by the Miller-Tydings Federal Enabling Act (amendment of 1937 to the Sherman Antitrust Act) and validation by the U. S. Supreme Court (Old Dearborn case, December 7, 1936).[38] In general the "fair trade" acts legalized contracts requiring the buyer to sell at or above the resale price set by the seller (for example, a drug manufacturer). Eventually a "non-signer clause" (California in 1933, later in other states) was added to require compliance of all distributors in an area where a pricing contract was effective, even though all had not signed the contract. This non-signer clause sparked periodic controversy during the ensuing years.

Although fair-trade laws are enacted for distributive occupations in general, pharmacy has received much of the credit—not always complimentary[39]—for the passage of many such laws, under the leadership of the National Association of Retail Druggists.

These fair trade laws are not simply legislative acts favorable to the interests of pharmacy. They are of profound general importance. They represent signs of a fundamental change in American public opinion as to the concept of liberty, the avowal that "the real difference between anarchy and an organized free society lies in the degree of individual restraint and in the kind of rules set up to insure mutual satisfaction in the economic relations of life." The period in which it seemed necessary "to protect the individual against the group" [i.e., the big corporations with monopolistic trends] apparently is being superseded in part by another "establishing, through Social Control, the protection of the group [i.e., here retail trade as a whole] against the unscrupulous individual."[40]

The Independent Pharmacy: Its Income and Competition

The small distributor's "unscrupulous" antagonist returned to the market place in a new guise, when the "seller's market" gradually disappeared after World War II. These low-margin distributors ("discount houses" and "supermarkets") found fair-trade restrictions increasingly galling.

After one supermarket operator named Schwegman obtained a decision by the U. S. Supreme Court (May 21, 1951) that a non-signer clause could not be enforced in interstate commerce, supporters of the fair-trade concept tried to repair the damage by securing passage of the McGuire Act (1952) in Congress.

Meanwhile, the state fair-trade acts have been challenged repeatedly. Often they have withstood constitutional tests; but in other states the non-signer clause has been found to be legally improper in some respect. Other harassments by opponents of price maintenance tended to weaken the effectiveness of fair trade after midcentury in various parts of the country.[41]

In a sense, fair trade has run counter to the American commitment to "free enterprise." Yet, it supports an equally traditional concern for the life-chance of small, independent entrepreneurs. This concern gained legislative strength as mass purchasing, mass distribution and mass promotion became linked into an increasingly efficient, powerful and impersonal mechanism for fulfilling consumer needs.

While such commercial trends seem to be remote from the professions, American pharmacy has been particularly vulnerable, being for decades only a part-time profession for a majority of practitioners. In the nonprofessional segment of his income-producing activities, the average pharmacist has a tradition of selling small inexpensive products, often not of the highest quality and subject to "bargain" merchandising. Even health products warranting a pharmacist's professional or technical service attracted price cutters. After all but a vestige of laboratory manipulations (about 4% of prescriptions in 1961) were withdrawn from American pharmacies into the large manufacturing laboratories, it became more difficult, despite the responsibilities inherent in prescription practice, for pharmacists to keep drugs as such isolated from commercial thought and ambition (among less thoughtful practitioners and non-pharmacist owners of pharmacies).[42]

Like the "pineboard drugstores" of the early part of the century, many early supermarkets used the technic of stocking a limited number of best-selling products, operating at the lowest possible cost, and making extreme price-cutting their principle. Others have gone farther by seeking out pharmacists willing to sell their services under grossly commercialized conditions, so that the name and the prescription service of a pharmacy might be exploited through flamboyant advertising. Such tactics became more widespread in the 1950's, bringing pressure especially on urban pharmacists who tried to maintain full professional services and the standards that have given pharmacy its standing as one of the health professions. Although threatening the economic base of professionally oriented establishments, there were signs that the exigencies of economic life and public reaction were setting severe limits on the development of "discounters" by the 1960's, in which some saw portents of their decline.[43]

As supermarket operators sought a pattern of survival, their "discounting" came to be reminiscent of the "loss leader" tactics of chain-store entrepreneurs who had pressed hardest on the independent pharmacist in earlier decades. Whereas the "supermarket" brought many kinds of small shops under one roof, the "chains" had emerged by linking together units of the same kind under many roofs but a single ownership. (This distinction has often been blurred in recent years, and large capital and high turnover are elements in common between the two types of enterprises, often giving them analogous characteristics.)

In large cities comparatively early there were pharmacists who owned two or even three drugstores in the community. However, they always considered themselves to be "independent" pharmacists, like the owners of a single establishment. The suggestion of Rorem and Fischelis that the term "chain stores" be used only for "four-store enterprises and sectional and national systems"[44] is certainly arbitrary but to some extent makes the term more meaningful.

The first "chains" of drugstores were established in England and Scotland, known there as company-pharmacies, and developed to a remarkable degree by 1900.[45] Probably the American movement in its later growth was stimulated by the English example. However, the first attempts before 1900 (e.g., Hegeman and Company of New York, Charles B. Jaynes of Boston, the Hall and Lyon Company of Providence, and Miss Cora Dow of Cincinnati) were doubtless the result of American conditions and not of any English example.

The rapid development of chain drugstores in America largely resulted from the work of two men: Louis K. Liggett, who (1907) had initiated the founding of the United Drug Company, and Charles R. Walgreen, who opened the first unit of the present chain in 1901.

By 1916 Liggett operated 45 drugstores and added to them the 107 drugstores of the Riker-Hegeman-Jaynes combination. In 1921 the Liggett concern had 229 establishments and by 1930 "touched its all-time peak of 672 stores." Grandiose plans of dominating retail pharmacy in the Anglo-Saxon world ripened. "Combining with various large manufacturers to form Drug, Inc., the concern extended its operations to England, building up Boots, Ltd., drugstores there. At the height of the boom of the late 1920's 1000 drugstores in the two countries came under this single ownership. The Boots stores were disposed of in 1933, and Drug, Inc. disbanded into several parts"[46] (see p. 268).

The Chicago pharmacist Charles R. Walgreen, Sr., the other leader in the chain-store development, had acquired 9 drug stores between 1901 and 1916. By 1922 his establishments numbered 29, then multiplied 4-fold within 5 years, and during the next 35 years multiplied 4-fold again (462 in 1961).

Since drug-chain managers have always preferred urban districts and the best situated places within them, chain drugstores naturally have sales volume very different from that of their independent competitors, on the average. While in 1935 "less than 4% of all independent drug stores did an annual business of over $50,000 . . . over 64% of chain stores did a business of over $50,000."[47]

A quarter century later, we find a drastic change, reflecting changes both in the American economy and in the style of operating community pharmacies. Among independent drugstores (1960) an estimated 77 per cent, compared with about 96.6 per cent among chain stores, had an annual business of over $50,000. The result of the aggressive mass-merchandising that is characteristic of multiple-unit management comes into bold relief for this more recent period only at higher volume levels. For example, 3 times as many chain stores took in over $125,000 annually as did independent stores (77.2% versus 26.5% of the total operating in each category).

Although the sharp expansion in dollar volume obviously has not been restricted to multiple-unit operations, the average chain unit did have twice as much volume as did its independent counterpart. That is, drugstores operating in chains of more than 3 units represented about 10 per cent of all pharmacy units but garnered about 22.5 per cent of the dollar volume. Equally significant is evidence that the chain store's proportional share has been stabilized at roughly a fourth of the total drugstore volume since the early 1930's.

The dollar volume of American community pharmacies totaled about $7.7 billion for 1960, twice what it was only 13 years earlier, and was estimated at nearly $8.5 billion for 1962. Of course, more than a third of this volume, even in independent pharmacies without fountains, has nothing to do with pharmacy. Although the average chain store distributed more health products and toiletries than the independent in all categories except prescriptions, the majority of the chain-drugstore sales had nothing

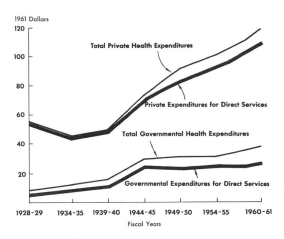

Health expenditures, private versus governmental, are charted during a 32-year period. At the end of the period private expenditures accounted for about three fourths of the total national expenditure on health and medical care, a proportion that has remained relatively constant since 1950. During the period, the aggregate expenditure for health care increased by about 700 per cent. However, this increase is only 146 per cent when calculated per capita and on the basis of a constant dollar. (From *Progress in Health Services* (H.I.F.) *12* (No. 1):1, 1963)

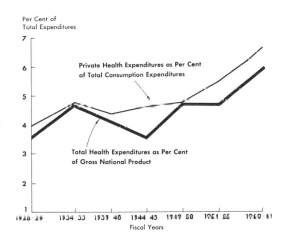

During the 32-year period depicted, all expenditures for health care as a proportion of the gross national product rose from 3.6 per cent to 5.7 per cent. During the same decades the portion of consumers' budgets spent for health increased from about 4 per cent to 6.6 per cent. Other industrialized nations spent roughly equal proportions of national income for all types of medical care as did the United States. (From *Progress in Health Services* (H.I.F.) *12* (No. 1):2, 1963)

to do with pharmacy or the health field. It is mainly this inexhaustible capacity of the chain-drugstore for efficient purveyance of variety-store merchandise that makes possible a dollar volume more than twice that of the average independent and that makes pharmaceutical service so inconspicuous in many "super-drugstores" that the term becomes incongruous and, to the public, even amusing.[48]

The Question of Ownership

The need for capital and for financial skill under these conditions tends to subordinate the importance attached to professional competence in the over-all operation and hence often attracts nonpharmacist ownership or control. Such a circumstance, in a field providing an important health service, was accepted as a serious public question in some sections of the country even earlier in the century. Several states (first New York and then Illinois, Michigan and Pennsylvania) attempted to prevent professional competition by nonprofessional persons, through restricting legally the ownership of pharmacies to registered pharmacists, following the continental European pattern. This was rendered ineffective after a decision of the United States Supreme Court (November 19, 1928) declaring the Pennsylvania law unconstitutional.[49]

Among the arguments presented in favor of pharmacist-ownership, J. H. Beal placed the psychological reality sharply in contrast with the legal fiction.[50] He emphasized the fact that the professional manager is expected to obey the directions of the nonprofessional owner and therefore, for cogent personal reasons, may not meet the legal responsibility imposed upon him. For this very reason the pharmaceutical legislation in Germany, for example, denied the right of widows and orphans, or of proprietors disabled by old age or long illness, to conduct their pharmacies personally or to exercise any influence on their management. Such pharmacies must be leased to registered pharmacists and must be conducted on the responsibility of the lessee.

Despite constitutional handicaps to such restrictions in the United States, the issue has remained alive, reinforced by some evidence that centering authority for the standards and the policies of pharmacy operation in the hands of pharmacists would be in the public interest.[51] However, the difficulties of doing so by State Board regulation alone were exemplified as recently as 1962 by a court case in Minnesota.[52] Some organizations have taken renewed interest in the question, believing that modified legal precedent and philosophy make the old court decisions no longer insurmountable obstacles.[53]

The issue has been somewhat confused by the fact that an increasing number of establishments legally defined as pharmacies are misbranded in that the main part of their operation has nothing to do with pharmacy. Such a circumstance led the Florida Supreme Court, for example, to strike down a statute requiring that a "re-tail drug establishment" be supervised by a pharmacist. The Court pointed out, in part:

It is only that part of the business of a retail drug establishment which deals with the preparation and sale of controlled drugs which affects the public health, as the legislature intended to safeguard it in the pharmacy statute. . . . To require that [other parts of] such operations be supervised by a licensed pharmacist merely because done in a storeroom which also prepares and sells controlled drugs does discriminate against the owners and operators of such establishments without valid reason therefor and we cannot sustain the statute which requires it.[54]

The degree to which pharmacy has been exploited commercially in the United States is perhaps historically unique among highly civilized countries; and while it seems too early to be able to evaluate the consequences of this circumstance, it does intrude even into these questions of legal control. For example, the Illinois Supreme Court looked back at the precedent-setting Liggett case (1928) and concluded that the chain "was conducting an ordinary business—namely, the operation of a drug store . . . ," while confirming, on a dental issue, that ". . . The law is well settled that the state may deny to corporations the right to practice professions and may insist upon the personal obligation of individual practitioners . . ."

So saying, the Court invoked a further idea that has recurred under many historical circumstances, to the effect that law makers "may deal with the different professions according to the needs of society in relation to each profession."[55]

To clarify and strengthen responsibility for pharmaceutical service by divorcing it from business enterprises of pharmacists, one statutory proposal (New Jersey, 1960) provided that "every registered pharmacy in this state shall be restricted to the sale of drugs, medicines, health aids and devices directly connected with health care as hereinafter defined."[56] Although the idea of thus devoting a pharmacy to activities related to the practice of pharmacy would have seemed an ordinary and traditional expression in various countries, within the

American context it has seemed too radical to be adopted in any of the 50 states up to this time.

Practitioners

A correlate of the American reluctance to confine the economic control of pharmacies to pharmacists is the reluctance to limit the number of pharmacies or pharmacists by legal regulation. Even informal limitations (e.g., difficulties of obtaining education or license, capital or credit) have not curbed the number of establishments or practitioners as much as in various other countries. Consequently, international estimates suggest (1962) that no country in the world has more pharmacists in relation to the population than does the United States.[57] The United States also has an unusually large number of pharmacies in relation to the number of people to be served, although there has been a tendency, since perhaps about 1900, toward a proportional decrease.

The growth in the national network of pharmacies has not shown any consistent relationship to the growth in population, because an elastic extension of nonprofessional functions has made it unnecessary, economically, for the supply of American pharmacies to bear any quantitative relationship to the demand for pharmaceutical services. Conversely, the "excess capacity," pharmaceutically speaking, of the average American pharmacy has permitted the growing demand for pharmaceutical service of recent decades to be absorbed without comparable increases in facilities, though pharmacists devote more of their time to the practice of their profession.

Historical information on trends in personnel and facilities remain inadequate and may never be satisfactory because of the fragmentary, uncertain nature of many of the statistics available for periods prior to World War II. Still earlier, before the late 19th century, our view of the size and the distribution of the profession is fogged by the lack of a stable definition of what constituted a pharmacist or a pharmacy before the passage of modern pharmacy laws.

One of the earliest quantitative reports on the development of community facilities is for Massachusetts, about 1850, when the number of drugstores in cities of 10,000 or more was 1 to 1,500 persons; in towns of about 6,000, the ratio was 1 to 2,000; and in "thickly settled districts," 1 to 3,000. Somewhat later statistics suggest that there had been no significant change. For example, as recently as 1930, estimates showed a ratio of 1 drugstore to 3,154 persons in rural districts, and 1 to 1,525 in urban districts.[58]

For the country as a whole in the half century before 1930, the available data suggest that the number of drugstores fluctuated rather narrowly at a ratio of about 1 drugstore to 1,850 to 2,250 persons. In the years between 1930 and 1947, such factors as the great depression, increased educational standards and the impact of World War II combined to increase the ratio from, roughly, 1 drugstore to 2,000 to 1 drugstore to 3,000 persons. From 1948 (when more consistent statistics begin to be available) to 1960, the number of persons served by each pharmacy continued to increase, from an estimated 2,930 to 3,360. The long-range trend toward an increased number of patrons makes this number seem large, until it is compared with other countries—such as (1962) an estimated 5,000 persons per pharmacy in Italy, 3,000 in France, 6,300 in Germany and 13,000 in Holland.

In terms of professional personnel, the increased patronage per American pharmacy since World War II has fostered some decrease in community pharmacies operated by only a single pharmacist from about 50 per cent to 40 per cent of the total number. During the same period (1948-1960) the number of pharmacies served by as many as 5 or more pharmacists remained stable at 1 to 1.5 per cent. The number of employed pharmacists (vs. pharmacist-owners) likewise has remained nearly constant, about 48 per cent of all practitioners licensed. The proportion of women as pharmacists remained relatively constant at 5 to 6.5 per cent, especially striking in view of the far larger proportion of women practicing pharmacy in various other countries.

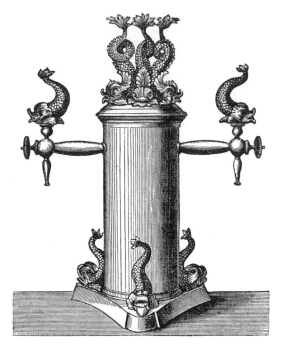

Nichols' Mineral Water Fountain typifies the simple counter device of the late 1850's which, by the end of the century, had developed into the elaborate soda fountain. The model shown has a double draft tube ornamented with dolphins disporting themselves. The top could be lifted off to repack in ice the block-tin coil of pipe inside the cylinder, for cooling the soda water. (From: Prices Current, for Druggists Only, T. Morris Perot & Co., Importers and Wholesale Dealers . . . Philadelphia, ca. 1858)

From available data in the early 1960's, Griffenhagen concluded that the United States had about 20 per cent of all pharmacists in the world (outside of Red China), serving less than 8 per cent of the world's population.[59]

The historical record testifies to the pressures of competition that once made a full-time profession for the average American pharmacist scarcely a realistic ambition. However, in a growing number of pharmacies, custom rather than sheer economic necessity accounts for the wide gamut of sidelines.

The Soda Fountain

Among side ventures unrelated to phar-macy it was the soda fountain that saved many drugstores from a more or less radical decline. It is a question of principle for American pharmacy, whether this rescue was to the advantage or disadvantage of the real task of the drugstore, its professional pharmaceutical service.

The development of the soda fountain as an integral and accepted part of the average American pharmacy seems to be unique in the world's pharmaceutical history. However, the manufacture of carbonated beverages as such was a European development, stemming from a fascination with the supposed medicinal value of natural mineral waters at spas. An English apothecary, Thomas Henry, is perhaps the earliest known producer of artificial mineral waters for public sale, albeit on a very small scale (sometime between 1767 and 1781). As early as the 1790's and through the 1820's, at least, "soda water" designated a particular type of carbonated water, in which soda was a medicinal ingredient, one of a class of therapeutic artificial mineral waters. Deletion of soda water from the 1831 edition of the U. S. Pharmacopeia perhaps signaled a shift of attention from its qualities as a treatment to that of a treat.

A citrus-flavored carbonated beverage was a European precursor of the fruit-flavored carbonated beverages of 19th-century America; but the ingenuity and the promotion that here popularized a wide variety of fizzy fruit drinks made them seem almost an American innovation. The U. S. Dispensatory gave recognition to such use in its first edition (1833), and a well-known drugstore (Smith and Hodgson in Philadelphia) was using fruit syrups by 1835.

While the famous chemist Benjamin Silliman of Yale University opened a "soda water concern" at New Haven in March, 1807, as did Joseph Hawkins at Philadelphia about the same time, the practical development and exploitation soon was taken up with particular effectiveness by pharmacists.[60] A former military pharmacist in the army of Napoleon, Elias Durand, operated in Philadelphia one of the first soda fountains in an American pharmacy (c. 1825), and the apparatus he later used for bottling under pressure "was his own invention and superior to any used in France."[61]

The dispensing of carbonated beverages by the glass from a small counter device soon became common in American drugstores. The more ornate fountains began to appear in the 1860's, gaining a prominent place in the average drugstore late in the century.

The soda fountain came into its own during the 80's of the 19th century, with the fight against the liquor business and with the passing of local and state legislation banning saloons and liquor stores. When national prohibition under the provisions of the Volstead Act became a fact (1919) the fountain business reached its climax. "From 1919 to 1929 new installations went on to the tune of $19,500,000 a year." By 1929, of the 54,745 independent drugstores, 31,813 had fountains; of the 3,513 drug chain units, 3,031 had fountains.[62] In 1935 drugstores took in $121 millions from fountains, including meals, accounting for 6.8 per cent of the total sales of meals for the whole country.[63]

Within a quarter century the total soda fountain volume increased 5-fold in American drugstores (about $600 millions), despite a decline in both the number and the proportion of drugstores with fountains. This decline was due largely to shortages of fountain personnel and materials during World War II, when about 1 fountain in 6 closed, many pharmacy owners finding meanwhile that the space could be used to better advantage. Estimates suggest (1960) that during three decades there has been a net drop in the number of pharmacies with fountain and food service from 58 per cent to about 46 per cent of the independent drugstores, and from 86 per cent to about 67 per cent of the drugstores in chains of more than 3 units. Thus it appears that a minority of American pharmacies (although nearly half) were operating soda fountains after midcentury.[64]

The soda fountain, now often expanded into a second-class restaurant, became so important a feature of the average American drugstore that in the imagination of many people the concept of a drugstore includes the fountain. How far American pharmacy drifted in this direction is strikingly illustrated by a story of a prominent Philadelphia pharmacist who operated a prescription pharmacy. He was asked to move to a new location in a physicians' office building. "The physicians who urged him to make the move added that of course they would expect him to provide a quick-lunch counter in his establishment to make it possible for the physicians in the building to conserve their time by running down to the soda fountain for a bite to eat."[65]

Growth and Character of Prescription Practice

Given the proper location, American pharmacists can earn a livelihood mainly from the profession for which they are educated. This has been evidenced, ever since the early 18th century, by a small core of pharmacies devoted almost entirely to services related to pharmacy (sometimes miscalled "ethical pharmacies").[66] Some of these pharmacies were well known for their exemplary professional standards as well as for their economic success (e.g., those of Marshall (1729-1825), owned for a century by members of the same family, of Durand (1825-1873), of Marshall's successors, Ellis and Morris, of Daniel B. Smith and other Philadelphia pharmacists).[67] American practical pharmacy can be proud that the men who laid the foundation for American scientific and professional pharmacy, Procter, Parrish, Grahame and others, have been investigators and teachers while still operating as practicing pharmacists.

In New York the shop of John Milhau (conducted by its founder from 1830 to 1869, and until 1903 by his son Edward L. Milhau) was one of the best-known representatives of the older American professional pharmacies. Like Durand of Philadelphia, John Milhau had received his pharmaceutical education in France.[68] In Boston the pharmacy of Theodore Metcalf (founded in 1837) became not only a well-known professional pharmaceutical institution but also the rendezvous of eminent American people and European visitors.[69]

The German influence on New York pharmacy evinced itself, as mentioned previously, in a number of professional pharmacies established by people of German descent, e.g., Alfred G. Dung, Adolph Heyl and George A. Cassebeer. Their pharmacies were "very popular prescription stores."[70]

Reporting his experience during a trip to the United States, Thomas Maben, a distinguished English pharmacist, wrote (1903), "The Germans practically monopolize the practice of pharmacy in New York, though, curious to say, some of the most prosperous establishments are conducted by Englishmen and Scotchmen." As examples of real pharmacies of Anglo-Saxon coinage, Maben named the establishments of Caswell, Massey & Co. of New York (tracing lineage from Wm. Hunter's pharmacy, founded 1752, at Newport, R. I.) and of Fraser and Company (founded in 1881). He calls the former "first-class prescription pharmacists" and attributes to the latter the honor of being "representative of the few retail drug establishments in the United States which realize in their operation the dreams of the educated, scientific pharmacists."[71] But many of those pharmaceutical establishments which considered themselves professional between 1870 and 1920 were old-fashioned drugstores, not professional pharmacies. It is the type of old druggist of whom L. K. Liggett ironically wrote that he sold all kinds of goods but "did not feature them," and displayed in his windows "festoons of dusty sponges, exhibits of cochineal bugs, rock sulphur and flyspecked cards announcing the 'Old Folks Supper' at the Methodist Church."[72]

While this somewhat fusty establishment can be disparaged from a later chrome-and-plastic vantage point, the fact remains that the late-19th-century pharmacy commanded considerable respect among the average citizenry. And the subsequent pharmaceutical literature is filled with apprehensions that new technologic and commercial currents would erode the professional foundations that a dedicated minority of earlier generations of pharmacists had helped to build.

Although having a professional function based on science, community pharmacies operated within the framework of business enterprise. As such they shared increasingly in the pressures felt by small specialty shops and family businesses during the present century. Under divergent influences, pharmacy tended to move off in all directions, becoming more varied than in other highly civilized countries.

On the one hand, some pharmacies have been incorporated into sprawling supermarkets, where prescriptions and other products related to health may require less than 5 per cent of the total floor area.[73] This infinitely variable mixture of pharmaceutical practice and variety-store merchandising has tended to cloud the "professional image" of pharmacy, especially when the entire establishment, and not just the pharmaceutical part, is labeled as a drugstore or pharmacy.

At the same time there has been a counter-trend toward more establishments that largely specialize in pharmaceutical services, including health-related supplies. In 1931 it was estimated that less than 1 per cent of all pharmacies (350 to 400) were "receiving 50 per cent or more of their total sales from their prescription departments"; and an informed opinion held that perhaps almost half of these had been opened within the previous 6 years.[74] Meanwhile, the number of professionally oriented American pharmacies has increased continuously, although there are differences of opinion about what constitutes a "professional pharmacy" and about what size and character of area will support one.

Already in 1935 one experienced analyst estimated that about 3,200 pharmacies seemed to be primarily interested in prescription practice (but not necessarily 50% of volume).[75] Twelve years later one professional journal believed that about 1 pharmacy of every 5 could be called "professionally minded," with nearly 700 specialized to the extent of dispensing at least 75 prescriptions a day.[76] The number of pharmacies dispensing that many prescriptions may have increased sharply during the next 15 years if a 1962 estimate is comparable that places the figure at about 8,600 pharmacies (16% of the total). A further conclusion was that almost 25 per cent of American pharmacies now derive at least half of their revenue from the prescription department,[77] in contrast with the 1931 estimate of only 1 per cent. However, another source contends that scarcely half as many pharmacies have such a large prescription practice.[78] Statistical disagreements have not been resolved, since sampling technics change from one investigator to another, and from one time to another, and sometimes have not been open to independent evaluation. However, there is agreement that the extent and the degree of professionalization has been growing in a widening sector.

Besides more pharmacies in which professional function dominates, especially after the depression of the 1930's, a sharp increase in prescription practice among community pharmacies in general can be seen. This often does not become superficially visible, first because excess capacity in prescription departments frequently has permitted a larger practice without much increase in floor space; and, secondly, because space devoted to other departments frequently has been increased even more, especially since World War II.

The sharply increased demand for pharmaceutical services cannot be accounted for on the basis of population growth alone. More effective drugs, economic prosperity, less dispensing by physicians and the tendency to prescribe individual drugs rather than compounds, probably all shared in increasing prescription totals.

The number of prescriptions dispensed in 1931 was estimated at "close to 165,000,000." Within 13 years the number had more than doubled (371 millions, representing a dollar volume of about $544 millions for 1948). After a like period, the number of prescriptions had approximately doubled again and the dollar volume nearly quadrupled (729 millions, yielding a dollar volume of about $2,219 millions for 1960). These prescriptions, which were divided about evenly between new prescriptions and refilled prescriptions, represented on the average about 28 per cent of the total dollar volume.[79]

Not only has prescription practice grown, but its character has changed profoundly since World War I, bringing far-reaching socioeconomic as well as professional consequences. This transformation can be illustrated by choosing among the prescription surveys three that are spaced at intervals of approximately 20 and 15 years. They will serve to illuminate a trend, if we pass by the question of comparability of exact figures, to look instead at the general magnitude and character of the change. Using samples supposedly representative of prescriptions nationally, these surveys were made approximately in 1926 (17,577 prescriptions), 1946 (13,125) and 1961 (149,438).

Within these 4 decades, a central function, with which the profession was closely identified both by patients and by practicing pharmacists themselves, was swept away by the combined effect of influences such as the final impact of the industrial revolution applied to pharmacy, the proliferation of individual drugs effective as therapeutic specifics, and the mass promotion of trade-named, ready-made prescription products. Still in the late 1920's up to 80 per cent of prescriptions were not of sufficiently "simple nature" to make a "broad knowledge of compounding" unnecessary. This figure was corroborated by a government study of comparable scope that found 75 per cent of prescriptions requiring "the special skill and knowledge of a trained pharmacist to compound" (1930-1931). Within 20 years only a third as many (26%) required some combination or manipulation of ingredients. And after another 15 years (1961) this proportion had dropped precipitously to 4 per cent of all prescriptions.[80]

As the compounding function moved from the prescription laboratory to the large-scale manufacturing laboratory, and expanding industrial research increased the number of drugs, an increasing number of different items was needed to dispense long runs of prescriptions, such as those surveyed. In the three illustrative surveys, the

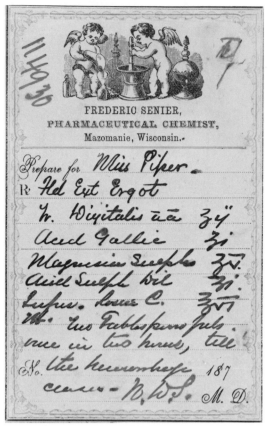

FREDERIC SENIER,
PHARMACEUTICAL CHEMIST,
Mazomanie, Wisconsin.

This prescription from the 1870's is typical of the compounding needed to dispense a majority of prescriptions received by practicing pharmacists until well into the present century.

number of pharmaceutically different products or preparations drawn upon to prepare the prescriptions rose from 1,973 to 2,400, and then to 3,300. However, only 411 of the 3,300 appeared 5 times or more in each 10,000 prescriptions. Of all the trade-named prescriptions (1961), about 64 per cent were for drugs made by 15 companies.

The massive shift away from a scientific or nonproprietary nomenclature toward the present practice in which each company creates a trademarked proprietary name of its own for a prescription drug occurred largely within the same time span (1920's to 1960). The analysis of prescriptions first showed 10 to 25 per cent prescribed by proprietary name, then 58 per cent, and finally about 88 per cent. Conversely, the

prescribing of U. S. Pharmacopeial drugs as such dropped from about 74 per cent, to 32 per cent, to 12 per cent, while National Formulary titles used in preparing these prescriptions started at only about 7 per cent of the total, then dropped to 3 per cent, and finally to only 0.8 per cent.[81] The victory of trademarks as names for drugs has been considered important by manufacturers, since it has been a stabilizing protection during a period of increasingly massive and competitive investment in both research and promotion.

These and other pharmaceutical changes were by no means peculiarly American; yet, pharmacy changed more erratically and quickly here than it did in some older countries, as it was buffeted in the freer American economy without having fully developed moorings of professional maturity and firm traditions, or the same degree of government protection as part of a public health system. Not well organized, unclear about the broader socioeconomic forces changing pharmaceutical practice, and harassed by new forms of competition both within the licensed network of pharmacies and outside it, the community pharmacist became less certain of his position and prospect—despite the upswing in demand for pharmaceutical services that became obvious by midcentury.

Dispensing Health Information

To reinterpret and bolster public understanding of pharmacists' professional function, cooperative projects were launched, such as National Pharmacy Week, a project initiated (1924) by the pharmacist Robert J. Ruth. This traditional observance has established a pattern and a time for stressing the service rendered by professional pharmaceutical work to the world in general and to the American people in particular,[82] although eventually it became obscured amid a welter of commercial "weeks" that crowd the American calendar.

Not only did the American Pharmaceutical Association try to prevent commercial exploitation of National Pharmacy Week itself, but it decided to shift the emphasis from simply telling about the pharmacist's professional service to an actual demonstration of the pharmacist's service in public health education. Under the leadership of Robert P. Fischelis, then the Association's Secretary, this objective was first made a reality (1947) by collaborating in the cancer-control program.

Said the President of the United States, Harry S. Truman,

It is particularly gratifying to note that pharmacists are endeavoring to use their close contact with the community to help control major diseases through public education in cooperation with private and governmental health agencies.[83]

A precursor program was the collaboration begun 8 years before (1940) with the American Social Hygiene Association to help to motivate those suffering from venereal diseases to undergo proper medical treatment.[84]

By 1948 the Association had adopted a long-range program of health education as official policy. Secretary Fischelis expressed the hope that

in the planning of new pharmacies and in the renovation of existing establishments, a section will be set aside for permanent use in storing and distributing authoritative health information . . . available continuously for good health and civic programs in all pharmacies.

In extending this kind of effort from a special "week" to a periodic but year-round program, cancer control again was made the theme. Said an official of the U. S. Public Health Service, the collaborating agency,

If pharmacists themselves are well informed, and if they use every opportunity to pass on their information to others, they have an extraordinary opportunity to make their establishments the health information centers of the entire community.[85]

This concept was of great potential value to pharmacists in creating good will, as well as in creating better health for the community; it attracted about 18,000 collaborating pharmacists, then faltered from insufficient supporting funds but remained alive as an objective through smaller scale, sporadic projects.

An opportunity to develop the foundation for such service on a more systematic basis came to the American Pharmaceutical Association in 1963 through a grant ($100,-800) from the U. S. Public Health Service "to evaluate the scope of the community pharmacy as a community health education center and formulate a procedure. . . ."

THE EQUIPMENT OF THE AMERICAN PHARMACY

Insofar as early American drugstores were general stores, their fixtures and equipment were those of such stores, supplemented by pharmaceutical equipment such as mortars, presses, sieves and funnels. Insofar as they had, or pretended to have, the character of a professional pharmacy, fixtures and equipment were mostly imported and represented the French, English or German style of the period.

Often the wholesale druggists and the drug importers dealt in drugstore fixtures and in pharmaceutical equipment. An advertisement in the *New York Weekly Post-Boy* (June 18, 1750) offered "to all Practitioners in Physick" drugs imported from London and "the utensils of a neat apothecary's shop." Effingham Lawrence of New York announced in the *New York Daily Advertiser* (October 5, 1789) that he had "received from Bristol, a large assortment of shop furniture of all kinds; large show globes, specie and stopper bottles . . . ointment, syrup and pill pots," etc. At the end of his "catalogue of the materia medica and of pharmaceutical preparations" (1817), the druggist Charles White of Boston offered "apothecaries shop furniture." In Philadelphia, Durand's pharmacy, which was regarded as "the handsomest drugstore in the Quaker City,"[86] brought its equipment from France (1825).

Some of this equipment of old-time American pharmacies has been preserved. Aside from miscellaneous collections, possibly the first instance of the preservation of an old-time drugstore as a museum unit is to be found in the 17th-century house of the Essex County Historical Society in Salem, Mass.

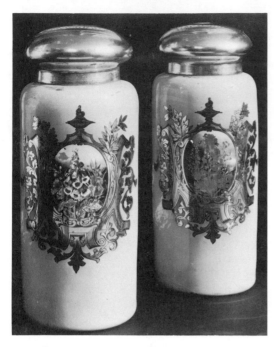

"Species" jars (above) were used in matched sets to hold stock quantities of compound powders and, especially later on, comminuted botanical drugs and chemicals. As species jars became outmoded in use, individual specimens often were retained to ornament a pharmacy, both in the United States and abroad. These glass jars usually were about 2 feet high, capped with a glass lid and richly ornamented with gold foil and colors. Because the 19th-century specimens shown lack drug names, they may have been made solely for ornament, although each cartouche does depict a medicinal plant. (Photograph from The Upjohn Pharmacy, museum reconstruction at Disneyland)

As an example of a colonial apothecary shop in its community setting, the Williamsburg, Va., restoration (1760-1776) holds particular interest. Another restoration interesting in its historical associations and setting is the pharmacy attached to the Ephraim McDowell house at Danville, Ky. Some colleges possess interesting or beautiful old pharmacy fixtures. For example, the Philadelphia College of Pharmacy and Science owns the fixtures and the furnishings of the drugstore of George Glentworth of Philadelphia, founded in 1812,[87]

and the Columbia University College of Pharmacy possesses pharmaceutical fixtures and equipment of the same period. The same era is represented by the Bringhurst shop exhibited at Mystic, Conn. (owned by the Smith, Kline and French Laboratories) and by the Stabler-Leadbeater pharmacy at Alexandria, Va.[88]

The historic apothecary shop of the physician and brigadier general of Revolutionary War fame, Dr. Hugh Mercer, at Fredericksburg, Va., has been maintained (since 1941) by the American Pharmaceutical Association (through "The Friends of Historical Pharmacy," a corporation comprised of all members of the Association). The building itself is believed to be the oldest extant in the United States that was used as a pharmacy. Another old pharmacy (Jo Mayer Collection) that became the property of the American Pharmaceutical Association is on permanent exhibit in the Smithsonian Institution, Washington, D. C. Imported from Germany by E. R. Squibb & Sons, it contains beautiful baroque fixtures (about 1750), while its contents (jars, bottles, apparatus, books, documents, etc.) date from the 15th to the 19th centuries.

An illustrated catalog of this magnificent collection has been published by G. Urdang and F. W. Nitardy (New York, 1940).

Quite a number of American pharmacies from the second half of the 19th century have been restored (see Appendix 5, under "United States"). One of the earliest period restorations of this type to be completed (1913) was brought together under the leadership of Edward Kremers and remains on exhibition at the State Historical Society of Wisconsin at Madison.

A restoration of this period holding still greater interest is "La Pharmacie Française" at New Orleans, housed in an earlier building (1823) actually used for his pharmacy by Louis J. Dufilho, one of the first pharmacists to be licensed under a pharmacy law of this country (see p. 164).

Modern developments in American pharmacy have brought forth as many types of fixtures and equipment as there are different types of drugstores or pharmacies: commercial or professional or mixed types, with or without soda fountains and luncheonettes, with the prescription department as the center of the establishment, or in the rear, or not visible at all.

Varied as these American drugstores and pharmacies have been, a great many of them, throughout their history, have used the old-fashioned Anglo-Saxon device of making obvious their character as pharmaceutical workshops with "show globes" filled with colored liquids and illuminated after dark by lights placed behind them.[89]

While each generation has left behind some artifacts as characteristic tokens of its history, the broader significance of an epoch ending can be seen in the new museum reconstructions of pharmacies from the late 19th and early 20th century. For in this period the community pharmacist was laying down his traditional tools for compounding drugs, which for centuries, though increasingly guided by science, had nevertheless served an art of the individual's own skilled hand. Then, primarily between the two world wars, these hand implements became little more than museum artifacts, being set aside to await the few prescriptions requiring their use.

Within the dispensing pharmacy, physical operations were subordinated to mental operations in a degree unknown through millenniums past. The new physical environment of the pharmacist had not yet taken final form; and in the early 1960's the automation of dispensing was discussed seriously for the first time, foreseeing a pharmacist practicing "at an electronic typewriter console wired to a dispensing machine" which would deliver the medication ready for labeling and visual check, automatically priced, invoiced and noted in inventory.[90] Whatever final form electronic "mind and muscle" take as equipment, it could affect the socioeconomic structure of the practice of pharmacy perhaps as much in the rest of the century as have the eventful decades already past.

WHOLESALE ESTABLISHMENTS

There is some doubt whether European professional pharmacies have emerged from the early general store or from the pharmaceutical work done by monks in the monasteries. Probably both conjectures are true. However, there is no doubt that in continental Europe dispensing pharmacy existed before the specialized wholesale drug trade came into being. The North American continent offers the paradoxical contrast that here the wholesale drug trade came first.

Like most paradoxes, this one surprises only when first presented. In Europe, with its comparatively early separation of medicine and pharmacy, the pharmacists from the 13th century on met the medicinal needs of the population. They were collectors of crude drugs and, on a small scale, manufacturers, buying limited amounts of imported drugs. It was not until the 17th century that the use of imported drugs had grown to a considerable extent, and not until the late 18th century that manufacturing on a large scale began to supersede the preparative work within the pharmacies. With this change, an organized wholesale trade in medicinals could establish itself.

This development could not take place in America. As stated previously, the medical and the medicinal needs of the populace in colonial times had to be met by the same persons. Although indigenous plants were collected and used, the official therapy of the colonies was that of Europe, more particularly that of England. This necessitated importation on a large scale. Hence, the wholesale drug trade was organized at an early date, since most American medicopharmaceutical practitioners wanted to employ the same pharmaceutical products that the pharmacists in Europe at that time usually prepared themselves. Thus it came about that American professional pharmacy became the legitimate offspring of the wholesale business. The country doctors had to be supplied with necessary drugs by someone in a not-too-distant town. An opportunity thus arose for locally restricted wholesale trade, usually in combination with retail pharmacy. This condition continued to a large extent until the Civil War. For example, it was not until 1868 that George A. Kelly of Pittsburgh disposed of his retail shops and devoted himself entirely to the wholesale business. Based on import, the American wholesale trade in drugs had its first centers in the great seaports, Philadelphia, New York, Boston, Baltimore and New Orleans. Later on the trade followed the inland waterways. Important establishments sprang up in cities farther south and west (such as Pittsburgh, Cleveland, Cincinnati, Detroit, St. Louis and Chicago and finally in California).

Some of the wholesale drug firms, founded between the end of the 18th century and the Civil War, are in existence today. The oldest of these was the Schieffelin Company in New York (founded 1794), which continued the wholesale part of its operation until 1963.[91] Henry H. Schieffelin, second in the long chain of members of the family heading the growing concern, was among the founders of the College of Pharmacy of the City of New York, its vice-president during the first 2 years of its existence (1829 and 1830), then president.

As new territories were opened and rapidly settled, canals and railroads built, and the telegraph invented, the opportunities for wholesale trade seemed to be inexhaustible. However, this picture of progress had its reverse side. The period was over in which the retail or sub-wholesale druggist traveled once or twice a year to "his" wholesaler "in the East" to purchase a large stock. Now the broker entered the picture. A new kind of competition started. The Civil War interrupted the development, but only to give way to a new boom. In 1866 a "review of the New York Market" described conditions as follows:

A great change in the business has taken place within the last few years. The means of communication are now so numerous and frequent, that the old regime of periodical business has in a large measure given way to smaller purchases and more frequent orders. . . . Another change . . . is the more prominent position given to brokers, a class of

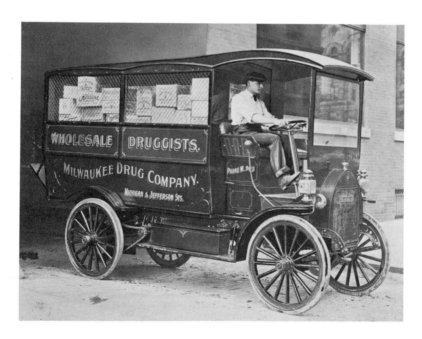

Ultra-modern lightning service was represented by this delivery truck when it was put on the road (about 1912); it is said to have been the first used by a wholesale druggist in Milwaukee. The entire development of drug wholesaling has been based primarily on quick supply of health products in small quantities drawn from diverse world-wide sources. (Photograph from George A. Moule, then Secretary of the Milwaukee Drug Company)

middlemen. We do not believe this service has any value to the small dealers who have established relations with the jobber, and which ought not to be disturbed except by his own choice.[92]

Tempted by short cuts to wealth, men rushed into business "imbued with the idea of 'getting there first.' "[93] A spirit of intolerance and discontent prevailed. Adulteration, short-weight and reprisals sometimes crept into business. In the wholesale drug field, destructive competition was the order of the day. Price, not quality, often governed the sale. In 1876 representative wholesale druggists of the Middle West met in Cincinnati and founded the Western Wholesale Druggist's Association, which later became the National Wholesale Druggists Association. The new organization was created to "correct excessive and unmercantile competition" and "remove, by concert of action, all evils and customs that are against good policy and sound business principles."[94] The Association has done a remarkable work. Its members have gained a key position in the drug trade, serving not only as a foremost supply agency for community pharmacy but as its advisor and promoter.

The expeditious pipeline for medicinal needs, provided by wholesale druggists to the country's network of pharmacists, brought a growth between 1930 and 1958 that approximately doubled the number of wholesaling drug merchants, of which about 3,000 were counted in 1958 (including both general-line and specialty-line houses). The total sales, about $2.8 billions (1958), had nearly quadrupled in 3 decades, paralleling the growth in dollar volume noted in community pharmacies. In the early 1930's more than two thirds of the entries on orders received ("line extensions") invoiced at under $2.00. As one would expect, low unit values have persisted (and undoubtedly will continue) in pharmaceutical wholesaling, although by 1950 the average "line extension" had risen to $3.37, and after another decade had reached $4.13.[95]

However, the wholesaling margin has been kept relatively low—both in relation to earlier decades and to certain other fields

of wholesaling—by various pressures. For example, wholesale houses that specialize in drugs and medical supplies, as contrasted with full-service wholesale druggists, had developed as a distinct movement within the field, of which their separate Pharmaceutical Wholesalers Association was one symptom. Moreover, especially since World War II, more manufacturers had been establishing branch depots in major cities, not only to supply wholesalers but to increase direct selling to pharmacists (often offering price inducements). While some drug manufacturers were by-passing the wholesale druggist, others were reducing the discounts allowed to the wholesaler for his services.

The various shifts in marketing practices produced economic uncertainties and readjustments in the drug distribution system. These were manifestations, one experienced editor-analyst inferred (1961), of a circumstance where pharmaceutical products had come to bear a disproportionate share of distribution costs involved in wholesale and retail operations in a commercialized system of pharmacy that embraced a vast range of disparate types of products. There seemed to be, in Editor Werble's view, a

serious doubt that a marketing system in which life or death therapeutic agents are used to carry part of the costs of distributing other less vital products can survive in our present stage of economic and social development.[96]

However, whatever competitive experiments might be tried, there seemed to be little question that the system would continue to hold a place and function for the wholesale druggist. In 1880 proprietaries were on the market in 2,700 different items and sizes. A few years later, this amount had almost doubled, and thereafter increased enormously. "The industry assumed that it had reached an absolute limit in 1916 when the wholesaler was able to list some 38,000 different items and sizes," but by 1933 the total was 60,000. "This has meant that the retailer . . . has become increasingly dependent on the 'stockroom' facilities extended by the wholesaler. Not even the best equipped manufacturer is prepared to make the instantaneous deliveries or to sell in the diminutive quantities stipulated by the neighborhood druggist in his average order."

MANUFACTURING PHARMACY

Manufacturing pharmacy in America has been repeatedly stimulated by wars. Born during the Revolution (1775-1783), it took the decisive step from childhood to manhood after and in consequence of the Civil War (1861-1865), and it became independent from Europe and dominant on the world market after World War I (1914-1918). World War II (1941-1945) made this dominance a generally accepted fact.

In 1778 the Apothecary General, Andrew Craigie, initiated and later on managed "a general laboratory" in which medicines for the needs of the military hospitals and the fighting army were prepared. Only 3 years after the war (1786), the firm of Christopher, Jr., and Charles Marshall, wholesale and retail druggists in Philadelphia, "entered quite extensively into the business of making muriate of ammonia and Glauber's salt,"[97] being probably the first to produce pharmaceutical chemicals in this country on a large scale.

The Philadelphia wholesale and retail druggists Samuel P. Wetherill and Company announced (*Poulson's Advertiser*, August 18, 1826) that they were "now engaged in manufacturing on a large scale a variety of paints and drugs." Among the advertised preparations of their own manufacture were "Tartaric Acid, Sup. Carb. of Soda, Rochelle Salt, Lunar Caustic, Red Precipitate, White Precipitate, Nitrate of Ammonia, Corrosive Sublimate, Blue Vitriol, Spirit of Hartshorn, Carbonate of Soda, Calomel, Sulphate of Quinine, Alcohol, Sulphuric Aether."[98]

In an advertisement (May, 1830) the Philadelphia wholesale and retail druggist John Elliott likewise offered "articles of his own manufacture." Among them were some of the products mentioned above. His advertisement also lists tartar emetic and Seidlitz salts.[99]

All these men were among the founders of the Philadelphia College of Pharmacy. John Farr also had been a member of the college since its founding. He established a manufacturing plant (1818), and the firm of Farr and Kunzi commenced the manufacture of quinine (1822). After the druggists Thomas H. Powers and William Weightman (the nephew of J. Farr) had become partners (1838) the firm name became John Farr and Company. Upon the death of Farr (1847) it was changed to Powers and Weightman. "The reputation of the house grew rapidly until it became the leading establishment of its kind in the country and perhaps in the world engaged in the manufacture of medicinal and other chemicals."[100] Although this statement represents the somewhat exaggerated tribute of an American author to early American industry, it proves the international recognition which this concern enjoyed at a time when American pharmaceutical industry in general was still in its infancy.

The next pharmaceuticochemical manufacturing plant to be founded at Philadelphia and to become of importance in the development of pharmaceutical chemistry in this country was that of Rosengarten and Sons (f. 1822). A year later the firm was the first to produce quinine sulfate in the United States. "They manufactured Morphine Salts in 1832, Piperine in 1833, Mercurials and Strychnine in 1834, Veratrine in 1835 and . . . Codeine, Bismuth and Silver Salts in 1836."[101] The trend toward consolidation after 1900 first brought about (1905) the amalgamation of Powers and Weightman with Rosengarten and Sons.[102] Finally, Merck and Company of New York consolidated (1927) with Powers-Weightman-Rosengarten Company of Philadelphia.[103]

In 1841 another well-known Philadelphia pharmaceutical manufacturer, the Smith, Kline and French Company, got its start. From a small pharmacy founded by George K. Smith, the enterprise gradually grew to its present importance.[104]

Before the Civil War, Philadelphia thus was the most important center for manufacturing prescription products, but not the only one even then.

Among the manufacturing laboratories still producing, some of the oldest are Caswell-Massey Co. Ltd. (beginning as a pharmacy) and Schieffelin & Co. of New York (beginning mainly as a wholesale house), the unusual Tilden Company, and The Wm. S. Merrell Co. of Cincinnati (f. 1828). This latter firm, as well as the firm of H. M. Merrell and Company of Cincinnati (which later became Lloyd Brothers), worked successfully in the so-called eclectic field (see p. 160) using indigenous plants as the basis of manufacturing.[105]

The Tilden Company likewise grew to importance in the field of eclectic medicine. The firm originated in the Shaker community at Lebanon, N. Y., organizing commercial production around 1847, when the Shakers themselves already had been marketing medicinal herbs for a quarter century. These religious sectarians had settled in Lebanon (1787) and originated "as a trade in this country the business of cultivating and preparing medicinal plants for the supply and convenience of apothecaries and druggists"[106] (about 1824).

Two Case Histories

Besides such specialized manufacturing plants, two of the prominent firms founded before the Civil War proved their usefulness and improved their business during the war to such an extent that they became leaders in the field. Therefore, these two firms, Frederick Stearns and Company of Detroit (absorbed by Winthrop in 1944) and E. R. Squibb & Sons of Brooklyn, will be discussed in some detail as typical examples of American development. The founders did more than create a prosperous business. By example and by incessantly emphasizing the ideal of purity, uniformity and reliability as the first and most important basis of manufacturing products for use in the fight against disease and death, they made this concept generally recognized. This implied more than an ordinary reform, since during the trying years in which these firms developed, honesty on the American scene had yielded largely to an unbridled mania for gain.

The manner in which Stearns started his work was characteristic. His original "laboratory" was a 12-foot by 12-foot back room in his pharmacy in Detroit (f. 1855). Without any capital on hand he could not manufacture a stock of preparations. "Samples were, therefore, prepared. These were shown to druggists on trips through the State of Michigan and, upon his return, the would-be manufacturer made up the goods for which he had received orders."[108] It was the Civil War, in which Stearns acted as medical purveyor for the Michigan troops, that caused the small laboratory of his pharmacy to develop into a plant covering the entire floor space of a four-story building and equipped with steam power, milling machinery, extraction apparatus, etc. Gradually the concern grew into an establishment known the world over. This success would have meant more to the owners of the firm than to pharmacy, had it not been the result of a new idea of general importance. This "new idea" (started in 1876 and fostered after 1879 by a house organ called the *New Idea*) was the creation of "popular non-secret family medicines," to counteract the branded nostrums whose composition often remained secret from pharmacists and laymen alike, thus giving free reign to increasingly massive and dishonest promotional schemes.

Disgusted with the rampant quackery of the time, Mr. Stearns resolved to offer a few simple preparations in popular-sized packages, bearing full directions for use and in addition a plain statement of the names and quantities of their ingredients. . . . Other druggists, lacking Mr. Stearns' manufacturing facilities, adopted the plan and had him manufacture and finish similar preparations for them, bearing their names. And from this beginning it spread over the country and within a few years had extended even to the Old World, so great was its popularity.[109]

The development of the Squibb laboratory differed from that of Stearns in much the same way as did the two men whose ideas were realized in the two plants. Stearns was the practical druggist, not without scientific knowledge, but led primarily by his practical sense and by his desire to improve the practice of pharmacy. Squibb was an educated physician who had served 5 years of pharmaceutical apprenticeship before he took up the study of medicine.[110] He had a firm knowledge of the practice of pharmacy, but he was led primarily by his scientific interests and his desire to improve the practice of medicine. Stearns had created new kinds of preparations and placed them at the disposal of pharmacists for over-the-counter sale primarily. Squibb found new ways to prepare purer and more reliable products and placed this improved medicinal armament at the disposal of physicians for prescribing, dispensing or direct application.

In the naval service (1847 to 1857) Squibb was first a surgeon and then (1852) assistant director of the pharmaceutical laboratory of the Navy. A year after his return to civilian life, Squibb was induced to establish (1858) a moderate-sized laboratory of his own by the Chief Medical Purveyor of the Army. However, it soon became evident that the medicinal wants of a peace-time Army of 25,000 men could not support even a laboratory of that size.

It was his medical friends who, recognizing the value to the medical profession of a manufacturer of his type, saved the young establishment from ruin in the first difficult years. From the very beginning, "the medical profession of Brooklyn took a great interest in the movement," and when on the evening of December 24, 1858, the laboratory building was entirely destroyed by fire, these physicians furnished Squibb the capital necessary to rebuild it.

Only 2 years later the Civil War broke out. "The needs of the army became very large, and additional buildings were hired and equipped. . . . In 1862 another site was purchased and a large and commodious laboratory was erected." The description of what went on in this four-story building, with hand operations by upwards of 50 employees, survives from an inspection ordered by the Surgeon General of the Army, giving us one of the most concrete and vivid contemporary accounts of the pharmaceutical industry at that time.[111] Squibb's earliest and most valuable contributions to medicine were the new meth-

ods developed by him for the preparation of pure ether and pure chloroform, resulting in products whose use almost completely rid anesthetization of the dangers which had been associated with it. One of Squibb's greatest services to pharmacy was his research work on percolation, the results of which he published for the benefit of the profession at large.[112]

It should be mentioned that Frederick Stearns, as well as E. R. Squibb, very actively supported the endeavor to elevate the general standard of American pharmacy. Stearns served the American Pharmaceutical Association as second vice-president (1856-57) and as president (1866-67), Squibb as first vice-president (1858-59), refusing to be elected president as he also declined the presidency of the American Medical Association.

Revolution in Technology

The manufacturers of the late 19th century not only applied but helped to develop the machine technics that eventually removed from community pharmacies their age-old function of making drug products. American contributions to percolation (notably by E. R. Squibb, J. I. Grahame and Wm. Procter, Jr., between 1845 and 1875) gave initial impetus to the development of processes of drug extraction that, although often adaptable to the prescription laboratory, were never considered very practicable by the majority of practitioners. The familiar hand plaster-iron gradually was laid aside after a Philadelphia pharmacist (Robert Shoemaker, 1838) "successfully developed a process for making plasters other than by hand and became a large manufacturer of this article."[113] Although sugar-coated pills, as well as gelatine capsules, were a French innovation of the 1830's, in America it was another Philadelphia pharmacist (William R. Warner, 1866) who became one of the first and certainly most successful of the large-scale manufacturers of sugar-coated pills.[114] Warner likewise introduced to American practice small pills ("parvules," 1879) that could be produced only on a large scale. Compressed and coated tablets pushed the production

of this form of medication still further beyond the range of the average prescription
laboratory. The first compressed-tablet machine in America, a simple hand punch, was
constructed by a Philadelphia druggist
(Jacob Dunton, 1864; similar to an English
invention by William Brockedon, 1843),
although the first automatic power machines
(single-punch and rotary) did not come
into use until 1874 to 1875.[115] The biologicals that came into use after the turn of
the century, and the antibiotics from the
1940's onward, were still less suited to
processing in a local pharmacy.

With each such innovation, the number
of large-scale drug manufacturers grew.
Although rather efficient apparatus for
small-scale manufacture became available,
few pharmacists outside hospitals could re-
sist the blandishments and the economies
proffered by mass-production laboratories.
Indeed, a substantial proportion of practicing pharmacists were not well prepared by
education for a modern manufacturing role
until after local production had become
scarcely feasible economically. Moreover,
successive changes in food and drug regulation during the present century made it
increasingly difficult for small-scale manufacturing laboratories to meet all legal and
scientific requirements.[116]

After the Civil War

After the Civil War the number of pharmaceutical manufacturing firms increased
rapidly. For example, Dr. S. P. Duffield
formed a partnership (1867) with H. C.
Parke under the firm name of Duffield,
Parke and Company, in Detroit which after
4 years became Parke, Davis and Company.
This firm, like most of its predecessors and
many of its successors, started with the production of only "a few chemicals," and "a
line of fluid extracts."

Frank O. Taylor relates,

The history of manufacturing pharmacy as
a whole and of Parke, Davis and Company
may be divided into four periods characterized by the most important activity of the
time, which periods are . . . as follows:
1. Formative Period, 1867-1874; 2. Botanical
Research Period, 1875-1882; 3. Standardiza-

tion Period, 1882-1894; 4. Biological Period,
1895 to present time.[117]

Since this was written (1915), at least
two more "periods" have been opened, that
of chemotherapeutic agents from about
1910; and that of antibiotics from about
1941. As early as 1902, Parke, Davis and
Company established its own research institute, one of the earliest in American
industry generally.

One after the other, pharmaceutical
manufacturing plants arose from modest beginnings to large establishments (c. 1860-
1880), some of them of world-wide importance. Often they traveled the same
course, from the preparation of galenicals to
the preparation of a few chemicals, pro-
gressing through research to a systematic
production of certain groups of chemicals,
biologicals, and antibiotics. Most of them
started with fluidextracts.

For example, when A. P. Sharp, Louis
Dohme and Charles E. Dohme, all graduates of the Maryland College of Pharmacy,
organized the firm of Sharp and Dohme
(1860) in Baltimore, "they first undertook
the manufacture of galenical preparations
and did not enter the field of chemical
manufacturing until 1886, when they began
the production of pure plant principles."
In 1929 the company acquired the H. K.
Mulford Company, in Philadelphia, thus
becoming the owner of one of the leading
producers of biological products in this
country.[118]

The small laboratory opened by the pharmacist and colonel of Civil War fame, Eli
Lilly, in Indianapolis (1876) "with cash
capital amounting to $700 and goods . . .
amounting to $600," started with the pro-
duction of "fluid extracts, elixirs, syrups, a
few wines and then new liquid pepsine
preparations."[119] Eli Lilly and Company
became the first American manufacturing
firm to establish a branch house (Kansas
City, Mo., 1882). "What is now known as
the scientific division had its beginning in
1886."[120] Not only was the founder of Eli
Lilly and Company an educated pharmacist, his only son and successor, Josiah K.
Lilly, graduated from the Philadelphia College of Pharmacy.

Most of the establishments mentioned, constituting important units of the great assets of American scientific and commercial life, have been founded by pharmacists, although the small laboratory of a pharmacy was not always the nucleus of the later plant.

The few firms that started systematic production of pharmaceutical chemicals shortly after the Revolutionary War did not have to face much American competition. Even after the great impulse exerted by the Civil War and its consequences, the establishments then emerging first devoted themselves, as previously shown, to the manufacture of galenicals.

In their further development until 1917 they concentrated on medicinal plant research and, finally, on the production of biologicals. The systematic synthesis and production of organic chemicals, particularly chemotherapeutic agents, came later. The reason was that in the second half of the 19th century, or at least after Kolbe's synthesis of salicylic acid (1874) and Knorr's preparation of antipyrin (1883) the field of pharmaceutical chemisty was dominated by the Germans. It required the exigencies of a third war to stimulate national pharmaceutical independence.

So far as there was American production of pharmaceutical chemicals before World War I, it was chiefly based on German research and conducted by people of German origin or at least German scientific education.

The firm of Rosengarten and Sons, for example, was founded by German-Swiss people and based essentially on German and partly on French discoveries. It held its own through a whole century, finally amalgamating with Merck and Company.

The Mallinckrodt Chemical Works of St. Louis is one of the few important American firms which specialized from the beginning in the manufacture of "pure chemicals for use in medicine, photography, and the arts." It was founded by three brothers of German descent (1867), two of whom "had just returned from a four years' residence in Germany where they completed their chemical education."[121]

Some large German firms had their own factories in the United States long before America entered World War I. For example, the American firm of Merck and Company had been started here as a branch of the old German mother concern (1891). Likewise, at the end of the 19th century the German essential-oil house of Fritzsche Brothers established laboratories in New Jersey. After the separation from the mother concern, and by virtue of its own scientific research, the American firm developed into one of the leading establishments of its kind in the world.

After World War I

Until World War I most products of the German pharmaceuticochemical industry were not manufactured in the United States, but only sold here under protection by American patents. The entrance of America into the war against Germany led to legislation to seize these patents and to make them available to American industry. *Chemical Industries* states,

The development of an American synthetic organic chemical industry was made possible by the late President Woodrow Wilson when he gave his approval to the organizing of The Chemical Foundation, Inc., to take over seized German chemical patents. Under the Foundation's charter, American manufacturers were enabled to use these chemical patents on equal terms and conditions. The use of these patents by American chemists was the beginning of a real effort to build up a 100 per cent self-contained synthetic organic chemical industry.[122]

What these spoils of war meant to American pharmaceutical industry, economically as well as in the quality of the chemicals manufactured here, becomes evident from the following quotation from a catalogue of the Abbott Laboratories in Chicago published in 1925.

For many years The Abbott Laboratories have manufactured fine medicinal chemicals; but this part of our business received a tremendous impetus during the World War, when we were asked by our Government to undertake the task of producing some of the synthetics formerly procurable only in Ger-

many. The difficulties of making organic medicinals in America have been and still are
very great but we are proud of the fact that
in spite of the technical complexity of the
problems to be dealt with, and in the face of
destructive competition from sources intent on
breaking the American chemical industry, we
have gone steadily forward.

In the list following these remarks, containing several compounds of German invention, mention is made of chlorazene,
dichloramine-T, arsphenamine, neoarsphen-
amine and sulpharsphenamine, as first made
in America by Abbott Laboratories, which
had been founded (1891) by a practicing
physician in Chicago.

For a still more obvious example of the
influence of the two World Wars (and of
postwar politics!) on the American phar
maceutical manufacturing industry, we may
consider the case history of Sterling Drug
Incorporated.[123] This steadily and rapidly
growing concern, amalgamating into its organization one firm after the other, got its
start as a partnership organized (1900) in
Sistersville, W. Va., for the purpose of
manufacturing an analgesic called "Neural-
gine." The founders were a pharmacist,
W. E. Weiss, and a friend of his, A. H.
Diebold, of Canton, Ohio. The concern
grew by adopting advertising as "a guiding
principle," and by "product diversification"
through purchase of other existing firms
(beginning with the J. W. James Company
in 1902 and the Sterling Remedy Company
in 1909), and in 1917 changed its corporate
name to Sterling Products, Incorporated.
There was progress, but it was slow. The
great chance for the firm came after World
War I, when the Alien Property Custodian
offered for sale the stock of the Bayer Company, Inc., of New York, "created by the
German Bayer Company to manufacture
and sell Aspirin, physicians' drugs and dyestuffs."

More than a hundred American firms
participated in the bidding at the public
auction (December 12, 1918). Sterling
topped all of them by a final bid of
$5,310,000. The Aspirin business was con-
tinued under the Bayer cross trademark,
while the Winthrop Chemical Company,

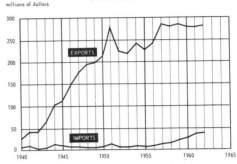

Source: U.S. Dept. of Commerce, U.S. Exports of Domestic & Foreign Merchandise (various annual issues).

Heavily dependent on drug imports
through the 19th century, the United
States became a major exporter of manufactured drugs only after the first World
War. The dramatic change shown in the
graph represents a ratio of exports to imports of more than 3 to 1 in 1925 compared with a ratio of 36 to 1 in 1952.
Although exports stabilized at a high
level after 1957, it may be seen that the
ratio has been narrowed by increasing
drug imports (valued by 1962 at approximately 277 million dollars in exports and
37 million dollars in imports). (Graph
from the Pharmaceutical Manufacturers
Association)

Inc., was organized as a new subsidiary to
manufacture the physicians' drugs which
had been acquired. The dye business "was
sold outright to another company." Trade-
mark difficulties were settled "through a
series of contracts with Farbenfabriken
vorm. Fried. Bayer & Company of Lever-
kusen, Germany, the former German owners
of American Bayer, and its successor, I. G.
Farben . . ." For a time Sterling became a
part of Drug Incorporated but resumed its
individual identity when (1933) this product of mass amalgamation was dissolved
"and its constituents went their several
ways." On this basis, expansion assumed a
rapid pace. The sales by Sterling in 1918
were $3,801,902; in 1944 they reached
$47,678,024, in 1957, $198,703,000 and in
1961, $229,199,000.

Early in 1941, "the company agreed to
cancel all contracts made by it or any of

its subsidiaries with I. G. Farben, and also to dissociate from its employment all persons who had any previous connection with Farben." After the canceling of all limiting contracts with the Germans (and of all German interests in any of the products of the company),

Sterling became the strongest competitor of I. G. Farben in the pharmaceutical markets of Latin America. . . . Winthrop's scientists cracked closely guarded German research secrets. It took them only a single year to learn how to make Atabrine on a commercial scale from raw materials available in the United States. . . . In 1942 the corporate name was changed to Sterling Drug Inc. and the corporate structure revamped through the absorption of 16 domestic subsidiaries into the parent organization . . . to assume more effective operation of an enterprise serving a multiplicity of professions, businesses, countries and peoples.

Concentration of Industry

Wars had laid the groundwork for this amazing development. The modern trend toward mammoth organization in industry at large has led also to a still-growing pharmaceutical edifice. With the growth seen in recent decades has come considerable restructuring of the pharmaceutical industry: heavier financial investments in the industry, notably from new outside sources, including the general public; more involvement of "outsiders" in the business of the industry, often through purchase or merger; an increased merger movement, especially vertically;[124] and, more recently, a diversification (especially amalgamation with producers of home remedies) by some companies formerly specializing in producing prescription drugs. Although the prescription-drug industry has not had as much of the market concentrated in the top companies as do many other industries, the 20 largest companies increased their share of the drug market from 63 per cent to 72 per cent between 1947 and 1956.[125] However, no single manufacturer has captured as much as 10 per cent of the drug market, and the number of manufacturing laboratories has grown slowly through the decades, with nearly 1,400 tabulated in 1954, as compared with about 1,100 in 1939; but

of these, only about 400 were plants with 20 or more employees.[126] Thus it can be seen that many small laboratories are still manufacturing, especially in the field of pharmaceutical preparations for a regional market. For example, 724 manufacturers of pharmaceutical preparations were employing, in 1954, fewer than 10 persons each (2,582 employees). Only 439 manufacturers employed more than 10 persons each, but their total employment numbered 73,969. In the same year 93 manufacturers of biologic products were tabulated (39 with fewer than 10 employees; 54 with more). There were 115 manufacturers of medicinal chemicals (also botanicals), of which 59 employed fewer than 10 employees, while 56 employed more than 10. However, the value of products produced by just 16 of these firms was 7 times that of all the other 99 combined.[127]

Cooperative effort and advancement of standards in the pharmaceutical industry are fostered through the Pharmaceutical Manufacturers Association ("P.M.A."), whose 140 members collectively produce about 90 per cent of the prescription drugs coming out of American laboratories. Of about 80 committees and subcommittees functioning in the P.M.A., more than half are involved in scientific matters to some degree. This organization was formed (1958) from two predecessor organizations.[128]

The American Drug Manufacturers Association (f. 1912) had attracted particularly the producers of "official and other nonsecret preparations to be dispensed by pharmacists on prescription, or to be used in compounding prescriptions." In 1931 member firms produced more than 80 per cent of all "druggists preparations."[129] Manufacturers who stressed the rising class of ready-made trade named prescription products had belonged either to this association or a second one, the American Pharmaceutical Manufacturers' Association (f. 1908), which tended also to attract the physicians' supply houses (making drugs packaged particularly for dispensing physicians). As conditions of drug manufacture and distribution changed over the years, the differences between the two associations became more diffuse and ill defined, while the duplication of efforts become more obvious, leading to their amalgamation in 1958 after more than 4 decades of separate existence.

The manufacturers of so-called patent medicines (not patented medicines!), i.e., "medicines . . . bearing coined names protected by trademarks and intended primarily for self-medication,"[130] are organized as the Proprietary Association of America (founded 1881). After 1938 the secret composition of most of these medicines was unmasked when a declaration of "the common or usual name of each active ingredient" was required by the revamped Federal Food, Drug and Cosmetic Act.

Production Volume

The value of the products prepared and sold annually by the pharmaceutical industry has been increasing steadily. Amounting to $51,000,000 in 1905, it multiplied more than 6-fold within a quarter century ($325,000,000 by 1929). Divided by classes of medication, the 1929 figures are $120,000,000 for "druggists' preparations," $56,000,000 for "ethical specialties" and $149,000,000 for "patent medicines" and other proprietaries sold to the general public,[131] while sales of cosmetics and toiletries amounted to $161,246,000.[132]

By 1947 (*Drug Topics* survey) consumers were spending an estimated $2,822,432,000 for all types of health products (in all types of stores). As to cosmetics, the industry estimated that in 1947 retail sales reached $744,000,000. In 1958, prescription-product manufacturers alone were estimated to have a volume of $1.8 billion (at producer's selling prices). By 1962 the estimate had soared past the $2 billion mark, with a distribution pattern of approximately three fifths to community pharmacies, one fifth to hospitals and one fifth to physicians (including 1.5% to other nonpharmacy community outlets).[133] While these figures are not directly comparable with those cited for the earlier period, there has been clearly a rather phenomenal increase in the production and the distribution of drug and cosmetic products.

Part of this increase is due to the expansion of the foreign market, especially between the end of World War II and 1957,

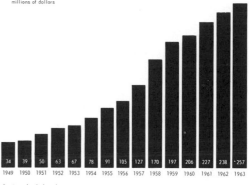

RESEARCH AND DEVELOPMENT OF U. S. PHARMACEUTICAL INDUSTRY, 1949-1963

millions of dollars

34	39	50	63	67	78	91	105	127	170	197	206	227	238	*257
1949	1950	1951	1952	1953	1954	1955	1956	1957	1958	1959	1960	1961	1962	1963

*estimated or budgeted

The graph illustrates the steady growth of expenditures by industry in the United States directed toward the discovery and the development of drugs intended primarily for prescription use by humans. The data represent firms distributing at least nine tenths of the prescribed drugs dispensed in the United States. Expenditures were for research performed or financed by the firms (including development of drugs through pilot-trial stage but not including marketing research and the like; and including overhead but not capital expenditures). The total research investment during the 15-year period exceeds $1.9 billion. (Graph from the Pharmaceutical Manufacturers Association)

during which time drug exports increased roughly 2½ times, far more than American exports in general.[134] Most of the large drug manufacturing plants in the United States have established footholds, subsidiaries and branches in other countries, not only in North and South America, Australia, Africa and the Near and the Far East, but in Europe as well. The United States, a country which long imported scientific ideas as well as most of the products based on them, has become an exporter of both. The drug industry prides itself on having taken a vigorous part in scientific development. Rapid development of research in and production of antibiotics has found the United States in the forefront, in close cooperation with English scientists, and much of the progress that has been made in the development of sulfonamides, vitamins, hormones and blood derivatives and blood substitutes is substantially based on original American research.

Importance of Industrial Research

Scientific research gradually became an integral part of pharmaceutical industry between the late 19th century and the years following World War I. After the first quarter of the present century, the fruits of such research decisively transformed drug therapy. The American industrial investment in this endeavor, about $60 million annually by 1951, increased nearly 4-fold during the ensuing decade, as competition in scientific terms continued to intensify. By the early 1960's the 23 largest pharmaceutical manufacturers had approximately 6,000 persons on their scientific staffs for research of one kind or another.

To support research adequately—a speculative and costly enterprise—has become increasingly difficult for smaller manufacturers. For example, among 86 manufacturing laboratories, it was found that a fourth of these firms (annual sales of more than $30 million each) had about 85 per cent of all the research employees and about 6 of every 7 of the scientific men employed by the 86 firms reporting.[135]

One indication of the yield from industrial research efforts of this magnitude comes from a study covering two decades. From 1941 to 1961 United States manufacturers originated at least 308 single chemical entities that were sufficiently useful to remain regularly available on prescription at the end of the period. These industry-originated drugs apparently represented 9 out of 10 medico-chemical entities solely of American origin. Among the additional medicinal chemical entities introduced by American firms but originated abroad (wholly or partly, 1941-1961, and still used), Switzerland, Germany and the United Kingdom evidently originated almost as many (about 18% of the total) as all other countries combined.[136] Since 1948 the number of single medicinal chemicals introduced nationally into prescription practice each year normally ranges between 30 and 50, although there are 10 times as many prescription products introduced (duplicates, mix-

tures, additional forms). Fewer than 100 American manufacturers participated in these innovations before the 1950's, but since then (to 1963) the number has varied between 100 and 130 companies.[137]

During the last 30 years American manufacturing pharmacy, as well as the legal and the educational standards of American pharmacy, has progressed quite as far as American medicine during the same period. As for proprietary medicines and their advertising, conditions have improved considerably, largely because of the unremitting efforts of the American Medical Association and other agencies in combatting pseudo-scientific pretenders in the health field and because of effects of the Wheeler-Lea Act. The remodeling of the Food, Drug and Cosmetic Act in 1938 and 1962, with rigid regulation of the labeling of drugs, medical devices, cosmetics and food-stuffs and of the introduction of new drugs on the market (dependent on examination of the claims and test data by the Food and Drug Administration) advanced standards of operation still further.

The pharmaceutical industry has given the dispensing pharmacist a more effective drug armamentarium. Conversely, it was community pharmacy that provided a nucleus for the development of industrial pharmaceutical manufacturing. And pharmacy has always given some of its best men to industrial pharmacy. The industry has good reason to foster the teamwork between dispensing pharmacy and manufacturing pharmacy and the continuance of the desire as well as the ability of the rising generation in pharmacy to aid the staffs of manufacturing laboratories. As for those in community and hospital pharmacies during this new era of drug production, Robert L. McNeil, speaking as president of the drug manufacturers, voiced a key concept:

In the face of rapid new developments he [the pharmacist] can become the source of expert drug knowledge for his busy colleague in the health professions—the doctor. To fulfill this highest professional function, the pharmacist should welcome all new additions to the medical armamentarium and should make every effort to keep building his vast foundation of drug information.[138]

Part Four

Discoveries and Other Contributions
to Society by Pharmacists

17: The American Pharmacist and Society

At this stage the term pharmacist does not need to be explained. What, though, do we mean by the term "society"? There are two main conceptions, the first being the discriminative designation of a group of people who represent, actually or supposedly, a cultural or financial standard higher than that of the common people; the other, a synonym for the social organism, the organization of peaceful and fruitful human relations. "Without this intersubjective intercourse mankind would remain a herd; with it they become a society."[1] It is service in this second kind of society by American pharmacists which is dealt with here.

THE PHARMACIST IN CIVIC LIFE

Philadelphians Set a Precedent

Pharmacists to whom the founding of the Philadelphia College of Pharmacy can be attributed set an early example of social contributions from the profession. The first president of the college, Charles Marshall, was active in the Society of Friends, carried on various civic activities and is said to have been "one of the picturesque figures of the Revolution on the patriot side . . ." and "a deep student of Latin and Greek."[2] The first vice-president, Peter Williamson, achieved the highest degree in American Masonry.[3] The second president, William Lehman, was an active member of the Pennsylvania legislature and one of the leaders of the Philadelphia Athenaeum (to which he left a bequest of $10,000).[4] The third president, Daniel B. Smith, "was elected a member of the Franklin Institute immediately after its organization in 1824 and was an incorporator of the Historical Society of Pennsylvania." He was elected a member of the American Philosophical Society (1829) and was also a member of the Academy of Natural Sciences. Furthermore, he was elected to the chairs of moral philosophy, English literature and chemistry at Haverford College (1834) and was made principal. He resigned to give increased attention to his pharmacy.[5] Henry Troth, whose energy did much to bring about the founding of the Philadelphia College of Pharmacy, is said to have been "one of the most progressive citizens of Philadelphia of his day . . . active in many philanthropic, business, and scientific organizations."[6] Later officers and teachers of the Philadelphia College of Pharmacy followed the example set by their early predecessors. The founding of the renowned Swarthmore College by the Society of Friends was largely due to the "personal exertions" of the pharmacist Edward Parrish, a professor at the Philadelphia College of Pharmacy (1864 to 1872). Parrish became the first president of Swarthmore College, and one of its buildings still carries the name "Parrish Hall."

To such men their profession of pharmacy must have seemed only a special aspect of their endeavor to render a particular service to society. This idea became more general as the professional status of pharmacy became more generally recognized. Thus American pharmacists participated to a remarkable extent in the development of American social life. People more and more took it for granted that the pharmacist was a well-educated man, whose advice and assistance were at the disposal of his fellow citizens. Often he grew up with his business, in his home town. It was only natural that he enjoyed the confidence of his fellow citizens and sometimes became the guardian of the general cultural development in his place of residence.

In rural districts and smaller towns, the

pharmacist has been now and again the mostly unpaid expert in questions requiring chemical and botanic knowledge. The method of the famous botanist G. H. E. Mühlenberg of asking "apothecaries . . . for the medicinal qualities and the trivial names of the officinal indigenous plants" he collected[7] has been followed in numerous noticed and unnoticed cases by other botanists as well as by laymen interested in botany, at least until pharmacists no longer needed to take such study so seriously in their own education and work. Probably most sizable communities can recall examples of a pharmacist's contribution to social welfare growing out of his professional knowledge and ethical commitments—such as the work that earned pharmacist Abraham Fleisher of Wyncote, Pa., a Presidential Citation for Meritorious Service to the Handicapped (1962).[8]

Historian of His Environs

Often the pharmacist became the historian of his parish, his city or even his state. A splendid example was the pharmacist Roy Bird Cook of West Virginia (1886-1961). Besides several pamphlets on historical subjects, Cook wrote *Family and Early Life of Stonewall Jackson* (1924) and other books. Although excelling the relatively dilettante endeavors of his colleagues, Roy Bird Cook can be considered the representative of American pharmacy in the great American historical movement. He never left practical pharmacy and devoted his talents to the history of pharmacy as well as fostering the profession's current progress. He wrote a noteworthy monograph on *The Rise of Organized Pharmacy in West Virginia* (1931; reprinted in the *Proceedings* of the West Virginia State Pharmaceutical Association, 1931), and a booklet entitled *The Annals of Pharmacy in West Virginia* (1946). When the University of West Virginia bestowed on him the honorary degree of Doctor of Laws, it was expressly declared that this honor indicated appreciation not only of the historian but also of the exemplary pharmacist.[9]

A similar example is the manufacturing pharmacist Eli Lilly, who wrote *Prehistoric Antiquities of Indiana* (1937) and a historical work on his own church, *The Little Church on the Circle* (1957) and engaged in other historical activities which earned a citation from the American Association for State and Local History. Mr. Lilly also demonstrated his conviction that "generosity should go beyond the limits of expediency," by the part he has played in many civic and philanthropic institutions.[10]

Humanitarian Endeavor

One of the least heralded of volunteer contributions has been humanitarian work by pharmacists, teamed with practitioners of the other health professions, in underdeveloped areas of the world. These representatives of the profession usually have served for little more than the satisfaction their work so richly yields. Often they leave secure positions at home to become part of a medical missionary team sponsored by one of the religious denominations. A secular counterpart, since the early 1960's, has been the scattering of pharmacists who serve in the Peace Corps.[11]

For various periods of duty, going back at least to 1910, American pharmacists have been working in field missions. Although at least some 30 individuals can be identified, their ministry to the poor and afflicted has been so unpublicized that we do not know how many more there have been. In addition to dispensing drugs, their work has included education, hospital management, drug manufacture and sanitation.[12]

Still another variant of such humanitarian service is exemplified in the voyages of the S.S. Hope. Practicing pharmacists across the country have contributed to this nonprofit private venture, pharmaceutical manufacturers donated millions of dollars in drugs, and pharmacists, together with other health personnel, have taken tours of duty on the ship to various parts of the world.[13]

THE PHARMACIST IN PUBLIC SERVICE

Pharmacy as a profession is and has to be public service; therefore, each pharmacist honestly serving his profession is a public servant. In general, however, the label "public servant" is restricted to persons holding public office, either by appointment or by election.

In the offices open to all citizens of the United States, pharmacists have always served in city, state and federal administrations, and many have served in legislatures of their states and in Congress. For example, in 1927 Georgia had no less than 9 pharmacists among its legislators. Idaho counted, at the same time, 3 senators and 3 representatives from the ranks of pharmacy. The Michigan legislature had 2 senators and 9 representatives who had been pharmacists.[14] In 25 states surveyed by the National Association of Retail Druggists (1945) not less than 51 pharmacists were serving in state legislatures. Furthermore, there were counted in the same states, without any pretense of completeness, 9 mayors or city commissioners with pharmaceutical backgrounds, a state treasurer, and many members of public health committees.[15] In 1955 a pharmacist was serving on the board of health in 23 states (including 16 states that made it mandatory).[16] When further inquiry was made in 1961, incomplete data showed 25 pharmacists on state boards of health, 38 in state legislatures or cabinets, and 25 as mayor of their cities.[17] Raleigh, North Carolina, offers an interesting example of the latter sphere of service, where pharmacists were mayors or other important municipal officials for more than two decades, excepting 2 or 3 years. "The people of Raleigh," wrote R. O. King, "recommend the 'pill rollers' to the world as honest, progressive, and efficient city officials."[18]

As early as 1860 a practicing pharmacist, John Gately Downey, was elected to the governorship of a state (California) by admiring fellow citizens, after his service as lieutenant governor. This pioneer and pharmacist had been the first person to establish a pharmacy in Los Angeles and "the first resident of Southern California to gain the highest position in the state. One of the lasting monuments commemorative of Downey's life is a town twelve miles southwest of Los Angeles which bears his

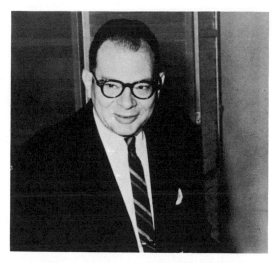

The former practicing pharmacist, Henry L. Giordano, during an interview following his selection (1962) as United States Commissioner of Narcotics. (Photograph from *Drug Topics* and Reni Photos)

name."[19] In more recent years the high office of governor has been occupied by men with pharmaceutical background in Arkansas, Arizona, Iowa, Maine and South Carolina. While these men had left the profession before entering politics, a pharmacist of Wisconsin who became governor (1947-51), Oscar Rennebohm, remained in the practice of his profession.

In Washington

At the federal level, apparently only one pharmacist has achieved the rank of membership in the President's Cabinet, David Henshaw of Boston. As Secretary of the Navy he served less than a year (1843-44), because the Senate, out of deference to Daniel Webster and other Whigs, did not accept his appointment. However, he did serve long enough to prove his eminent qualifications, introduce a system of strict accountability for handling Navy funds and materials, and argue for the annexation of Texas. Henshaw had been an enterprising pharmacist, starting his own pharmacy at the age of 21. Within 13 years his clientele had grown to one of the largest in Boston

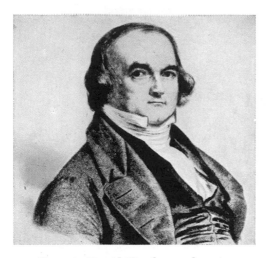

Druggist David Henshaw, who was appointed to the Cabinet of President Tyler, had given up the world of drugs for the world of politics and entrepreneurist adventure. (J. Am. Pharm. Assoc. 24:858, 1935)

pharmacy. In addition, he had become a banker, one of the directors of a railroad, and the founder and owner of a newspaper (*Boston Statesman*)![20]

At the rank of ambassador, Pharmacist Teodoro Moscoso of Puerto Rico (b. 1910) first served as United States representative to Venezuela, then was appointed by President Kennedy as U. S. Coordinator of the Alliance for Progress (1961), with the rank of Assistant Secretary of State. Moscoso (a member of Rho Chi, U. Michigan) served as the first president of the Colegio de Farmacéuticos de Puerto Rico (f. 1938), while president of the Puerto Rican-American Drug Co. He gained prominence as the administrator (1942-1961) of the highly successful "operation bootstrap" program for the economic development of Puerto Rico.

In Congress, pharmacists from time to time have taken their place alongside leading citizens from other walks of life in governing the country. Two recent examples are the representative and the senator who introduced the Durham-Humphrey amendments (1951) to the Federal Food, Drug and Cosmetic Act. Carl T. Durham had been a practicing pharmacist in North Carolina for 30 years before his election to Con-

gress (1938), where he served with distinction for 22 years. Actually, his political career began in 1922, as town councilman, and thereafter he held a continuous succession of public offices until he reached Washington. There he became noted particularly for his work as chairman of the Joint Committee on Atomic Energy of the United States Congress.

The second pharmacist, almost 20 years Durham's junior, has served in the United States Senate since 1948. Hubert H. Humphrey, the son of a pharmacist, practiced in the family pharmacy for 4 years before taking further studies to prepare for a career in public service and politics. His 3 years as mayor of Minneapolis served as a springboard to Washington, where he became an energetic and articulate senator and (under the Kennedy administration) assistant majority leader of the Senate.[21]

THE PHARMACIST IN THE ARMED FORCES

The frequent election of pharmacists to political office proves the confidence that the public has in them, in their ability and common sense, which doubtless is related to the part that pharmacy plays in the life and the minds of the people. But what of the role that pharmacy has been assigned in the armed forces of the United States? Here things have changed much since the Revolutionary War, to the detriment of pharmacy until comparatively recent periods.

In the Revolutionary War the apothecary serving in the army of the patriots in his professional capacity held a rank equal to that of the surgeon, being a commissioned officer. This remained unchanged in the War of 1812. H. George Wolfe, who has described the situation of American military pharmacy (and medicine) from the Revolutionary War until 1821,[22] has this to say about pharmacy during the War of 1812:

Economizing peacetime congressmen had not allowed the Army to utilize the experience which the medical [and pharmaceutical] officers had gained during the Revolutionary War. . . . It was not until 1813—when nine months of war had vastly aggravated the situation—that

Congress took action. An act of March 3 provided that . . . a physician and surgeon general, as well as an apothecary general be appointed, with annual salaries of 2,500 and 1,800 dollars respectively. Dr. Francis LeBarron, a former Navy and Army surgeon was chosen for the position of apothecary general.

More than a year later, a man whose former activities had been of a pharmaceutical nature was appointed assistant apothecary general of the United States Army. This man was James Cutbush.

The "Rules and Regulations for the Army" issued on May 1, 1813 . . . provided . . . detailed information about the new uniform which was identical for all officers of the medical department and quite ornate. It was not until December, 1814, that the War Department clearly defined the duties of the various types of medical officers. Concerning the "Apothecary General and his assistants" it was stated that they were "to receive and take charge of all hospital stores, medicines, surgical instruments and dressings, bought by the Commissary General of Purchases" and that they were to "account to the Supt. General of Military Supplies for all expenditures of the same." They were further directed "to compound and prepare all officinals and put up and issue medicines, etc., in chests or otherwise, conformably to requisitions."

. . . After the war's end . . . by an act of March 3, 1815 Congress reduced the Army to a minimum. . . . To the Secretary of War, this seemed to imply the end of the Hospital Department and the necessity of discharging the physician and surgeon general, the assistant apothecaries general and many other officers. Yet significantly, the President directed in May, 1815, that the apothecary general and two assistants be retained in the "Military Peace Establishment of the United States." The office of "Physician and Surgeon General," however, was abolished, and the Apothecary General became the ranking Officer of the Medical Department until 1818. In that year there was appointed the first officer to bear the present title of "Surgeon General."

. . . In 1818, the office of the "commissary general of purchases" was abolished by the Army. Consequently, "that portion of his duties which pertained to the Medical Department" was transferred to the apothecary general and his assistants. . . . General Orders from the War Department, issued in Septem-

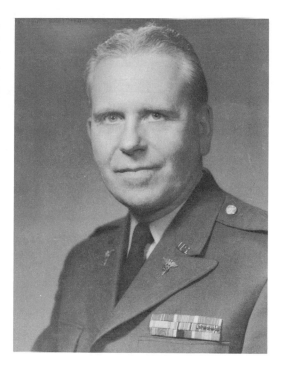

A former practicing pharmacist in Minnesota and Wisconsin, Bernard Aabel (b. 1907) is representative of those of his profession who have made distinguished contributions to governmental and military service. He has headed a major departmental unit in the Army Surgeon General's Office; he served in the American Embassy at Helsinki (military attaché); he became Deputy Commander, then Commander at the largest military medical installation during the Korean War. Later, Col. Aabel was responsible for procurement of Regular career officers for all 6 corps of the Army Medical Service Corps (64 allied specialties). He was serving the Central Intelligence Agency before becoming Director (1962) of the Department of International Health of the American Medical Association. (Photograph from the U. S. Army)

ber 1818, outline the new—and the old—duties at great length [cited in full in Wolfe's meritorious paper].

In March, 1821, Congress had once more reduced "the military peace establishment of the United States." The budget did not allow for retention of the following grades, among others: assistant surgeons general, apothecary general, assistant apothecaries general. The holders of these offices were unceremoniously discharged.

In the long period between 1821 and 1861 there was not much need for a regular pharmaceutical service in the insignificant army and navy of the United States. Moreover, pharmacists evinced little interest in this service.

It is significant that the existence of something like a pharmaceutical service in the armed forces of the United States was not recorded and commented on by the representatives of organized American pharmacy before 1862 when the editor of the *American Journal of Pharmacy* commented:

Occasionally, for many years, apothecaries have been employed on some of our naval vessels to facilitate the duties of the surgeons; but from the fact that no rank attaches to the position, we are told, it is but little sought after, as the "surgeon's mate" is socially ill situated on ship-board. We are not aware, that the apothecary has heretofore been employed in the medical department of the "regular" army of the United States. . . . To make this service more effective, it should be separated sufficiently from that of the surgeon to give a distinct standing and rank to the pharmaceutist, as in the French army, with clearly defined duties, that his proper self-respect, and ambition to be eminent in his sphere, may have ample room for display. Unless such an arrangement can be made it is not probable that the better class of graduates in pharmacy would seek positions of this kind.[23]

A law of May 20, 1862, created a special group of pharmaceutical professionals in the military service by authorizing the Secretary of War "to add to the Medical Department of the Army, Medical Storekeepers, not exceeding six in number, who shall have the pay and emoluments of Military Storekeepers of the Quartermaster's Department, who shall be skilled Apothecaries or Druggists."

The duties of these men were "under the direction of the Surgeon General and Medical Purveyors, with the storing and safe keeping of medical and hospital supplies, and with the duties of receiving, issuing and accounting for the same according to

regulations." These "U. S. Army Storekeepers were granted the pay and the allowances of a first lieutenant of the Army but no actual rank."[24]

This small group of pharmacists must be considered rather a civil than a military addition to the Army. It was in a similar civil rather than a military rôle that John M. Maisch served the United States during the Civil War by conducting the laboratory of the United States Army at Philadelphia after 2 years of collaboration with the manufacturer and former United States Navy Surgeon E. R. Squibb.

Insofar as pharmacists were engaged in their professional rôle within the regular military service of the Army and the Navy, they ranked as Hospital Stewards.[25]

With the close of the Civil War, serious attempts to better the position of the military pharmacists seem to have ended. In 1894, we find for the first time, among the committees of the American Pharmaceutical Association, a "Special Committee on the Status of Pharmacists in the Army and Navy of the United States."[26] In the following year, this Committee reported a detailed survey concerning the regulation of the pharmaceutical service in the armies of all civilized countries, and 2 proposals for a legal change of the status of pharmacists serving in the United States Army and Navy.[27]

As early as 1898, the Committee could report a first success, and it may be assumed that the Spanish-American War provided the necessary favorable atmosphere. In the Navy the situation complained of during the Civil War still prevailed, and the naval apothecary had no legal status at all. Therefore, the endeavor of the Committee was centered on this question as the most urgent one. It succeeded, to the extent that the Hale Bill for the first time recognized pharmacists as representatives of a special profession with just claims to an appropriate designation, rank and pay. The bill established a Hospital Corps of the United States Navy consisting of "pharmacists, hospital stewards, hospital apprentices, and for this purpose the Secretary of the Navy is empowered to appoint twenty-five pharmacists with the rank, pay and privileges of warrant officers."[28] In 1902, the pharmaceutical "hospital stewards" too were granted the title of pharmacist.[29]

A significant sequel came only a year after New York passed a bill assigning a pharmacist to each regiment of the New York National Guard, with the title of pharmacist and the rank of first lieutenant in the State of New York.[30] This bill was repealed because of the alleged inadequate "social standing of pharmacists."[31]

The year 1903 in some ways was a landmark in the relations between official pharmacy and the agencies in which pharmacists were or should be working professionally as public servants. At the meeting of the American Pharmaceutical Association the United States Navy and the Department of Agriculture were represented by delegates. The United States Army declined to be represented, stating that "the position of pharmacist or apothecary does not exist in the Army," that "there are some graduates of pharmacy and many others competent to fill prescriptions . . . among our Sergeants . . ." and that "the Sergeant must be first a soldier, the dispensing of the 'ready-prepared tablets' or compounding of the 'simple medicines required' being only 'one of his secondary duties.' "[32]

No further progress was made until 1916, when two new grades, Master Hospital Sergeant and Hospital Sergeant, were created in the United States Army. In the Navy "the pay and allowances that are now or may hereafter be allowed a lieutenant in the United States Navy" were granted to the Chief Pharmacist on the active list.[33]

After World War I

The experiences of World War I, in conjunction with the increasing educational requirements for pharmacists, began to become effective by 1922. According to a letter of the Surgeon General there were at this time "about fifteen commissioned officers of the Medical Department [meaning the Medical Administrative Corps established in 1920] who are pharmacists, these being commissioned . . . in the grades of captain, first and second lieutenants" beside 69 pharmacists "already commissioned in

the Medical Administrative Reserve."[34] Two years later the number of pharmacists in the Reserve section of the medical service had increased to 89, and "twenty-five commissions have been granted with a rank above that of Captain in the Sanitary Corps."[35]

In the same year a bill was passed, then vetoed by the President, but finally became law in 1926, concerning governmental service "based upon the established principles of a profession or science and which requires professional, scientific, or technical training, equivalent to that represented by graduation from a college or university of recognized standing." With this law the requirements for pharmacists as applicants for professional public service were clearly defined.

The difficulties which had to be overcome did not come mainly from outside the profession. Once pharmaceutical education was on an equal footing with that of other professions, the pharmacist could expect a commensurate position in governmental service.

In 1936, a bill finally made graduation from a recognized 4-year school of pharmacy a prerequisite for appointment to the Medical Administrative Corps, appointees receiving the grade of second lieutenant. The number of these Regular Army pharmacist-officers, who had to pass an examination before appointment, was limited to 16. The development was epitomized in a report to the American Pharmaceutical Association (1937):

Ten years ago, pharmacy was still listed as a sub-profession. . . . To-day, pharmacy is recognized fully as a profession; pharmacists are classified in the professional as well as the sub-professional groups under the Civil Service. . . .[36]

This change was crowned by two acts of Congress creating a special Pharmacy Corps of the United States Army (act of July 12, 1943), and putting pharmacists in the United States Public Health Service on the same plan as other officers of the service (1944).

The Pharmacy Corps was created as a separate unit against the advice of the ad-

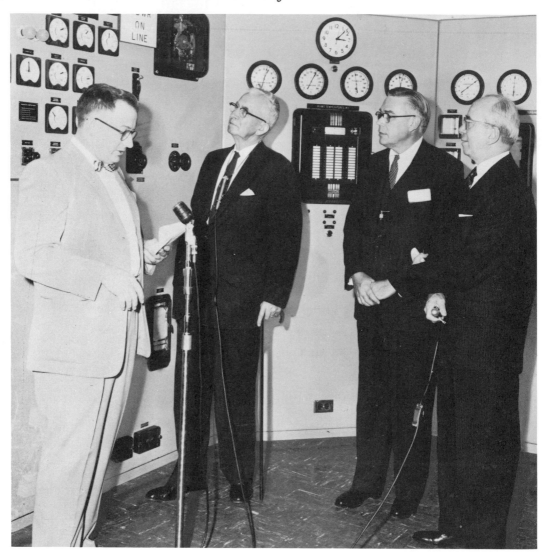

The pharmacist in civic life is exemplified by Congressman Carl T. Durham of North Carolina (second from left), shown about to throw the switch starting the experimental boiling-water reactor at Argonne National Laboratory (1957). Durham, who was serving as chairman of the Joint Committee on Atomic Energy, is accompanied by Lewis L. Strauss (far right), then chairman of the Atomic Energy Commission. (Photograph from Argonne National Laboratory and *Drug Topics*)

ministration of the Army Medical Department. In the opinion of the Surgeon General and his staff, it was only by cooperation with the other medical auxiliary groups within one administrative unit that the greatest benefit could accrue from the services of well-educated military pharmacists. Since the education of the pharmacist makes him acquainted with a range of sciences and their applications in a way not paralleled by any other single profession, the qualified pharmacist has been regarded by some as the coordinator par excellence of services rendered by medical auxiliary groups.

It was largely for this reason that, with

the consent of organized pharmacy (given after the demands of pharmacy were satisfactorily met), a Medical Service Corps in both the Army and the Navy was established by law (August 4, 1947) bringing increased opportunities for pharmacists in commissioned rank and for proper development of military pharmacy. (With the advent of this new administrative structure the separate and chronically controversial Pharmacy Corps was abolished.)

The highest rank to be achieved by a pharmacist in the Army is that of Colonel, in the Navy that of Captain. The Army Medical Service Corps had as its first Chief a pharmacist, Colonel Othmar F. Goriup. In the Navy at that time, Commander W. Paul Briggs was the highest ranking pharmaceutical officer, guiding the development of the pharmaceutical service of the U. S. Navy Bureau of Medicine and Surgery. With the upward stabilization of the pharmaceutical activities and rank in the United States Navy, the titles of "Pharmacists' Mate" as the designation of enlisted Hospital Corps personnel, and of "Pharmacist" as the designation of Warrant Officers were finally abandoned (neither title presupposing graduation in pharmacy).[37]

In 1962 the Navy had 43 billets for pharmacy officers, although additional pharmacists were serving as officers in other related fields; the Army had 93 pharmacy officers authorized, plus a number of civilian pharmacists practicing in Army hospitals; while the Air Force had 252 commissioned pharmacists in various professional, scientific and administrative services.[37a]

Veterans Administration

Although not a part of the armed forces of the United States, the Veterans Administration may be referred to at this time. Since World War II it has developed into an important organization in which pharmaceutical activities play an essential part. Due to the initiative and the clear-mindedness of Commander W. Paul Briggs, Director of Pharmacy Service in the Veterans Administration through 1947, this service developed admirably within the veterans' hospitals and was brought into harmony with the interests of pharmacy in general.

In the Veterans Administration, by 1953, 450 qualified pharmacists were practicing under Civil Service appointments in some 165 hospitals and other posts (615 in 1962). Inpatient or outpatient pharmaceutical facilities had been developed in every state, but these have been supplemented by contract-service from private hometown pharmacies. Despite periodic controversy over regulations governing the "hometown" service, millions of prescriptions have been thus dispensed to veterans with service-connected disabilities.

Organizationally, pharmacy functions in the Veterans Administration "on a level with the other professional specialties," with a Director of Pharmacy Service (since 1954, the pharmacist Vernon O. Trygstad), who is responsible to the Chief of Professional Services. An Assistant Director of Pharmacy Service has program responsibility, aided by pharmacy specialists in specific fields such as drug standards, personnel and operating procedures; while other pharmacists function as field supervisors of pharmacy operations. This professional level has been reached only since 1946 (under Public Law 293, 79th Congress).[38]

PHARMACISTS IN THE PUBLIC HEALTH SERVICE

The United States Public Health Service originated in an act (July 16, 1798) creating the "Marine Hospital Service" for sick and disabled seamen. As additional duties fostering general public health were gradually imposed on this agency, its designation evolved into the "United States Public Health Service" (1912).

Beginning in 1897, graduation in pharmacy became a requirement for those appointed to pharmaceutical duties. When the U. S. Public Health Service was further authorized (1930) to commission pharmacists, comparable to the commissioning of medical officers, it became a precedent that has since benefited pharmacists in other branches of government service.[39]

The duties and, still more, the performance of these men never have been limited to strictly pharmaceutical activities. They always have been both managerial and professional and have included quarantine procedure, supply and research. It is significant that one of the most remarkable pharmaceutical officers in the Public Health Service, Benjamin Holsendorf (d. 1944) devoted the greater part of his more than 40 years of service to a successful study of rat infestation of ships and its prevention. In an article on the rôle of the pharmacists in the Public Health Service as individuals and as a group the U.S.P.H.S. pharmacists George F. Archambault, Thomas A. Foster and Raymond D. Kinsey have said of recent developments:

In 1944 the new Public Health Service Act lifted the promotion limitation and pharmacists can now be promoted to the director grade, which corresponds to an Army Colonel. . . . There was established in 1945 a Pharmacy Service with a Senior Pharmacist officer as its full-time chief. This pharmacy unit functions as part of the Hospital Division . . . which in turn is part of the Bureau of Medical Services. . . . The Service Senior Regular Corps pharmacist officer has been assistant to the chief of the Bureau since early 1944 . . .[40]

The three pharmacists here quoted are among the most distinguished who have served the United States Public Health Service. Raymond D. Kinsey became (1949) the first pharmacist to receive the rank of Director (equivalent to Army colonel); and, subsequently, Thomas A. Foster and George F. Archambault both were likewise promoted to Director. Foster, originally a community pharmacist in Alabama, worked up through the ranks (since 1933) to become Chief of Supply and Procurement for the entire service. On assignments with the Office of Defense Mobilization and in other government activities he rendered distinguished pharmaceutical service. Pharmaceutical progress in the Division of Hospitals has been steady under the administration of George F. Archambault, pharmacist-lawyer from Massachusetts, who entered the Public Health Service (1947) to become Chief of the Pharmacy Branch

and (since 1959) to represent the Service in all pharmaceutical activities.[41]

By 1954 every pharmaceutical function in the Public Health Service was being "carried out by either a commissioned pharmacist or a Civil Service civilian pharmacist." This recognition has proved to be more difficult to achieve in the armed forces, which have shown a chronic preference, whenever circumstances permit, to induct pharmacy graduates in the enlisted ranks under Selective Service.

Pharmacists have been employed (104 regular and 85 reserve officers, 1962) at U.S.P.H.S. posts in hospitals, clinics, quarantine and supply stations, Indian Affairs clinics, prisons, state health services and in the Washington office of the Surgeon General.[42]

Any review of recent progress of pharmacy in government service, civil as well as military, would be incomplete without mentioning the effective support given by the pharmacist Carl T. Durham, former representative in Congress for North Carolina.

INDIVIDUAL PHARMACISTS IN GOVERNMENTAL SERVICE

There always have been individual pharmacists in public service with authority and pay commensurate with the high standard of their special work. The work referred to here is not pharmacy as such, although it draws on pharmaceutical knowledge and experience as well as other specialized training. Of the responsibilities assigned to such men, a few examples must suffice:

Lyman F. Kebler, who did meritorious work as Chief of the U.S.D.A. Drug Division (forerunner of the Food and Drug Administration) was not only a pharmacist but had the degree of Doctor of Medicine as well and was a chemist of recognized training and experience.

Frederick B. Power was head of the Phytochemical Laboratory of the United States Department of Agriculture (1916-1927), was a member of the National Research Council, and has been so far the only American pharmacist elected to the

National Academy of Science. Power was a chemist and pharmacist whose knowledge secured him a unique position and recognition as an international authority.

Oswald Schreiner, the first pharmacy student to earn the Doctor of Philosophy on the basis of graduate work in a school of pharmacy of an American university (1902, Wisconsin), became Chief of the Soil Fertility Division of the U. S. Department of Agriculture.

Frederick W. Irish, a former community pharmacist (1921-31), entered government service as a chemist, first for the Food and Drug Administration and then for the Federal Trade Commission. Since 1951 Mr. Irish has been Chief of the Commission's Division of Scientific Opinions.

Henry L. Giordano left the practice of pharmacy to devote his career to government service in the Bureau of Narcotics (1941). Rising through the ranks, he became Deputy Commissioner, and since 1962 has administered the entire program of narcotics control as the U. S. Commissioner of Narcotics.

Still other pharmacists have made notable contributions to the control of narcotics and

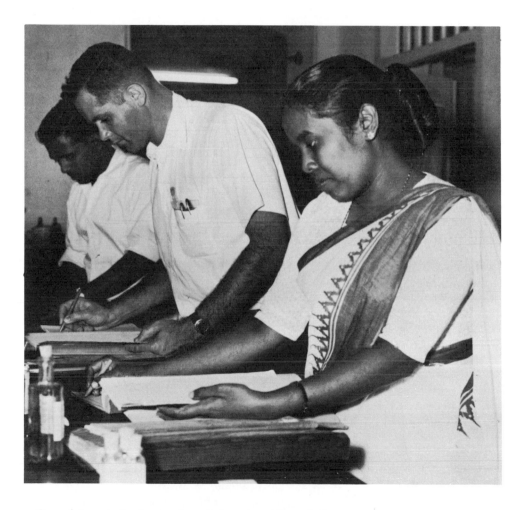

One of America's pharmacist-missionaries, Albert S. Bauman of Ohio (center), brings the pharmacy's records up to date with the aid of two Indian associates at the day's end in Vellore. The work of such pharmacists epitomizes a humanitarianism traditionally associated with all health professions. (Photograph from A. S. Bauman)

addiction, such as Joseph M. Bransky, who served the Bureau of Narcotics for 43 years, both in this country and abroad. He was honored by the government of Japan for his aid in restoring order in the distribution of narcotics after World War II and in organizing the present Japanese Pharmaceutical Association. Mr. Bransky has been lauded for the "unique sense of personal dedication which he gave his public trust."

A still different type of distinctive service by individual pharmacists is exemplified in Robert C. Gasen, a former community pharmacist from Illinois. The French government decorated him with the highest grade of the Order of Public Health, honoring the caliber of his medical supply work while attached to the Civilian Affairs Section of Allied Force Headquarters in Algiers, during World War II. Mr. Gasen later served with the U. S. Foreign Economic Administration.[43]

PHARMACEUTICAL EMERGENCY SERVICE

The rise of pharmaceutical education produced a growing number of men offering the necessary scientific knowledge as well as the experience and the administrative talents needed in governmental agencies dealing with drugs and regulations concerning their production and distribution. In recent times, officials coming from pharmacy have been such men as Frank A. Delgado, who for a decade was chief of the Drug Section in the Bureau of Foreign and Domestic Commerce and, during the war, headed the Drugs and Fine Chemicals Unit of the OPA* Chemicals and Drugs Branch (1941-1943), subsequently serving as medical supply officer for the Office of Foreign Relief and Rehabilitation. Indeed, the war brought a group of men from pharmacy into government posts to help deal with the special problems created in medical supply, a group perhaps most notably represented by Robert P. Fischelis as director of the Chemicals, Drugs and Health Supplies Division of the WPB† Office of Civil-

* Office of Price Administration.
† War Production Board.

ian Requirements (later Secretary of the American Pharmaceutical Association), and Fred J. Stock as chief of the Drugs and Cosmetics Branch of the WPB Chemicals Bureau.

Besides the public service performed in the daily routine of a profession, or in fulfilling the obligations of a public office, there is a third service dictated by emergency, which requires above all a special human quality and an unqualified readiness to help. In the great floods which this country has experienced, now and again, American pharmacists have proved themselves equal to such tasks, as the dramatic and tragic episodes of 1936 illustrated:

Their selfless loyalty to the public trust will furnish a bright chapter in that grim tale of destruction and misery. . . . They worked by candle and lamplight in unheated stores with ice water slopping over their boot-tops. They braved treacherous currents in calling for and delivering prescriptions by boat. They saved biologicals, first-aid supplies, flashlights, and foodstuffs. . . . They gave unstintingly of their professional knowledge, helping bacteriologists test water and food. . . . They manned relief centers. . . . They fought a successful battle for others against a rampant, hostile nature . . . .[44]

This role of the pharmacist in combatting nature's disasters finds a logical extension in civil defense against the threat of manmade disasters. While every pharmacist has a potential role to play locally, selected pharmacists help to provide the leadership for preparedness within a larger framework, such as pharmacist Arnold H. Dodge, Chief of the U.S.P.H.S. Health Resources Branch in the Division of Health Mobilization (a field of work he entered in 1955). Of such responsibilities, the Surgeon General of the U. S. Public Health Service, Leroy E. Burney, has said:

Because we recognize the planning abilities and diversified competencies of the pharmacist, we are presently placing heavy reliance on our headquarters pharmacists to develop plans and operational programs in the field of emergency medical supply, availability, stockpiling, distribution and utilization. However, it is only through disaster preparedness efforts of all pharmacists as members of the health profession team that we can hope to establish a firm basis for emergency medical care programs of the type anticipated under a post-nuclear attack situation.[45]

THE PHARMACIST IN LITERATURE

Only a few pharmacists have attained more than local fame in American literature. A discriminating examination perhaps would leave only one member of the profession whose writing was comprehensive and valuable enough to give him a place among American novelists: John Uri Lloyd. The versatility of this man seems miraculous. Not only did he work in many different fields but he attained a rank of considerable importance in all of them.

In fiction Lloyd may be grouped with those authors whose books always have found a hearty reception and a broad distribution, not so much because of their literary values, although they have not lacked such values, but as recognition of the sound philosophy of life, the knowledge of human nature, and the genuine love for justice on which they are built and which they inculcate.

The first book of fiction published by Lloyd, *Etidorhpa, or the End of the Earth* (1895), which went through no less than 18 editions up to 1936, represents a scientific vision of literary as well as informative value. In addition he wrote *The Right Side of the Car*, the story of a sentimental journey (1897); *Stringtown on the Pike*, a folklore study of Kentucky (1900); *Warwick of the Knob* (1901) and *Redhead* (1903), both based on the feudal past of Kentucky; *Scoggins* (1904), a peculiar story of an early and undying love; *Felix Moses, the Beloved Jew* (1930), the story of a Jewish peddler who fought in the Confederate Army during the Civil War, and *Our Willie*, which is set in the hills of Boone County, in old Kentucky.

Each [book] rapidly became a best seller and continued to be reprinted year after year. The demand for his books grew rapidly until suddenly he found himself confronted with the choice of turning author or sticking to pharmacy. He chose the latter course.[46]

The combination of historian and poet, perhaps typical of the literary pharmacist, was also characteristic of the Chicago pharmacist Edwin Oscar Gale (1832-1913) who conducted his pharmacy until his 66th year. He published *Reminiscences of Early Chicago* and a booklet of poetry, *Falling Leaves*, which had more than a local audience.[47]

In 1942, a practicing pharmacist, Shine Philipps of Big Spring, Texas, wrote *Big Spring*, a "biography" of his home town as the story of the simultaneous birth and growth of his pharmacy as well as of the community.

One man coming from pharmacy wrote his name with indelible ink into the history of American literature: O. Henry (to call him by his real name, William Sidney Porter, 1862-1910), the author of short stories that rank as classics of their kind. He had learned pharmacy in his home town of Greensboro, N. C., in his uncle's pharmacy, became licensed as a pharmacist in North Carolina, and had worked for 2 months in a drugstore in Austin, Texas. He became a bookkeeper, a bank clerk, and, finally (on a charge involving bank funds), the inmate of a penitentiary. It was here that O. Henry, who never admitted that he was guilty of the crime, returned to pharmacy and "was placed in the hospital as night drug clerk."[48] On the 85th anniversary of the birth of the writer-pharmacist, the Greensboro Historical Museum Society dedicated a memorial room, including a rare collection of O. Henryana and a recreated section of the old "Dr. Porter's Drugstore." E. P. Herman maintained that

O. Henry was an "A No. 1 druggist," and even when he became famous as an author he never forgot his pharmaceutical training. Over and over again in his short stories we find references to drugs and pharmacy. Many of his best tales have a distinct pharmaceutical flavor.[49]

Another distinguished pharmacist, Ivor Griffith (1891-1961), former president of the Philadelphia College of Pharmacy and Science, was a down-to-earth philosopher and optimist, who published two volumes entitled *Lobscows* (1939) and *To the*

Lilacs, containing many of his poems, essays, speeches and random thoughts, which are, to quote from the *Philadelphia Inquirer,* indicative of "a man of gentle humor, quiet faith and deep humanity."

A meritorious translation of *Oedipus the King,* a masterpiece of the ancient Greek dramatist Sophocles, was published (1946) by Nathan E. Truman, a practicing pharmacist in Bainbridge, N. Y. A small booklet of verses (1950) testified further to his poetic mind.

Book-loving pharmacists are, naturally, much more numerous than their book-writing colleagues.[50] There were, for example, two American pharmacists who not only revered poetry but devoted themselves to the memory of poets whom they particularly loved: the pharmacist Joseph Jacobs of Atlanta, whose poetic idol was the gifted Scot Robert Burns, and William Alfred Speck of New York (later of New Haven), who greatly admired the great German poet, Johann Wolfgang Goethe. They did much to foster admiration for these writers.

It is because of Jacobs' love for the poetry of Burns that America could boast of a unique Burns Club founded in 1896. This club, open to all lovers of the poet, has on its grounds the only replica of the original cottage of Burns.[51] Jacobs' private collection of all the editions ever published of the works of Burns is open to the public once a month.

The collection of items connected with the life and work of Goethe was begun by the pharmacist Speck when, as only a 15-year-old boy, he bought a complete set of Goethe's works. At the age of 49 he sold his pharmacy, which he had inherited from his father, in order to devote his time exclusively to the study and the collection of the work of Goethe.

In 1913 Mr. Speck gave up his business and promptly transferred his collection to New Haven, depositing it with the Yale University Library. He was made its Curator during the extent of his life. The collection then numbered 6,000 unique, rare, and costly items. At his death on October 9, 1928 the collection had mounted to roundly 20,000 items . . . Collecting was the nimbus of his life; to know and to live by Goethe was its profound significance . . . To instruct was his greatest delight . . . On German-English literary relations during the Goethe period he had no peer.[52]

Another pharmacist-bibliophile of discrimination, Josiah K. Lilly, Jr. (1893-   ), the father of Eli Lilly previously mentioned, collected "20,000 first editions, thousands of manuscripts"—many of them precious documents in the history of science—then conveyed the treasure to the University of Indiana.[53]

These unique accumulations and their transmission to the public domain make the avocation of such pharmacists an asset to the nation.

There have been not a few American pharmacists who likewise (although more modestly) have attempted to make their own devotion to literature and philosophy fruitful for other people.

Various autobiographic sketches published in the pharmaceutical journals, and as separate pamphlets, have often been imbued with poetry and philosophy. One of the finest attempts of a pharmacist to open to his friends the world that gave so much inspiration to him was a volume assembled by the Chicago pharmacist Henry Biroth, whose own poetic talent is evidenced by articles and poems scattered through the pharmaceutical journals. He did not publish a collected edition of his own writings but preferred to make an anthology of what great contemporaries had said, in the simplest and most beautiful way, concerning the essential principles of humanity. The book bears the title *Tolerance in Religion: Liberal Thoughts of Modern Thinkers* (1913) and the following no less significant motto: "There is a religion behind all religions, and that is, Love and Charity in all things."

Finally, two men coming from pharmacy may be mentioned whose literary work secures them a place among the writers, not of fiction, but of general cultural subjects. These men are Sir Henry Wellcome and James Henry Breasted.

The American pharmacist Henry S. Wellcome, whose mercantile genius made him one of the founders and the great leader of Burroughs, Wellcome and Company, one of the most important pharmaceutical concerns in the world, wrote, when he was 34 years old and amidst the difficulties of carving out a business career, a work of some 500 pages on the Indians of Alaska. In this book, *The Story of Metlakahtla* (1887), he paid his tribute to the American Indians, whom he regarded as "the noblemen of God's primitive peoples."

In his later life Sir Henry Wellcome was more the promoter of cultural and scientific writings than an author himself. His discovery of several Ethiopian archaeologic sites in the Upper Nile region, and the excavations carried on under his personal supervision, rank first among his contributions to our knowledge of the past. The Wellcome medico-pharmaceutical museum and library in London, referred to at another place, are among the most important of their kind internationally.

It was in the field of ancient cultures, especially that of Egypt, that James Henry Breasted, a graduate of the Chicago College of Pharmacy (class of 1886), achieved world-wide recognition. His *History of Egypt* is a classic in its field. It has become one of the most popular books of its kind and has been published in many languages and even in an edition for the blind. As to the history of pharmacy and medicine,

Breasted has assured for himself a permanent place through his masterful translation into English of the Edwin Smith Papyrus (see p. 9).

Promoters of art, and collectors who made their hobbies a source of delight to a multitude of men, were two other American large-scale manufacturers who came from pharmacy. Pharmacist Frederick Stearns (see p. 287) presented this country with one of the world's most complete collections of musical instruments, now the cherished property of the University of Michigan. Josiah K. Lilly (see p. 422) developed the greatest collection of Fosteriana in the world, thus perpetuating the memory of "Stephen Foster, America's Troubadour," in the composer's native city, Pittsburgh.[54]

The part of American pharmacy and pharmacists in the life of the nation naturally could not fail to attract the attention of various writers of fiction. More or less accurately portrayed, dealt with as a type or as a remarkable individual, the American pharmacist is met again and again in novels and short stories, whether as the protagonist or as a modest background figure.[55]

How people visualize the American pharmacist and his part in the American scene is suggested also by his portrayal in various motion pictures.[56]

18:   Contributions by Pharmacists to Science and Industry

As has been shown in the earlier chapters, the profession of pharmacy has produced many scholarly representatives who applied to their calling the results of research in the sciences on which pharmacy rests. These representatives (usually teachers or authors of textbooks) and their activities have been pointed out as part of pharmaceutical history in the countries concerned. Had they done nothing more, pharmacy as a profession would have led but a parasitic life. Fortunately for the calling, some of them made fundamental contributions to science. It is their story that is to be told here.

Writers on pharmaceutical history tend to claim as representatives of pharmacy anybody and everybody who has spent even a brief period in this field. Thus Justus Liebig has been claimed for pharmacy, though he spent only 10 months as an apprentice in the pharmacy at Heppenheim. Humphry Davy is another of whom it has been said that he was "an apothecary's clerk at the beginning of his career."[1] The facts are that Davy spent 3 years as an apprentice to an apothecary-surgeon, John Borlase, who had a large practice in Penzance.[2] The young man availed himself of the opportunity thus offered to conduct chemical experiments. No doubt he assisted in the preparation of remedies, but he can scarcely be regarded as having been a pharmacist. It has been a custom among French writers on the history of pharmacy to claim men who taught at educational institutions of pharmacy.[3] Claude Louis Berthollet, Louis Pasteur[4] and Louis Jacques Thénard were not genuine representatives of pharmacy. The eminent Swedish chemist Joens Jacob Berzelius did not "first earn his living as apothecary."[5]

So many facets of science and technology have in fact been sustained by contributions coming from pharmacy that there is no need to claim or debate borderline instances.* The men and women to be mentioned here as pharmacists either practiced as such for a time or held a full legal qualification to practice pharmacy if and when they wished to do so. Hence we may speak of contributions coming from pharmacy, or contributions by pharmacists, even if in later life they devoted themselves to some specialized branch of scientific endeavor. Indeed, during the course of the 19th century, further specialization in education and effort became practically a prerequisite for memorable scientific achievement. The "pharmacist" thus often tends to become obscured in the modern context of science, even though the original profession of such creative men and women influenced, in widely divergent ways and degrees, their life choices and contributions.

GENERAL CHEMISTRY

Ferdinand Hoefer points out, in his famous *La Chimie*, that the "first materials of chemistry . . . were to be met with in the shops of the smithy, the enameler, the painter, in the boutique of the pharmacopolist or druggist, as a matter of fact in the practice of all the useful arts, including the culinary art. In other words, science is born of the needs of life."[6] At the close of the Middle Ages metallurgy flourished in central Europe. It was in mining localities and from the miners that Paracelsus acquired much of his chemical knowledge. A wealth of chemical knowledge, processes and apparatus is to be found in the *De Re Metallica* of George Agricola (1494-1555), physician and for a time an official geolo-

* Discoverers mentioned in this chapter are not from pharmacy unless so identified.

312

gist and metallurgist of the mining industry of Bohemia; in the *Alchimia* of Andreas Libavius (1540-1616), physician and later a teacher in Saxony; and in writings reflecting the comprehensive life work of Johann Rudolf Glauber (1604-1670).[7]

What the chemists of the postrenaissance period needed was not so much additional empiric knowledge as a more satisfactory theory than that of the four elements of the Greek thinkers, or that of the three "principles" attributed to Paracelsus. Even the unifying phlogiston theory suggested by the German physician Johann Joachim Becher (1635-1682) and elaborated by Georg Ernst Stahl (1660-1734) served only for a comparatively short period, for it was the product of speculation based on unsatisfactory explanations of observed phenomena, rather than on exact experiment. A sounder hypothesis was made possible by the discovery of oxygen—by men who died unaware of the importance of their discovery and with unshaken belief in the phlogiston theory.

The qualitative period of chemical history is sometimes divided into two equal periods: the iatrochemical period and the phlogistic period. A survey of these two subperiods reveals as representatives of the former more physicians than pharmacists, while those of the latter were more often pharmacists. The classical experimental researches of Lavoisier and their correct interpretation were made possible by phlogistonists, of whom two were pharmacists.

In 1774, the French pharmacist Bayen reported before the Paris Academy of Science on *un fluide elastique* which escaped when mercuric oxide was heated.[8] The credit for the independent discovery of this substance is commonly given to the English clergyman Joseph Priestley, who called it "life-air," and to the German-Swedish pharmacist Carl Wilhelm Scheele, who designated it "fire-air." Lavoisier later misnamed it oxygen ("acid former"), although he knew it was a base former as well. Thus two pharmacists helped to lay the foundation for the antiphlogistic theory, which cleared the way for the rapid progress of chemistry during the 19th century.

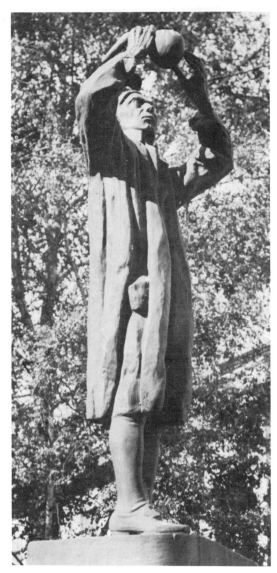

Carl W. Scheele of Sweden retains his place, after two centuries, as one of the great pharmacists of all time. This bronze statue by Milles at Köping (unveiled in 1912) shows the modest practitioner and experimenter in an attitude quite different from that of the glamorized monument at Stockholm. (Photograph from T. Lindham, Farmacevitiska Föreningen)

Ancient Greek philosophers had conceived the atom as something which could not be further divided. In 1661, Robert Boyle in his *Sceptical Chymist*, defined an element as a substance which could not be

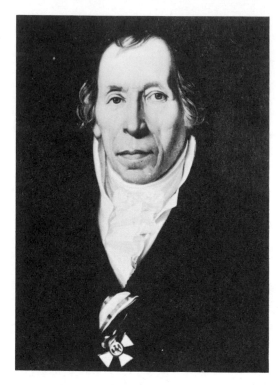

Pharmacist Martin H. Klaproth was called "Europe's greatest analytical chemist" by Berzelius. Like much of his research, his discovery of uranium (1789) was made in the laboratory of his pharmacy in Berlin. (Photograph from the Edgar Fahs Smith Collection, University of Pennsylvania; from an oil portrait in the Deutsches Museum, Munich)

resolved into simpler substances. About 50 years later, the French pharmacist Etienne-François Geoffroy presented his attempt to define the specific relationship existing between different substances. His chemical relationship table (published in 1718 in the *Mémoirs* of the Paris Academy of Science) represents an early attempt at a clarification of the principles of chemical affinity.[9]

Twenty-five years later Guillaume François Rouelle,[10] also a French pharmacist, solved the problem of the nature of salts, a problem which had baffled the best chemical minds for centuries. He defined a salt as the product of the union of an acid with a base (1744).[14] Soon thereafter, Lavoisier, a student of Rouelle, defined an acid as the product of the union of a nonmetal with

oxygen, and a base as that of the union of a metal with oxygen. Thus was laid the foundation of the chemistry of the early decades of the quantitative period, the chemistry of acids, bases and salts.

Just as the *"tables de rapports"* of the French pharmacist Geoffroy served as the starting point of numerous speculations, so the grouping of analogous elements as "triads" by Johann Wolfgang Döbereiner (1780-1849), a German pharmacist, was destined to become the forerunner of the periodic table of the elements.

But even before Döbereiner conceived his triads (papers 1817, 1829; the atomic weight of the middle element was the arithmetic mean of the sum of atomic weights of the two extremes), another pharmacist had pronounced a mathematical rule. Joseph Louis Proust (1754-1826) pointed out, as a result of numerous investigations, that the elements combine with one another in definite proportions, which are constant. When the nonpharmacist John Dalton (1766-1844) demonstrated the law of simple, constant and multiple proportions, it was based partly on the experimental statements of Proust.

Almost of equal importance was the discovery of the 4 halogens—chlorine, iodine, bromine and fluorine: the first by Scheele (1774), the second by Courtois (1811), the third by Balard (1826) and the fourth by Moissan (1886). All of these men came from the ranks of pharmacy. This group of elements, individually important in themselves, brought about the overthrow of Lavoisier's oxygen theory of acids and thus gave rise to concepts that played so important a rôle in the development of the new chemistry, concerning acids, bases and salts. Also, chlorine, iodine and bromine constituted one of Döbereiner's groups of triads which, as already pointed out, with Newland's octaves (1864), became the foundation for the periodic system constructed by D. I. Mendelejeff and J. Lothar Meyer.

As is well known, the metallic elements potassium and sodium, magnesium, calcium, strontium and barium were first isolated by Sir Humphry Davy, the father of electrochemistry; however, the preparatory work leading toward their discovery had been done by German pharmacists. Thus derivatives of sodium and potassium, and magnesium, calcium and barium had been studied by Andreas S. Marggraf (1709-1782); those of barium by Carl W. Scheele; and, lastly, those of strontium by Martin H. Klaproth (1743-1817).

Klaproth has been acclaimed as one of the most gifted discoverers. He owed his discoveries, not to accident, but to his extraordinary skill in both qualitative and quantitative analysis.[12] Although he did not isolate any of the elements enumerated above in a pure state (unlike Davy, he did not have the tools to effect their isolation) he has been credited with the discovery of uranium (1789), zirconium (1789) and cerium (1803). In addition, he has to his credit the verification of the elemental character of tellurium, strontium, titanium, chromium and yttrium.[13] However, it must be mentioned that cerium was discovered simultaneously and independently by Berzelius and Hisinger. Although Klaproth's announcement of the discovery of chromium was made several months later than that of Vauquelin (1797), the credit for its isolation nevertheless goes to pharmacy; for Louis N. Vauquelin came from the ranks of French pharmacy.

Elemental carbon, both as charcoal and as diamond, has been known since antiquity, although its elemental nature was not suspected at that time. However, the discovery of some of the most important properties of amorphous carbon was made by pharmacists. The German pharmacist Karl Gottfried Hagen[14] explained the adsorptive quality of powdered charcoal as a physical property (1793-94). Whereas the German-Russian pharmacist Tobias Lowitz experimented exclusively with vegetable charcoal, the French pharmacist P. C. Figuier published (1810) his results with animal charcoal, proving the latter to be superior to the vegetable variety in several instances. Lastly, the French pharmacist Tuéry demonstrated the antidotal properties of charcoal to the skeptical members of the French Academy of Medicine by swallowing a gram of strychnine after having previously taken 15 grams of charcoal.[15]

The list of pharmaceutical discoverers of elements does not end with Klaproth. In 1844, the German pharmacist Heinrich Rose (1795-1854) announced the discovery of a new element which he named niobium. Some claim that it was but a rediscovery of columbium, which had been isolated from columbite by the English chemist Charles Hatchett. However, the prevailing opinion is that Hatchett did not discover niobium but tantalum, which is closely related to niobium and is commonly associated with it. (Columbium designates this element in the United States, whereas niobium, the name given to it by Rose, has been used in all other countries.)

The great Danish physicist Hans Christian Oersted (1777-1851), who paved the way for the isolation of metallic aluminum and established the laws of electromagnetism, worked as a youth in the pharmacy of his father and even managed, for a short time, a pharmacy in Copenhagen.

Elemental fluorine not only was discovered by the pharmacist Henri Moissan, but it was made known to the world before a pharmaceutical group, the *Société de pharmacie de Paris*.[16] Moissan, then professor at the Ecole Superieure de Pharmacie de Paris, came like Balard, Courtois and Scheele from the ranks of pharmacy. For his research he was awarded a Nobel Prize (1906). It was also a pharmacist, A. S. Marggraf who (1768) obtained hydrogen fluoride by distilling fluorspar with sulphuric acid. The resulting product attacked the glass retort he had used. Then, in checking Marggraf's results, Scheele made the same mistake. Johann Carl Friedrich Meyer, owner of a pharmacy in Stettin, in a detailed communication advised Scheele to use lead instead of glass.[17] With this modification in the apparatus, the real nature of hydrogen fluoride could be revealed.

In like manner, discovery of the halogen derivatives is attributed in no small part to pharmacists. Thus Antoine Balard (1802-1876), who had isolated bromine, also studied its compounds. The pharmacist

George Simon Serullas studied derivatives of iodine as well as those of bromine. He prepared both iodoform (1822) and ethyl-bromide (1827). If the discovery of iodoform is attributed to Serullas without question, that of chloroform has been claimed by three individuals: the American physician Guthrie, the German chemist Liebig and the French pharmacist Eugène Soubeiran (1797-1858). According to Max Speter, who made a thorough study of this question, it was the German pharmacist Friedrich Moldenhauer who first obtained (1830) a product which he, like Guthrie, regarded as a "chloric ether." Both Liebig and Soubeiran, however, pronounced the product obtained by them (1831) to be a new compound. The pharmacist Soubeiran correctly recognized it as a compound of carbon, hydrogen and chlorine, whereas Liebig overlooked its hydrogen content. The correct formula was assigned to it by J. B. A. Dumas, who replaced the designation "formyl chloride" with "chloroform."[18]

Research on halogens and their derivatives was not new to Dumas. While he was working in a Geneva pharmacy he was requested to look for iodine, which had been isolated by Courtois, in sponges. A local physician, Dr. Coindet, desired to use it as a specific against goiter. Dumas was successful; and he suggested that the iodine be used in the form of an alcoholic tincture or as potassium iodide (or combination of iodine and aqueous potassium iodide). With the publication of these results, Dumas made his first appearance in print.[19] Although Dumas left the profession, he was always grateful to pharmacy. Wherever opportunity offered, whether as Senator of France or as Secretary of Agriculture, he promoted pharmacy.

The chemical work of Louis Nicolas Vauquelin, who also came from pharmacy, was not restricted to the halogens and their derivatives. He discovered cinchonic acid (1806), lecithin (1811), daphnin (1817) and cyanic acid (1818). More than that, his laboratory became a practical school of chemistry, from which emerged a number of prominent chemists, who followed in his footsteps.[20] The famous Liebig, who is commonly credited with having established the first chemical laboratory at a university, worked for a time in the laboratory of Vauquelin.

Like Vauquelin, the pharmacists Marggraf and Klaproth did not owe their chemical reputation to restricted work in a narrow chemical field. Marggraf has been designated[21] "the second father or renewer of chemistry." No less an authority than Berzelius, himself one of the greatest analysts, pronounced Klaproth "the greatest analytical chemist" of Europe.

A characteristic of Marggraf was that he never was content with having solved a specific problem; he tried in addition to find out all about it, regardless of its immediate practical value. He also avoided the fanciful generalizations so common during his time. He worked out an inexpensive method for the preparation of phosphorus and of phosphoric acid, thus providing the basis for important industries. He prepared and described phosphorus pentoxide and demonstrated that phosphorus is contained in urine as phosphates. When he first prepared potassium cyanide, he also showed its property of forming double salts with those of the heavy metals and gave to chemistry the ferrocyanides and ferricyanides as reagents for iron. His discovery of sugar in the sugar beet is one of the rare accomplishments which, influencing industry, have shaped the national economy. The use of ethyl alcohol as the solvent for extraction of the raw material paved the way for a new technic, as did his use of the microscope in the examination of the sugar crystals.

The exactness so characteristic of the experimentation of Marggraf is, likewise, typical of the experimental work of Klaproth. Like Marggraf, he published nothing without having thoroughly verified his findings. Unlike many of his contemporaries, if not most of them, he not only published his results but also gave in detail the methods by which they were obtained, thus making his technic available to others. In a way, this was revolutionary. The policy eventually curtailed drastically the publication of questionable research.

Many manipulations which appear self-evident to the analytical chemist of today originated from Klaproth. He was the first to point out the necessity of drying at a definite temperature before weighing and to ignite precipitates until constant weight was obtained. He also took into account the contaminations resulting from grinding hard minerals in iron mortars, prior to analysis. He realized the importance of analysing salts to determine the exact composition of precipitates, and he devised many efficient methods for preparing analytical reagents.[22]

Marggraf had been thoroughly educated as a pharmacist and for several years assisted his father in the latter's pharmacy in Berlin. However, when 30 years of age, he became connected with the Royal Society of Berlin (known later as the Royal Prussian Academy of Science) and discontinued the practice of pharmacy. Klaproth, on the other hand, accomplished most of his remarkable experimental work in the laboratory of his pharmacy while busily engaged as a pharmaceutical practitioner. It was not until he had reached the age of 57 years that he sold his pharmacy in order to devote his entire time to research and teaching.

The author of the article about Klaproth in *The Laboratory*, quoted above, refers to his hero as "the forgotten chemist." Since all histories on chemistry give Klaproth his due, this designation is scarcely correct; but it does apply to a contemporary, Tobias Lowitz.[23] Like Klaproth, he accomplished most of his results in a pharmacy, the laboratory of the Imperial Russian Court Pharmacy in St. Petersburg (Leningrad). Here he served first as apprentice and then as assistant and, from 1776 until his death, as manager. This long experience was interrupted only by a 3-year absence, which he spent at the University of Göttingen in his native city.

Lowitz discovered mono- and trichloroacetic acids (1793). He first prepared absolute alcohol and pure ether (1796). He first employed the specific gravity test as a means of determining purity. He was the first to employ the seeding of solutions to induce the crystallization of the solutes. However, possibly his most important contribution to mankind was the discovery of the decolorizing and deodorizing property of charcoal (1785). Fully aware of the importance of this discovery, he made a thorough investigation of the subject. As early as 1794, he could report to the Russian navy that he was able to make impure water fit to drink. He introduced charcoal

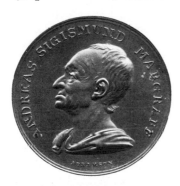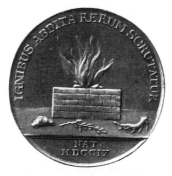

"Hidden things he searches out by fires," proclaims the Latin motto on a medal honoring a research pharmacist of the 18th century. The allusion to fire symbolizes the art of chemistry, since fire seemed to be the indispensable tool in probing the secrets of the three natural kingdoms, which are represented before the chemist's hearth by a stone (mineral), a branch (vegetable) and an antler (animal). The obverse side shows a portrait of Pharmacist Andreas S. Marggraf, born the son of a pharmacist (1709), who discovered sugar in the sugar beet and advanced qualitative analysis.

into the alcohol distilleries to remove fusel oil and developed other uses.

As this survey shows, there is scarcely a field of general chemistry without some important enrichment brought about by pharmacists. Thus it is only natural that they have also contributed to the development of chemical apparatus. The introduction of the microscope as a means of chemical research by the pharmacist Marggraf has already been mentioned. Less well known is the fact that it was the French pharmacist Nicolas LeFebvre (1610-1674) who introduced the use of the thermometer into chemistry. The French pharmacist Antoine Baumé created with his hydrometers (or aerometers) (1768) the possibility of an easy and fairly exact determination of the density (specific gravity) of liquids, a method widely used up to the present. The German pharmacist Carl Friedrich Mohr (1806-1879) gave to volumetric analysis most of its auxiliary implements, among them the Mohr-pinchcock. The specific-gravity balance, likewise bearing his name, has been an important piece of laboratory apparatus. At the end of the 19th century the pharmacist Ernst Beckmann (1855-1923) presented chemistry with two different pieces of apparatus for the determination of boiling points and freezing points. Finally, the modern micromethods to a considerable extent owe their development and present status to pharmacists. The Austrian pharmacist Richard Wasicky (1884-   ), an honorary member of the American Pharmaceutical Association, constructed an apparatus for continuous extraction of micro-quantities of solids.[24] One of Wasicky's pupils, the Austrian pharmacist Ludwig Kofler (1891-   ), invented a melting-point apparatus for use on a microscope (in collaboration with Hilock, one of his students).[25] Since 1940 Wasicky has been teaching at the University of São Paulo, Brazil, and systematically investigating the pharmacologic and the pharmacognostic aspects of the Brazilian flora. Finally, it was Wilhelm Carl Böttger (1871-1949) a man who started his career as a German pharmacist, to whom the world of chemistry

is indebted for fundamental studies of potentiometric volumetric analysis and of the application of physicochemical laws to analytic problems.[26]

PHYTOCHEMISTRY

The vegetable kingdom, up to the 19th century, supplied more materia pharmaceutica than did the mineral and the animal kingdoms combined. The romance of these items produced a particular charm, but later insight into their chemical constitution was even more intriguing.

The pharmacist Nicolas Lémery supposedly was the first (in his *Cours de chimie*, 1675) to attempt to list separately from other drugs the vegetable substances whose chemical nature was supposedly known. However, there are mentioned in this division of Lémery's treatise only a few individual chemicals: camphor, flowers of benzoes (benzoic acid) and sugar were almost the only ones. Even oil of turpentine (mostly pinene) could scarcely be regarded as an organic chemical.

The isolation of constituents of plant drugs was a goal to be sought zealously. In this endeavor pharmacists played an important role. The art of distillation of aromatic spirits and waters and, subsequently, of volatile oils was of importance in the practice of pharmacy, particularly during the phlogistic period of chemical history. Just as the distillation of aromatic waters (supposed to represent the quintessence of the plants) led to the isolation of volatile oils, so the storage and the observation of the volatile oils led to the isolation of the so-called camphors. Thus Caspar Neumann, administrator of the Prussian Court Pharmacy, in 1719 observed thyme camphor (thymol), and the pharmacist Johann Christian Wiegleb (1732-1800), discovered mace camphor (myristic acid) in 1774.

Each observation constituted a notable contribution to the list of the few individual organic chemicals then known. The discovery of *Oelsüss* (i.e., glycerin) by Scheele, while making lead plaster, is a well-known instance. The French pharmacist Joseph Louis Proust isolated mannitol (1806). He also has leucin, gliadin and hordein to his credit.

Of far greater significance was the recognition of the acid character of the "flowers of bonzoes." Their name had been derived from the production by the dry method of sublimation. It was in the process of preparing the "flowers" by the wet method (extraction of gum benzoes with milk of lime, and precipitation of the acid from its calcium salt by means of hydrochloric acid) that Scheele recognized their acid character.

The application and the extension of this method led to the discovery of several new plant acids: tartaric acid (1769), citric acid (1784) and malic acid (1785). It also enabled him to demonstrate the wide distribution of oxalic acid in the vegetable kingdom. Scheele also obtained oxalic acid upon oxidation of sugar with nitric acid, an accomplishment of no mean significance later on, when the study of the structure of organic molecules by means of the "Abbau" method revealed many secrets of organic chemistry.[28]

During infancy organic chemistry leaned heavily on its older sister, inorganic chemistry, and formulated its theoretic concepts accordingly.

In 1805 and 1806 the German pharmacist Friedrich Wilhelm Sertürner published his first papers about his work on opium leading to the discovery of what he then called the *principium somniferum* (somniferous principle). Shortly before (1803) the French pharmacist Charles Louis Derosne had reported on a crystalline precipitate—later considered to be a mixture of morphine and narcotine—isolated by him out of the same raw material. Derosne stated that small amounts of the new substance exerted the same physiologic effect as much greater quantities of the raw material, opium. It was likewise before the first publication of the findings of Sertürner that another Frenchman, the nonpharmacist Armand Seguin, reported (1804) a new *"matière végéto-animale toute particulière"* (a very peculiar vegetable-animal material). But this report was not published until 1814. In contrast with Derosne and Seguin, Sertürner recognized immediately the alkaline character of the substance that he had found and the fundamental importance of this fact. However, his first statement received no attention. It was not before the appearance, in 1817, of his comprehensive publication, *Über das Morphium, eine neue salzfähige Grundlage . . .* in Gilbert's *Annalen der Physick*, that the real character of Sertürner's discovery and, hence, its full significance, was recognized.

Here the salifyable property of this "plant base" was emphasized, and the organic analog to the inorganic base was supposed to have been found. It formed salts with organic acids (morphine acetate) as well as with inorganic acids (morphine hydrochloride). Thus organic systematics were supplied with a theory of acids, bases and salts, analogous to the inorganic classification. How this classification later gave way to the recognition of the alcohols as the true bases of organic chemistry is another story. It is sufficient here to point out that as a technic had enabled Scheele to isolate a number of plant acids, so the new technic of Sertürner enabled others to isolate plant bases from other drugs.

The very name alkaloid, "alkali-like," coined (1818) by the German pharmacist K. F. W. Meissner, is suggestive of the rôle these substances played in organic theory and systematics. During the next 10 years no less than 10 alkaloids were isolated from vegetable drugs. To Joseph Pelletier and Joseph B. Caventou, two Parisian pharmacists, the world has been indebted for the discovery of strychnine (1818) and brucine (1819), colchicine (1819) and, above all, quinine and cinchonine (1820).

The history of alkaloids is a story by itself. Here only a few additional milestones may be mentioned. Pelletier and Dumas isolated narceine (1832) and thebaine (1833). The pharmacist F. F. Runge had isolated caffeine from the coffee bean (1821). A year later the same alkaloid was isolated independently by Pelletier, Caventou and Robiquet. The pharmacist Pierre Jean Robiquet had previously isolated nar-

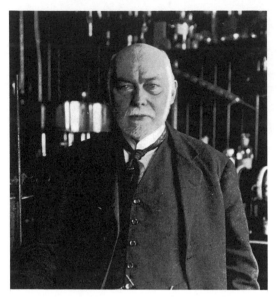

Frederick Belding Power, an American pharmacist who became a distinguished plant chemist, earned the Ebert Prize, the Flueckiger Medal, the Hanbury Medal and many other honors. (Photograph from the American Pharmaceutical Association)

cotine (1817) and reported codeine (1832). The pharmacist Rudolph Brandes had isolated atropine in an impure state. Later, the pharmacist Philipp Lorenz Geiger, with the cooperation of the nonpharmacist Hesse, obtained it in a pure state. They also isolated aconitine. Moreover, Geiger prepared pure coniine (1831), previously isolated by the nonpharmacist Carl Giesecke in an impure condition. The pharmacist Georg Franz Merck discovered papaverine; and the pharmacist F. Gaedcke isolated "small needle-shaped crystals" from "erythroxylon coca" (1855), a mixture of coca alkaloids, according to R. Zaunick. Finally the young pharmacist Albert Niemann, a student of the great chemist Wöhler, succeeded in isolating pure cocaine from coca leaves (1860). This promising young scientist died (not quite 27 years of age) only 1 year after receiving, on the basis of his work on cocaine, his degree of Doctor of Philosophy.

The pharmacist E. Jahns synthesized arecoline (1890), an alkaloid which, with arecaidine and guvacine, he had isolated

from the areca nut. These results he accomplished in the small laboratory of his pharmacy in Göttingen. It was the same pharmacy in which young Albert Niemann had served his apprenticeship (from 1849 to 1853). Likewise, the German pharmacist Ernst A. Schmidt isolated scopolamine (1890). The German-American pharmacist, Ferdinand F. Mayer, may be credited with development of the so-called "Mayer's reagent for alkaloids" (mercuric potassium iodide test solution).[30]

Naturally, pharmacists have interested themselves in the study of glucosides as well as of alkaloids. The pharmacist Rudolph Brandes isolated delphinine (1817), and the pharmacist Kahler discovered santonin (1830). Possibly no drugs afforded greater difficulty in the unraveling of their constituents than digitalis and ergot. In the early study of both, pharmacists played a conspicuous part, although the decisive work in both cases was done by a nonpharmacist, the great Swiss chemist, Arthur Stoll.

Important basic work in the study of essential oils was done by Sir William Tilden[31] (1842-1926), a pharmacist in the true sense of the word. He introduced nitrosyl chloride as a useful reagent for terpenes in the seventh decade of the 19th century.

In the United States Frederick B. Power[32] (1853-1927) increased our knowledge of the volatile oils as well as other constituents of plants in a remarkable series of researches. Having begun his investigations in F. A. Flueckiger's Pharmaceutical Institute at the University of Strassburg, Power continued them at the Philadelphia College of Pharmacy and at the University of Wisconsin. As Scientific Director of the Laboratory of Fritzsche Brothers, in Passaic, N. J., and later as Director of the Wellcome Research Laboratory in London, he, with his colaborers, published an epoch-making series of papers on phytochemical subjects. By no means least of these is his study of chaulmoogric and hydnocarpic acids, which not only contributed to the fight against leprosy, but made necessary a revised definition of the fatty acids. Upon Power's return to the United States, his phytochemical work was continued in the Bureau of Chemistry of the Department of Agriculture in Washington, and resulted in his election as a member of the National Academy of Science. At the University of Wisconsin his work on essential oils was continued by Edward Kremers (1865-1941), a disciple of Power as well as of Wallach.

It would scarcely be appropriate to refer to Flueckiger without at least mentioning Daniel Hanbury of London (1825-1875), Alexander Tschirch of Bern (1856-1939) and Hermann Thoms of Berlin (1859-1931). All these men, who did meritorious work in examining and isolating plant contents, came from pharmacy. Flueckiger owned a pharmacy for some years, and Thoms managed one.

PHYSIOLOGIC CHEMISTRY

Physiologic chemistry has been defined in a somewhat restricted sense as the application of chemistry to the study of the normal processes of the human body. In a broader sense, it covers the normal processes of all animal life, and the term may even be applied to the normal processes of plant life. Today its use has been largely replaced by biochemistry, which includes both.

Particularly in France, where clinical technology has been closely associated with pharmacy, many of the pharmacists who rise to the level of real scientific research have shown a bent toward the biologic aspects of chemistry. Such pharmacists in the early 19th century often studied medicine for advanced training. "This does not mean," Berman points out, "that these pharmacists practiced medicine, that they were clinicians, or that they had surrendered their identity as pharmacists, as the examples of Bouchardat, Méhu, Mialhe, Chatin, and Virey illustrate."[32a]

Indeed, for some 23 years Apollinaire Bouchardat (1806-86) had practiced hospital pharmacy while he conducted versatile investigations. His work in hygiene influenced the French etiologic approach to medicine. His research on diabetes provided the basis for what has been called "the most rational method of treatment up to his time."

In the opinion of the distinguished American biochemist, E. V. McCollum, the hospital pharmacist Camille Méhu (1835-87) "made one of the most important discoveries in the entire history of protein investigations,"[32a] notably that proteins precipitate from solution without changing their nature when saturated with ammonium sulfate.

Another French pharmacist, Louis Mialhe (1807-86), isolated ptyalin and demonstrated the action of this enzyme on starch, among other contributions to physiologic chemistry. A contemporary who practiced hospital pharmacy in Paris for some 33 years, Gaspard A. Chatin (1813-1901) developed a micro-method for measuring iodine, on the basis of his studies of the iodine content of plants. He also advanced the view that a lack of iodine caused endemic goiter (1851-52).[32a]

One of the most important products of animal metabolism, urea, was discovered (1773) by the French pharmacist Hilaire Marie Rouelle (brother of G. F. Rouelle, previously mentioned). Another French pharmacist, Vauquelin, was one of the group of scientists who made a special study of this substance, which has played an important role, not only in physiologic chemistry, but also in the theory of vitalism.

H. M. Rouelle, furthermore, was the first to recognize the iron content of blood. The pharmacist Antoine Baumé first pronounced milk an emulsion. Of the ten eminent early physiologic chemists who, according to Lieben, made important contributions to the study of milk, no less than six were pharmacists (Geoffroy, Baumé, Rouelle, Parmentier, Vauquelin and Scheele).[33] Among other observations, Vauquelin noticed that the addition of acid prevents fermentation.

The discovery of sugar in beets by the pharmacist A. S. Marggraf has already been mentioned. Proust isolated grape sugar from grape juice, and for a time was credited with discovering this substance. However, the pharmacist Tobias Lowitz had isolated it from honey 14 years earlier in pure crystalline form. Henri Braconnot, a phar-

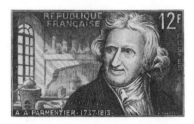

Commemorative postage stamps have been issued to help honor some of the pharmacists whose scientific contributions became significant. Pictured on this French issue is J. A. A. Parmentier, perhaps best remembered for his discoveries in the field of food chemistry.

macist in Strassburg previous to his appointment as a professor at Nancy and director of the Botanical Garden, was the first to obtain grape sugar by treating sawdust with sulphuric acid, thus laying the foundation for an important chemical industry (1819). In addition, he discovered pectin and pectic acid (1824) and dextrin (1833). As early as 1820, he had obtained glycocoll, the first amino acid resulting from the hydrolysis of albumen with the aid of a mineral acid.[34]

The amino acid leucine had previously (1819) been discovered by the pharmacist Joseph L. .Proust, whom Lieben regards as an "exact analyst" and as "one of the early albumen and nutrition investigators."[35] The first to characterize albumen was the English apothecary William Thomas Brande (1788-1866). The albumen reagent, an acetic acid solution of mercuric chloride in potassium iodide, was designed by the French pharmacist Charles Joseph Tanret (1847-1917), in the laboratory of his Troyes pharmacy.

It was pharmacist Scheele who first recognized the acid reaction of normal urine,[36] and it was his French colleague Proust who taught the prevention of the spontaneous fermentation of urine, which renders it alkaline and thus unfit for analytic tests by reagents. In the elaboration of the numerous reagents and methods employed in the analysis of urine, pharmacists or men trained in pharmacy have participated suc-

cessfully. It may suffice to call attention to the inventor of Fehling's solution (1850), which is used for the detection of inverted sugar in the blood as well as in urine. Hermann v. Fehling practiced pharmacy for about 8 years before he gave up his profession in order to devote his life to scientific research.

To conclude these examples of contributions made by pharmacists to physiologic chemistry, mention should be made of two men whose work was of greatest importance: the Frenchman Claude Bernard (1813-1878) and the German Max v. Pettenkofer (1819-1901). Both men started their early careers as pharmacists but later studied medicine. Whereas Bernard, at an early date, devoted himself exclusively to scientific research, Pettenkofer spent his life as pharmacist-in-ordinary to the King of Bavaria and director of the Royal Bavarian Court Pharmacy besides being professor of hygiene and director of the first Hygiene Institute at the University of Munich. Their medical work certainly may not be claimed by pharmacy. However, their development as physiologic chemists no doubt was influenced by their early activities in the pharmaceutical laboratory. Pettenkofer at least has stated his indebtedness to pharmacy for his acquisition of accuracy in work and manual skill and for the prevention of scientific one-sidedness.

INDUSTRY

Scientific research has supplied the basis of industry in general and of special industries in particular to such an extent that each attempt at recounting the work of scientists and its effect on the development of industry of necessity entails some repetition.

Thus several industries, among them the manufacture of explosives (nitroglycerin), owe their existence to the discovery of glycerin by Scheele, mentioned earlier. Another discovery of Scheele, that of chlorine, became a basis for the bleaching and laundry industry. The importance of Scheele's discovery of the fruit acids, especially citric acid, for the foodstuffs industries (especially the production of beverages) is obvious. The decolorizing and purifying power of charcoal, discovered by Lowitz, plays an important part in the process of production in a number of industries.

A few words more may be devoted to the discovery of beet sugar by Marggraf, already mentioned, since the discovery has become a part of world history. It was Napoleon, in the course of his attempt to bar England from trading with those parts of continental Europe then under French domination, who recognized the importance of Marggraf's discovery in liberating Europe from the English monopoly in cane sugar. Furthermore, Napoleon appreciated the possibility, inherent in this discovery, of making sugar a general foodstuff for all, instead of a luxury for the rich. The famous Napoleonic edict (January 15, 1812), which became the basis of the further development of the beet sugar industry, made provision for the training of 100 young people in the manufacturing of sugar, apprentices "to be chosen among the students of pharmacy, of medicine and of chemistry."[37]

Discoveries of pharmacists not yet mentioned also may be considered as of worldwide importance. The discovery of catalysis by the pharmacist Johann W. Döbereiner and the finding and characterizing of aniline in coal tar by the pharmacist Friedlieb F. Runge were of vital significance.

The scientific and industrial values of both discoveries proved to be almost immeasurable. In 1816, Döbereiner already had found that alcohol could be changed to acetic acid through catalysis by platinum. He obtained aldehyde in the same way. His memorable pamphlet was titled *"Über Neu Entdeckte Höchst Merkwürdige Eigenschaften des Platins"* (about recently discovered highly peculiar qualities of platinum). In the year of publication (1823), now fully aware of the technical as well as of the scientific bearing of his invention, he constructed his famous tinder box. This was based on the catalytic capacity of spongy platinum to bring the hydrogen generated in the box into chemical union with oxygen from the air, hence to ignition. Döbereiner explained in detail the principles of its function and its manufac-

ture. The historian of chemistry, H. Kopp, has commented appreciatively about the scientific unselfishness of this pharmacist:

What science and practical life owe to this invention [of catalysis] is known. With the employment of it for the construction of his so widely used tinder box Döbereiner presented it to his contemporaries, while frequently the practical employment of scientific discoveries of much less importance has been used as a private speculation in order to gain riches.[38]

The number of industries using, if not entirely dependent on, the process of catalysis—a term coined by Berzelius (1835)—is very large. A notable example is the "contact process" for the preparation of sulfuric acid. The entire industry of artificial fats, margarine, etc., is based on the coagulation of liquid oils to solid fats of the desired consistency by catalytic hydrogenation processes.

F. F. Runge published (1834) his classic essay *"Über Einige Merkwürdige Produkte der Steinkohlendestillation (Kyanol, Pyrrol, Leukol, Carbolsäure, Rosolsäure und Brunolsäure),"* discoveries that included aniline (i.e., the "kyanol" of Runge) in coal tar. Thus the ground was laid for the entire industry of dyestuffs and synthetic organic remedies, using the aniline derived from coal tar as raw material. Runge's discovery of carbolic acid furnished the essential germicide for Lister's surgical antisepsis. Like Döbereiner, Runge was fully aware of the importance of his discoveries and took the first steps to prove them practically. He was the first to observe (1834) the blue color of aniline after the addition of chloride of lime and to find that by treating aniline with other oxidizing substances, dark green to black dyestuffs can be obtained. "He already had in his hands the emeraldin and the aniline black, so eminently important until to-day."[39] Furthermore, Runge gave the first impetus to the processing of cottonware with sulfonized oils and was the first to produce the oxidation product of aniline on the textiles themselves. Because of this, some historians see in Runge the first to recognize and employ practically the principles of capillarity. The statement of Kränzlein that this pharmacist opened a new epoch with his discoveries is uncontested. "The world," says Kränzlein, "can consider Runge the first inventor of coal tar dyestuffs without by this taking away anything of the immortal fame gained in the same field by A. W. Hoffmann and his pupils, and especially by W. H. Perkin."[40]

The genius of F. F. Runge was not exceeded, although perhaps almost paralleled, by another pharmacist, Adolf Frank (1834-1916), whose inventions establish him as the founder of several industries and who became, on the basis of his scientific findings, an industrialist himself. Frank invented (1882) the process of purifying water by filtration through infusorial silica (Berkefeld filter). Together with Caro, he discovered the possibility of binding free nitrogen to calcium carbide and thus laid the basis for the calcium cyanamide industry. The development of the calcium carbide and acetylene industry is to a large extent due to the technical inventions of this pharmacist, who likewise is considered to be one of the founders of the German potassium salts industry. Frank's studies on enamel and glasspastes laid the groundwork for the modern mosaic industry.[41]

It was a similar combination of scientific genius and commercial and administrative talent that made the pharmacist Fritz Hofmann (1866-1956) one of the leading figures in modern chemical industry. His world fame derives from his successful work in the synthesis of caoutchouc (preceded by the manufacture of isoprene from turpentine by the English pharmacist William Tilden). This achievement was rewarded by a flood of honors—among them the Emil Fischer Medal, the highest proof of appreciation that organized German chemistry has to offer. In addition, Hofmann did much work in other fields of chemical research, including pharmaceutical chemistry. The following extract from a letter written by Hofmann conveys an idea of the man and his work. Having reported about his 6 years spent in practicing pharmacy and in pharmaceutical and post-graduate study and, finally, his appointment as a member of the staff of the Elberfelder Farbwerke (later the center of I. G. Farbenindustrie), Hofmann continued as follows:

In Elberfeld I became director of the pharmaceutical scientific laboratory and vice-president of the concern. *My collaborators and I invented a long row of well-known synthetic remedies which belong until the present to the medicinal armamentarium.* Besides my activity in the pharmaceutical field the problems I worked on were those of the chemistry of perfumes, the chemistry of fermentation, that of light, and finally the search for chemical means against plant-diseases and vermin. . . . By 1909 I had succeeded in the synthesis of caoutchouc in the laboratory of the Elberfelder Farbenfabriken. . . . In Elberfeld I founded and conducted for six years the Institute for Chemotherapy which later under the leadership of Professor Hörlein reached the highest degree of perfection . . . and presented the world with Germanin, Plasmochin, etc.[42]

Hofmann remembered gratefully his work as a practicing pharmacist, to which he felt indebted for the general skill "which became so helpful to me in my later work."

"My collaborators and I invented a long row of well-known synthetic remedies." This statement by Hofmann is revealing. It reminds us why, in recent history, the invention of remedies usually has not been so closely connected with the name of single individuals as it was in earlier times. In this epoch of mass problems and mass production, even invention has become a matter of organization rather than of isolated genius. Yet, this organized research also requires men of ingenuity, talent and even genius, with ambition and vision as well as skill. There is no doubt that in this army of relatively anonymous workers on the problems of joint research the contingent of people coming from pharmacy is still an important one. This has been proved now and again when, in cases like that of Hofmann, the impact of exceptional results has removed the obscurity that subordinates the individual research worker within the group of workers or within the complex of innovations from diverse laboratories on which a notable advance often depends.

Dulcine (phenetidine-urea), discovered by the pharmacist Hermann Thoms in the last decade of the 19th century, is 220 times as sweet as the sugar discovered in beets by Marggraf or that derived from sugar cane. This was a fact startling enough to end the anonymity of the inventor, although the discovery was made by Thoms while in the service of an industrial laboratory.[43]

That dimethylamino-antipyrine (pyramidone) was a result of researches of the pharmacist Friedrich Stolz (1860-1936) became known when the new substance gained general appreciation.[44] The honor of succeeding in the synthesis of epinephrine (i.e., synthetic suprarenine) is shared by Stolz and the chemist Franz Flaecher.[45]

Sometimes an individual pharmacist, besides making an important scientific discovery outside of industry, has succeeded in utilizing it. E. Ritsert, a pharmacist who practiced in Frankfort-on-the-Main, found (1888) that the acetanilide then on the market was not chemically pure and invented a special process for manufacturing a pure product. In pursuing his private research, he prepared (1890) p-aminobenzoic-acidethylester (benzocaine), which he called Anaesthesin because of its anesthetic effect. He made this product the basis of a factory of his own. Not only has benzocaine been used extensively the world over in external and internal therapy, but modern substitutes for cocaine, among them procaine, have been built on the basis of the invention by pharmacist Ritsert. Concluding a kind of autobiographic report, Ritsert wrote:

I state with satisfaction that my observations . . . have laid the ground for an entire group of remedies of greatest importance. Even more satisfaction I take in the fact that, although being a pharmacist relying completely upon myself and without the means and the aid of big institutes or chemical plants, I was able to overcome all difficulties encountered and to carry the results of my work to victory.[46]

One of the most successful workers in the field of chemotherapy (i.e., the direct attack on the morbific agents in the cells, by chemical substances having specific effects), the Frenchman Ernest F. A. Fourneau (1872-1949) came from the ranks of pharmacy, for quite a while combining his research activities with his service in his pharmacy. The internal arsenic compound Stovarsol was a child of Fourneau's genius. He bared the secret of the effective drug Germanin by duplicating it with a preparation called Fourneau 309. From the Fourneau laboratories at the Pasteur Institute, as the fruit of Fourneau's initiative and under his guidance, came the important discovery that the astonishing effect of the German drug Prontosil was due to the sulfonamide part of the complex molecule. Furthermore, from the same place and under the same circumstances, there emanated the first group of chemicals to earn the title of antihistamine agents, some of them carrying Fourneau's name.[47]

As indicated in preceding chapters, modern pharmaceutical industry is to a great extent derived from community pharmacies. In Germany the laboratories of pharmacies developed in so many cases into industrial plants, which later on gained wide and sometimes international recognition, that it does not seem exaggerated to call German community pharmacy the nucleus or seedbed for the German pharmaceutical industry.[47a] In other countries the situation has been similar, except that often instead of the laboratory of a pharmacy becoming a manufacturing plant, pharmacists have founded industries without using a pharmacy as a foundation.

As shown in the chapter on economics, however, there are in the United States several examples of pharmacies having served as nuclei for large present-day manufacturing laboratories. Furthermore, the success of some of the American pharmaceutical plants owned by pharmacists was sometimes to a significant extent due to the personal scientific research of their owners, e.g., Alfred Dohme of Sharp and Dohme, and Henry A. B. Dunning of Hynson, Westcott and Dunning.

MISCELLANEOUS

Wherever we glance over the pages of the book of science, we meet the phenomenal figure of the pharmacist Carl Scheele. In describing researches concerning chemical effects due to the spectrum, the historian Friedrich Dannemann wrote:

Already Scheele had proved that the parts of the spectrum show different chemical effects (1777). Knowing that silver chloride gets gradually blackened if exposed to light, he brought a piece of paper prepared with silver chloride into the spectrum and observed that it blackened much quicker under the influence of violet than by exposure to other colors. *This simple experiment may be considered the beginning of the spectral photography so highly developed in our days.*[48] [Italics added.]

The physicist who later (1801) proved the existence of chemically efficient rays beyond the violet, Johann W. Ritter, had worked in a pharmacy for 4 years before he devoted himself exclusively to science and became one of the best-known physicists of his time.[49] In the experiments by which he established with certainty the more powerful chemical effect of the rays—later to be called "ultraviolet" rays—he used Scheele's method of testing the differences in the rapidity of the destruction of silver nitrate.[50]

Early in the 18th century, a former practicing pharmacist, Johann Friedrich Böttger, who supposedly knew the alchemical mystery of the transmutation of base metals into gold, presented the precious invention of the manufacture of porcelain to the covetous King August of Saxony, who kept him a prisoner. About this chemical invention Ferchl and Süssenguth wrote, "The greatest progress came to the European ceramic industry with the re-invention of the genuine Chinese porcelain, which we owe to the apothecary clerk Johann Friedrich Böttger."[51]

Of the many pharmacists who devoted themselves to botany, the "lovable science," we can mention here only six eminent men: the German Oskar Brefeld (1839-1925),[52] the Frenchmen A. L. A. Fée (1789-1874) and Emile Bourquelot (1851-1921), the Englishmen Edward Morell Holmes (1843-1930) and George Claridge Druce (1851-1932), and the German Ferdinand v. Müller (1825-1896).[53]

Of Brefeld's contribution to his special field of botany, J. R. Green wrote that "The work of Brefeld included a very careful study of the biology of many of the fungi and the nature of their dependence upon external conditions, together with the effect of the latter upon their pleomorphy and their reproductive processes."[54] It was Brefeld who introduced the method of cultivation into mycologic research. Likewise, it was in the field of mycology that E. Bourquelot contributed fundamental scientific and practical information. A. L. A. Fée was one of the foremost cryptogamists of his time and also gained world-wide recognition by his excellent historical research on antique materia medica and botany, especially his *Commentaires sur la botanique et la matière de Pline*, commenting on about 1,000 plants.[55]

The German Ferdinand v. Müller, educated as a pharmacist as well as in the science of botany, emigrated to Australia and became that continent's greatest botanist; he recorded his studies of the flora of Australia in 40 volumes. His advice was very influential in the agricultural and horticultural development of his adopted country. One of Müller's services was his advice that the eucalyptus tree should be cultivated in the Mediterranean countries, South Africa and the United States, as a means of saving the soil from erosion. Thus he has been credited with preserving and even creating wide areas in which human and animal life may prosper.

While the French and German pharmacist-botanists mentioned above have devoted the greater part of their lives to academic research, after having completed their pharmaceutical education, their English colleagues E. M. Holmes and G. C. Druce for a considerable time combined the practice of pharmacy with their scientific pursuits. Holmes has been regarded as "probably the greatest expert on economic botany of his time,"[56] and Druce as "the greatest British field botanist of his day."[57]

Pharmacists even may be mentioned among the pioneers of modern aeronautics. A French pharmacist, Pilâtre de Rozier, was the first human being who dared to make a balloon ascension (1783). Furthermore, he invented a new type of balloon, the so-called *rozière,* replacing the *montgolfière.* De Rozier was killed in a flight over the English channel.[58] Thus the first flyer as well as the first victim of aeronautics was a pharmacist. Moreover, it was a Dutch pharmacist and chemist, Johann P. Minkelers who first replaced hot air or hydrogen in balloons with illuminating gas (1785), in whose manufacture he was a pioneer.

One of the first scientists, if not the first who tried to examine experimentally the physical phenomena connected with aeronautics was likewise a pharmacist. Only one year afer Pilâtre de Rozier's first flight, the young pharmacist M. H. Klaproth ventured a flight in a *montgolfière* balloon, armed with instruments for the determination of air pressure, etc. (1784). But the balloon was torn and rose only to a height of 10 meters, and thus the flight was without scientific results. More fortunate was the Brazilian pharmacist Paulo Seabra (1899-), who has done remarkable research on the biologic and the psychological effects of high-altitude flying. Moreover, one of the prerequisites to high-altitude flight itself was the invention of apparatus for oxygen inhalation by the French pharmacist Stanislas Limousin.[59]

CONCLUSION

Both contemporaries and posterity have shown their appreciation and gratitude toward many of the men mentioned in this chapter. Monuments have been erected and medals have been coined in honor of many of the great pharmacists. In Stockholm and in the small town of Köping, statues commemorate the modest pharmacist Scheele, who passed his life in his profession while serving the world in his laboratory.

In Paris for more than 40 years, from 1900 until its destruction by the Nazis, one monument united in bronze the figures of Caventou and Pelletier, the two pharmacists whose joint work presented the world with so many important alkaloids, including quinine.[60] Their undying renown is indicated by the fact that a second public monument

to the same pharmacists has been erected on the same spot.

Sertürner is commemorated by tablets in Paderborn, Einbeck and Hameln, the places where this pharmacist practiced his profession, in Neuhaus where he was born and within the University of Münster. The bust of Klaproth adorns the peristyle of the University of Berlin, close to the busts of the brothers Alexander and Wilhelm v. Humboldt. The bust of another pharmacist, A. S. Marggraf, on the wall of the building in Berlin which once housed the laboratory of the Royal Prussian Academy of Science, bears witness to his work there for the benefit of humanity.

In Melbourne, Australia, the statue of the pharmacist-botanist F. v. Müller looks down rows of eucalyptus trees, *his* trees. In Canada, a monument in Quebec and a tablet in Annapolis Royal honor the memory of the pharmacist Louis Hébert (see p. 137).

All gratitude and honors naturally are given to the individuals, rather than to the profession which these men practiced or in which they were trained. Yet every profession has some part in the bent of the efforts and the values of the work of its sons.

This survey of contributions by pharmacists to science and industry has necessarily been restricted to representative facts, findings and experimental work of significant importance, and no person has been admitted on the basis of literary work alone. Even with this restriction, there is a need to select from among an abundance of individuals and scientific deeds. Such an abundance can scarcely be accidental. It must have some basis. Perhaps this basis can be found in the fact that hardly any other profession is committed like pharmacy to the study and the utilization of a number of sciences, and at the same time is closely connected with the desires and the needs of the daily life of society. From this arises an incentive to high attainment in the sciences, and a dedication to work for the benefit of mankind.

The members of the profession derive pride from the deeds of their great colleagues. The younger generation may take these deeds and these men as models and as evidence of the opportunities open to everyone who attempts to honor his profession and himself in it. The world in general, and legislation and public opinion, should take cognizance of what pharmacy really means. Thus becomes clear a rational basis for public recognition and protection of pharmacy, to help to assure the maintenance of professional vigor and creative spirit.

If we do not wish to lose the great men and deeds that emerge from pharmacy, we must cultivate the ground from which they spring.

Notes and References

1. ANCIENT PRELUDE

1. Artelt, W.: Studien zur Geschichte der Begriffe "Heilmittel" und "Gift," Studien zur Geschichte der Medizin 23:7, 1937; Meyer-Steineg, Th., and Sudhoff, K.: Geschichte der Medizin im Ueberblick, p. 9, Jena, 1921.

2. Srivastava, G. P.: History of Indian Pharmacy, 2nd ed., vol. 1, Calcutta, 1954, (when published, volume 2 will cover the period since 1600). See also the review by Berman, A.: Bull. Hist. Med., 29:578, 1955. For a summary of some principal facets of classic therapeutics in China and India, see the second edition of Kremers and Urdang: History of Pharmacy, Philadelphia, Lippincott, 1951, pp. 3 to 6 (hereafter referred to as Kremers and Urdang, 2nd ed.). For more information see, for example, from a medical viewpoint: Zimmer, H. R.: Hindu Medicine, 3rd Ser., no. 6, Inst. Hist. Med., Johns Hopkins Univ., Baltimore, 1948; and Müller, R. F. C.: Grundsätze altindischer Medizin, vol. 8, Acta Historica Scientiarum Naturalium et Medicinalium, Kopenhagen, 1951. The latter includes commentary on Charaka's Samhita, whose classic text has been published at least twice in English. On medical services in ancient China: Hume, E. H.: The Chinese Way in Medicine, Baltimore, 1940; Wong, K. C. and Wu, L.-T.: History of Chinese Medicine, Tientsin, 1932; Huard, P. and Wong, M.: La Médecine chinoise, au cours des siècles, Paris, 1959, Evolution de la matière médicale chinoise, Janus 47: 3, 1958, and such German works as those by Franz Huebotter and Gottfried Schramm. There is a comprehensive history of Japanese pharmacy as such (in Japanese) by Simizu (or Shimizu), Tootaroo: Nihon Yakugakushi, Tokyo, 1949.

3. Jastrow, M.: The medicine of the Babylonians and Assyrians, Proc. Roy. Soc. Med. 7:109, 1913.

4. Temkin, O.: Beiträge zur archäischen Medizin, Kyklos 3:90, 1930.

5. Artelt, W.: op. cit., p. 33; Temkin, O.: op. cit., p. 133.

6. Thompson, R. C.: The Assyrian Herbal, London, 1924; On the Chemistry of the Ancient Assyrians, London, 1925; Urdang, G.: Pharmacy in ancient Babylon-Assyria, Palestine and Egypt, Am. J. Pharm. Ed. 7:50, 1943.

7. Castiglioni, A.: A History of Medicine, p. 39, New York, 1941.

8. Levey, M.: Chemistry and Chemical Technology in Ancient Mesopotamia, p. 149, Amsterdam, 1959. (Transliterated words have been omitted from the quotation.) An excellent source of information based on the original documents. [See also, Levey, M.: A Sumerian medical text from Nippur of the 3rd millennium B.C., Actes du VIII Congres International d'Histoire des Sciences Collection de Travaux de l'Academie . . . No. 9:843, 1956; and Kramer, S. N.: First pharmacopeia in man's recorded history, Am. J. Pharm. 126:76, 1954.]

9. Ibid., p. 151.

10. Sigerist, H.: A History of Medicine, vol. 1, Primitive and Archaic Medicine, p. 484, New York, 1955. Probably the best account in English of Babylonian and Egyptian medicine.

11. Meissner, B.: Babylonien und Assyrien, p. 359, Heidelberg, 1925. Von Oefele refers to the "pasisu" in a letter to Hermann Schelenz.

12. Castiglioni, A.: op. cit., p. 38.

13. Dawson, W. R.: Magician and Leech, p. 128, London, 1929.

14. Temkin, O.: Recent publications on Egyptian and Babylonian Medicine, Bull. Inst. Hist. Med., Johns Hopkins Univ., 4:247, 341, 1936. The names and the estimated dates of the main medical papyri as listed by Temkin are: Kahun, gynecology (also veterinary fragment), c. 1900 B.C.; Edwin Smith, surgery, c. 1550; George Ebers, medicine and pharmacy, c. 1500 B.C.; Hearst, formulary, c. 1500 B.C.; and between 1350 and 1100 B.C., London 10059, drug therapy and incantations; Berlin 3038 (Brugsch major), therapeutics and fertility tests; Berlin 3027 (Brugsch minor; edited by Erman), diseases, therapy

and incantations for childbirth and infants. In addition the short Chester Beatty (BM 10686) papyrus, c. 1200 B.C., is a formulary for anal diseases. See also, Sigerist: History, 298-318 et passim; Leake, C. D.: The Old Egyptian Medical Papyri, Lawrence, 1952.

15. Grapow, H.: Untersuchungen über die altägyptischen Papyri, I. Teil. Mitt. vorderasiatisch–ägyptische Gesells. *40*:(1), 1935.

16. Ebbell, B.: The Papyrus Ebers, Copenhagen, 1937.

17. Temkin, O.: Isis *28*:126, 1938.

18. Leake, C. D.: Ancient Egyptian therapy, Ciba Symposia, *1*:311, 1940, referring to both the Ebers and the Hearst papyri.

19. Ebbell: *op. cit.*, p. 38.

20. Quantitative measurement in the medical papyri, and drug measurements in particular, is discussed by Leake: Medical Papyri, pp. 18-33.

21. Ebbell: Papyrus, p. 19; cf. p. 29.

22. Sigerist: History, p. 303. For the Smith papyrus, see Oriental Institute Publications, Volumes 3 and 4: "The Edwin Smith Surgical Papyrus," James H. Breasted, translator and editor, Univ. Chicago Press, 1930.

23. Dawson, W. R.: Studies in ancient materia medica, Am. Drug. *73*:22, 1925.

24. Besides present-day flora and ecology, numerous historical asides may be found in Fahmy, I. R.: The medicinal plants of the Middle East, Lebanese Pharm. J. *4*:12, 1956.

25. Thompson, C. J. S.: The Mystery and Art of the Apothecary, pp. 11, 12, London, 1929.

26. Breasted, J. H.: A History of Egypt from the Earliest Times to the Persian Conquest, p. 113, London, 1921.

27. Jonckheere, Frans: Le Preparateur de remèdes dans l'organisation de la pharmacie égyptienne, Publication No. 29, Institut für Orientforschung, Deutsche Akad. Wiss. Berlin, pp. 160-161, et passim, Berlin, 1955. In examining past views in the light of evidence, the author specifically argues against attributing pharmaceutical connotations to "Urma" and to "ph-armaki." With regard to the formulas for unguents and perfumed preparations that have been found inscribed on the walls of Ptolemaic temples, the author concludes that these are archival type-formulas for cult ceremonies and festival rituals, without therapeutic purposes. Likewise, the "laboratory" rooms excavated within the walls of the sanctuary, but outside the sacred chambers proper, must have required "pharmaceutical" or "chemical" types of knowledge for their operation, but Jonckheere asks for evidence showing that their products were put to therapeutic use. (See, *ibid.*, pp. 151-157.)

28. Sigerist, History, 343.

29. Grapow, H.: Die ägyptischen medizinischen Papyri, Munich Med. Wochenschr. *82*:135, 958, 1002, 1935.

30. Thompson, C. S. J.: *op. cit.*, p. 24.

31. Especially rich and reliable sources of information about Greek temple medicine are, Kerenyi, Ch.: Le Medecin divin: promenades mythologiques aux sanctuaires d'Asclepios, Basle, 1948, and Edelstein, E. J., and Edelstein, L.: Asclepius. A Collection and Interpretation of the Testimonies, 2 vols., Baltimore, 1945.

32. Osler, William: The Evolution of Modern Medicine, p. 69, New Haven, 1923.

33. Oliver, J. R.: Greek medicine and its relation to Greek civilization, Bull. Inst. Hist. Med., Johns Hopkins Univ. *3*:623, 1935.

34. Edelstein, L.: Peri Deron, und die Sammlung der Hippokratischen Schriften, Berlin, 1931.

35. Jones, W. H. S.: Hippocrates, vol. 1, p. 21, London, 1923.

36. Wootton, A.: Chronicles of Pharmacy, p. 78, London, 1910.

37. Jones, W. H. S.: The Doctor's Oath, Cambridge, England, 1924.

38. Tschirch, A.: Handbuch der Pharmakognosie, Leipzig, 1910, 1. (Abt. 3): 1271-1290.

39. Crateuas' drawings are contained in part of the famous Vienna Codex of Dioscorides' writings on crude drugs. It was once possessed by Juliana Anicia, daughter of an emperor of the Western Roman Empire (Anicius Olybirius, 512 A.D.).

40. The Greek Herbal of Dioscorides: John Goodyer, trans., 1655; Gunther, R. T.: ed., Oxford, 1934; Hafner, New York, 1959 (reprint); see also Cohen, M. R., and Drabkin, I. E.: A Source Book in Greek Science, New York, 1948.

41. Albutt, T. C.: Greek Medicine in Rome, p. 380, London, 1921.

42. Brock, A. J.: Galen on the Natural Faculties, p. ix, London, 1916.

43. Thompson, C. J. S.: *op. cit.*, p. 35.

44. Pliny, Natural History, bk. 34, ch. 25

(Bostock-Riley edition, vol. 6, p. 195; and footnotes 1, 21, p. 143; and 15, vol. 3, p. 357).

45. For a discussion of some of the evidence and difficulties of interpretation, see Dann, G. E. *in*: Zur Geschichte der Pharmazie No. 1, 1954, pp. 5 and 6 (Beilage der Deutschen Apotheker-Zeitung), based on: Tergolina in Raccolta di scritti in onore di Giulio Conci a cura di A. E. Vitolo (Pisa, 1953). Some comments in Pliny's Natural History on the *seplasiarii*, as cited by Ernst Stieb, may be found at 34.25 (6:195 of the Bostock-Riley edition) and 33.58 (6: 143); see also in the Bostock-Riley edition, note 1 at 6:195, note 21 at 6:143, and note 15 at 3:357. One of the most comprehensive sources of information is Schmidt, A.: Drogen und Drogenhandel in Altertum, Leipzig, 1924; the passages of special pharmaceutical interest have been translated into English (see Urdang, G.: Pharmacy in ancient Greece and Rome, Am. J. Pharm. Ed. 7:160, 1943).

46. Spencer, W. G.: Celsus De Medicina, vol. 2, pp. xv-lxvii, Cambridge, (Mass.) 1938.

47. Marx, F.: Prolegomena, Corp. Med. Lat. 1, Leipzig, 1915; Castiglioni, A.: Aulus Cornelius Celsus as a historian of medicine, Bull. Hist. Med. 8:857, 1940; Meinecke, B.: Aulus Cornelius Celsus— plagiarist or artifex medicinae? Bull. Hist. Med. 10:288, 1941.

48. Schelenz, H.: Geschichte der Pharmazie, p. 165, Berlin, 1904; Schonack, W.: Die Rezeptsammlung des Scribonius Largus, Jena, 1913; Rinne, F.: Scribonii Largi "Compositiones," Dorpat, 1892.

49. Chem. and Drug. 106:804, 1927.

50. Singer, C.: From Magic to Science, 178, 179.

51. For lists of the plants mentioned by Pliny see Wittstein: Die Naturgeschichte der Caius Plinius Secundus, Leipzig, 1881, and Fée: Commentaires sur la botanique et la matière médicale de Pline, Paris, 1883. For Pliny's chemical knowledge, see Bailey, K. C.: The Elder Pliny's Chapters on Chemical Subjects, 2 vols., London, 1929 and 1932. For a historic paper of great pharmaceutical interest, see Stieb, E. W.: Drug adulteration and its detection, in the writings of Theophrastus, Dioscorides and Pliny, Journal Mondial de Pharmacie 2:117, 1958.

52. A masterly English translation and commentary may be found in: Adams, F.:

The Medical Works of Paulus Aegineta, London, 1844-1847; see also Berendes, J.: Paulos' von Aegina, des besten Arztes sieben Bücher, Leiden, 1914.

2. THE ARABS AND THE EUROPEAN MIDDLE AGES

1. Hitti, P. K.: History of the Arabs, p. 174, London, 1937.

2. Baas, J. H.: Outlines of the History of Medicine and the Medical Profession, Handerson, H. E., trans., p. 220, New York, 1889.

3. Campbell, D.: Arabian Medicine and its Influence on the Middle Ages, vol. 1, p. xi, London, 1926.

4. Sarton, G.: Introduction to the History of Science, vol. 1, p. 611, Baltimore, 1927.

5. Ranking, G. S. A.: The life and works of Rhazes, 17th Internat. Congr. Med. 23: 237, 1914; Campbell, D.: *op. cit.*, pp. 60-102.

6. Chem. and Drug. 106:808, 1927.

7. Campbell, D.: *op cit.*, p. 71.

8. Ruska, J.: Die Alchemie Al-Razi's, Der Islam 22:319, 1935.

9. Das Buch der Alaune, p. 12, Berlin, 1935.

10. Sarton, G.: *op. cit.*, p. 709.

11. Meyer-Steineg, Th., and Sudhoff, K.: Geschichte der Medizin in Ueberblick, p. 160, Jena, 1921.

12. Urdang, G.: Zur Geschichte der Metalle in den Amtlichen Deutschen Arznei- büchern, pp. 14, 15, Mittenwald, 1933.

13. Osler, William: Incunabula medica, p. 36, Oxford, 1923.

14. Hamarneh, S. K., and Sonnedecker, G.: A Pharmaceutical View of al-Zahrawi (Abulcasis) in Arabic Spain, Leiden, 1963 (pending publication).

15. Sarton, G.: *op. cit.*, 2, p. 663, Baltimore, 1931. For detailed information, see: Von Sentheimer, J.: Grosse Zusammenstellung über die Kräfte der bekannten einfachen Heil- und Nahrungsmittel von Abu Mohammed Abdallah ben Ahmed aus Malaga bekannt unter dem Namen Ebn Baithar, 2 vols., Stuttgart, 1840 and 1842, or Leclerc, L., trans., Traité des Simples, par Ibn el-Beither, 3 vols., Paris, 1877-1883.

16. For the materia medica of Maimonides, and a multilingual key to medieval drug terminology, see Meyerhof, Max, ed. and trans.: Un Glossaire de Matière Médicale de Maimonide . . . , Mémoires présentés a l'Institut d'Égypte, Vol. 41, 1940. For

an excellent general evaluation of Arabic writings on drugs, see Meyerhof's four essays in: Ciba Symposia 6:1847-1876, 1944.

17. Reisman, D.: The Story of Medicine in the Middle Ages, p. 64, New York, 1935. The compiler of "Maimonides' Oath" was Marcus Hertz (1747-1803), whose German was translated into Hebrew by Isaac Euchel. Among other Arabic writers that deserve mention are Ibn Sarabi (Serapion, Jr., 11th or 13th century), whose *Liber de medicamentis simplicibus* . . . was an essential part of the medieval literature of pharmacy (see Guigues, P.: Les noms arabes dans Sérapion *Liber de simplici medicina*, Paris, 1905); also, Abu Marwan Ibn Zuhr (ca. 1092-1162, called Avenzoar), whose *al-Taisir*, a treatise on practical medicine, interestingly describes the methods of preparing medicines. Probably both of them lived in Arabic Spain.

18. Meyer-Steineg, Th., and Sudhoff, K.: *op. cit.*, pp. 156, 225, 255.

19. Ruska, J., and Kraus, P.: Der Zusammenbruch der Jabir Legende, Beilage zum dritten Jahresbericht des Forschungsinstituts f. Geschichte der Naturwiss. in Berlin, 1930.

20. Ruska, J.: Arabische Giftbücher, Fortschritte der Med. 50:524, 1932.

21. For further information in English, see Taylor, F. S.: The Alchemists, London, 1953; see also: Holmyard, E. J.: Alchemy, Harmondsworth, 1957 (now in paperback Pelican, A348).

22. Ruska, J.: Das Buch der Alaune, p. 11.

23. Hamarneh, S. K., citing 'Ali Abu al-Hasan al-Quifti: Ikhbar al-'Ulama bi Akhbar al-Hukama, pp. 74 and 248, Cairo, 1908.

24. Hamarneh, S. K., citing Aḥmad 'Isā: Tarikh al-Bimāristānāt fī al-Islām, p. 203, Damascus, 1939.

25. Hamarneh, S. K.: The rise of professional pharmacy in Islam, Med. Hist. 6:63, 1962.

26. *Ibid.*, 61 f. The information and the conclusions about Arabic practice of pharmacy conveyed here, including Arabic references, rest almost entirely on this article by Hamarneh and on his Ph.D. thesis: Some Pharmaceutical Aspects of al-Zahrawi's *al-Tasreef* about 1000 A.D., University of Wisconsin, 1959 (especially Chapter I; unpublished).

27. Campbell, D.: *op. cit.*, p. xii.

28. Fort, G. F.: Medical Economy During

the Middle Ages, p. 137, New York, 1883.

29. Meyer-Steineg, Th., and Sudhoff, K.: *op. cit.*, p. 172.

30. Buck, A. H.: The Growth of Medicine from the Earliest Times to about 1800, p. 238, New Haven, 1917.

31. Sigerist, H. E.: The medical literature of the early middle ages, Bull. Hist. Med. 2: 32, 1934.

32. Castiglioni, A.: (Krumbhaar, E. B., trans.) Italian Medicine, pp. 10, and 3, New York, 1932.

33. Buck, A. H.: *op. cit.*, p. 187.

34. Sigerist, H. E.: *op. cit.*, p. 33.

35. *Ibid.*, p. 40.

36. Singer, C.: From Magic to Science, p. 185, New York, 1928.

37. Extracts from the work of Pliny were compiled for practical use in the so-called *Plinius Valerianus* and in a *breviarium*, known as *Medicina Plinii* or *Plini Secundi Junioris de medicina libra*. This breviarium "almost literally plagiarized Scribonius." The Pseudo-Apuleius and other contemporary or earlier compilations are the sources of the book *De medicamentis physicis, empiricis ac rationalibus*, written by a high Roman official of Celtic origin, Marcellus of Bordeaux (A.D. 410), who describes, in addition to drugs of ancient classic literature, many medicaments in popular use by his people, the Celts. About 200 years later a learned Bishop, Isidore of Seville (570-636), wrote his famous encyclopedia, a part of which was devoted to medicine. In this treatise "especially Caelius has been plundered." (Meyer-Steineg, Th., and Sudhoff, K.: *op. cit.*, pp. 171 and 174.)

38. Campbell, D.: *op. cit.*, p. 106.

39. The monasteries of Luxeuil (France), Fulda and Reichenau (Germany), St. Galls (Switzerland) and Bobbio (Northern Italy) were some of their stages. At Reichenau in 825 a German abbot, Walahfried, wrote his *Hortulus*, a Latin poem on plants growing in that district, which became famous not only as poetry but also as an excellent description of the appearance and the medicinal virtues of the plants. The intense devotion to medical and pharmaceutical treatment of patients in St. Galls is attested by the plan of a new monastic building, dating from 820. (The building itself was never erected.) It provides not only an infirmary or

hospital for the sick, but also a large *armarium pigmentariorum,* i.e., a special room for the preparation and storage of medicines; and a *herbularius,* i.e., a garden for the cultivation of medicinal plants, the names of which are mentioned in the plan.

About 25 years earlier (794 or 795) the so-called *Capitulare de villis* was promulgated by Louis the Pious (not by the Emperor Charlemagne, as was assumed before the researches of Dopsch). This edict orders and regulates the planting and raising of herbs and vegetables, useful medicinally and otherwise, in all the gardens appurtenant to the royal domain in Aquitania (Southern France). It is important for pharmacy because it represents the first official acknowledgment of the importance of the cultivation of medicinal plants in Western Europe north of the Alps. (Meyer-Steineg, Th., and Sudhoff, K.: *op. cit.,* pp. 175 and 176.)

40. Singer, C.: *op. cit.,* p. 188.
41. Meyer-Steineg, Th., and Sudhoff, K.: *op. cit.,* p. 177.
42. Garrison, F.: An Introduction to the History of Medicine, p. 147, Philadelphia, 1929.
43. Sigerist, H. E.: *op. cit.,* p. 28.
44. Castiglioni, A.: *op. cit.,* p. 14.
45. Campbell, D.: *op. cit.,* p. 123.
46. According to Paul Dorveaux (Le livre des simples médecines, Paris, Société française de l'histoire de la médecine, 1913, p. xvi), the *Circa Instans* is only a revised, corrected and considerably augmented edition of Constantine's treatise (*De Gradibus Simplicium*).
47. Lutz, Alfons: Der verschollene frühsalernitanische Antidotarius magnus in einer Basler Handschrift aus dem 12, Jahrhundert und das Antidotarium Nicholai, Acta Pharmaciae Historica, 1959, No. 1 (an important paper based on Ms. D/III/14 in Basler Universitäts-Bibliothek); on the Antidotarium Nicholai, cf. Van den Berg, W. S.: Eene Middelnederlandsche vertaling van het Antidotarium Nicolai Leiden, 1917. The three *Antidotaria Nicolai,* most historians now would agree, may be distinguished as follows:

(a) Antidotarium Nicolai Salernitani: oldest of the three (written about 1250?).

(b) Antidotarium Nicolai Myrepsi: the most comprehensive of the three formularies; written in the 14th century by Nicolaus Myrepsus (also called Alexandrinus), a native of Alexandria living at Byzantium

(c) Dispensatorium ad aromatarios: presumably written by Nicolaus Praepositus, at Lyon, about 1500 (not a second treatise of the so-called Nicolaus Salernitanus, as previously thought). (Wickersheimer, E.: Nicolaus Praepositus, ein französischer Arzt ums Jahr 1500, Arch. f. Geschichte d. Med. 5:302, 1912.)

A later version written in the 14th and 15th centuries appeared incompletely in French translations, which have been edited and commented on (Dorveaux, P.: L'antidotaire Nicolas, Paris, 1896).

48. Meyer-Steineg, Th., and Sudhoff, K.: *op. cit.,* p. 205. A Latin inscription on the title page indicates that the *Regimen Sanitatis* was prepared by the entire school of Salerno for an English king; but Singer considers this too typical of royal ascriptions prevalent, at the time, for achieving greater sale of copies, to be considered alone as convincing evidence. (Singer, C.: *op. cit.,* p. 247.)
49. Campbell, D.: *op. cit.,* p. 126.
50. Hariz, J.: La part de la médecine arabe dans l'évolution de la médecine française, Paris, Université de Paris, Thèse, 1922.
51. Häfliger, J. A.: Die Fachbücherei der Mittelalterlichen Apotheker Basels, Pharm. Acta Helv. 2:140, 1927.
52. Osler, W.: *op. cit.,* p. 19; Meyer-Steineg, Th., and Sudhoff, K.: *op. cit.,* pp. 225-61.

3. CONCEPTS AND MEDICAMENTS BECOME MODERN

1. A scholarly and extensive discussion of this legal milestone in the history of the pharmacist—based on collation and translation of early documents—has been published by W.-H. Hein and K. Sappert: Die Medizinalordnung Friedrichs II (Bd. NS 12, Veröffentlichungen Internat. Gesellsch. Geschichte der Pharmacie), Eutin, 1957. The authors conclude that the main pharmaceutical provisions of the edict were promulgated sometime between 1231 and 1240. (pp. 17-18 and 98) Cf. Adlung, A., and Urdang, G.: Grundriss der Geschichte der deutschen Pharmazie, p. 7, Berlin, 1935. The date of the edict concerning the separation of pharmacy from medicine in the Two Sicilies is given variously in earlier literature (1224, 1231,

1240 and 1241). It has to be kept in mind that the edict was not an isolated legislative act but part of comprehensive legislation to regulate the hygienic conditions of the Southern Italian kingdom, and was started already under the Norman King of Sicily, Roger II, the grandfather of Frederick II. The opinion that the edict concerning the separation of pharmacy from medicine marks the end of this serial legislation, and was promulgated in 1240, was expressed by Huillard-Bréholles in his *Historia diplomatica Friderici Secundi* (Paris, 1854, vol. 4).

2. Häfliger, J. A.: Das Apothekenwesen Basels, p. 31, Mittenwald, 1938.

3. Adlung, A., and Urdang, G., *op. cit.*, p. 52.

4. Neuburger, M.: History of Medicine (English translation), Oxford, 1925, vol. 2, part I, p. 2.

5. Stillmann, J. M.: Paracelsus, p. 45, Chicago, 1920.

6. In the medical field the Greek originals did not replace the medieval Greco-Arabic treatises immediately or extensively. Meyer-Steineg, Th., and Sudhoff, K.: Geschichte der Medizin in Überblick, pp. 247-271, Jena, 1821.

7. Stillmann, J. M.: *op. cit.*, p. 106.

8. Meyer-Steineg, Th., and Sudhoff, K.: *op. cit.* p. 275. For further information, the most meaningful book is by Pagel, W.: Paracelsus: An Introduction to Philosophical Medicine in the Era of the Renaissance, Basel, 1958.

9. Multhauf, R.: Medical Chemistry and "The Paracelsians," Bull. Hist. Med. *28*: 101, 1954.

10. The effect of drugs was explained (in this case mercury bichloride and mercurous chloride) by adherents of the iatrochemical or the iatrophysical theory in the way described by George Urdang: The early chemical and pharmaceutical history of calomel, *in* Chymia, pp. 99-101, Philadelphia, 1948.

11. Garrison, F. H.: An Introduction to the History of Medicine, p. 314, Philadelphia, 1929.

12. Sigerist, Henry E.: The Great Doctors, p. 293, New York, 1933.

13. ———: Man and Medicine, p. 248, New York, 1932.

14. ———: The Great Doctors, p. 343.

15. For a concise evaluative biographic article, see Cowen, David L.: Ehrlich the

man, the scientist, Am. J. Pharm. Ed. *26*: 4, 1962.

16. Fleming, Alexander: Chemotherapy, Yesterday, To-day and To-morrow, p. 6, Cambridge, England, 1946.

17. Domagk, G.: Entwicklung der Chemotherapie in den letzten 25 Jahren und Ausblick in die Zukunft, Münch. medizin. Wschr. *100*:2, (reprint) 1958.

18. Osborne, G.: Chemical compounds in the official compendia, Am. J. Pharm. Ed. *26*: 22, 1962.

19. Tishler, M.: Impact of Research on Medicinal Chemistry (Division of Medicinal Chemistry, Am. Chem. Soc.), p. 14, (mimeograph) 1959.

20. On the early history of antibiotics, see the special issue, J. Hist. Med. *6*: No. 3, 1951. On Gosio and other precursors of Fleming, see the article by J. Brunel, p. 295.

21. Welch, H.: Pharmacology of antibiotics, J. Hist. Med. *6*:348, 1951.

22. Sigerist, H. E.: Man and Medicine, p. 252; Adlung, A., and Urdang, G.: *op. cit.*, pp. 361-380.

23. One of the best sources of information on homeopathic pharmacy is: Steinbichler, E.: Geschichte der homöopathischen Arznei Bereitungslehre in Deutschland bis 1872 (Bd. NS 11, Internat. Gesellsch. Geschichte der Pharmazie), Eutin, 1957.

24. Ackerknecht, E. H.: A Short History of Medicine, pp. 131 f., New York, Ronald, 1955.

25. Meyer-Steineg, Th., and Sudhoff, K.: *op. cit.*, p. 321.

26. Sigerist, H. E.: Man and Medicine, p. 247.

27. ———: The Great Doctors, pp. 175-184.

28. *Ibid.*, pp. 185-190.

29. Meyer-Steineg, Th., and Sudhoff, K.: *op. cit.*, p. 416.

30. In the 15th century the English physician Howel, in his formulary, recommended "cod oil" in the preparation of a "cere cloth," a kind of cerate to be used on wounds. About 1730, Norwegian fishermen and farmers found that cod-liver oil cured rickets (Brauer, P.: Die Geschichte des Lebertrans. Neue homöopathische Zeitung 9:437, 1934). In 1770, the English physician Thomas Percival recommended the oil against rheumatism. However, there was no theoretic explanation of the effect of the oil, and the scientific world hesitated to acknowledge it. In 1837 the pharmacist Hopfer de l'Orme in Hanau found iodine in cod-liver oil (Schelenz, H.: Geschichte

der Pharmazie, p. 811, Berlin, 1904); and an explanation of its beneficial effect was based on this discovery. The oil entered the pharmacopeias but as time went on it again fell into disrepute. There was an abundance of other iodine preparations, and according to contemporary theories there was nothing in the iodine content of the oil to explain the peculiar effect attributed to it. Hence it was regarded as of no greater value than other fats and distinguished from them merely by the special disadvantage of bad taste (Kofler, L.: Das Vertrauen zur Arznei im Wandel der Zeiten. Die Vorträge der Hauptversammlung, Basel; Gesellsch. für Geschichte der Pharmazie, p. 138, Mittenwald, 1934).

31. Facsimile of the first edition of the Pharmacopoeia Augustana, with Introductory Essays by Theodor Husemann, E. Kremers, ed., Madison, Wis., 1927.
32. *Ibid.*, p. xxix.
33. Urdang, G.: The Pharmacopoeia Londinensis of 1618, p. 81, Madison, Wis., 1944.

4. THE DEVELOPMENT IN ITALY

1. Conci, G.: Pagine di Storia della Farmacia, p. 245, Milan, 1934.
2. Schelenz, H.: Geschichte der Pharmazie, p. 313, Berlin, 1904.
3. *Ibid.*, p. 155.
4. Thompson, J. W.: Economic and Social History of Europe in the Later Middle Ages, vol. 1, p. 26, New York, 1931.
5. *Ibid.*, vol. 2, p. 5.
6. Ciasca, R.: L'Arte dei Medici e Speziali, Florence, 1922 and 1927; Staley, E.: The Guilds of Florence, London, 1906; Davidsohn, R.: Geschichte von Florenz, Berlin, 1896-1927.
7. Thompson, J. W.: *op. cit.*, vol. 2, p. 227.
8. Heyd: Geschichte des Levantehandels im Mittelalter, Stuttgart, 1879.
9. Staley, E.: *op. cit.*, pp. 256, 257, 265.
10. *Ibid.*, p. 273.
11. In Verona a guild of the pharmacists (*la magnifica arte degli speziali*) is mentioned in 1221 (Conci, G.: *op. cit.*, p. 241). In Milan the *Paratico apothecariorum spetiariorum et aromatariorum* was founded about 1300. In Piacenza the *speziali* constituted a guild in the 13th century. In Venice (*ibid.*, p. 279) we again find physicians and pharmacists joined in the *capitolare medicorum et spetiatiorum*, founded in 1258. In 1565, the pharmacists parted

company with the physicians and formed the *Collegio degli speziali*. Conci (*ibid.*, p. 297) mentions additional pharmaceutical guilds in Monza, Como, Cremona, Siena, Mantua, Volterra, Lucca, Pistoia, Pisa, Perugia, Bologna and Padua.
12. Poce, M.: Pagine storiche sul nobile collegio chimico-farmaceutico, Roma, 1931.
13. Davidsohn: *op. cit.*, 2, 215.
14. Rosenthaler, L.: Die Drogenliste der Pergolotti, Schweiz, Apoth. Ztg. 60:89, 1922. In regard to the drugs involved in this trade, information may be gained from *La practica della mercatora*, written in the 14th century by the Florentine, Pergolotti, an employee of the Baldi, the great Florentine merchants.
15. Heyd: *op. cit.*
16. Conci: *op. cit.*, p. 291.
17. Schelenz: *op. cit.*, p. 364.
18. Staley, E.: *op. cit.*, p. 241.
19. Pedrazzini, C.: La Farmacia Stroica et Artistica Italiana, Milan, 1934. Häfliger, J.: Pharmazeutische Altertumskunde, pp. 27-39, Zürich, 1931.
20. For a comprehensive list see Appendix 5 and George Griffenhagen: Pharmacy Museums, Madison, Wis., 1956. In his older list Josef Häfliger (*ibid.*) mentions the "*Sammlung Jo Mayer*" Wiesbaden, calling it "the most important German private collection." This collection was bought in 1932 by E. R. Squibb & Sons, and about a decade later was presented by the firm to the American Pharmaceutical Association. It is now in the United States National Museum (Smithsonian Institution), in Washington, D. C. The contents of the collection have been described by George Urdang in a booklet entitled *The Squibb Ancient Pharmacy*, New York, 1940.
21. Rosenthaler, L.: Die Drogen des Puti, Pharm. Ztg. 75:1439, 1930.
22. Castiglioni, A.: Italian Medicine, p. 55, New York, 1932.
23. Ullersperger, J. B.: Geschichtsumriss der Pharmacie im Königreiche Italien, Neues Repertorium für Pharmacie (Buchner, L. A., ed.) 21:1872, 291.
24. Conci: *op. cit.*, p. 301.
25. ———: *op. cit.*, p. 283. The last year for the sale or the abandonment of old hereditary and salable privileges was 1943 (law of 1913), although in 1946 this term was prolonged for some specified cases.
26. Urban, E.: Apothekengesetzgebung im Ausland. Thom's Handbuch der prak-

tischen und wissenschaftlichen Pharmazie, vol. 1, p. 203, Berlin, 1924.

27. Thompson, C. J. S.: The Mystery and Art of the Apothecary, p. 129, London, 1929; Zimmerman, L.: Saladini de Asculo Serenitatis Principis Tarenti Physici Principalis Compendium Aromatariorum, Leipzig, 1919.

28. Schelenz: *op. cit.*, p. 334.

29. *Ibid.*, p. 337.

30. Schumacher, B.: Das Luminare Majus von Joannes Jacobus Manlius de Bosco 1536, Mittenwald, 1936.

31. Schelenz, *op. cit.*, p. 407.

32. Conci: *op. cit.*, p. 138. One of Sgobbi's predecessors, the German-born Georg Melich, wrote a "practice" of pharmacy, the *Dispensatorium medicum,* of which the first edition in Italian was published in Venice in 1574, the last in Latin translation in Germany in 1657.

33. *Il giornale di farmacia e di chimica,* Torino, founded in 1852, and the *Bollettino chimico-farmaceutico,* Milan, founded in 1861 under the title *Bulletino farmaceutico.* In 1906 the *Corriere dei farmacisti, Milan,* made its appearance. Since 1945 the *Corriere* has been issued as the official *Organo degli Ordini dei farmicisti e delle associazioni sindacali di categoria.*

34. The most definitive paper to date on the question of the "first pharmocopeia," and the *Nuovo receptario* particularly, is by Alfons Lutz: Studien über die pharmazeutische Inkunabel 'Nuovo Receptario' von Florenz, Bd. 13 NS, Internat. Gesellsch. für Geschichte der Pharmazie, Stuttgart, 1958. The title of the Florentine book was later changed to *Ricettario* and finally, in 1567, to *Ricettario fiorentino,* under which name it was reissued until 1789. Although the first edition is dated 1498, Lutz shows that by our calendar it would have been printed January 21, 1499.

35. The *Antidotarium Bononiense* (1574) in Bologna, the *Pharmacopoea Bergamensis* (1580) in Bergamo, the *Antidotarium Romanum* (1583) in Rome, the *Pharmacopoea Veneta* (1618) in Venice, the *Antidotarium Messanense* (1629) in Messina, the *Antidotarium Neopolitanum* (1649) in Naples, the *Pharmacopoea Ferrariensis* (1725) in Ferrara, the *Pharmacopoea Taurinensis* (1736) in Turin, the *Pharmacopoea Sardoa* (1773) in Sardinia, the *Formulario farmaceutico* (1791) in Genoa,

and lastly the *Pharmacopoea Parmiensis* (1823) in Parma.

36. Urdang, G.: Pharmacopoeias as witnesses of world history, J. Hist. Med. Allied Sci. 1:47, 1946. For a general discussion of the history of pharmacopeias, including a chronologic international list of the various editions (but by no means limited to "official pharmacopeias"), see Volckringer, J.: Evolution et unification des formulaires et des pharmacopées, Paris, 1953.

37. Other chairs for medical botany followed at Bologna (1534), Mondovi (1561), and Turin (1566).

5. THE DEVELOPMENT IN FRANCE

1. Hein, W. H., and Sappert, K.: Die Medizinalordnung Friedrichs II (Bd. NS 12, Internat. Gesellsch. für Geschichte der Pharmazie), pp. 76-78, Eutin, 1957, referring to F. Prevet and quoting a parchment manuscript, the "Petit Thalamus," found in the municipal archive in Montpellier.

2. Bouvet, M.: Histoire de la pharmacie en France, Paris, 1937, p. 226.

3. *Ibid.*, p. 252.

4. *Ibid.*, p. 227.

5. Hein, W., and Sappert, K.: *op. cit.*, p. 76.

6. Bouvet, M.: *op. cit.*, p. 60.

7. *Ibid.* p. 61.

8. *Ibid.*, p. 236.

9. *Ibid.*, p. 71.

10. *Ibid.*, p. 74.

11. *Ibid.*, p. 253.

12. Personal communication from Dr. Louis Irrissou. He reports that the main importance of the edict of Villers-Cotterets rests on the fact that it made the French language (as spoken in and near Paris) compulsory for official documents, thus reducing the other languages spoken in France at this time, especially Provençal, to mere dialects and discouraging the use of Spanish, English and German by the population of areas bordering on one of the countries concerned.

13. Dorveaux, P.: Le livre des simples médecines, p. xx, Paris, 1913.

14. Bouvet, M.: *op. cit.*, p. 64.

15. *Ibid.*, pp. 280-284. It was later ruled that pharmacists who wanted to practice the trade of a spicer could qualify by preparing a special spicer's "masterpiece" (1581), a kind of practical examination. The rights of the competing groups were

further adjusted in parliamentary ordinances of 1629, 1689, 1734 and 1742.

16. Personal communication from Dr. Louis Irrissou.

17. In 1957 there remained about one herboristerie to every thirteen pharmacies. (Laurent, J.: La Pharmacie en France: Etude de Géographie Economique, p. 208, Paris, 1959. The legal bases of French pharmacy had been the royal declaration of 1777 and the law of 1803, which were replaced by the law of September 11, 1941, as amended May 23, 1945.

18. Bouvet, M.: *op. cit.*, pp. 218-224.

19. *Ibid.*, p. 42.

20. *Ibid.*, p. 213.

21. *Ibid.*, p. 265, 266. Champier's initial libel was called *Myrouel des apothicaires et pharmacopoles* (1532). It was followed by the *Déclaration des abus et tromperies que font les apothicaires* (1553) by the physician Sébastian Collin (pseudonym: Lisset Benancio), and a lampoon by the physician Jean Surrelh, *L'apologie des médecins contre les calomnies et grands abus de certain apothicaires* (1558). A pharmacist at Lyon (Bernard Palissy?), writing under the pseudonym Pierre Brailler, published a *Déclaration des abus et ignorance des médecins* (1557), then fired the other barrel, *Articulations sur l'apologie de Jean Surrelh* (1558).

22. *Ibid.*, p. 267.

23. *Ibid.*, pp. 301-307.

24. Philippe, A.: Histoire des apothicaires, pp. 221-234, Paris, 1853; Bouvet, M.: Histoire de la Pharmacie, pp. 355-357.

25. White, F. A.: French pharmaceutical societies, Amer. Drugg. *71* (No. 9):11, 1923.

26. Humbert, G.: L'ordre des pharmaciens français, Bull. Féd. Int. Pharm. *21*:155, 1947.

27. Authorized by Article 571 of the Code de la Santé Publique, as reported in a personal communication from M. Bouvet and H. Bonnemain, February 23, 1962. The area of Paris and the Seine, with a ratio of about 2,800 to 1, does not yet conform entirely to the general regulation.

28. Bouvet, M.: *op. cit.*, pp. 149, 150.

29. *Ibid.*, p. 138.

30. Deno, R. A.: Pharmacy in France, J. A. Ph. A., Prac. Pharm. Ed. *12*:164, 1951.

31. Lesur, J.: Pharmacists and Biological Analysis, (mimeograph) 1961, 11 pp.

32. Bouvet, M.: *op. cit.*, pp. 66, 310-317.

33. Pegurier, G.: The supervision of pharmacy in France, Chem. and Drugg. 79:483, 1911.

34. Green, D. S.: American Assistant Trade Commissioner at Paris, as quoted in Am. Drugg. *74*:17, 1926.

35. Revue d'histoire de la pharmacie 3:204, 1932.

36. Heger, H.: Apothekerbilder, 2, pp. 88-92, Vienna, 1919. Sellier, Ch.: La Pharmacie Centrale de France, Paris, 1903.

37. Bouvet, M.: *op. cit.*, p. 108.

38. *Ibid.*, pp. 78-79.

39. *Ibid.*, pp. 95, 96.

40. Centenaire de l'Ecole supérieure de pharmacie de l'Université de Paris, pp. 9, 10, Paris, 1904.

41. Bouvet, M.: *op. cit.*, pp. 88, 89.

42. For details of the development see Centenaire: *op. cit.*

43. All four years may be taken at one of the Facultés de Pharmacie (Paris, Montpellier, Nancy, Strasbourg), at one of the Facultés mixtes de Médecine et de Pharmacie (Bordeaux, Lille, Lyon, Toulouse, Alger), or at one of the Ecoles de plein exercice de médecine et de pharmacie (Angers, Clermont-Ferrand, Limoges, Nantes, Rennes, Tours), or three years at one of the Ecoles préparatoires de médecine et de pharmacie (Amiens, Besançon, Caen, Dijon, Grenoble, Poitiers, Reims, Rouen) followed by a fourth year at one of the above-mentioned institutions. (Personal communication from Hans Dieckmann, 1953.)

44. Based on an enactment of May 4, 1937, as modified at various times meanwhile. Personal communications from M. Bouvet and H. Bonnemain, February 23, 1962, and from Hans Dieckmann, 1953. The diploma based on these examinations opens all kinds of pharmaceutical activity to the pharmacist, except that he must be 25 years old to become owner or manager of a pharmacy. He may continue with graduate study and research leading to the degree of *Docteur de l'Université de . . . mention pharmacie,* which is considered to correspond with the Ph.D. A still higher degree of *Docteur d'Etat* is expected of those aspiring to positions such as full professorships.

45. Jean de Ruelle (Latinized, Ruellius) published in 1536 his *De natura stirpium.* The Parisian Jacques du Bois (Latinized, Sylvius) issued in 1541 his *Methodus medicamenta componendi,* and in 1548 his *Pharmacopoeiae, libri tres,* which was translated

into French by André Caille. In 1556 G. Rondelet of Montpellier published his famous *Materia medica*.

46. Cordonnier, E.: Sur le plus ancien traité de pharmacie rédigé en francais, *L'enchirid ou manipul des mirapoles,* de Michel Dusseau (1561), Janus 5:471.

47. For example, the pharmacist Thibaut Lespleigney wrote a versified description of drugs (1537). Joseph du Chesne (Latinized, Quercetanus), physician-in-ordinary to King Henry IV, may be mentioned here as a zealous partisan for Paracelsian ideas, which are reflected in his *Pharmacopoea dogmaticorum restituta* (1603).

48. Titles and dates of some of the outstanding works of this period are the *Pharmacopée royale* of Moise Charas (1676); *Traité de la chymie* (also as *Cours de chymie*) of N. Lefebvre (1660); *Cours de chymie* (1675), *Traité universel des drogues simples,* and *Pharmacopée universelle* (1697) of Nicholas Lémery; *Elémens de pharmacie* of A. Baumé (1672); *Manuel du pharmacien* of J. F. Demachy (1788); and the *Tractatus de materia medica* of E. F. Geoffroy (1741, posthumously).

49. Next was the *Formulaire de Blois* (1634); then the first *Codex medicamentorum seu pharmacopoeia Parisiensis* (1638); followed by the *Pharmacopoeia Lillensis* (1640) and the *Pharmacopoeia Burdigalensis* (1643) and others, the last local standard appearing in Lyons (1778).

50. On the history of the French journals from 1665 to 1860 see especially Guitard, Eugène. Deux Siècles de presse au service de la pharmacie, Paris, 1913.

  In 1809 the *Bulletin de pharmacie* was founded. In 1814 its title was changed to *Bulletin de pharmacie et des sciences accessoires* (one year later the word "bulletin" was replaced by "journal"). After 1842 it had been known as the *Journal de pharmacie et de chimie*. In 1942, this time-honored scientific mouthpiece of French pharmacy merged with the *Bulletin des sciences pharmacologiques* (established in 1899), into the *Annales pharmaceutiques françaises*, which has become the organ of the Académie de Pharmacie since the establishment of the latter in 1946.

  Among well-known French pharmaceutical journals which have been discontinued mention is merited by *Le répertoire de pharmacie,* founded in 1844. It was merged in 1926 with *L'union pharmaceutique,* a journal issued since 1869 by the French cooperative mentioned above, the *Pharmacie centrale de France,* as an "organe des intérêts scientifiques, pratiques et moraux de la profession." This journal was a victim of the troubled times of 1940. *La pharmacie française* has a special place as the journal of French students of pharmacy since 1896.

51. André-Pontier, L.: Histoire de la pharmacie pp. 21-53, Paris, 1900.

52. Bouvet, M.: *op. cit.*, pp. 368-416.

53. *Ibid.*, p. 411.

54. Berman, A.: The Scientific Tradition in French Hospital Pharmacy, Am. J. Hosp-Pharm. *18*:110, 1961.

55. *Ibid.*, p. 113.

56. Balland, A.: Les pharmaciens militaires français, p. 2, Paris, 1913.

57. *Ibid.*, p. 5.

58. Berman, A.: *op. cit.*, p. 117.

59. Bouvet, M.: *op. cit.*, pp. 370, 371.

6. THE DEVELOPMENT IN GERMANY

1. Häfliger, J. A.: Das Apothekenwesen Basels, pp. 77, 113-115, 125, 126; Mittenwald, 1938; and Schelenz, H.: Geschichte der Pharmazie, p. 531, Berlin, 1904.

2. Schmitz, R.: Das Apothekenwesen von Stadt- und Kurtrier, Frankfurt/Main, 1960.

3. Adlung, A., and Urdang, G.: Grundriss der Geschichte der deutschen Pharmazie, pp. 38-42, Berlin, 1935. The archives in Zerbst preserve a *privilegium*, dated as early as 1303, showing that the Margrave Otto IV of Brandenburg-Landsberg granted Pharmacist Walther, Jr., a salable, hereditary and exclusive right to practice in Prenzlau.

4. *Ibid.*, pp. 42-45.

5. *Ibid.*, pp. 45-47, 497.

6. *Ibid.*, pp. 9, 40; Schelenz, H.: *op. cit.*, p. 465. In the 15th century, for example, such pharmacies were maintained by Lüneburg and Braunschweig and in the 16th century in other north-German cities, such as Güstrow, Hamburg, Hannover, and Hildesheim. (Arends, D., and Schneider, W.: Braunschweiger Apotheken-register 1506-1673, p. 18, Braunschweig, 1960.

7. Adlung, A., and Urdang, G.: *op. cit.*, pp. 47, 48.
8. Apotheker-Jahrbuch, Stuttgart, 1951 and 1962; and Ehrenstein, E.: Pharmacy in West Germany, Amer. Prof. Pharm. *26*: 729, 1960.
8a. Klie, W.: 700 Years of Pharmaceutic-System in Germany (mimeograph), n. p., n. d. (c. 1960), p. 3.
9. Adlung, A., and Urdang, G.: *op. cit.*, p. 3.
10. *Ibid.*, p. 101.
11. See, for example, *ibid.*, pp. 532-542.
12. Flückiger, Fr. A.: Die Frankfurter Liste, Arch. d. Pharmazie, 201: 433-464, 508-521, 1872; Das Nördlinger Register, Arch. d. Pharmazie, *211*:96-115, 1887.
13. Adlung, A., and Urdang, G.: *op. cit.*, pp. 346-361. Valid for more than a decade in the West German republic is an edition of the "Deutschen Arzneitaxe" first effective 1 May 1952 and amended by regulation (e.g., 3 February 1961).
14. *Ibid.*, pp. 117-129.
15. Based on a personal communication from Wolfgang Schneider, 16 May 1962.
16. Adlung, A., and Urdang, G.: *op. cit.*, pp. 131-152.
17. *Ibid.*, p. 132.
18. Berendes, J.: Das Apothekenwesen, Stuttgart, 1907, p. 169.
19. Adlung, A., and Urdang, G.: *op. cit.*, pp. 134, 135.
19a. For an American assessment of West German pharmaceutical education in the 1950's see, Sonnedecker, G.: Studying Pharmacy in West Germany, Am. J. Pharm. Ed. 22:169, 1958. and Burckhalter, J. H.: Doctoral and Postdoctoral Study in Germany, Am. J. Pharm. Ed. 22:18, 1958.
20. *Ibid.*, pp. 411-421.
21. *Ibid.*, pp. 412, 413, 417.
22. *Ibid.*, p. 413.
23. *Ibid.*, p. 418; Urdang, G.: Goethe and Pharmacy, Madison, Wis., 1949.
24. Adlung, A., and Urdang, G.: *op. cit.*, p. 405.
25. Ferchl, Fritz: Illustrierter Apothekerkalender, Mittenwald, Stuttgart, Berlin, 1925-1939, and the post-war continuation edited by Wolfgang-Hagen Hein; Zur Geschichte der deutschen Apotheke, Berlin, 1933-1942; and Die Apotheke von der Gotik bis zum Biedermeier, Mittenwald, 1920. Beautiful pictorial evidence further supporting this statement, as well as an ex-cellent photograph of the Renaissance pharmacy at Lemgo, may be seen in: Hein, W. H.: Die Deutsche Apotheke; Bilder aus ihrer Geschichte, p. 58, et passim, Stuttgart, 1960.
26. An incident illustrating their resourcefulness occurred during the prolonged German operations in East Africa during World War I. A military pharmacist, Schulze, succeeded in manufacturing sufficient amounts of quinine from cinchona trees in the Usambara district to ward off malaria; otherwise the prolonged resistance of the troops would not have been possible. (Adlung, A., and Urdang, G.: *op. cit.*, p. 279.)
27. Here are some of the best known examples: The *Buch der Natur* by the cleric Conrad von Megenberg (1309-1374) is the first natural history in German. The *Arzneibuch* of a supposed physician named Ortolff von Bayrlandt is a compilation of Latin medical books of his time, written at the beginning of the 15th century. The *Gart der Gesuntheit*, also called the little *Hortus sanitatis*, probably was written by the physician Joh. Wonnecke of Caub and published in 1485. (Schelenz, *op. cit.*, pp. 326 and 327) These books were followed by the so-called large *Hortus sanitatis* (1491), an anonymous comprehensive work in Latin (Fischer, H.: Mittelalterliche Pflanzenkunde, pp. 95-109, Munich, 1929); a distillation book by the surgeon Hieronymus Brunschwig, who lived from about 1450 to before 1512 (*ibid.*, pp. 109-113); the herbals of the so-called "fathers of botany"; Otto Brunfels (1488-1534), Hieronymus Bock (1498-1554), and Leonhart Fuchs (1501-1566); and also the herbals of Adam Lonicerus (1528-1586) and Johann Theodor who was called Tabernaemontanus (1520-1590). (Nissen, C.: Die botanische Buchillustration, Geschichte und Bibliographie, Stuttgart, 1951).
28. Fischer, H.: *op. cit.*, p. 109.
29. It was republished with annotations by Joachim Camerarius in 1588, B. Verzasha in 1678, and Ph. Zwinger in 1696. All three were physicians.
30. By 1647 Wecker's book had appeared in nine Latin and two French editions. The book is curious for its special chapter on excrements used as medicaments, which stemmed from primitive medicine and old superstitious beliefs about the nature of

disease. Excrementa now came into new vogue—reflecting the lack of critical attitudes and of reliable technics for evaluating materia medica—and reached a climax with the book *Dreckapotheke*, published by the physician Paullini in 1696.

31. Schroeder's book was published in Latin in 1641 and translated not only into German but also into English, under the title The Complete Chymical Dispensatory.

32. Gugel, K. F.: Johann Rudolph Glauber 1604-1670, Leben und Werk, Würzburg, 1955.

33. In 1740 the Praelectiones chymicae of the pharmacist Caspar Neumann were published posthumously. This book, based on his own experiments, represented a much more critical spirit than the book of Schroeder and became very popular. In 1777, J. Ch. Wiegleb (1732-1800) published his *Deutsches Apothekerbuch* (German practice of pharmacy). One year later, in 1778, J. F. A. Goettling (1755-1809) published his *Einleitung in die Pharmazeutische Chemie* (introduction to pharmaceutical chemistry). Between 1778 and 1782, K. G. Hagen in Koenigsberg (1749-1829) published his *Lehrbuch der Apothekerkunst* (textbook on the practice of pharmacy), which until the middle of the 19th century was the most-used book in the scientific education of the apprentices. In 1790, Joh. Bartholomaeus Trommsdorff began his long series of textbooks on pharmacy, among them his *Handbuch der pharmazeutischen Warenkunde*, the first textbook on pharmacognosy written in German, and his *Allgemeines pharmazeutisch-chemisches Wörterbuch oder die Apothekerkunst in ihrem gesamten Umfange* (pharmaceutico-chemical dictionary or the art of pharmacy in its entire extent). In 1792, Hermbstaedt (1760-1833) published his *Katechismus der Apothekerkunst* (catechism of the art of the apothecary) and, in 1795, Westrumb (1751-1819) published his *Handbuch der Apothekerkunst fuer Anfaenger* (textbook on pharmacy for beginners). The pharmaceutical textbooks written by German pharmacists in the 19th and the 20th centuries are too numerous to permit even the naming of a selection.

34. Bleyer, B.: Aus den Anfängen der pharmazeutischen Lehreinrichtungen an den deutschen Universitäten, Arch. Pharmazie *272*:359, 1934.

35. Adlung, A., and Urdang, G.: *op. cit.*, p. 147.

36. Vershofen, W.: Die Anfange der chemisch-pharmazeutischen Industrie, Bd. 1, Berlin-Stuttgart, 1949; Bd. 2, Aulendorf, 1952; Wirtschaftsgeschichte der chemisch-pharmazeutischen Industrie, Aulendorf, 1958.

37. Lutz, A.: Das Nürnberger Dispensatorium des Valerius Cordus vom Jahre 1546, die erste amtliche Pharmakopöe, *in* Festschrift z. 75. Geburtstag von Ernst Urban, pp. 107-125, Stuttgart, 1949. Cf., Urdang, G.: The Development of Pharmacopoeias, p. 9, New York, 1950. See also Winkler, L.: Die älteste deutsche Pharmakopoea von Valerius Cordus, Mittenwald, 1934. We cannot expect agreement on "first" pharmacopeias without a definition held in common. A more meaningful focus is that there *were several* kinds of attempts in several places to give force to drug standards, suggesting a recognized need by the mid-16th century going beyond an isolated, local concern.

38. In the 17th century, particularly notable was the series of Augsburg pharmacopeias (for example, 1613, 1640 [for the first time with a Mantissa hermetica], 1684, etc.). The Cologne pharmacopeia appeared in a new edition in 1627, the Nuremberg in 1612 and 1666. A Facsimile of the First Edition of the Pharmacopoeia Augustana was published by the State Historical Society of Wisconsin in 1927.

39. Seven editions followed under the title *Dispensatorium Borusso-Brandenburgicum*, the title signalizing the fact that the duchy of Prussia had been made a kingdom (1701), and the electorate of Brandenburg had been assigned second place in the union of the two states. When the Holy Roman Empire of the German Nation disappeared (1806), additional state pharmacopeias were published in Württemberg (1741, 1750, 1754, 1760, 1771, 1785, 1798), Braunschweig (1777), the Palatinate (1764, 1802), Hessia (1806), and in the hierarchic principalities of Fulda (1787, 1791), Münster (1739) and Würzburg-Bamberg (1778, 1782, 1796). Dispensatories of municipalities were issued in the same period in Bremen (1792), Hamburg (1716, 1768, 1772) and Regensburg (1727, 1737).

40. It was supplemented by a collection of official formulas published in a *Catalogus medicamentorum compositorum*. Up to

1722 all subsequent editions of the *Augustana* remained in force. In 1729, the first Austrian pharmacopeia printed in Austria appeared under the title *Dispensatorium Pharmaceuticum Austriaco-Viennenense*. This book lived through six further editions, until 1770. In 1774, there appeared the *Pharmacopoeia Austriaco-provincialis*. The name signified that Austria was but one of the many provinces of the Empire. The last editions of this treatise were issued in 1794 (Latin) and 1795 (German). It was followed in 1812 by the first *Pharamacopoea Austriaca* (Zekert, Otto: Oesterreichische Pharmakopoeen, Pharm. Monatshefte *12*:2, 22, 55, 75, 1931). Again this name is significant. Now Austria was no longer one of the constituents of the Holy Roman Empire of the German Nation. It had become a separate unit, one of a new empire embracing all the countries belonging to the Austrian line of the princely house of Habsburg, to the exclusion of most of the German states. The ninth edition of the *Pharmacopoea Austriaca* appeared in 1961.

1. Urdang, G.: Zur Geschichte der Metalle in den amtlichen deutschen Arnzeibüchern, pp. 36-38, Mittenwald, 1933.

2. Adlung, A., and Urdang, G.: *op. cit.*, pp. 308, 309, 331, 332.

3. According to R. Folch y Andreu, the situation in Spain was the reverse. In Spain the galenical pharmacopoeias were prepared by pharmacists who, when chemicals for internal use were introduced into the official books, were replaced by physicans. (Die Prae-hispanischen Offizinellen Pharmakopoeen. Die Vorträge der Hauptversammlung der Gesellschaft für Geschichte der Pharmazie in Basel, 1934, pp. 212-223, Mittenwald, 1934.

. Adlung, A., and Urdang, G.: *op. cit.*, pp. 333, 334.

. Schneider, W.: Vorgeschichte der ersten Pharmacopoea Germanica, Pharm. Ztg. *104*:495, 519, 1085, 1959.

. In regard to the development of pharmaceutical journalism in Germany, see Adlung, A., and Urdang, G.: *op. cit.*, pp. 259-271.

. Among them was *Gehlen-Buchner's Repertorium für die Pharmacie* (1815). Subject to frequent changes were the *Annalen der Pharmacie* (which first appeared in 1832), combining Haenle-Geiger's *Magazin für Pharmacie* (founded in 1823) with the *Archiv des Apothekervereins im noerdlichen Teutschland* (founded in 1822; first issued two years previously as *Pharmaceutische Monatshefte*). In 1834 *Trommsdorff's Journal* was merged with the *Annalen*. However, the *Archiv* regained its independence under the title *Archiv der Pharmacie* (1835). Woehler, in his capacity as one of the editors, suggested that the original title *Annalen der Pharmacie* be changed to *Annalen für Chemie und Pharmacie*. After the death of Liebig the word pharmacy was dropped. Since 1874 this lost child of pharmacy has borne the title *Justus Liebig's Annalen der Chemie*. (Schneider, W.: Justus von Liebig und das *Archiv der Pharmazie*, Arch. Pharm. *286*:165, 1955.)

48. Schneider, W.: 100 Jahre Pharmazeutische Zentralhalle, Pharm. Zentralhalle *98*:330, 347, 1959.

49. ————: 100 Jahre Deutsche Apotheker-Zeitung. Vom Pharmaceutischen Wochenblatt aus Württemberg über die Suddeutsche Apotheker-Zeitung zur Deutschen Apotheker-Zeitung, D. Apoth. Ztg. *101*:761, 1961.

50. Geschichte des Apothekenwesens in Nürnberg 1722; Brunner, L.: Dreihundertjahrfeier des Collegium Pharmaceuticum Norimbergense, Stuttgart, 1932.

51. In 1794 the Berliner Apotheker Konferenz, in 1798 the Magdeburger Apotheker Konferenz, and in 1808 the Erfurter Kraenzchen followed.

52. After the governmental change in 1933 the Deutscher Apothekerverein became first the Standesgemeinschaft Deutscher Apotheker, and in 1935 the Deutsche Apothekerschaft.

53. In regard to the German pharmaceutical associations, see Adlung, A., and Urdang, G.: *op. cit.*, pp. 259-271.

54. After being under the jurisdiction of the leader of the totalitarian Deutsche Apothekerschaft from 1934 to 1945, the Pharmazeutische Gesellschaft began a reorganization in 1947.

55. After 1933 the *Apotheker-Zeitung* became known as the *Standeszeitung Deutscher Apotheker* and after 1934 as *Deutsche Apotheker-Zeitung*. Having disappeared at the end of the war (1945), it revived in 1949, to be merged (1950) with the *Süddeutsche Apotheker-Zeitung*. The *Jahresbericht der Pharmazie*, published

annually since 1841, has been issued since 1906 by the Apothekerverein.

56. The "Gremien" in Austria—the first of which was the "Wiener Apotheker Gremium" (1723)—were unofficial associations but had official approval. In Saxony similar compulsory bodies entrusted with the same tasks were founded in 1865 under the name Pharmazeutische Kreisvereine.

57. Such Kammern have existed in Brunswick since 1865, in Prussia since 1901, in Baden since 1906, in Hessia since 1923, in Wuertemberg since 1925, in Thuringia since 1926 and in Bavaria since 1927. Later, in the totalitarian organizing of the whole life of the German people into groups guaranteeing the desired political character and indoctrination, the Reichapothekerkammer, based upon the Reichapothekerordnung, came into existence (1937). Thus an official and compulsory pharmaceutical body for the "ethical" affairs of all German pharmacists was created. All pharmacists, even those not in active service, had to belong to the Kammer and were submitted to a rigid control. The leader of the Deutsche Apothekerschaft was also president of the Reichapothekerkammer, exerting a far-reaching power over the professional and, in part, even the private activities of German pharmacists.

58. Hügel, H.: Pharmazeutische Gesetzeskunde, 9th ed., Stuttgart, 1962.

7. THE DEVELOPMENT IN BRITAIN

1. Adlung, A., and Urdang, G.: Grundriss der Geschichte der deutschen Pharmazie, pp. 190-192, Berlin, 1935.
2. Trease, G. E.: The "Spicer-Apothecary" of the Middle Ages, The Future Pharmacist, No. 26 (Summer):54, 1957, clarifies the evolution and the function of the different groups; see, also: The Spicers and Apothecaries of the Royal Household in the Reigns of Henry III, Edward I and Edward II *in* Nottingham Mediaeval Studies 3 and 19, 1959. The early spicer (or speciarius) dealt in a variety of commodities that Trease found to include spices and crude drugs, prepared medicines and sweetmeats, sugar, rice, dried and candied fruits, perfumes, dyestuffs, alum and a limited number of other chemicals, as well as cotton thread, silk and paper.

3. For a good general account of this period, see Whittet, T. D.: "Part 6. England and Wales" from his series on the evolution of pharmacy in Britain (in mimeograph form as of 1961).
4. Thompson, C. J. S.: The Mystery and Art of the Apothecary, pp. 86-100, London, 1929; Chem. & Drugg. *108*:855, 1928; Gilmour, J. P.: The origin of British Pharmacy, Quart. J. Pharm. & Pharmacol. 5: 425, 1932; Kirkby, W.: The Supply of Physic, Chem. & Drugg. *117*:234, 1932. Some prominent 14th century apothecaries mentioned by Thompson (some of them having come from France) were Henry (also Richard) Montpellier, Roger de Frowicke, Pierre de Montpellers, Coursus de Gangeland, and J. Falcand de Luca.
5. Barrett, C. R. B.: Society of Apothecaries of London, p. xv, London, 1905.
6. Pharm. J. *116*:437, 1926.
7. Barrett: *op. cit.*, p. xvi.
8. Thompson: *op. cit.*, p. 180.
9. Barrett: *op. cit.*, pp. 42-49, 79-83, 267-293.
10. At this time it established a special naval stock. "Practically a company and distinct from the Laboratory, the funds were raised in a similar way, that is by money borrowed on bond and by share taken to a fixed amount by the Livery." (Barrett: *op. cit.*, pp. 102 and 119.) In 1811 and for 10 years previously drugs supplied to the navy averaged annually about $100,800. The supply of drugs to the East India Company averaged about $90,350 annually. (*Ibid.*, p. 176.) Considering the change in the purchasing power of English as well as American currency, these figures must be multiplied to compare with present-day values.
11. Bell, J., and Redwood, T.: Historical Sketch of the Progress of Pharmacy in Great Britain, London, 1880, p. 11.
12. Thompson: *op. cit.*, p. 273.
13. *Ibid.*: p. 275. A detailed account of the controversies is in Mullet, C. F.: Physician vs. apothecary, 1669-1671, Scientific Monthly *49*:558, 1939.
14. Barrett: *op. cit.*, p. xvii.
15. Thompson: *op. cit.*, p. 278.
16. Wootton, A.: Chronicles of Pharmacy, I, pp. 152-154, London, 1910; Bayles, H.: The Rose Case, Chem. & Drugg. *133*:9, 1940. See, furthermore, Leake, C.: Percival's Medical Ethics, pp. 112-119, Baltimore, 1927.

17. Pharm. J. *116*:457, 1920.
18. Bell and Redwood: *op. cit.*, p. 64, and personal communication from T. Douglas Whittet, January 1962. The Apothecary Society's control of medical education in England and Wales continued until the General Medical Council was formed in 1859.
19. Thompson: *op. cit.*, p. 280; see also, "The title of chemist and druggist," Chem. & Drugg. *105*:90, 1926.
20. Ferguson, T.: The apothecary in Scotland, Chem. & Drugg. *116*:695, 1932; Wilbert, M. I.: John Morgan, Am. J. Pharm. *76*:6, 1904; Pharm. J. *161*:23, 1948.
21. Whittet, T. D.: From Apothecary to Pharmacist, Ireland; and, From Apothecary to Pharmacist, Scotland (mimeograph version), London, 1961.
22. Barrett: *op. cit.*, p. 224.
23. Bell and Redwood: *op. cit.*, p. 98.
24. *Ibid.*: pp. 116-119.
25. *Ibid.*: pp. 216-218.
26. Pharm. J., *116*:458, 1926.
27. *Ibid.*: *130*:549, 1933.
28. The principal acts regulating the practice of pharmacy in Northern Ireland are the Pharmacy and Poisons Act (Northern Ireland, 1925) and the Medicines, Pharmacy and Poisons Act (Northern Ireland, 1945). The corresponding acts in Eire are the Pharmacy Act (Ireland, 1875) and the Pharmacy Amendment Act (Ireland, 1890).
29. Personal communication from T. Douglas Whittet, January 1962.
30. Pharm. J. *116*:566, 1926. In an amendment to the Dental Practitioners Bill of 1878, initiated by the Pharmaceutical Society, the British government provided that druggists should be registrable who had practiced dentistry in conjunction with pharmacy. A large group of druggists in this way became dentists.
31. Gamble, F. W.: The Conference, Chem. & Drugg. *99*:129, 1923.
31a. National Pharmaceutical Union 1921-1946, London, 1946 (20 pp.) contains historical notes and a summary of functions.
32. Chem. & Drugg. *75*:136, 1909.
33. Among these were The Chemist (1840-1858); *The Chemical Gazette* (f. 1842), which merged with *The Chemical News* in 1859; *The Annals of Chemistry and Practical Pharmacy* (1842-1843); *The Pharmaceutical Times* (1846-1849); An-nals of *Pharmacy and Practical Chemistry* (1852-1854) (Bayles, H.: Six journals for chemists, Chem. & Drugg. *146*:244, 1944). Typical of the erratic evolution that often makes journal bibliography perplexing (and suggestive of changes occurring on a broader historical stage) is the journal founded in 1884 as the *British and Colonial Druggist,* which became the *British and Colonial Pharmacist* (1915), then the *British and Overseas Pharmacist* (1952), next broadening its scope to *British and Overseas Pharmacy and Medicine* (1958), moving further into medicine as the *Chemotherapy Review* (1960), and now appearing (since 1961) as the *Medical Observer and Chemotherapy Review.*
34. Chem. & Drugg. *108*:855, 1928.
35. Barrett: *op. cit.*, p. xxxiv.
36. Bell and Redwood: *op. cit.*, p. 21; Barrett: *op. cit.*, p. 132; Chem. & Drugg. *105*:198, 1926.
37. Ferguson: *op. cit.;* Chem. & Drugg. *116*: 696, 1932.
38. Thompson: *op. cit.*, pp. 162, 166, 167.
39. *Ibid.*: p. 263. In Scotland, more of the pharmacies retained a dignified appearance, Whittet believes (personal communication, 1962).
40. Kopp, H.: Geschichte der Chemie, 1843; reprint, I, p. 163, Leipzig, 1931.
41. Wootton: *op. cit.*, I. p. 365.
42. *Ibid.*: p. 141; Thompson: *op. cit.*, pp. 266-268.
43. Pharm. J. *116*:437, 1926.
44. Ferguson: *op. cit.*, Chem. & Drugg. *116*: 697, 1932.
45. Barrett: *op. cit.*, p. xxxii.
46. *Ibid.*: pp. 5, 103, 197.
47. Bell and Redwood: *op. cit.*, pp. 104, 167, 175.
47a. Fairbairn, J. W.: Pharmaceutical education in Great Britain—a comparative study, Am. J. Pharm. Ed. 22:1, 1958.
48. The degree of Bachelor of Pharmacy may be taken at the universities of Leeds, London, Nottingham and Wales, and the Bachelor of Science in Pharmacy at the universities of Glasgow and Manchester. The London degree may be taken "externally" through several provincial technical colleges. The University of Edinburgh is establishing a degree in pharmacy; and the University of Liverpool offers a degree stressing pharmacology that is recognized by the Pharmaceutical Society. Technical

colleges that give courses of instruction qualifying for the examinations of the Pharmaceutical Society are in Aberdeen, Birmingham, Bradford, Brighton, Bristol, Cardiff, Leicester, Liverpool, Plymouth, Portsmouth and Sunderland.

49. Other reciprocal arrangements made by Great Britain include Australia, New Zealand and South Africa.

50. Report of the Committee on the General Practice of Pharmacy, Pharm. J., Sept. 30, 1961; reprint pamphlet, p. 9. This Report in general is a significant document concerning the character and the outlook of British pharmacy.

51. The discussion of recent British pharmaceutical education draws heavily upon personal communications with T. Douglas Whittet of London (1962). On the earlier period, see Sage, C. E.: School of Pharmacy of the Pharmaceutical Society of Great Britain, Pharm. Era, Dec. 31, 1896, pp. 869-871.

52. Urdang, G.: Pharmacopoeia Londinensis of 1618, Madison, Wis., 1944, pp. 24, 77-81.

53. *Ibid.*: pp. 36, 54; Wootton: *op. cit.*, 2, pp. 2-4, 61-64. Wootton speaks of 1028 simples in the second issue of the London Pharmacopoeia of 1618. He takes this number from Munk (The Rolls of the Royal College of Physicians of London, 1878, 3, p. 376) who counted only the individual paragraphs and not the different drugs sometimes listed in the same paragraph; as a result, his numbers are too low.

54. Urdang, G.: *op. cit.*, pp. 61-63.

55. Wootton: *op. cit.*, 2, pp. 64-69. Editions of the London Pharmacopoeia were published in 1617, 1650, 1677, 1721, 1746, 1788, 1809, 1824, 1836 and 1851.

56. An excellent paper, with definitive bibliographic information, is by Cowen, David L.: The Edinburgh pharmacopoeia, Medical History 1:123, 340, 1957; see also his guide: Library Holdings of the Edinburgh Pharmacopoeia (mimeograph) Rutgers University, 1957, 14 pp., surveying libraries in twelve countries. Cowen identifies the twelve editions as published in 1699, 1722, 1735, 1744, 1756, 1774, 1783, 1792, 1803, 1817, 1839, 1841.

57. Bell and Redwood: *op. cit.*, p. 329.

58. A volume of *Additions* was issued in 1874. New versions were published in 1885 (with an *Addendum* in 1890) and in 1898. In 1900 and thereafter, there ap-
peared an *Indian and Colonial Addendum* which was incorporated into the *Pharmacopoeia* of 1914. The *Pharmacopoeia* issued in 1932 showed for the first time the influence of a closer cooperation with the Committee on Revision for the *United States Pharmacopoeia.* Addenda were published in 1936, 1940, 1941 (two), 1942, 1943 and 1945.

59. Barrett: *op. cit.*, p. 157, 168.

60. Bell and Redwood: *op. cit.*, p. 208.

61. *Ibid.*: p. 329; see also, Urdang, G., and Sonnedecker, G.: "Authoritative English-language drug compendia supplementing pharmacopoeias," Food Drug Cosmetic Law J. 8:485, 1953.

62. Anon.: Side-lights on English pharmacy 1550-1650, Chem. & Drugg. 120:720, 1934; and Singer, C.: Sketches in the history of English medicine, Chem. & Drugg. 112:800, 1930.

63. Thompson: *op. cit.*, p. 150.

64. Bell and Redwood: *op. cit.*, p. 14.

65. Kirkby, W.: A quack of the seventeenth century, Pharm. J. 84:255, 1910.

66. Kremers, E.: William Lewis, J. A. Ph. A. 20:1204, 1931.

67. Bell and Redwood: *op. cit.*, p. 163.

68. The investigations of T. Douglas Whittet of London permit a more adequate documentation of British pharmaceutical contributions to science than heretofore; see also, e.g., Schofield, M.: A pharmacist turned chemist, Pharm. J. 160:22, 1948.

69. Cripps, E. C.: Plough Court, pp. 25-51, London, 1927.

70. Chem. & Drugg. 114:749, 1931; 116:711, 1932; 118:667, 1933; 120:732, 1934; 124:737, 1936. See furthermore the article by, Anon.: Established one hundred years, Pharm. J. 146:153, 1941, and the anniversary publications by Howard, Geoffrey E., Howards 1797-1947, Ilford, 1947, and by H. J. Baker: The History of Duncan, Flockhart & Co., Edinburgh, 1947.

8. SOME INTERNATIONAL TRENDS

1. Schelenz, H.: Geschichte der Pharmacie, Berlin, 1904, p. 432.

2. Thompson, C. J. S.: The Mystery and Art of the Apothecary, London, 1929, p. 233.

3. Personal communication from Howard Bayles of England.

4. Schelenz: *op. cit.*, p. 579.

5. Wootton, A.: Chronicles of Pharmacy, 1, pp. 319-322, London, 1910.

6. Encyclopaedia Britannica, 11th ed., vol. 20, p. 903, 1901.

7. Langenhan, H. A.: Liquor potassii arsenalis. Bull. Univ. Wis., Ser. No. 1153, Gen. Ser. No. 936. The English patent law of 1852, which required preliminary disclosure, began an era of real invention, as is shown by patents granted in the years 1854-1856: use of glycerin in cosmetics (1854, No 85, John Henry Johnson); capsules (1855, No. 824, Jules Denoual); first aniline dye (1856, No. 1984, William Henry Perkin); use of "paraffine" in hair oils and ointments (1856, No. 2945, Charles Humphrey). (Chem. & Drugg. *124*:758, 1936)

   A so-called "medicine-stamp" act (1783) imposed the requirement of a license on any person selling medicines, unless he had "served a regular apprenticeship to any surgeon, apothecary, druggist or chemist," and introduced simultaneously a tax on all medicines that were sold by a person so licensed, or sold under letters patent. In 1785 the form in which the tax was levied was altered; in 1802, a law defined the requirements more exactly. Increasing difficulty of administrative interpretation, combined with a progressive fall in revenue from licenses and stamps, led to the passing in 1941 of the Pharmacy and Medicines Act. (Chem. & Drugg. *136*:316, 1941; personal communication from Howard Bayles; see also, Bouvet, M.: Les commissions de contrôle des spécialités pharmaceutiques au 18e siècle, La pharm. française, *27*:7-17, 1923).

8. Inlow, E. B.: The Patent Grant (Johns Hopkins U. Studies in Historical and Political Science, Series 68, No. 2), pp. 36-38, 13 and 18, Baltimore, 1950.

9. Fischelis, R. P.: What is a patent or proprietary medicine? Am. J. Pharm. Ed. *2*: 163 f., 1938.

10. Schechter, F. I.: The Historical Foundations of the Law Relating to Trade-Marks, pp. x and 19-21, New York, 1925.

11. The History of Pharmacy in Pictures, commissioned by Parke, Davis & Company, recreates in painting No. 7 a general impression of the scene as Lemnian earth was being made into one of the very earliest "trademarked" drugs. (This and other paintings in the series created by the artist Robert Thom in collaboration with George Bender may be consulted in various printed forms.)

12. XI. Congrès international de la pharmacie: Compte rendue, La Haye (The Hague), 1913, pp. 143-153; Chem. & Drugg., Year Book, p. 382, London, 1945.

13. Schechter: *op. cit.*, pp. 139-141 et passim. The various national laws have been revised repeatedly. The first American law had to be re-enacted in 1876 to make it constitutional, and was subsequently revised in 1881, 1905, 1920, and 1946.

14. For a readable handbook on the purposes, provisions, and legislative history, see Toulmin, H. A., Jr.: The Trade-Mark Act of 1946, Cincinnati, Ohio, 1946. 224 pp. and 1947 Supplement.

15. Wilbert, M. I.: On the problem of proprietary and trade names, Proc. A. Ph. A. *51*:529, 1903.

16. Editorial. On the promotion of drugs, N. Eng. J. Med., *263*:44, 1960.

17. National Pharmaceutical Council, Statements on Generic Equivalency, New York, p. 1-2 (loose-leaf service).

18. Archambault, G. F.: Are trade names for single drug entities and "official" preparations really necessary to insure quality drugs? Am. J. Hosp. Pharm. *17*:502 f., 1960.

19. For representative discussion, e.g., see: Section of industrial pharmacists: trade marks and free names for medicinal substances, Journal Mondial de Pharmacie [F.I.P.] *3*:331, 1960; What's in a name? [a symposium], J. A. Ph. A., n.s. *1*:92, 1961; Leake, C. D.: Economic aspects of drug names, Am. J. Hosp. Pharm. *18*:443, 1961; Drug terminology and the urgent need for reform, N. Eng. J. Med. *263*: 21, 1960; for one of the best demonstrations of limitations of the idea of "therapeutic equivalency," see Levy, G., and Nelson, E.: Pharmaceutical formulation and therapeutic efficacy, J.A.M.A. *177*: 689, 1961.

20. Adlung, A., and Urdang, G.: Grundriss der Geschichte der deutschen Pharmazie, p. 200, Berlin, 1935.

21. *Ibid.*: pp. 211-218.

22. Urdang, G.: Pharmacy's position under regulated community medicine, J. A. Ph. A. *27*:702, 1938; Urdang, G., and Murphy, J.: Position of Pharmacy in Sickness Insurance, pp. 14-20, Madison, Wis., 1942.

23. A brief discussion of possible influences is included in Sonnedecker, G.: Govern-

ment health insurance—in historical perspective, J. A. Ph. A., n.s. 2:654, 1962.

24. Farman, C. H., and Hale, V. M.: Social Security Legislation Throughout the World, Social Security Administration, Bureau Report No. 16, Washington, D. C., 1949, 176 pp. Pharmaceutical coverage is not identified separately in Farman's 1954 report: Old-Age, Survivors, and Invalidity Programs Throughout the World, Social Security Administration, Bureau Report No. 19; and Follmann, J. F., Jr.: Trends in the future of voluntary health insurance, Proceedings, 1961, Ann. Conf. County Med. Soc. Officers (reprint), p. 6.

25. Sulzbach, W.: German Experience with Social Insurance, p. 7, New York, 1947.

26. Eckstein, H.: The English Health Service; Its Origins, Structure, and Achievements, p. x, Cambridge, Mass., 1958. For a good concise survey with special reference to pharmacy, see The British National Health Service, London (Pharmaceutical Press), 1961, 22 pp.

27. Linstead, H. N.: Pharmacists and machines, J. A. Ph. A. 2:346, 1962.

28. On the initiative of a pharmacist, Sir William Glyn-Jones, who was a member of Parliament, the act (1911) contains a clause which prohibits "arrangements for the dispensing of medicines being made with persons other than persons, firms, or bodies corporate entitled to carry on the business of a chemist and druggist under the provision of the Pharmacy Act." (Pharm. J. *131*:60, 1933.)

29. Bull. Féd. Internat. Pharm. 7:57, 1926.

30. Hauser, V.: The Impact of Sickness Societies on Retail Pharmacy (mimeographed), p. 4, Internat. Pharm. Fed. London, 1955.

31. See, e.g., Field, M. G.: Doctor and Patient in Soviet Russia, Cambridge, Mass., 1957.

32. Follman, J. F., Jr.: Trends . . ., *op. cit.*, pp. 3 f.; and, The Cost of Medical Care, p. 153, Geneva, 1959.

33. For the period up to World War II, a particularly good source of information is Anderson, O. W.: The Health Insurance Movement in the United States; A Case Study of the Role of Conflict in the Development and Solution of a Social Problem (unpublished Ph. D. thesis, Univ. of Michigan, Ann Arbor, 1948); see also his Family Medical Costs and Voluntary Health Insurance, a Nationwide Survey, New York, 1956. A rich source of eco-

nomic and sociologic information on contemporary American medical care is the variety of publications from the Health Information Foundation (New York and, from 1962, Chicago), under grants from pharmaceutical industry.

34. On the slow emergence of a concept and understanding of addiction, see Sonnedecker, G.: Emergence of the concept of opiate addiction, J. Mondial Pharm., No. 3, 1962, pp. 275-290 and No. 1, 1963, pp. 27-34.

35. Terry, C. E., and Pellens, M.: The Opium Problem, New York, 1928, is rich in historical information. See Renborg, B. A.: International Drug Control, Washington, D. C., 1947 (276 pp.) for an excellent historical account and the situation current in the 1940's.

36. The 12 Congresses have been held as follows: Braunschweig, 1865; Paris, 1867; Vienna, 1869; St. Petersbourg, 1874; London, 1881; Brussels, 1885; Chicago, 1893; Brussels, 1897; Paris, 1900; Brussels, 1910; The Hague, 1913; Brussels, 1935. After 1935, it appears that the International Congress, in its old sense, was supplanted by the "General Assemblies" of the International Federation. To clarify this organizational question a special Commission of the Council recommended in 1956 that the international congresses may be considered to be comprised of all meetings and their manifestations concerning the Federation's work, both professional and scientific. The general or professional part includes the General Assembly, a body organized to act for the constituent societies (Ordinary Members); the part programmed by the Scientific Sections has been presented (since 1958) as an International Congress of Pharmaceutical Sciences (annually, the 21st at Pisa in 1961). The plan is to hold a specialized symposium in conjunction with the General Assemblies of the F.I.P., and in alternate years to hold a scientific congress of broad scope.

The General Assemblies convened since the founding of the Federation, biennially when international conditions permit, have been held as follows (designated by a numbering separate from the pre-1912 Congresses):

1. The Hague 1912
2. Ghent 1913
3. Brussels 1922

4. London 1923
5. Lausanne 1925
6. The Hague 1927
7. Paris 1928
8. Stockholm 1930
9. Brussels 1935
10. Copenhagen 1937
11. Berlin 1939 (not held)
12. Zurich 1947
13. Amsterdam 1949
14. Rome 1951
15. Paris 1953
16. London 1955
17. Brussels 1958
18. Copenhagen 1960
19. Vienna 1962

37. An excellent summary and critical commentary on the early Congresses was published by Hoffmann, Fr.: The international pharmaceutical congresses, Am. J. Pharm. 73:315, 373, and 431, 1901; see also Oldberg, O.: The international pharmaceutical congresses, Western Drugg. 15:24, 1893.

38. "History of the Federation," *in* Official Handbook, 16th General Assembly, Féd. Internat. Pharm., London, 1955, pp. E17-19, has been mainly drawn upon here. See also Sonnedecker, G.: One world for pharmacy? Modern Pharmacy 41 (No. 3): 12, 1956; also J. A. Ph. A. 21:1070, 1932, and Bull. Féd. Internat. Pharm. 12:22, 1931.

39. Reinstein, J. A.: The history and objectives of the International Pharmaceutical Students' Federation, J. Am. Pharm. Assoc., Prac. Pharm. Ed. 19:88 f., 1958. For operational details of the pharmacy student exchange program, see Samuels, J. D.: International Pharmaceutical Students' Federation, J. A. Ph. A. n.s. 2:355 f., 1962. The A. Ph. A. authorized full membership of the Student Section in 1957; the earlier associate membership of the Association's University of Wisconsin Branch apparently was the first American participation by an organization.

40. Hampshire, C. H.: The International Pharmacopoeia of the World Health Organization, Bull. Féd. Internat. Pharm. 24:123, 1950-51.

41. Power, Fr. B.: Unification of potent medicaments, Am. J. Pharm. 75:1, 1903.

42. Hampshire, C. H.: Interim report of the Technical Commission of Pharmacopoeial Experts, League of Nations, Bull, Health Org. 12:112, 1945-46.

43. Miller, L. C.: An International Pharma-copoeia, Food Drug Cosmetic Law J. 8: 299 f., 1953. See also the series of articles in.: Bull. Féd. Internat. Pharm. 24:123, 1950-51; and Rasmussen, H. B.: fifty years' endeavor to create an international pharmacopoeia, Bull. Féd. Internat. Pharm. 24:20, 1950-51.

44. For good discussions from different viewpoints, see Miller, L. C.: International non-proprietary names, The Trade-Mark Reporter 43:133, 1953; and Levy, M. W.: Who authorized it?, The Trade-Mark Reporter, 229.

45. These six Pan-American Congresses have been held as follows:
    (1) Havana, Cuba, 1948;
    (2) Lima, Peru, 1951;
    (3) Sao Paulo, Brazil, 1954;
    (4) Washington, D. C., 1957;
    (5) Santiago, Chile, 1960;
    (6) Mexico City, Mexico, 1963

46. Orfila, A.: Manuscript address in the Edward Kremers Archive, Univ. of Wisconsin (filed C36 [h] III), p. 1.

47. Haddad, A. F.: The first Middle East Pharmaceutical Conference, Lebanese Pharm. J. 4:221, 1956.

48. Versuch einer Geschichte des Apothekenwesens in der freyen Reichsstadt Nürnberg, Nuremberg, 1722, and facsimile edition, Nuremberg, 1932.

49. Urdang, G.: Wesen und Bedeutung der Geschichte der Pharmazie, pp. 7-25, Berlin, 1927.

50. Of American bibliographic guides, see particularly Sonnedecker, G., Hoch, J. H., and Schneider, W.: Some Pharmaco-Historical Guidelines to the Literature, Madison, Wis., 1959 (also in Am. J. Pharm. Ed. 23:143, 1959); note also Sonnedecker, G., and Berman, A.: Some Bibliographic Aids for Historical Writers in Pharmacy, Madison, Wis., 1958, 15 pp.

51. Pharm. Ztg. 41:183, 1896; 42:765, 775, 783, 1897.

52. Häfliger, G.: Pharmazeutische Altertumskunde, pp. 27-38.

53. Griffenhagen, George: Pharmacy Museums, Madison, Wis., 1956; for a country-by-country guide, see also Appendix 5; American Pharmacy's Historical Collections, Madison, Wis., n.d. (in revision, 1963) provides a pocket guide to the traveler; for more detail and references, see Early American Pharmacies, Washington, D. C., 1955 (also serially in J. A. Ph. A., Prac. Pharm. Ed. 14-15, 1953-54).

54. When surveyed in 1951. For an analysis, see Sonnedecker, G.: A survey of the status of history of pharmacy in American pharmaceutical education, Am. J. Pharm. Ed. *16*:21, 1952, and more recently, Grosicki, T. S.: History of Pharmacy in the Five-Year Program, Am. J. Pharm. Ed. *27*: 237, 1963.

55. Urdang, G.: Section on historical pharmacy [A. Ph. A.], Am. J. Pharm. Ed. *17*: 389, 1953. The A. Ph. A. further expressed its respect for history when it established the Friends of Historical Pharmacy, Inc. (1941) to preserve the apothecary shop of the physician and Revolutionary War hero, Hugh Mercer, at Fredericksburg, Virginia. The Association has also given consistent support and encouragement to the American Institute of the History of Pharmacy.

56. On George Urdang (1882-1960) and his work, see issues No. 2 and 3 of Volume 5 (1960) of Pharmacy in History [AIHP]; on Edward Kremers see Urdang, G.: Edward Kremers (1865-1941): reformer of American pharmaceutical education, Am. J. Pharm. Ed. *11*:631, 1947. On the Institute, see Stieb, E. W.: American Institute of the History of Pharmacy: Through Two Decades, Madison, Wis., 1961.

57. Urdang, G.: The pharmaceutico-historical movement, Am. J. Pharm. Ed. *16*:214, 1952.

58. Brans, P. H.: Les organisations mondiales d'histoire de la pharmacie, Arch. Internat. d'Hist. d. Sciences, No. 26, p. 51, 1954. The International Academy of the History or Pharmacy holds sessions alternately in association with meetings staged by the *Internationale Gesellschaft für Geschichte der Pharmazie* and by the *Union Mondiale des Sociétés d'Histoire Pharmaceutique*. The *Union Mondiale*, in turn, holds its meetings in association with the *Fédération Internationale Pharmaceutique*. It should be noted that since the *Gesellschaft* added the adjective "international" to its name (1949)—and is Englished as "International Society"— some confusion arose among Americans as to its activities in relation to the "World Union" and the "International Academy." The *Gesellschaft* has "Landes-gruppe" in various European countries and is international in its aim and outlook, although it remains heavily Germanic. Its members are individuals, whereas the World Union is a federation of societies for the history of pharmacy. How the international aspect of pharmaco-historical activities can best be served, organizationally, probably will be clarified and simplified as experience is gained in supranational collaboration.

59. Linstead, Hugh: Pharmacists and machines, J. Am. Pharm. Assoc. n.s. *2*:376, 1962.

9. THE NORTH AMERICAN COLONIES

1. Morgan, J.: The Birth of the American People, p. 54, New York, 1930.

2. *Ibid.*: pp. 32, 33.

3. *Ibid.*: p. 166. "Pennsylvania remained culturally more German than English until the revolutionary era." According to Franklin about one-third of the inhabitants of Pennsylvania, at the time of the revolution, were Germans.

4. Kremers, E.: Drugs of North American Indians, Pharm. Rev. *23*:130, 1905; Youngken, H. W.: The Drugs of the North American Indians, Am. J. Pharm. *96*:485, 1924; *97*:158, 257, 1925; Corlett, T. W.: The Medicine Man of the American Indian, p. 318, New York, 1935.

5. Roys, R. L.: Ethno-botany of the Maya, Pub. No. 2, Mid. Am. Res. Ser., Tulane University, New Orleans, 1931.

6. Cruz, M. de la: The Badianus Manuscript; an Aztec Herbal of 1552, Introduction, translation and annotations by Emily Walcott Emmart, Baltimore, 1940. See also, Standley, P. C.: The Flora of Yucatan, Pub. No. 279, Field Mus. of Nat. Hist., Chicago, 1930.

7. Weinland, J. L.: Some U.S.P. drugs used by early Central American Indians, Purdue Pharm., 11, No. 2, pp. 6-8; No. 3, p. 3.

8. Such as the Englishmen William Wood (New England's Prospect, London, 1634; reprinted in 1635 and in 1639 in London, in 1764 and in 1865 in Boston) and John Josselyn (New England's Rarities, London, 1672, reprinted in 1865; An Account of Two Voyages to New England, London, 1674, reprinted in Boston in 1834 and in 1869; both books reprinted in abstract as Bulletin 8 of the reproduction series of the Lloyd Library, edited by H. W. Felter); Peter Kalm, a Swede (Report of his travels, in the Swedish Acad-

emy of Sciences, 1753-1763; summary by Fr. Hoffmann in Pharm. Rev. *16*:260, 1898); J. D. Schoepf, a German (Reise durch einige nordamerikanische Staaten, Erlangen, 1788; summary by Fr. Hoffmann in Pharm. Rev. *16*:296, 1898; Schoepf's Materia Medica Americana reprinted as Bulletin 3 of the reproduction series of the Lloyd Library, with an introduction by Edward Kremers); André and Francois-André Michaux, Frenchmen (Travels between 1793 and 1796, reprinted in Thwaites: Early Western Travels, vol. 3; summary in Pharm. Rev. *23*:53, 1905. Fr.-A. Michaux: Journal of 1802, Paris, 1804 and 1808, trans. into English in 1805; reprinted in Thwaites: Early Western Travels, vol. 3; summary in Pharm. Rev. *23*:86, 1905); and the Americans: Thaddeus Mason Harris (Journal of a Tour, made in 1803; reprinted in Thwaites: Early Western Travels, vol. 3; summary in Pharm. Rev. *23*:92, 1905; of special interest is the account of "Seneca Indian Oil" [petroleum]); Thomas Nuttall (Journal of 1819, Philadelphia, 1821; reprinted in Thwaites: Early Western Travels, vol. 13; summary in Pharm. Rev. *26*:19, 1908); Benjamin Smith Barton (Collections for a Materia Medica of the U.S.A., Philadelphia, 1798 and 1804); and Peter Smith, the so-called "Indian Doctor" (The Indian Doctor's Dispensatory, Cincinnati, 1812; reprinted as Bulletin 2 of the reproduction series of the Lloyd Library). The studies of H. S. Smith among the Wisconsin Indians include comprehensive lists of drugs. (Milwaukee Pub. Mus. Bull. vol 4, No. 1, 1923, p. 14; vol 4, No. 2, 1928, p. 184; vol 4, No. 3, 1932, p. 348; vol. 7, No. 1, 1933, p. 32). See furthermore the list of similar publications in the Index-Catalogue of the Library of the Surgeon-General's Office, U. S. Army, vol 6, 1885, p. 815; also second series, vol. 2, 1902, p. 876; and Smithsonian publications of the Bureau of American Ethnology: Bourke, I. G.: The Medicine-Men of the Apache, 9th annual report, p. 443; Gilmore, M. R.: Use of Plants by the Indians of the Missouri River Region, 33rd annual report, p. 43; Swanton, J. R.: Religious Beliefs and Medical Practices of the Creek Indians, 42nd annual report, p. 473; Densmore, Fr.: Uses of Plants by the Chippewa Indians, 44th an-

nual report, p. 275; J. Mooney and Fr. M. Olbrechts, The Swimmer Manuscript, i.e., Cherokee Sacred Formulas and Medical Prescriptions, Bulletin 99; W. W. Robbins, J. Peabody Harrington and B. Freire-Marreco, Ethnobotany of the Tewa Indians, Bulletin 55.

Because of the careful collection of information and later pharmacologic screening, particular interest attaches to a study of some 200 medicinal plants used by the Paiute, Shoshone and Washoe tribes of Nevada, reported by Train, P., Henrichs, J. B., and Archer, W. A.: Medicinal Uses of Plants by Indian Tribes of Nevada (Contributions Toward a Flora of Nevada, No. 45), United States National Arboretum, Washington 25, D. C., rev. ed., 1957.

9. Krafka, Jos., Jr.: An account of the attempt of the Society of Apothecaries to establish the drug trade in colonial Georgia, J. A. Ph. A. *28*:616, 1939.

10. Richtmann, W. O.: A history of the cultivation of medicinal plants in the U. S., J. A. Ph. A. *9*:816, 1920.

11. Stuenzer, K.: Die Schrift des Monardes über die Arzneimittel Amerikas, Halle, 1895.

12. Cowen, D. L.: America's Pre-Pharmacopoeial Literature, p. 28, Madison, Wis., 1961.

13. Hartwich, C.: Die Bedeutung der Entdeckung von Amerika für die Drogenkunde, Berlin, 1892.

14. Haggis, W. A.: Fundamental errors in the early history of Cinchona, Bull. Hist. Med. *10*:417, 568, 1941.

15. Lib. I, Chaps. 25 to 75: Historia de las Indias, by Las Casas, printed for the first time in 1875-1876 *in* the Coleccion de documentos ineditos para la historia de España.

16. Major, R. H.: Select letters of Christopher Columbus, Hakluyt Society, No. 2, 1847.

17. Cowen, D. L.: Colonial laws pertaining to pharmacy, J. A. Ph. A. *23*:1242, 1934.

18. Birkett, H. S.: The History of Medicine in the Province of Quebec, 1535-1838, New York, 1908.

19. Thwaites, R. G.: Jesuit Relations, p. 155, 1897.

20. Bradley, Th. J.: The first pharmacist in North America, J. A. Ph. A. *25*:628, 1936.

21. Kremers, E.: History of American pharmacy, Am. Drugg. *68*:10, 1920.
22. Liot, A.: Les apothicaires dieppois du 16 au 19 siècle, Chap. 4, Ronen, 1912.
23. Parkman, F.: History of La Salle, Boston, 1892; Sayre, L. E.: Orvietan or Theriac, Amer. Drugg. & Pharm. *44*:71, 1904.
24. Lafitau, J. F.: Mémoire, La plante du Ginseng de Tartaire en Canade, Paris, 1718.
25. Duffy, J., ed.: The Rudolph Matas History of Medicine in Louisiana, pp. 87-89; 117, Baton Rouge, 1958.
26. Cable, G. W.: The Grandissimes, New York, 1912.
27. Morgan: *op. cit.*, p. 119.
28. Ward, Chr.: New Sweden on the Delaware, p. 134, Philadelphia, 1938.
29. Johnson, A.: The Instruction for John Printz, Governor of New Sweden, p. 30, Philadelphia, 1930.
30. New Netherland Register: *1*:89, 1911.
31. Shrady, J.: Med. Reg. of New York *25*:233, 1887; and New Netherland Register *1*:26, 1911.
32. Shrady: *op. cit.*, pp. 232, 233.
33. Raubenheimer, H.: Early American pharmacy, Med. Life *33*:57, 1926.
34. Morgan: *op. cit.*, p. 38.
35. Blanton, W. B.: Medicine in Virginia in the Seventeenth Century, pp. 8, 9, Richmond, 1930.
36. *Ibid.*: pp. 30, 31.
37. *Ibid.*: p. 116.
38. *Ibid.*: pp. 24-26.
39. Viets, H. R.: Some features of the medicine in Massachusetts during the Colonial period, 1620-1770, Isis *23*:389, 1935.
40. Judd, S.: History of Hadley, pp. 438-444, Springfield, Mass., 1905.
41. Bradley, W. T.: Medical practices of the New England aborigines, J. A. Ph. A. *25*:146, 1936.
42. Reprint with comments, Badger Pharmacist No. 15, 1937; Kremers, E.: American Pharmaceutical Documents, 1643 to 1780, Madison, Wis., 1944.
43. Viets: *op. cit.*, p. 392.
44. Browne, C. A.: Some relations of early chemistry in America to medicine, J. Chem. Ed. *3*:268, No. 3.
45. *Ibid.*: pp. 270, 271, 273.
46. Drug list of King Philip's War: Badger Pharm., No. 25, 1939.
47. Bradley, W. T.: Giles Firmin, Sr., J. A. Ph. A. *26*:250, 1937.
48. Holmes, Oliver Wendell: Works, Medical Essays, vol. 9, pp. 312-369, Boston, 1895.
49. Wilbert, M. I.: The beginnings of pharmacy in America, Am. J. Pharm. *79*:400, 1907.
50. Cowen, D.: Colonial laws pertaining to pharmacy, J. A. Ph. A. *23*:1236, 1934. The quotations are from the act of 1646.
51. Griffenhagen, G.: Bartholomew Browne, Pharmaceutical Chemist of Salem, Massachusetts, 1698-1704, Essex Institute [Mass.] Historical Collections, January 1961, pp. 19-30; summarized in Pharmacy in History 7:1, 1962.
52. Viets: *op. cit.*, p. 397.
53. *Ibid.*: p. 403. Viets erred in stating that Gardiner "established the first apothecary shop in 1744" in New England.
54. Norris, G. W.: Early History of Medicine in Philadelphia, p. 603, Philadelphia, 1886.
55. Pharm. Era *33*:200, 1920.
56. Van Doren, C.: Benjamin Franklin, p. 128, New York, 1938; Wilbert, M. I.: Benjamin Franklin, Am. J. Pharm. *78*:219, 1906.
57. Van Doren: *op. cit.*, p. 429.
58. Wilbert, M. I.: Beginnings of American pharmacy, Am. J. Pharm. *79*:400, 1907.
59. Troth, S. A.: A retrospect of pharmacy, Am. J. Pharm. *77*:426, 1905.
60. Smith, D. B.: Christopher Marshall, J. Phil. Coll. Pharm. *2*:255, 1830; Ellis, E. T.: The story of a very old Philadelphia drugstore, Am. J. Pharm. *75*:57, 1903; England, J. W.: First Century of the Philadelphia College of Pharmacy, p. 28, Philadelphia, 1922.
61. The Squibb Message *1*:112, 1923.
62. Schoepf, Joh. D.: Reise durch einige nordamerikanische Staaten, p. 121, Erlangen, 1788.
63. The quotation is taken from David L. Cowen's article, "Colonial laws pertaining to pharmacy," J. A. Ph. A. *23*:1236, 1934. The Virginia Act of 1736 was first published as chapter 10 of the acts of 1736. (At a General Assembly . . . continued to the fifth day of August—1736) (Williamsburg, 1736), p. 26. Cowen says furthermore: "Various authorities have erroneously dated this act as 1636. See Wickes, 'History of Medicine in New Jersey' (Newark, 1879), page 54; F. H. Garrison, An Introduction to the History of Medicine (Philadelphia, 1914), pages 233, 682; *Ibid.*, 1929 ed., pages 304, 824; and LaWall (4000 Years of Pharmacy), pages 331, 571. . . . Wickes cites as his authority the 'Half Yearly Compendium of Medical

Science,' Jan. 1878 (page 66). This, however, gives the date correctly as 1736." The mistake of Wickes, obviously a mere slip of writing or printing, in this way became perpetuated.

According to Cowen, the reference to a New Jersey act of 1664 as the "earliest law regulating apothecaries in the new world" (LaWall, C.: 4000 Years of Pharmacy, p. 572, Philadelphia, 1927) is baseless. The first assembly ever convened in New Jersey met May 26 to 30, 1668.

64. Cowen, D. L.: Colonial laws pertaining to pharmacy, J. A. Ph. A. 23:1241, 1934.
65. This early history of the hospital by Franklin once again has become readily available through a reprint edition, with an introduction by I. Bernard Cohen, Baltimore, 1954.
66. Wilbert, M. I.: John Morgan, Am. J. Pharm. 76:5, 1904.
67. *Ibid.*: p. 9; see also Kredel, F. E., and Hoch, J. H.: Early relations of pharmacy and medicine in the United States, J. A. Ph. A. 28:704, 1939; Blanton, W. B.: Medicine in Virginia in the Eighteenth Century, pp. 12, 32, Richmond, 1931.
68. See Austin, R. B.: Early American Medical Imprints: A guide to works printed in the United States 1668-1920, Washington 25, D. C., 1961, for bibliographic information on early American pharmaceutical literature and on libraries where copies may be found. Concerning the American editions of the British books by Culpeper, David L. Cowen has published a valuable article: The Boston editions of Nicholas Culpeper, J. Hist. Med. 11:156, 1956.

10. THE REVOLUTIONARY WAR

1. Duncan, L. C.: Medical Men in the American Revolution, Carlisle Barracks, Pa., 1936, p. 187; Eberle, E. G.: Hugh Mercer, J. Am. Pharm. A. 15:424, 1926; Waterman, J. M.: With Sword and Lancet, Richmond, Va., 1941.
2. Duncan, L. C.: *op. cit.*, p. 24.
3. ———: *op. cit.*, p. 77.
4. ———: *op. cit.*, p. 105.
5. ———: *op. cit.*, p. 18.
6. Shrady, John: Med. Reg. New York, 19: 194, 1881.
7. Balland: Les pharmaciens militaires français, Paris, 1913, pp. 9, 89.
8. Bouvet, Maurice: Histoire de la pharmacie de France, Paris, 1937, p. 331. Other French compatriots who, at one time or other, served as pharmacists in Rochambeau's army were Jean Baunach, Berry, Dessenis, Gourdon, Claude-Charles Humbert, Benjamin Magenc, Maheux and Vancalbeck (or Vancattelech), as given by Bouvet in his unique work: Le service de santé français pendant la Guerre d'Indepéndance des Etats-Unis (1777-1782), Paris, 1934, p. 38.
9. Duncan, L. C.: *op. cit.*, p. 22.
10. ———: *op. cit.*, p. 40
11. Shrady, John: Med. Reg. New York, 18: 190, 1880; Duncan, L. C.: *op. cit.*, p. 40.
12. The medical directors who succeeded (and denounced) each other (see Gibson, James E.: Dr. Bodo Otto, and the Medical Background of the American Revolution, Springfield, Ill., p. 185) were Benjamin Church, John Morgan, William Shippen, and John Cochran (Duncan, L. C.: *op. cit.*, pp. 61, 78, 79, and 276; see also Wilbert, M. I.: John Morgan, Am. J. Pharm. 76:1, 1905).
13. Duncan, L. C.: *op. cit.*, p. 60.
14. Gibson, J. E.: *op. cit.*, p. 106.
15. Duncan, L. C.: *op. cit.*, p. 194.
16. ———: *op. cit.*, p. 239. In a "list of medical men who took a part in the American revolution" (containing about 1,400 names but considered incomplete), the following entries are of pharmaceutical interest:

    1. Apothecaries general: Andrew Craigie (Mass.); C. Henry Flagg (S. C.), who served first as a surgeon; Giles; Israel Root (Conn.); Josiah Root (Conn.).

    2. Assistant Apothecary General: William Johonnot (France).

    3. Apothecaries: John Crane (S. C.) and B. John Cutting (N. Y.); Joseph Prescott (Mass.) who served first as a surgeon's mate.

    4. Deputy Apothecaries: Evan Lewis (S. C.) and Patrick Carnes (S. C.).

    5. "Continental druggist": William Smith (Pa.).

    6. Individuals "furnishing medicine": Aubury, Robert Bass, Benjamin Dyar, Lothrop, Isaac Thom, Samuel Treatre and George Wood.

    7. Individuals concerned with saltpetre: Christian Vaught, who "made saltpetre"; Robert Harris, who "made powder"; and Josiah Gilman, who was "inspector of saltpetre" (p. 379).
17. Duncan, L. C.: *op. cit.*, p. 159.

18. ———:*op. cit.*, p. 41.
19. Kebler, L. F.: Andrew Craigie, J. Am. Pharm. A. *17*:66, 1928. Later, when Morgan succeeded Church as medical director, it seems probable that Craigie was transferred for a short period, rather than being forced "out of office" temporarily, as Kebler inferred.
20. Duncan, L. C.: *op. cit.*, pp. 330, 331.
21. Gibson, J. E.: *op. cit.*, p. 155.
22. ———: *op. cit.* p. 153.
23. Kebler, L. F.: *op. cit.*, p. 173.
24. Griffenhagen, George: Drug Supplies in the American Revolution, Paper 16 in Contributions from the Museum of History and Technology, United States National Museum, Bulletin 225, Washington 25, D. C., 1961, and also separately; see pp. 130-133.
25. This quotation and most of the information given on drug supply in the Revolution is taken from Griffenhagen, *Ibid.*, pp. 129 f., *et passim.* On the pharmaceutical content of the "standardized field boxes," see also Gibson, James E.: Dr. Bodo Otto, and the Medical Background, p. 167; and on a drug inventory of the general hospital (1775) by Craigie, see Kebler, *op. cit.*, p. 73.
26. Gahn, B. W., and Kebler, L. F.: Dr. William Brown, J. Am. Pharm. A. *16*:1090, 1927.
27. Berman, Alex: The Beth Holim Formulary of London (1749). Am. J. Hosp. Pharm. *17*:24, 1960.
28. Badger Pharmacist, Nos. 22 to 25, 1938; Kremers, E.: American Pharmaceutical Documents, 1643-1780, Madison, Wis., 1944; Adlung, A., and Urdang, G.: Grundriss der Geschichte der deutschen Pharmazie, Berlin, 1935, pp. 4 and 317; Urdang, G.: Zur Geschichte der Metalle in den amtlichen deutschen Arzneibüchern, Mittenwald, 1933, p. 40.
29. Published by Rho Chi (Eta) in the Badger Pharmacist, Nos. 22 to 25, 1938 (Lititz Pharmacopoeia) and Nos. 27 to 30, 1940 (Coste's compendium); and re-published as part of Kremers, Edward (ed.): American Pharmaceutical Documents, 1643-1780, Madison, Wis., 1944. In addition, a facsimile of the original Latin text of the Lititz Pharmacopoeia was published as a separate pamphlet by the American Pharmaceutical Association, Washington, D. C. (no date), 32 pp. (reprinted from England, Joseph: The First Century of

the Philadelphia College of Pharmacy, Philadelphia, 1922).

11. YOUNG REPUBLIC AND PIONEER EXPANSION

1. Wilbert, M. I.: Some early botanical and herb gardens, Am. J. Pharm. *80*:412, 1908; and sections on natural history and botany in Struik, Dirk J.: Yankee Science in the Making, Boston, 1948, and Hindle, Brooke: The Pursuit of Science in Revolutionary America 1735-1789, Chapel Hill, 1956.
2. Maisch, J. M.: G. H. E. Muehlenberg als Botaniker, Pharm. Rund. *4*:123, 1886.
3. *Ibid.*: p. 124.
4. Bull. Lloyd Libr., Repro. Ser. No. 1.
5. *Ibid.*: Repro. Ser. No. 4.
6. Maisch, J. M.: *op. cit.*, p. 123.
7. Wilbert, M. I.: *op. cit.*, p. 413.
8. Bull. Lloyd Libr., Repro. Ser. No. 7, p. 15; details about Thomson remedies, p. 75.
9. Berman, A.: Botanico-Medical Movement (dissertation), p. 319.
10. Berman, Alex: The Impact of the Nineteenth Century Botanico-Medical Movement on American Pharmacy and Medicine (unpublished Ph.D. dissertation), University of Wisconsin, Madison, 1954, p. 91. See also Berman's excellent published papers, such as Bull. Hist. Med. *25*:405-428 and 519-538, 1951 (on original Thomsonians); J. Hist. Med. *11*:133-155, 1956 (on neo-Thomsonians); and Bull. Hist. Med. *30*:1-25, 1956 (on their scientific aspirations).
11. *Ibid.*: pp. 321 and 324.
12. Wilder, Alex: History of Medicine, New Sharon, Maine, 1901, p. 453.
13. *Ibid.*: p. 430.
14. *Ibid.*: p. 439.
15. Berman, Alex: C. S. Rafinesque (1783-1840): a Challenge to the Historian of Pharmacy, Am. J. Pharm. Educ. *16*:411-415, 1952.
16. Bull. Lloyd Libr., Repro. Ser. No. 7, p. 75.
17. Wilder, Alex: *op. cit.*, p. 1; Packard, F. R.: History of Medicine in the United States, New York, 1931, p. 1227; Shafer, H. B.: The American Medical Profession, 1783-1850, New York, 1938, pp. 201, 210.
18. Rice, Ch.: Notes about Certain Vegetable Drugs, Bull. Lloyd Libr., No. 12, p. 43.
19. Mayo, C. A.: The Lloyd Library and Its Makers, Bull. Lloyd Libr., No. 28, p. 31.

20. Shafer: *op. cit.*, p. 211. The regulations were issued in New York in 1760; New Jersey, 1772; Massachusetts, 1781; and New Hampshire, 1791.
21. Shafer: *op. cit.*, p. 214.
22. Brewer, W. A.: Reminiscences of an old pharmacist, Pharm. Rec. *4*:326, 1884. Young, James Harvey: The Toadstool Millionaires: A Social History of Patent Medicines in America before Federal Regulation, Princeton, 1961, appears to be the best book of its scope.
23. Shrady, John: Med. Reg. N. Y. *22*:245, 1884.
24. Shrady, John: Med. Reg. N. Y. *24*:264, 1886. A good insight into the kind and the amount of drugs usually imported by American druggists may be found in two invoices (1785) concerning shipments of drugs from London to the Marshall brothers and to M. Bartram, both of them druggists in Philadelphia. Reproductions of these invoices with comments are available (Kremers, E.: Two invoices of 1785, J. Am. Pharm. A. *20*:682, 1931). They supplement the authentic Colonial lists of drugs previously mentioned—the "receipts" used by John Winthrop, Sr., Locke's drug list, the *Lititz Pharmacopoeia* and Le Coste's *Compendium*. Together, they make possible a comparative study of the drugs used in the North American settlements until the close of the 18th century.
25. Sadtler, S. P.: Influence of pharmacists on the development and advance of modern chemistry, Am. J. Pharm. *93*:197, 1921.
26. Ellis, E. T.: The story of a very old Philadelphia drugstore, Am. J. Pharm. *75*:57, 1903; W. A. Brewer, Sr., *op. cit.*, pp. 210, 232, 255, 282, 304, 326, 348, 410, 424, 442, 460, 475, 494.
27. LaWall, C. H.: The founding of the Philadelphia College of Pharmacy and Science, Am. J. Pharm. *93*:172, 1921; Arny, H. V.: Pharmacy 100 years ago, Am. J. Pharm. *93*:188, 1921.
28. Cowen, D. L.: Louisiana, Pioneer in the regulation of pharmacy, Louisiana Hist. Quart. *26*:5, 1943.
29. *Ibid.*: pp. 7, 8, 10, and 11.
30. *Ibid.*: p. 9 (Gibson's Guide and Directory of the State of Louisiana and the Cities of New Orleans and Lafayette for 1838).
31. *Ibid.*: p. 10.
32. Hoch, J. H.: The first American board of of pharmacy, Am. J. Pharm. *104*:750, 1932.
33. Ellis, E. T.: *op. cit.*, p. 59.
34. Shrady, John: Med. Reg. N. Y. *17*:178, 1879.
35. England, J. W.: The First Century of the Philadelphia College of Pharmacy, Philadelphia, 1922, p. 55.
36. Arny, H. V.: *op. cit.*, p. 184.
37. Shrady, John: Med. Reg. N. Y. *25*:243, 245, 1887; and Kredel, F. E., and Hoch, J. H.: Early relation of pharmacy and medicine in the United States, J. Am. Pharm. A. *28*:796, 1939.
38. Sharpless, Isaac: Two Centuries of Pennsylvania History. Philadelphia, 1900, p. 239.
39. Lindley-Hawes-Schneider-Quaife: The Ordinance of 1787 and the Old Northwest Territory, Marietta, Ohio, 1937, p. 31. In the resolutions of October 6, 1780, concerning reorganization of the medical department of the army it is stated that the several officers of the medical staff also "shall at the end of the war be entitled to a certain provision of land, in the proportion following: the Apothecary the same as a Lieutenant-Colonel. Assistant Apothecary the same as Major." (Kebler, L. F.: Andrew Craigie, J. Am. Pharm. A. *17*: 172, 1928.)
40. Lindley-Hawes-Schneider-Quaife: *op. cit.*, p. 30.
41. Sigerist, H. E.: American Medicine, New York, 1934, p. 58.
42. Cf.: An American physician-apothecary of 1793. Pharm. Era *48*:298, 1915.
43. Sealsfield, George: Lebensbilder aus der westlichen Hemisphaere; more specifically in the chapter: Ein Nachtstück am untern Mississippi; and Thwaites, R. G.: Early Western Travels, vol. 4; Pharm. Rev. *23*: 15, 1905.
44. Kremers, E.: The history of American pharmacy, Am. Drugg. *68*(May), 1920; Badger Pharmacist No. 5, 1930.
45. Lindley-Hawes-Schneider-Quaife: *op. cit.*, p. 82.
46. *Ibid.*: p. 65.

12. THE GROWTH OF ASSOCIATIONS

1. Davenport, B. F.: History of the Massachusetts College of Pharmacy, p. 7, Cat., Mass. Coll. Pharm. 1882-83.
2. England, J. W.: The First Century of the Philadelphia College of Pharmacy, p. 46, Philadelphia, 1922.
3. *Ibid.*: p. 54.

4. *Ibid.*: p. 356.
5. LaWall, C. H.: The founding of the Philadelphia College of Pharmacy and Science, Am. J. Pharm. *93*:175, 1921.
6. *Ibid.*: p. 63.
7. Kremers, Edward: The teaching of pharmacy during the past 50 years, Drugg. Circ. *51*:61, 1907.
8. England, J. W.: *op. cit.*, p. 352.
9. ————: *op. cit.*, pp. 114, 357; Am. J. Pharm. *45*:513, 1875.
10. *Ibid.*: p. 373; W. Procter, Jr., Necrology, Am. J. Pharm. *18*:315, 1846.
11. England, J. W.: *op. cit.*, p. 57.
12. *Ibid.*: p. 72.
13. *Ibid.*: p. 70.
14. *Ibid.*: p. 71.
15. Marshall, E. C.: Early History of the Massachusetts College of Pharmacy, Quart. Bull. Mass. Coll. Pharm. *3*:9, 1911.
16. Davenport, B. F.: *op. cit.* p. 8.
17. Marshall, E. C.: *op. cit.*, p. 10.
18. *Ibid.*: p. 15.
19. Robbins, D. C.: Address, Alumni Association Representative, New York College of Pharmacy, 1872.
20. A centennial history was published by Wimmer, C. P.: The College of Pharmacy of the City of New York, New York, 1929, supplemented by Ballard, C. W.: A History of the College of Pharmacy, Columbia University, New York, 1954.
21. Proc. A. Ph. A. *7*:87, 1858.
22. The Graduate, p. 18, Cincinnati College of Pharmacy, 1925.
23. Am. J. Pharm. *26*:380, 1854.
24. *Ibid.*: p. 381.
25. Proc. A. Ph. A. *7*:86, 1858.
26. Am. J. Pharm. *37*:157, 1865.
27. Meyer Brothers' Drugg. *39*:48, 1918.
28. Am. J. Pharm. *37*:158, 1865.
29. Day, W. R.: The School of Pharmacy, Illinois Alumni Record, 1921.
30. Among these were the Richmond Pharmaceutical Society, founded in 1852 (Am. J. Pharm. *24*:385, 1852), which later on adopted the name Richmond College of Pharmacy (Proc. A. Ph. A. *8*:104, 1859) and was revived in 1873 as the Richmond Pharmaceutical Association (Am. J. Pharm. *45*:575, 1873), "a social scientific union in Boston" (Proc. A. Ph. A. *6*:74, 1857) which was reorganized as the Boston Druggist's Association in 1875 (Drugg. Circ. *51*:171, 1907); the Pharmaceutical Association of Washington City (Proc. A. Ph. A. *6*:6, 1857); and the San Francisco Pharmaceutical Association, which was founded in 1858 (Proc. A. Ph. A. *7*:88, 1858) and died out in 1860 (Proc. A. Ph. A. *9*:67, 1860). Such city organizations were founded, disappeared and revived again and again all over the country. In large cities pharmaceutical associations existed at that time and continue to exist, which were organized because of very different motives. In New York City, a multiplicity of such associations strives for cooperation in an organization founded in 1910 under the name of New York Pharmaceutical Conference and reorganized, in 1935, as the New York Pharmaceutical Council. There are no fewer than 14 local pharmaceutical groups affiliated with the Council, among them the New York German Apothecaries' Society and the New York Italian Pharmaceutical Association J. A. Ph. A. *26*:369, 1937). The New York organization of Chinese druggists does not consist of licensed pharmacists.
31. Adlung, A., and Urdang, G.: Grundriss der Geschichte der deutschen Pharmazie, p. 417, Berlin, 1935. In the small German principality of Baden, for example, 30 physicians and 20 pharmacists left their native country after the defeat of the uprising.
32. Eberle, E. G.: Old druggists in Texas, Drugg. Circ. *51*:187, 1907.
33. Mayo, C. A.: The Lloyd Library and its makers, Bull. Lloyd Library, No. 28, p. 10, 1928. See Article XI, par. 2 of the Society's by-laws of October 1, 1851. In 1852 the *Leserverein* changed its name to *Deutscher Pharmazeutischer Verein* and, in 1875, to *Deutscher Apotheker-Verein von New York*.
34. Am. J. Pharm. *28*:90, 1856.
35. Schleussner, C. F., and Lehman, R. S.: History of the German Apothecaries Society, p. 24, New York Deutscher Apotheker Verein, New York, 1926.
36. Proc. A. Ph. A. *53*:74, 1905; *54*:21, 93, 1906.
37. On the development of professional fraternities in American Pharmacy see, e.g., Brown, L. N.: A brief history of Phi Delta Chi fraternity, J. A. Ph. A. *11*:351-352, 1922; Knox, J. W. T.: Historical sketch of Phi Chi fraternity, Proc. A. Ph. A. *52*:439, 1904; Bliss, A.: A brief history of the Kappa Psi fraternity, J. A. Ph. A. *11*:352, 1922; Bowers, R. A., and Cowen, D. L.: Rho Chi Society; Development of the

Honor Society of American Pharmacy, ed. 2, Indianapolis, 1961; Boonshoft, Jerome, and Kirschner, Robert: 40 Years of AZO; A Complete and Factual History of the Events and Activities of Alpha Zeta Omega Pharmaceutical Fraternity, n.p., 1960; Bonow, E. R.: The Pearl of Kappa Epsilon [Madison, Wis.], 1951; Bonow, E. R.: The history of professional pharmaceutical fraternities for women, Am. J. Pharm. Ed. *18*:410-413, 1954.

38. Am. J. Pharm. *40*:88, 1868.
39. Am. J. Pharm. *50*:460, 1878; Proc. A. Ph. A. *28*:586, 1880.
40. Proc. A. Ph. A. *29*:536, 1881.
41. Am. J. Pharm. *26*:475, 1890; Proc. A. Ph. A. *40*:1107, 1892.
42. Am. J. Pharm. *52*:382, 1880.
43. Proc. A. Ph. A. *32*:26, 1884.
44. Drugg. Circ. *51*:116, 1907; Proc. A. Ph. A. *50*:40, 1902.
45. Cowen, D. L.: The New Jersey Pharmaceutical Association, New Jersey J. Pharm. *18*:(No. 12) 16, 17, 1945.
46. Am. J. Pharm. *43*:280, 1871.
47. *Ibid.*: p. 329. Another type of medical influence may be seen in the reorganization of the West Virginia association (1881). Among the pharmacists thus active were "a number of physicians who maintained stores in various localities." (Proc. West Virginia State Pharm. Assoc., p. 34, 1931.)
48. The list in Drugg. Circ. *51*:115, 1907, has been corrected and completed from various sources; e.g., see West. Drugg., Extra, *15*:39, 1893; H. M. Whelpley: Pharm. Era *16*:887, 1896; C. W. Holmes: Am. Drugg. & Pharm. Rec. *36*:194, 1900; West. Drugg. *24*:209, 1902.
49. For example, in Michigan (1883), Mississippi (1891), where pharmacy laws were enacted in 1885 and 1892, and in West Virginia (1881) and Maine (1890), where pharmacy laws were amended in 1882 and 1891.
50. Proc. A. Ph. A. *15*:18, 1867.
51. Am. J. Pharm. *45*:329, 422, 1873.
52. Proc. A. Ph. A. *46*:1128, 1898.
53. Elliott, E. C. (ed.): The General Report of the Pharmaceutical Survey, p. 56, Washington, D. C., 1950.
54. Drugg. Circ. *51*:100, 1907.
55. Shafer, H. B.: The American Medical Profession, 1783-1850, p. 230, New York, 1936. As to the medical influence on legislation concerning the adulteration of drugs,

see Nitardy, F. W.: Notes on early drug legislation, J. A. Ph. A. *23*:1122, 1934.
56. Drugg. Circ. *51*:100, 1907.
57. Am. J. Pharm. *23*:290, 1851.
58. *Ibid.*: *24*:85, 1852.
59. *Ibid.*: *24*:86, 1852.
60. For further information about the prominent part played by William Procter, Jr., in the founding of the American Pharmaceutical Association, see Urdang, George: College of pharmacy associations, Am. J. Pharm. Ed. *17*:334, 1944.
61. Am. J. Pharm. *25*:13, 1853.
62. England, J. W.: *op. cit.*, p. 127.
63. Am. J. Pharm. *26*:290, 1854.
64. Hoffmann, F.: A retrospect of the development of American pharmacy and the American Pharmaceutical Association, Proc. A. Ph. A. *50*:122, 1902. A history of the pharmaceutical codes of ethics has been published by C. H. LaWall in J. A. Ph. A. *10*:895-961, 1921.
65. J. A. Ph. A. *11*:728, 1922; Yearbook of the Am. Pharm. Assoc., beginning with 15 (1925); the Code of Ethics was last revised extensively in 1952.
66. J. A. Ph. A. *1*:928-929, 1079-1084, 1912.
67. Cf. Constitution and By-laws of the American Pharmaceutical Association, Washington, D. C.: [1961], p. 2 (current version available from Association on request). The interpretation of the objectives was discussed by the chairman of the House of Delegates in 1958, Lansdowne, J. W.: Seven objectives, J. A. Ph. A. (Pract. Ed.) *19*:728, 1958.
68. The Proceedings of the American Pharmaceutical Association and, since 1912, the Journals are the most satisfactory sources of the history of the Association. Short surveys are published in anniversary numbers of several pharmaceutical journals. Reference may be made to: C. L. Diehl, Pharm. Era *16*:878, 1896; Drugg. Circ. *51*:100, 1907; F. Hoffmann, Retrospect, Proc. A. Ph. A. *50*:100, 1902; J. H. Beal, Address, J. A. Ph. A. *16*:799, 1927.
69. On Remington and the founding of the Sections see Proc. A. Ph. A. *35*:472 f. and 485, 1887. The best single source on the history of the Sections is: The Sections of the American Pharmaceutical Association —A Symposium, Madison, Wis., 1953 (also in Am. J. Pharm. Ed., vol. 17, No. 3, 1953).
70. Drugg. Circ. *51*:73, 1907; Maisch, John M.: Die Conference der Fachschulen der

"Colleges of Pharmacy," Pharm. Rundschau *1*:182, 1883; and Sonnedecker, Glenn: The conference of schools of pharmacy—a period of frustration, Am. J. Pharm. Ed. *18*:389-401, 1954.

71. Kraus, E. H.: American Association of Colleges of Pharmacy, J. A. Ph. A. *14*:981, 1925; and Sonnedecker, Glenn: The section on education and legislation, Am. J. Pharm. Ed. *17*:371-375, 1953.

72. *Notes and Journal* of the N.A.R.D., Am. J. Pharm. Ed. *13*:358-375, 1949; The National Association of Retail Druggists, Drugg. Circ. *51*:104, 1907.

73. Boards of pharmacy, Drugg. Circ. *51*:137, 1907; see especially, National Association of Boards of Pharmacy 1904-1954, Madison, Wis., 1955 (also in Proc. N.A.B.P., 1954).

74. J. A. Ph. A. *16*:842, 1927.

75. J. A. Ph. A. *16*:842, 1927; Swain, R. L.: The principles of law enforcement, J. A. Ph. A. *21*:1319, 1932; Dretzka, S. H.: Proc. Natl. Assoc. Bds. Pharm. 1944, pp. 170 f., and 1949, pp. 94 and 110-113.

76. J. A. Ph. A. *28*:938, 1939. The "conference" was preceded by the Association for the Advancement of Professional Pharmacy in New York in 1939; J. A. Ph. A. (Pract. Ed.) *2*:334, 1941.

77. Stieb, E. W.: American Institute of the History of Pharmacy—Through Two Decades, Madison, Wis., 1961.

78. J. A. Ph. A. (Pract. Ed.) *2*:177, 1941. The General Report of the Pharmaceutical Survey 1946-49, Washington, D. C., 1950, p. 47 f.; also gives reliable sketches on other national organizations.

79. Urdang, George: The precedents of the N.A.R.D. and its founding fifty years ago, Am. J. Pharm. Ed. *13*:358, 1949.

80. General Report of the Pharmaceutical Survey, p. 51.

81. Kelly, E. F., and Dargavel, John: Report on historic A.Ph.A.- N.A.R.D. Conference, J. A. Ph. A. (Pract. Ed.) *4*:394, 1943; also, Second annual A.Ph.A.-N.A.R.D. Conference, J. A. Ph. A. (Pract. Ed.) *6*:13, 1945.

82. While the A.Ph.A. maintained an aloof silence publicly, the deep split that occurred is suggested by the bitter denunciations under such raucous headlines as "Druggists sold down the river. Plotters use A.Ph.A. in betrayal . . .," (N.A.R.D. Journal 73:730 f., 1951); see also Misguided and weasel opposition, N.A.R.D.

Journal 72:1499, 1950; Destructive confusion confounded, *ibid.*, 72:1835, 1950; and Fischelis of the A.Ph.A. aligns himself with manufacturers against N.A.R.D. bill, *ibid.*, 73:808 and 826-836, 1951. Hurling such adjectives as "inane" and "befuddled," the latter article scarcely left anyone in doubt that "coordination" and joint conferences were at an end.

83. Berman, Alex: The American Society of Hospital Pharmacists—a tribute, Am. J. Hosp. Pharm. *19*:212, 1962; Austin, E. C.: Training hospital pharmacists, Drugg. Circ. *65*:87-88, 1921.

84. Berman, Alex: *op. cit.*, p. 213; see also, Ten years of the American Society of Hospital Pharmacists, Bull. Am. Soc. Hosp. Pharm., vol. 9, No. 4, 1952.

85. General Report of the Pharmaceutical Survey, p. 39.

86. Bowersox, C. H.: Drug clerks' organizations, Pharm. Era *45*:272 f., et passim, 1912; C. H. Bowersox of Cleveland, O., to Frank J. Steele of Greenwich, Conn., April 18, 1935 (copy in Kremers Reference Files, University of Wisconsin); see also the Association's journal, National Drug Clerk, e.g., Jan. 1927, p. 28; and Drugg. Circ. 57:162, 1907.

87. General Report of the Pharmaceutical Survey, p. 186.

88. Pharm. Era *16*:901, 1896; Harding, H. B.: Proprietary articles, Am. Drugg. & Pharm. Rec. *36*:190, 1900; Drugg. Circ. *51*:112, 1907.

89. For sketches on the manufacturing organizations see the General Report of the Pharmaceutical Survey, pp. 42, 46 and 53; on the founding of the N.A.M.M.P. see Drugg. Circ. *56*:158, 1912; and on the A.P.M.A. see Maltbie, B. L.: A Quarter Century of Progress in Manufacturing Pharmacy, New York, 1937.

90. Pharm. Era *16*:896, 948, 1896; Drugg. Circ. *51*:110, 1907; Proc. Nat. Wholesale Drugg. Assoc., especially 1924, p. 28, and A History of the National Wholesale Druggists Association, from Its Organization to 1924, New York, 1924.

91. The association was formed by buying clubs of retail druggists.

92. Some national examples not discussed in another context in this book would be the American Society of Pharmacognosy (f. 1959), Plant Science Seminar (f. 1923; see Claus, E. P.: A brief history of the Plant Science Seminar, Am. J. Pharm. Ed. *17*:433-436, 1953), Metropolitan Drug

Association Secretaries, Friends of Historical Pharmacy (f. 1941, primarily to maintain the Hugh Mercer Apothecary Shop; see General Report of the Pharmaceutical Survey, p. 48), National Drug Trade Conference (f. 1913; see, *ibid.*, p. 51). National Conference of State Pharmaceutical Association Secretaries (f. 1927; *ibid.*), National Pharmaceutical Council (f. 1953; J. A. Ph. A. (Pract. Ed.) *15*:28 and 214, 1953), Association of Food and Drug Officials of the United States (f. 1897; before 1938 titled American Dairy, Food and Drug Officials), National Conference on Pharmaceutical Research (1920-1941; see J. A. Ph. A. *12*:623, 1923).

Associations that thus far remain largely regional in their scope include the American College of Pharmacists (f. 1944), American Congress of Pharmacists (f. 1960) [Drug Topics, May 9, 1960, pp. 12 and 62], Drug, Chemical and Allied Trades Section of the New York Board of Trade (voting membership restricted to firms within 75-mile radius of New York City), Society of Doctors of Pharmacy (mainly California), and Jewish Pharmaceutical Society of America (mainly New York area).

93. Francke, D. E.: Editorial: American pharmacy's federation—false hope or bright future, Am. J. Hosp. Pharm. *19*:209, 1962. The far-reaching decision taken by the Association at the 1962 meeting was reported: J. A. Ph. A. n.s. *2*:270 and 281, 1962.

13. THE RISE OF LEGISLATIVE STANDARDS

1. Duffy, John: The Rudolph Matas History of Medicine in Louisiana, Baton Rouge, 1958, vol. 1, pp. 326-327.
2. Cowen, D. L.: America's first pharmacy laws, J. A. Ph. A. *3*:168, 1942. Key legal issue was a provision that the New York College of Pharmacy should bring suits and itself receive the $150 penalty from the convicted.
3. Cowen, D. L.: Louisiana, pioneer in the regulation of pharmacy, Louisiana Hist. Quart. *26*:334, 1943.
4. Charter of the City of Louisville of 1851, and Ordinances of the City, Louisville, 1869, p. 431.
5. Proceedings of the American Pharmaceutical Association, 1868, Philadelphia, 1869, p. 370.
6. Laws of Pennsylvania, 1866, Harrisburg, 1866, p. 679.
7. Am. J. Pharm. *44*:137, 1872; Apothecaries' Union of New York City, Report of the Executive Committee, New York, 1871; Pharm. Rev. *21*:465, 482, 1903; *22*:31, 155, 1904.
8. Proc. A. Ph. A. *20*:150, 1872.
9. Cowen, D. L.: America's first pharmacy laws, J. A. Ph. A. *3*:162-169, 214-221.
10. *Ibid.*: pp. 162-166.
11. *Ibid.*: pp. 166-167.
12. *Ibid.*: pp. 167-168. An interesting sidelight of the legislative history in Georgia was the provision for the licensing of "Botanic or Thomsonian apothecaries" in an 1847 act.
13. *Ibid.*: p. 168.
14. Cowen, D. L.: A roster of the licensed apothecaries of Louisiana, J. New Orleans Coll. Pharm. 8:3-4, 20-21, 1943.
15. Cowen, D. L.: America's first pharmacy laws, J. A. Ph. A. *3*:214.
16. Hoch, J. H.: The first American board of pharmacy, Am. J. Pharm. *104*:752, 1932.
17. Cowen, D. L.: America's first pharmacy laws, J. A. Ph. A. *3*:169.
18. *Ibid.*: p. 215.
19. Partial lists of early state laws on adulteration and poison are to be found in Cowen: Lousiana, pioneer in the regulation of pharmacy, Louisiana Hist. Quart. *26*:334, 335.
20. Some facts on early poison legislation are given by Wilbert, M. I.: The evolution of laws regulating the sale and use of poisons, J. A. Ph. A. *1*:1259-1261, 1912.
21. Proc. A. Ph. A. *17*:51, 1870.
22. Beal, J. H.: The evolution of pharmacy laws in the United States, Am. Drug. & Pharm. Rec. *36*:179, 1900.
23. Am. J. Pharm. *44*:137, 1872.
24. Kremers, Edward: The history of American pharmacy, Am. Drugg., *68*(No. 5): 14, 1920.
25. Am. J. Pharm. *44*:137, 1872.
26. Beal, J. H.: A general form of pharmacy law, Proc. A. Ph. A. *48*:309, 1900; Pharm. Rev. *18*:203, 1900.
27. As to pharmaceutical activities left to general merchants by the state pharmacy acts, see Robert Fischelis: A survey of state pharmacy laws with reference to the sale of drugs and medicines by several merchants. J. A. Ph. A. *20*:1331, 1931.
27a. Sonnedecker, Glenn: The birth of the National Association of Boards of Pharmacy

fifty years ago, in National Association of Boards of Pharmacy 1904-1954, Madison, Wis., 1955, pp. 23-33; also published in Proceedings of the National Association of Boards of Pharmacy, 1954.

28. Wiley, H. W.: Education of a Hoosier, Indiana Mag. Hist. *24*:94 f., 1928.

29. Editorial, Bull. A. Ph. A. *5*:391, 1910.

30. Editorial, Pharm. Era *14*:512, 1895.

31. For the evidence and judicious accounts of the complex background to the law, see Anderson, O. E., Jr.: The Health of a Nation; Harvey W. Wiley and the Fight for Pure Food, Chicago, 1958; and Wilson, Stephen: Food and Drug Regulation, Washington, 1942.

32. Report of committee on drug reform, Bull. A. Ph. A. *5*:655, 1910.

33. See, e.g., Proc. A. Ph. A. *55*:241, 1907, and Bull. A. Ph. A. *4*:467, 1909.

34. Wallace, J. C.: The chairman's address, J. A. Ph. A. *1*:939, 1912. For an account of one segment of the state endeavors in this field before Federal legislation, see Sonnedecker, Glenn, and Urdang, George: Legalization of drug standards under state laws in the United States of America, Food, Drug, Cosmetic Law J. *8*:741-760, 1953; also article on legal aspect—Sonnedecker, Glenn: The section on education and legislation of the American Pharmaceutical Association, Am. J. Pharm. Ed. *17*:362-383, 1953.

35. Dunn, C. W.: Our food and drug law, with some observations on its major statute, Food, Drug, Cosmetic Law J. *9*:385, 1954. The only other major statutes controlling interstate commerce are the Interstate Commerce Act (1887) and the Sherman Antitrust Act (1890). Dunn calls the 1938 Food and Drug Act "of profound legal importance, in itself and as a modern administrative law; and because it . . . makes an extreme use of the congressional power over interstate commerce, to regulate intrastate commerce as well." Administration of the Federal law at first was placed with the U. S. Department of Agriculture's Bureau of Chemistry (from 1927 part of a Food, Drug and Insecticide Administration; from 1930 as the Food and Drug Administration). After revision of the law, the FDA was transferred, executively, to the Federal Security Agency (an agency absorbed into the present Department of Health, Education, and Welfare). [*ibid.*, p. 385]

36. Senate Document No. 124, 75th Congress, 2d Session; this report on a case is reprinted in Herrick, A. D., and Smith, A. E.: New Drugs, p. 157, New York, 1946.

37. "Editorial" [E. F. Kelly, Secretary], J. A. Ph. A. *27*:369, 1938; see also Winne, A. L. E.: Proc. Natl. Assoc. Bds. Pharm., p. 58 f., 1938.

38. Veldee, M. V.: Federal regulation. II. U. S. Public Health Service, J. A. Ph. A. *8*:161-163, 1947.

39. Herzog, S. A.: Durham-Humphrey—two years after, Food Drug Cosmetic Law J. *10*:119-128, 1955.

40. See, Hearings Before the Subcommittee on Antitrust and Monopoly of the Committee on the Judiciary, United States Senate, Eighty-Sixth Congress, Second Session: Administered Prices in the Drug Industry, Washington, D. C., 1961, especially parts 14 through 26; see also, "Report" on same to the Eighty-Seventh Congress, First Session, Report 448, Senate.

41. For a factual review of events leading to enactment of the Drug Amendments of 1962 (signed October 10), see Stempel, Edward: The impetus of thalidomide on drug legislation and regulation, Am. J. Pharm. *134*:355-364, 1962. For the provisions of the enactment and discussions of possible implications in practice, see J. A. Ph. A. n.s.2:638-646, 1962; and on the thalidomide aspect particularly, FDC Reports *24*:No. 32 (Aug. 6) and No. 33 (Aug. 13), 1962.

42. On the erratic evolution of our understanding of addiction, see Sonnedecker, Glenn: Emergence of the concept of opiate addiction, J. mondial Pharm., opiate addiction, part 1, J. mondial Pharm. No. 3 (Sept.-Dec.), pp. 275-290; part 2, J. mondial Pharm. No. 1 (Jan.-Mar.), 1963, pp.27-34.

43. On this Committee's work, see Proc. A. Ph. A. *49*:465, 1901; *50*:567-574, 1902; *51*:471, 1903.

44. Supplemental Federal acts have included the Narcotic Drugs Import and Export Act of 1922 (revising the Act of 1909), the Marihuana Tax Act of 1937 (subsequently placed in the Internal Revenue Code), the Opium Poppy Control Act of 1942, Public Law 729 of 1954 (an

amendment important to practicing pharmacists), and the Narcotic Control Act of 1956 (which provides remarkably punitive penalties for unlawful sale or possession of narcotic drugs and marihuana). With few exceptions, state laws substantially follow a model issued in 1932 as a "Uniform State Narcotic Law," with the joint backing of medical, pharmaceutical and government agencies.

45. Drug Topics, p. 2, col. 1, Dec. 17-31, 1962.

14. THE DEVELOPMENT OF EDUCATION

1. Wilbert, M. I.: The beginnings of pharmacy in America, Am. J. Pharm. 79:406, 1907.
2. LaWall, C. H.: The founding of the Philadelphia College of Pharmacy and Science, Am. J. Pharm. 93:169, 1921.
3. Hoch, J. H.: Dr. Lewis Mottet's projected Institute of Pharmacy, J. A. Ph. A. 27:1260-61, 1938.
4. Wolfe, H. G.: James Cutbush—author, teacher, apothecary general, Am. J. Pharm. Ed. 12:89-125, 1948.
5. LaWall, C. H.: op. cit., p. 170.
6. Kremers, Edward: The Old Northwest Territory and Pharmaceutical Education, p. 7, Purdue University, Lafayette, Indiana, 1934.
7. England, J. W.: The First Century of the Philadelphia College of Pharmacy, p. 463, Philadelphia, 1922.
8. Proc. A. Ph. A. 3:14, 1854; Am. J. Pharm. 26:388, 1854.
9. Am. J. Pharm. 18:148, 1846.
10. England, J. W.: op. cit., p. 143.
11. Ibid.: p. 404.
12. Wilbert, M. I.: John M. Maisch, Am. J. Pharm. 75:356, 1903.
13. Osborne, G. E.: David Stewart, M.D., first American professor of pharmacy (1833-1899), Am. J. Pharm. Ed. 23:219-230, 1959; see also Meyer Bros. Drugg. 17:200, 1896.
14. Parrish, Edward: American pharmacy, Am. J. Pharm. 26:216, 1854.
15. Sonnedecker, Glenn: American Pharmaceutical Education Before 1900, unpublished dissertation, Ph.D., University of Wisconsin, Madison, 1952, Pt. 2, p. 461 ff., and Urdang, George: The part of doctors of medicine in pharmaceutical education, Am. J. Pharm. Ed. 14:516-

556, 1950. See also Kremers, Edward: The teaching of pharmacy during the past fifty years, Drugg. Circ. 51:68, 1907.
16. Day, W. B.: The school of pharmacy, Alumni Rec., University of Illinois, p. xxvi, 1921.
17. England, J. W.: op. cit., p. 147.
18. Ibid.: p. 406.
19. Shafer, H. B.: The American Medical Profession 1783-1850, p. 43, New York, 1936.
20. Am. J. Pharm. 44:189, 1872.
21. Ibid.: p. 233.
22. Am. J. Pharm. 19:256, 1847.
23. Sonnedecker, Glenn: op. cit., p. 115. About the same time some pharmacy was taught at the neighboring University of South Carolina, but it had a tenuous connection because of exigencies of the reconstruction period; and apparently there were no graduates until 1886. The first place where pharmacy instruction began within a general college program (1865) probably was Baldwin University, a small institution in Berea, Ohio
24. Proc. A. Ph. A. 19:425, 1871.
25. Comparative data on practical experience requirements in 54 countries are given by Dieckmann, Hans: Geschichte und Probleme der Apothekerausbildung, in erster Linie in Frankreich und Deutschland, pp. 187-195, with commentary, 121 ff., Frankfurt a/M, 1954.
26. Proc. A. Ph. A. 19:96, 1871.
27. Ibid.: p. 47.
28. Letter of J. O. Schlotterbeck, written November 12, 1906.
29. Pharm. Rev. 21:362, 1903.
30. Am. J. Pharm. 41:472, 1869.
31. Proc. Am. Assoc. Coll. Pharm., p. 27, 1926.
32. Blauch, L. E., and Webster, C. L.: The Pharmaceutical Curriculum, p. 16, Washington, D. C. A few schools continued 3-year courses optionally until as late as 1939.
33. General Report of the Pharmaceutical Survey, p. 230, Washington, D. C., 1950.
34. Brady, E. S.: The six-year program, Am. J. Pharm. Ed. 17:448, 1953, and 26:62, 1962. A 6-year (Pharm. D.) program was adopted by the University of California in 1956, and by the University of Michigan (particularly for hospital pharmacy) in 1962.
35. Urdang, George: Edward Kremers (1865-1941), reformer of American pharma-

ceutical education, Am. J. Pharm. Ed. *11*: 650, 1947.

36. Green, M. W.: Progress and problems in graduate instruction in pharmacy, Am. J. Pharm. Ed. *19*:467 ff., 1955; and General Report of the Pharmaceutical Survey, p. 110.

37. Sonnedecker, Glenn: American Pharmaceutical Education Before 1900, pp. 113-120.

38. The comparative comments are based upon Scoville, W. L.: Proc. Am. Conf. Pharm. Facul., p. 17, 1905; General Report of the Pharmaceutical Survey, p. 68; and Directory Supplement, J. A. Ph. A. (Scient. Ed.) *45*:40, 1956. States not yet having a school of pharmacy (1962) were Alaska, Delaware, Hawaii, Maine, Nevada, New Hampshire and Vermont.

39. On the rise and demise of the Syllabus Committee, and the subsequent development, see: Blauch, L. E., and Webster, G. L.: The Pharmaceutical Curriculum, pp. 18-27.

40. Sonnedecker, Glenn: *op. cit.*, pp. 282-287.

41. Pharm. Era *16*:384, 1896.

42. Proc. West Virginia Pharm. Assoc., p. 341, 1931. See also Cook, R. B.: The Annals of Pharmacy in West Virginia, pp. 31 ff., Charleston, 1946.

43. Pharm. Era *17*:499, 1897.

44. Proc. A. Ph. A. *54*:200, 1906.

45. For example, see the account of subsequent diploma peddling by the "dean" of pharmacy at the erstwhile "Lincoln-Jefferson University": "Teacher of pharmacy." The unsavory story. . . . J. A. Ph. A. (Pract. Ed.) 7:196-202, 1946.

46. The Apothecary *1*:4, 1891. Purchasers of Oldberg's book could obtain guidance through sets of questions sent by the author periodically. Earlier Oldberg had issued (1885) for the same home-study purpose an *Outline of a Course of Study in Practical Pharmacy*.

47. Christensen, H. C.: What legal difficulties may we get into when we abolish assistant registration, Am. J. Pharm. Ed. *1*:44 and 47, 1937. A comprehensive survey of the question of the assistant pharmacist and its historical development is given by John Grover Beard in J. A. Ph. A. *15*: 119, 1926. A case study of the "cram school" technic can be found in the article entitled "Teacher of pharmacy . . ." J. A. Ph. A. (Pract. Ed.) 7:196-202, 1946.

48. Oldberg, Oscar: The principles of university and school extension applied to pharmaceutical studies, The Apothecary *1*:3, 1891.

49. The seven that did were in Connecticut, Florida, Massachusetts, Minnesota, New Jersey, South Dakota and Texas.

50. General Report of the Pharmaceutical Survey, pp. 231 f.

51. *Ibid.* Through the initiative of Sylvester H. Dretzka, then State Board Secretary, Wisconsin had a particularly viable program, beginning in 1937, which included an itinerant instructor.

52. Cf. Cowen, D. L.: Notes on pharmaceutical training in New Jersey before 1900, Am. J. Pharm. Ed. *12*:303, 1948; and Parrish, Edward: The preliminary education of apprentices, Proc. A. Ph. A. *20*: 178, 1872.

53. At Purdue a "good common school education" or an equivalent examination and 2-year apprenticeship were required in 1884 (Lee, C. O.: The first courses in pharmacy, Am. J. Pharm. Ed. *4*:60, 1940). At Michigan those with practical experience could defer the examination covering preliminary education and receive other concessions (Annual Announcement . . . Michigan, 1887-88, pp. 8-10; see also Pharm. Rundschau 5:128, 1887).

54. Bastin, E. S.: Pharmacal education, West. Drugg. *10*:403, 1888.

55. Sonnedecker, G.: American Pharmaceutical Education Before 1900 (unpublished Ph. D. thesis, University of Wisconsin), pp. 264 f.

56. Beal, J. H.: Report on preliminary education requirement, Proc. A. Ph. A. *46*:548, 1898.

57. By-laws of the American Conference of Pharmaceutical Faculties, in: Proc. Am. Conf. Pharm. Fac., pp. 45, 46, 1906.

58. Blauch, L., and Webster, G.: The Pharmaceutical Curriculum, pp. 14 f. on this point and the development of prerequisites in the present century.

59. Mayo, C. A.: The prerequisite law in New York, Bull. Pharm. *18*:502, 1904.

60. England, J. W.: The First Century of the Philadelphia College of Pharmacy, p. 182; The status of prerequisite laws and pharmaceutical licensure, Am. J. Pharm. *93*: 539, 1921.

61. Hynson, H. P.: Historical notes on degrees in pharmacy, Drugg. Circ. *51*:80, 1907.

62. Scoville, W. L.: American Pharmaceutical Colleges, p. 16, Am. Conf. Pharm. Faculties, 1905. Ten years later (1915) the School of Pharmacy of Northwestern University still offered a 1-year course leading to the degree of Graduate in Pharmacy. The degree of Pharmaceutical Chemist was awarded after a second year of study. Before the American Conference of Pharmaceutical Faculties (1918) A. Koch reported, "The Ph.G. degree is conferred by 39 institutions for a two-years' course, and by one school after 4 years; the degree of Bachelor of Science in Pharmacy by 20 schools for a four-years' course, by one for three years and by one for two years; the Doctor of Pharmacy degree by three schools for three years, by one for four years, by three schools for six years and by one for a seven-years' course. The Master of Pharmacy degree is conferred by one school for three years, and the Master of Science in Pharmacy by three schools for a five-years' course." (Proc. Am. Conf. Pharm. Fac., p. 44, 1918)

63. The foregoing discussion is based on the following article and the sources there cited: Sonnedecker, Glenn: The Conference of Schools of Pharmacy—a period of frustration, Am. J. Pharm. Ed. *18*:389, 1954; on Maisch, see Pharm. Rundschau *1*:193, 1870.

64. Proc. A. Ph. A. 38:243 f., 1890.

65. A copy of Dr. James H. Beal's *Memoirs* was put at the disposal of the author of this book by his son, Dr. George D. Beal.

66. Proc. Am. Conf. Pharm. Fac. pp. 7 and 8, 1902.

67. General Report of the Pharmaceutical Survey 1946-49, pp. 70 f. and 214 ff. Standards were first published by the Council in 1937, revised in 1942, then again in 1945. As a temporary measure after World War II the Council used a classification system in rating schools (A, B, C, Y) but has been able to return to a simple designation of "accredited" (or nonaccredited). A list of accredited schools may be obtained on request to the Council at 77 West Washington St., Chicago 2, Ill.

68. National Wholesale Druggists' Association Year Book for 1948, pp. 477-494.

69. A. F. P. E.—Foundation for the Future, p. 4, Washington, D. C., 1955, and announcement of the Foundation (mimeograph), Washington, D. C., March 27, 1963.

70. Charters, W. W.: Basic Material for a Pharmaceutical Curriculum, p. v, New York, 1927.

71. *Ibid.*: p. xiii.

72. Proc. Am. Assoc. Coll. Pharm., p. 24, 1927.

73. J. Am. Ph. A. *16*:351, 1927.

74. J. A. Ph. A. (Sci. Ed.) *32*:368, 1943.

75. Am. J. Pharm. Ed. 7:574. 1943; 8:245, 246, 1954.

76. Findings and Recommendations, Pharmaceutical Survey, *op. cit.*, p. 6.

77. Lyman, R. A.: The American Institute of the History of Pharmacy and the Pharmaceutical Press (mimeograph address), p. 5, Madison, Wis., 1942.

15. THE ESTABLISHMENT OF A LITERATURE

1. Trans. New York M. Soc., p. 131, 1807-1831.

2. England, J. W.: The First Century of the Philadelphia College of Pharmacy, p. 94, Philadelphia, 1922.

3. Trans. Coll. Phys. Phila.: Ser. 3, 9:101, 1887.

4. Collections for an Essay towards a Materia Medica of the United States, read before the Philadelphia Medical Society, February 21, 1798, and published in the same year; the second part was published in 1804. See reprint in Bull. Lloyd Libr. vol. I, Part 1, p. 32 and Part 2, p. 6.

5. Proc. Conn. Med. Soc.: reprint; p. 191.

6. *Ibid.*: p. 196.

7. U.S.P., 1820, p. 10.

8. Alden, E.: Historical Sketch of the Origin and Progress of the Massachusetts Medical Society, Mass. Med. Soc. Comm. 6:56, 1838.

9. Pharmacopoeia, Mass. Med. Soc., Boston 1808: p. v.

10. The Medical Repository, New York, 5, 1808.

11. Pharmacopoeia, Mass. Med. Soc., p. v.

12. Burrage, W. L.: A History of the Massachusetts Medical Society, 1781-1822, p. 75, Norwood, Mass., 1923.

13. Minutes Med. Soc. South Carolina, 1808.

14. U.S.P., 1820, p. 19.

15. Minutes Med. Soc. South Carolina, 1808.

16. Niles, F. H.: The Massachusetts Pharmacopoeia of 1808, J. A. Ph. A. *25*:542, 1936.
17. Pharmacopoeia Nosocomii Neo-Eboracensis: p. v.
18. *Ibid.*: p. vi.
19. *Ibid.*: p. vi.
20. *Ibid.*: p. vi.
21. *Ibid.*: p. vii.
22. *Ibid.*: p. ix.
23. *Ibid.*: p. iii.
24. *Ibid.*: p. vi.
25. Am. Med. & Philos. Reg. *4*:602, 1814.
26. Kebler, L. F.: S. L. Mitchill, J. A. Ph. A. *26*:908, 1937. Kebler states that the correct spelling of the name is Mitchill and not Mitchell.
27. U.S.P., 1820: p. 5.
28. Trans. New York State M. Soc. p. 112 and 130, 1807-1831.
29. U.S.P., 1820: p. 9. The first two circulars of the Committee were issued on March 4 and November 21, 1818.
30. Kebler: *op. cit.*, p. 912; Selwyn-Brown, A.: The Physician Throughout the Ages, vol. 1, p. 801, New York, 1928.
31. U.S.P. XI, 1937: p. xix.
32. On the founding and the men who participated see, Sonnedecker, Glenn: The men who participated in the founding convention, pp. 13-15, et passim, and also historical articles by others, in Founding of the United States Pharmacopeia 1820; Dedication of a Painting . . ., New York, 1957.
33. Trans. Coll. Phys. Phila.: Ser. 3, 9:135, 1887.
34. *Ibid.*: p. 135.
35. U.S.P., 1820; p. 15.
36. Trans. Coll. Phys. Phila.: *loc. cit.*
37. Eberle, E. G.: A Copy of Proof Sheets U.S.P. I, Am. Pharm. Assoc., Baltimore, 1932. The copy preserved is the one assigned to Dr. DeButts and apparently returned by him with his suggestions to the chairman. (It was reproduced by E. C. Eberle and thus made generally available.)
38. U.S.P., 1820: p. 26.
39. *Ibid.*: p. 22.
40. Phil. J. Med. & Phys. Sci. *2*:367, 1821.
41. Spalding, J. A.: The Life of Dr. L. Spalding, p. 363, Boston, 1916.
41a. The first edition of the U. S. Pharmacopeia was changed more for the second issuance than had been thought before the study by Laurence D. Lockie, *The Second (1828) Edition of the Pharmacopeia of the United States* (mimeograph, Section on Historical Pharmacy, American Pharmaceutical Association, 1958; 5 pp.). Lockie reported that type was re-set, the copyright changed, typographical errors corrected, 3 changes made in the materia medica lists, and 7 changes made in procedural directions.
42. *Ibid.*: pp. 363, 364.
43. For information on the schism and the two second editions, see J. Phila. Coll. Pharm. *3*:64-65 and 68, 1832; U.S.P., 1830: title page and pp. 3-6; U.S.P., 1831: pp. vii, ix, xxix; Trans. Coll. Phys. Phila.: Ser. 3, 9:135, 1887.
44. On early pharmaceutical cooperation, see England, J. W.: *op. cit.*, p. 96; Trans. Coll. Phys. Phila.: *loc. cit.*; U.S.P., 1831: pp. xiv and xxviii.
45. Am. J. Pharm. *14*:122, 1842; see also England, J. W.: *op. cit.*, p. 120; Thrush, M. C.: U.S.P. and its predecessors, Drugg. Circ. *51*:46, 1907.
46. U.S.P., 1873: pp. xiii and xviii.
47. Proc. A. Ph. A. *24*:631-33 and 646, 1876.
48. Am. J. Pharm. *49*:209, 1877.
49. Trans. Am. Med. Assoc. *28*:109, 1877.
50. Proc. A. Ph. A. *25*:538, 1877.
51. Proc. A. Ph. A. *26*:668, 879, 1878.
52. Am. J. Pharm. *54*:638, 1882. The book appeared in October 1882, but in a reprinting necessary the next year the title page was re-dated 1883.
53. U.S.P., 1893: p. xxvi. On pre-1906 drug standards, see Sonnedecker, G., and Urdang, G.: Legalization of drug standards under state laws in the United States of America, Food Drug Cosmetic Law J. 8:753, 1953.
54. U.S.P., 1905: p. xxv, and later editions: A facsimile reprint of the Certificate of Incorporation was published in Pharm. Rev. *18*:546, 1900. The first three paragraphs were reprinted in Urdang, G.: Pharmacy's Part in Society, p. 13, Madison, Wis., 1946.
55. Proc. A. Ph. A. *38*:263, 1890.
56. U.S.P., 1905: p. xxxi.
57. *Ibid.*: p. xxxix.
58. U.S.P., 1936: p. xxix.
59. *Ibid.*: p. xxx.
60. U.S.P., 1916: xliii.
61. Succeeding Remington for the unexpired term of office was the pharmacist Charles H. LaWall, professor at the Philadelphia College of Pharmacy.

62. U.S.P., 1936: p. xxxiv.

63. Cook, E. F.: The new Pharmacopoeia, J. A. Ph. A. *14*:864, 1925.

64. Pharmacopoeial Board of Trustees, U.S.P.: J. A. Ph. A. *28*:1011, 1939. The U.S.P. once observed, "No funds are received from either government or private sources, although the conservatively estimated monetary value of the talent and time contributed from these sources exceeds the actual expense of the revision activities." (Preface, U.S.P. XV, 1955, p. xiii.)

65. U.S.P., 1936: p. xiv.

66. *Ibid.*: p. xi; p. xiii; a harbinger of U.S.P. reference standards was the offer in U.S.P. X (1926, p. 4) from the Bureau of Chemistry of the U.S. Department of Agriculture to "supply standard substances conforming to the pharmacopoeial requirements" in biologic assays.

67. U.S.P., 1942: p. xxv (preface).

68. This decision was to "become effective in time for the 1950 Convention." The amendment to the by-laws providing for the full-time director was among the changes inaugurated by the adjourned meeting of the Pharmacopeial Convention held in Cleveland, Ohio, in 1942.

69. Am. Prof. Pharm. *15*:435-439, 470, 1949. As temporary quarters, the Pharmacopeia had purchased a building in Philadelphia and established offices there in 1945.

70. Miller, L. C.: Stewardship of our legacy *in* Founding of the United States Pharmacopeia 1820, p. 30, New York, 1957.

71. For a good discussion of the changing circumstances and Latin usage, see Urdang, G.: The place of Latin in the official standards of pharmacy, Bull. Natl. Form. Comm *12*:201-220, 1944.

72. U.S.P. XV, 1955: p. xi (preface).

73. U.S.P. XVI, 1960, pp. xvi and xxvii.

74. Holland, A. H., Jr.: The road ahead *in* Founding of the United States Pharmacopeia 1820, p. 37, New York, 1957.

75. The nine editions are dated 1806, 1810, 1814, 1818, 1822, 1825, 1827, 1830, and 1831. On early dispensatories of America and related works see Cowen, D. L.: America's Pre-pharmacopoeial Literature, pp. 19 ff, Madison, Wis., 1961.

76. J. Phila. Coll. Pharm. *4*:94, 1833.

77. Alden, E.: *op. cit.* (note 8), p. 57. The four editions were 1810, 1813, 1817, and 1821.

78. The eleven editions edited jointly by Wood and Bache appeared in 1833, 1834, 1836, 1839, 1843, 1845, 1847, 1849, 1851, 1854 and 1858.

79. Wood, H. C., Jr.: The history of the U.S. Dispensatory, J. A. Ph. A. *20*:792, 1931.

80. Since the 15th edition, additional editions have appeared in 1888 (16th), 1894 (17th), 1899 (18th), 1907 (19th), 1918 (20th), 1926 (21st), 1937 (22nd), 1943 (23rd), 1947 (24th) and 1960 (25th). The consistent popularity and distinction of the *Dispensatory* represents a long and successful cooperation between the editors previously mentioned and their publishers. Grigg and Elliot of Philadelphia published the first 8 editions. Then Lippincott—at that time called Lippincott, Grambo and Company—bought out Grigg and Elliot. For more than a century (from 1851, the 9th edition, until the present) the book has been published by Lippincott.

81. Further editions appeared in 1884 (3rd), 1889 (4th), and 1894 (5th), the latter reprinted with a supplement in 1896.

82. Am. Drugg. & Pharm. Rec. *24*:195, 1894.

83. Cowen, D. L.: The Boston editions of Nicholas Culpeper, J. Hist. Med. *11*: 156-165, 1956.

84. For bibliographic clarification, see Cowen, D. L.: America's Pre-pharmacopoeial Literature, pp. 20 f.

85. The editions of King's *American Dispensatory* that represent actual revisions are dated 1864, 1870, 1889 and 1900.

86. See, for example, Steinbichler, Eveline: Geschichte der homöopathischen Arzneibereitungslehre in Deutschland bis 1872, Eutin, 1957.

87. England, J. W.: The First Century, pp. 72, 73.

88. Proc. A. Ph. A. *6*:81, 1857; 7:230, 1858.

89. Am. Drugg. *15*:199, 1886.

90. U.S.P., 1882: p. xxx.

91. Proc. A. Ph. A. *34*:558, 1885.

92. *Ibid.*

93. Sonnedecker, G., and Urdang, G.: Legalization . . . (note 53), p. 754.

94. Cook, E. F.: J. A. Ph. A. *30*:469, 1941; and Powers, J. L.: *ibid.*, p. 477.

95. Quotation from Preface, National Formulary, 8th ed., p. xi. The numbered editions of the National Formulary, to-

gether with the year in which they became effective ("official") are: 1st, 1888; 2nd, 1896; 3rd, 1906; 4th, 1916; 5th, 1926; 6th, 1936; 7th, 1942; 8th, 1947; 9th, 1950; 10th, 1955; 11th, 1960. (For the first 3 editions, before there was a date of "officiality," the year of publication is listed.)

96. Powers, J. L.: Trends in official drugs and a preview of the new National Formulary (VIII), Bull. Natl. Form. Comm. *14*:124 f., 1946; see also, Osborne, G. E., and Lee, C. O.: Graphic story of official galenicals, Bull. Natl. Form. Comm. *15*:185-204, 1947.

97. J. A. Ph. A. *1*:168, 366, 505, 637, 760, 1307, 1912; *4*:1178, 1915; Lascoff, J. L.: The value of the recipe book to the pharmacist, J. A. Ph. A. *16*:714, 1927. See also the Historical Introduction in the respective *R. B.* editions.

98. New and Non-official Remedies, 1909, pp. 9 and 10.

99. *Ibid.*

100. *Ibid.*: p. 5.

101. In the title of the book by Redwood and Procter, Mohr has been erroneously given the Christian name Francis.

102. Am. J. Pharm. *21*:120, 1849.

103. *Ibid.*: p. 213.

104. England, J. W.: The First Century, p. 403.

105. Am. J. Pharm. *28*:10, 1856.

106. Am. J. Pharm. *27*:574, 1855.

107. In 1859, a 2nd edition and in 1864 a 3rd edition appeared. In this latter the title *Introduction to Practical Pharmacy* was changed to the less specific title *A Treatise on Pharmacy*. The reason for dropping the word "practical" is to be found in the enormous increase in theoretical and scientific matter. After the death of Parrish in 1872, Thomas S. Wiegand published a 4th edition in 1874 and a 5th edition in 1884.

108. The editions of 1885, 1889, 1894, 1905, 1907 and 1917 appeared under the editorship of the original author. Among the many collaborators, E. Fullerton Cook and Charles LaWall, assistants to Remington in the Philadelphia College of Pharmacy, were the most active. Thus it was only natural that after the death of Remington (1918), these two men, more particularly Cook, edited the next (7th) edition, which appeared in 1926, and the 8th edition, issued in 1936.

After the death of LaWall in 1937, Cook chose Eric W. Martin as his partner in the task of editing a 9th edition of Remington's *Practice of Pharmacy* (1948). Martin continued as editor-in-chief for the 12th edition, which appeared in 1961.

109. Am. J. Pharm. *60*:270, 1888.

110. Pharm. Rundschau *6*:148, 1888.

111. Am. J. Pharm. *66*:556, 1894.

112. A 2nd edition appeared in 1901, a 3rd in 1906, a 4th in 1910 and a 5th in 1916. One year later, in 1917, Charles Caspari, Jr., died. The editorial task of revision was taken over by E. F. Kelly, long assistant and associate of Caspari on the faculty of the Maryland College of Pharmacy. Kelly, in addition to continuing the work, returned to the original intent of making a concise book. The 6th revision, published in 1920, with its 954 pages, still retained the volume to which the book had gradually grown. However, the 7th edition (1926) was condensed to 615 pages, and the 8th edition (1939) to 553 pages.

113. The 2nd edition appeared in 1917, the 3rd in 1926, and the 4th, edited by Arny with the collaboration of R. P. Fischelis, in 1937. A noteworthy feature of Arny's *Principles* was its comprehensive bibliography at the end of each chapter, giving direct reference to the literature covered in the text.

114. Glenn L. Jenkins was senior editor for the 9th edition appearing in 1957. A more concise competitor, which has not survived, was an "outline of a systematic course of study for the novice in extemporaneous compounding" by J. H. Beal, titled *Prescription Practice and General Dispensing: an elementary treatise for students of pharmacy* (1908). It is one of those rare books which respect self-drawn limits. An interesting attempt to meet the needs of "students of medicine and of pharmacy who desire to acquire a complete knowledge of what a prescription was, is, and should be" (preface to the 4th, 1917, edition) was made by Otto A. Wall, Ph.G., M.D., in his book *The Prescription, Therapeutically, Pharmaceutically, Grammatically, and Historically Considered.* The 1st edition appeared in 1888. The most popular book devoted exclusively to the problem of incom-

patibilities was published by Edsel A. Ruddiman in 1897 under the title *Incompatibilities in Prescriptions*. A 2nd edition appeared in 1900, a 3rd in 1908, a 4th in 1917, a 5th in 1925 and a 6th in 1936.

115. Among them L. E. Sayre's *Organic Materia Medica and Pharmacognosy* (1894), and more recently textbooks by Youngken (first edition in 1922) and by Mansfield (first edition in 1926). The *Textbook of Pharmaceutical Botany* by Heber Youngken was issued from 1914 until 1951, in 7 editions. Much used by students of pharmacy were Bastin's *Elements of Botany*, first published in 1887, the name of which was later changed to *College Botany*, and the books of Henry Kraemer, *Applied Economic Botany* and *Scientific and Applied Pharmacognosy*, both first published in 1915. Based on the 3rd edition of Kraemer's book, E. N. Gathercoal and E. H. Wirth published their *Pharmacognosy* (ed. 2, 1947). A modern view is represented by Robertson Pratt and Heber W. Youngken, Jr., in *Pharmacognosy* (ed. 1, 1951), and Emil Ramstad in *Modern Pharmacognosy* (ed. 1, 1959).

116. John Uri Lloyd's *Chemistry of Medicines* had appeared in 1881. In 1884, William Simon published the 1st edition of his *Manual of Chemistry*. In 1887, Oscar Oldberg and John H. Long published a *Laboratory Manual of Chemistry, General and Pharmaceutical*. In 1894, an *Elementary Course in Inorganic Pharmaceutical Chemistry*, written by F. J. Wulling, appeared, and in 1895 S. P. Sadtler and H. Trimble published their *Textbook of Chemistry for the Use of Pharmaceutical and Medical Students*.

Several pharmacists wrote books on analytic chemistry, one of the first being the *Manual of Chemical Analysis, as applied to the examination of medicinal chemicals*, published by Frederick Hoffmann in 1873 (1883, ed. 2). In 1885 Trimble's *Handbook of Analytical Chemistry* appeared. Of books of more recent vintage, the following are exemplary: E. V. Lynn, *Organic Chemistry, with Applications to Pharmacy and Medicine* (1941); G. L. Jenkins and others, *Quantitative Chemistry* (1931; ed. 3, 1949);

G. L. Jenkins and W. H. Hartung, *The Chemistry of Organic Medicinal Products* (1941; ed. 3, 1949); L. M. Parks, Paul J. Jannke, Loyd E. Harris, John E. Christian, *Inorganic Chemistry in Pharmacy* (1949).

117. England, J. W.: The First Century, p. 100; see p. 278 of the same book for a history of the journal; also Am. J. Pharm. 76:223, 1904.

118. The *New York Journal of Pharmacy* (1852-1854) of the New York College of Pharmacy was revived several times and under different titles. The *Journal and Transactions of the Maryland College of Pharmacy* (1858-1862), *The Pharmacist* (1868-1885) of the Chicago College of Pharmacy, and *The Apothecary* (1891-1897) of the Illinois College of Pharmacy all had only a short existence.

119. Sonnedecker, G.: The Journal [of A.Ph.A.] is born, J. A. Ph. A., n.s. *1*: 744-5 and 776-7, 1961.

120. Sonnedecker, G.: Two decades of progress with the American Journal of Hospital Pharmacy, Am. J. Hosp. Pharm. *19*:215-225, 1962.

121. Other state associations which soon journalized their proceedings are those of Texas (1926), Maryland (1926), New Jersey (1928) and Wisconsin (1933). More rapid was the development of journals of county and city associations (Meyer, M. M.: The pharmaceutical journals in the U.S., unpublished Master of Science thesis, University of Wisconsin, 1934. The geographic list was published in the J. A. Ph. A. *22*:424, 1933). Sometimes the development went another way: In February, 1927, there appeared the first number of *The New York Pharmacist*, "Official Journal of the N. Y. Pharmaceutical Conference, Inc.," which in July, 1932, became the organ of the New York State Pharmaceutical Association as well. The title changed (1935) to the *New York State Pharmacist*, becoming exclusively the official organ and property of the New York State Pharmaceutical Association. Some of these publications disappeared after a time, became merged with independent commercial journals, or continued as such with changed names. Among local association journals still extant, the *Chicago*

Retail Druggist's Association (C.R.D.A.) News and the *Philadelphia Association Retail Druggist's Bulletin* (1901) are noteworthy, among 13 local journals identified in the "Third Annual Pharmaceutical Directory," J. A. Ph. A. n.s. 3:36, 1963.

122. Noteworthy among the private journals that at some time served an association officially have been the *Modern Druggist* (1912), official journal of the Louisiana and Mississippi pharmaceutical associations; the *Southeastern Drug Journal* (1926), official journal of the Florida, Georgia, South Carolina, Alabama and Tennessee pharmaceutical associations; and the *Rocky Mountain Druggist* (1888), official journal of the Colorado Pharmacal Association, the Wyoming Pharmaceutical Association, the Denver Retail Druggists Association and the Allied Drug Travelers of Colorado (Kassner, H. C.: How we learn, Am. Drugg. 88:284, 1933. See also the statements of Meyer, M. M.: *op. cit.,* pp. 216, 254, 352, 364).

123. Meyer, M. M.: *op. cit.,* p. 10. See also J. A. Ph. A. 22:424, 1933.

124. The old *Pacific Drug Review* (1888-1961, thereafter called *Western Pharmacy*) and the *North Western Druggist* (f. 1892) showed particular strength; also serving the far West are the *Rocky Mountain Druggist* (f. 1888) and *West Coast Druggist* (f. 1928, combining *Stirring Rod,* f. 1906, and the *California Retail Drug Journal,* f. 1915). The Middle West has been similarly served by *Midwestern Druggist* (f. 1925) and the *Central Pharmaceutical Journal* (f. 1947); the South is served by the *Southern Pharmaceutical Journal* (f. 1908) and the *Southeastern Drug Journal* (f. 1926); and in the East *The Apothecary* (founded, 1888, as *The New England Druggist*) and the *Mid-Atlantic Apothecary* (replacing, 1953, the *Mid-Atlantic Pharmacist,* f. 1951).

125. Hoffmann, F.: A century of American pharmaceutical literature, Amer. Drugg. & Pharm. Rec. 36:164, 165, 1900.

126. Kassner, H. C.: *op. cit.,* p. 280.

127. It was edited by Hoffmann and Edward Kremers until 1900; and from 1901 to 1909, by Kremers. In 1909 it was consolidated with the *Midland Druggist,* remaining alive under the title *Midland Druggist and Pharmaceutical Review* until 1926. At this time the title was changed to *Interstate Journal.* The *Pharmaceutical Review* became the cradle of another monthly, which completed the coverage of information, the *Pharmaceutical Archives.* There appeared 6 volumes between 1898 and 1903. Discontinued for more than 30 years, the *Archives* was revived in 1936, to be discontinued again in 1945. The *Review* published surveys and abstracts. The *Archives,* a child of the ideals and the endeavor of Edward Kremers, was devoted exclusively to the publication of more lengthy original papers.

128. There existed in 1875 a *Deutsch-Amerikanische pharmaceutische Zeitung,* for pharmacists and druggists as well as for physicians of German origin, published in Belleville, Ill. In New York the *Apotheker-Zeitung* appeared from 1880 to 1933 (beginning 1895, it was the official organ of the New York German Apothecaries Society). From 1885 to 1897 this Society published the *Monatsblatt des New Yorker deutschen Apothekervereins,* which was revived in 1934. Other foreign language publications, though short-lived, were the *Gaceta medico-farmacéutica de Nueva York* (1892-1898); *Monitor medico-farmacéutico* (1883); *Revista americana de farmacia* (1895-1921) (Meyer, M.: *op. cit.,* p. 14). *Pharmacy International* (in English) since 1947 and *El Farmacéutico* (in Spanish) since 1925 are private journals designed to serve pharmacy abroad and to promote international trade. *La Farmacia moderna* is a similar publication in Spanish issued in the United States (f. 1945).

129. *The Philadelphia Druggist and Chemist,* founded in 1878, changed its name a year later to the *Monthly Review of Medicine and Pharmacy* (1879-1882) and was followed in 1895 by a *Monthly Retrospect of Medicine and Pharmacy,* also published in Philadelphia (1895-1902). In New York a journal with the title *Physician and Pharmaceutist*—from 1871 on, *Pharmacist*—was published from 1868 to 1879. In 1879 the journal changed its name to *Physician and Pharmacist and the Bulletin of the Medical-Legal Society;* a few months later, dropping the word *Pharmacist,* it

was continued as the *Physician and Bul-letin of the Medico-Legal Society.*

130. Kassner, H.: *op. cit.,* p. 280.

131. These publications served those engaged in making and marketing drugs. The firms, in turn, produced a periodical literature of "house organs" designed to interest practicing pharmacists, hence provide a vehicle for promoting the company concerned. Perhaps the first such house organ of substance was the vigorous *New Idea* published (1879-1924) by Frederick Stearns and Company of Detroit (a firm absorbed by Winthrop). Following Stearns by a year, Meyer Brothers and Company of St. Louis transformed their price list into a house organ (1880), the *St. Louis Drug Market Reporter,* which survives today as the *Meyer Druggist.* Meanwhile, house organs have appeared in almost every type and format of pharmaceutical periodical known. To discuss them in a text, where we do not have space even to mention some important independent and association journals, would go too far; some additional details may be found in the previous (2nd) edition, pp. 397-399.

132. J. A. Ph. A. 22:424, 1933.

16. ECONOMIC AND STRUCTURAL DEVELOPMENT

1. England, J. W.: The First Century of the Philadelphia College of Pharmacy, p. 28, Philadelphia, 1922; Ellis, E. T.: The story of a very old Philadelphia drugstore, Am. J. Pharm. 75:57, 1903.

2. Proc. A. Ph. A. 2:24-42, 1853; 3:34, 1854; 50:124, 125, 1902.

3. Jenkins, G. L., Osborne, G. E., and Lee, C. O.: Hoosier Pharmacy *in* Russo, D. R.: One Hundred Years of Indian Medicine, 1849-1949, Chapter 14, p. 142, Indianapolis, 1944.

4. Drugg. Circ. 51:181, 1901.

5. *Ibid.*

6. Leach, J. G.: History of the Bringhurst Family, pp. 39, 41, 52, Philadelphia, 1901.

7. *Ibid.*: p. 52.

8. Parchen, H. M.: Early days of Montana pharmacy, Drugg. Circ. 51:191, 1907.

9. Bull. Pharm. 16:100, 1902.

10. Besides France, Holland and Switzerland especially have practiced for many dec-

11. Proc. A. Ph. A. 48:462, 1901.

12. Bull. Pharm. 18:267, 1904.

13. Rorem, C. R., and Fischelis, R. P.: The Costs of Medicine, p. 207, Chicago, 1932. In regard to the drug purchases of medical practitioners, see p. 92.

14. Young, J. H.: Pioneer nostrum promoter: Thomas W. Dyott, J. A. Ph. A. n.s. 1:290, 1961.

15. Liggett, L. K.: Pharmacy in the past 25 years, Pharm. Era 47:52, 1914.

16. Mason, H. B.: A remarkable pharmacy, Bull. Pharm. 18:144, 1904.

17. *Ibid.*: p. 229.

18. Drugg. Circ. 51:149, 1907.

19. Amer. Drugg. & Pharm. Rec. 41:328, 344, 1902.

20. Rorem and Fischelis: *op. cit.,* p. 74; and Rexall Drug and Chemical Co., Annual Report, p. 7, 1961.

21. Rexall Drug and Chemical Co., Annual Report, pp. 1, 4, 17, and 22, 1962.

22. Amer. Drugg. & Pharm. Rec. 47:115, 275, 1905.

23. Rorem and Fischelis, *op. cit.,* p. 74.

24. *Ibid.*: p. 75.

25. Drugg. Circ. 51:149, 1907.

25a. Among them we find the New York Consolidated Drug Company "doing business as a regular wholesale institution" and turning over "its $60,000 capital stock about ten times a year"; the Brooklyn Consolidated Drug Company, the Calvert Drug Company of Baltimore; the Washington Wholesale Drug Exchange; and the Philadelphia Wholesale Drug Company (Drugg. Circ. 51:149, 1907). The last-mentioned company, founded in 1886 under the name "Apothecaries' Union, Limited," and one of the oldest American retail druggists' buying clubs, was "so successful as virtually to monopolize the wholesale drug business in Philadelphia," its sales to its 800 members and to other retail dealers in 1930 exceeding $12,000,000.

26. Rorem and Fischelis, *op. cit.,* p. 126.

27. There existed at that time buying clubs of larger importance in 13 cities: Philadelphia, Baltimore, Washington, Providence, New York, Rochester, Buffalo, Cincinnati, Indianapolis, St. Louis, Kansas City, Atchison and Minneapolis. In addition, Weld mentions "a company in Cleveland with branches in Chicago,

Columbus, and Detroit, which operates in a similar manner to that of the co-operatives, but which is owned and operated largely as a private enterprise." (Weld, L. H. D.: Cooperative buying by retail druggists, Drugg. Circ. *61*:120, 1917.)

28. Rorem and Fischelis, *op. cit.*, p. 126.
29. *Ibid.*: p. 128.
30. *Ibid.*: pp. 127, 128. Founded as Olcott and McKesson in New York (1833), the name changed to McKesson and Robbins, Inc. in 1853.
31. Road to Market; 125 Years of Distribution Service [by McKesson & Robbins], 1833-1958, New York, 1958. The corporation's growth is all the more remarkable in view of the scandal of fraudulent mismanagement discovered in 1938 (see, e.g., McKesson breakdown, Drug & Cosmetic Ind. *43*:683-685, 1938; and *ibid.*, *44*:37, 1939).
32. Drugg. Circ. *50*:70, 1906.
33. Drugg. Circ. *51*:105, 1907.
34. N.A.R.D. J. *52*:629, 1931.
35. A decree entered in the United States Circuit Court for the District of Indiana, May 9, 1907, under the Sherman Anti-trust Act, declared all the essential and effective measures of the agreement to be illegal.
36. Drugg. Circ. *51*:434, 1907.
37. N.A.R.D. J. *52*:629, 1931.
38. Wilson, Stephen: The background and operation of the Pennsylvania fair trade law in the drug trade, J. A. Ph. A. *28*:541, 1939.
39. Statement of Maurice Mermey . . . at public hearing, Wednesday, May 25, 1955, before the Special Sub-Committee in Connection with the Study of the Anti-Trust Laws of the Committee on the Judiciary of the U. S. House of Representatives, mimeograph, Bureau of Education on Fair Trade, New York, 1955, p. 3; and, Are we heading for a federal price-fixing law?, Consumer Reports, May, 1958.
40. Parsons, L. C.: Some economic and social implications of fair trade legislation, J. A. Ph. A. *28*:539, 1939.
41. The account of recent developments in fair trade is based largely upon Helfand, W. H.: The fair trade movement (unpublished paper), American Institute of the History of Pharmacy, 1962.
42. On price-cutting of prescriptions, for ex-

amples see Drug News Weekly, pp. 4 and 5, April 11, 1962, and other issues of this tradepaper. On compounding that survives, see: Market Research Report, Abbott Laboratories (mimeographed), North Chicago, p. 1, July 26, 1962.
43. Weekly Pharmacy Reports, *12* (No. 2): 3, January 14, 1963.
44. Rorem and Fischelis, The Costs of Medicine, p. 85.
45. Mason, H. B.: A new economic order in pharmacy, Proc. A. Ph. A. *49*:470, 1901.
46. Stephenson, H.: Drug store, Am. Drugg. *88*:224, 1933.
47. Delgado, F. A.: Chain and independent drug store, J. A. Ph. A. *26*:931, 1937; N.A.R.D. J. *69*:1424, 1947.
48. Drug Topics' Drug Trade Marketing Guide, New York, 1961, pp. 10, 12, et passim; also Chain Store Age (Drug Store Manager's Edition), June 1950 [Silver Jubilee Issue], pp. J5 and 14 ff.; and Olsen, in Drug Topics, p. 75, April 8, 1963.
49. Pharm. Era *65*:355, 1928.
50. Beal, J. H.: Directing the trend of evolution in pharmacy, Pract. Drugg. *48*:14, Sept. 1930; Rorem and Fischelis, *op. cit.*, p. 181.
51. Powers, W. E.: Address of the president, Proc. Natl. Assoc. Bds. Pharm., pp. 29 f., 1956.
52. Snyder's Drugstores vs. Minnesota State Board of Pharmacy, District Court, Second Judicial District, File No. 324715, 17 Dec. 1962.
53. Greenberg, Emil, and Sharenow, I. L.: The Constitutional Basis of a Pharmacy Ownership Law (mimeographed), p. 11, 1962; and Mellon, L. P.: Legislation, can it effectively limit practice of pharmacy to pharmacists?, J. A. Ph. A. n.s. *2*:647, 1962.
54. State of Florida vs. Leone, 118 S. 2d 781, as quoted by Leonard F. Mellon in J. A. Ph. A. n.s. *2*:648, 1962.
55. *Ibid.*: p. 650.
56. *Ibid.*: p. 649, quoting a proposal drafted by Judge Andrew Salvest, attorney (1960) for the New Jersey board of pharmacy.
57. Griffenhagen, George: A "U.N." of Pharmacy (mimeographed address, Am. Pharm. Assoc., Philadelphia Chapter, 1963), pp. 19 and 21.
58. Data extracted from the Era Druggists

Directory and the Statistical Abstracts of the United States.

59. Appreciative acknowledgment is made to Paul O. Williams of the University of Wisconsin for comparative analysis of data for 1948 to 1960 during his graduate studies in pharmacy administration at the University of Wisconsin. The statistics used are mainly from annual surveys reported in the Proceedings of the National Association of Boards of Pharmacy. Griffenhagen is quoted from his Philadelphia address, *loc. cit.*, p. 18. Community pharmacy was included in a business census by the U. S. Bureau of the Census 7 times in 33 years since 1929; while these data are useful, they are complicated by the inclusion of non-pharmacies that sell a certain range of packaged drugs, in all but two of the surveys, plus vagaries of definition.

60. Riley, J. J.: A History of the American Soft Drink Industry, pp. 3, 6, 9 f., 52-57, Washington, D. C., 1958. This carefully written volume includes information on the scientific as well as the commercial background, and on the European as well as American developments.

61. Youth of the fountain, Amer. Drugg. 88:75, 208, Oct. 1933; Procter, W.: E. Durand, Am. J. Pharm. 45:513, 1873; J. W. England: *op. cit.*, pp. 357, 514.

62. Amer. Drugg. 88:214, Oct. 1933.

63. Delgado, F. A.: *op. cit.*, p. 929.

64. Drug Topics' Drug Trade Marketing Guide, New York, 1961, pp. 57 f., and N.A.R.D.-Saturday Evening Post: The Independent Druggist, Report No. 1, p. 61, Philadelphia, 1945.

65. Rorem and Fischelis, *op. cit.*, p. 65. Similar expectations by physicians and laymen that the pharmacist will provide food service is cited by Delgado, F. A.: The Professional Pharmacy, ed. 2, p. 1, Washington, 1935.

66. The application of this term to any business to the exclusion of others is wrong. All business should be conducted on an ethical basis. The commercialization of the drugstore, as distinguished from professionalization, is not necessarily unethical.

67. England, J. W.: *op. cit.*, pp. 101-114.

68. Drugg. Circ. 51:89, 167, 1907.

69. Mason, H. B.: The Metcalf pharmacy in Boston, Bull. Pharm. 22:279, 1908.

70. Drugg. Circ. 51:167, 1907.

71. Am. Drugg. & Pharm. Rec. 42:132, 134, 1903.

72. Liggett, L. K.: Pharmacy in the past 25 years, Pharm. Era 47:51, 1914.

73. For example, when Walgreen Drug Stores acquired the three units of Globe Discount City, each unit covered "over 100,000 square feet," of which the prescription department measured about 20 by 20 feet; and other "departments common to drugstores" (including toys and tobacco) measured about 3,000 square feet. (Walgreen enters discount house field . . . , Drug Topics, p. 12, 9 April 1962).

74. Jordan, C. B.: Address, J. A. Ph. A. 20:812, 1931.

75. Delgado, F. A.: The Professional Pharmacy, p. 1.

76. Am. Prof. Pharm. 11:905, 1945.

77. Olsen, P. C.: What pharmacy graduates should know . . . , Drug Topics, p. 75, 8 April 1963.

78. The concentration of high-volume prescription practice in a much smaller number of pharmacies is cited from surveys by manufacturers' representatives for the journal *American Professional Pharmacist;* see The Clark-O'Neill Indicia, vol. 5, p. 4, Feb. 1963. A striking claim by *American Professional Pharmacist* (although not corroborated by Olsen's data) is that approximately one third of the American community pharmacies were providing about three fourths of all prescriptions dispensed. (e.g., Am. Prof. Pharm., July 1961, p. 34, n.; Business Publications Audit of Circulation; and personal communication from editor I. Rubin, 15 August 1961). For Olsen's vigorous rebuttal, see Drug Trade News, p. 4, April 6, 1959.

79. Drug Topics, p. 2, 25 April 1949, and Drug Topics' Drug Trade Marketing Guide, p. 28; and Delgado, F. A.: Prescription Department Sales Analysis in Selected Drug Stores, p. 1, Department of Commerce, Washington, D. C.

80. Charters, W. W., *et al.*: Basic Material for a Pharmaceutical Curriculum, p. 19, New York, 1927; cf. Delgado, F. A., and Kimball, A. A.: Prescription Department Sales Analysis in Selected Drug Stores, p. 22; Elliott, E. C. (ed.): The General Report of the Pharmaceutical Survey, pp. 220-228, Washington, D. C.,

1950; and "1961 prescription survey," Abbott [Laboratories] Market Research Report (mimeographed, 26 July 1962).

81. Charters, W. W.: *op. cit.*, pp. 259 f.; Delgado and Kimball: Prescription Department Sales Analysis, pp. 31 and 35; Mordell, J. S.: The Prescription Study of the Pharmaceutical Survey, pp. 11 and 261 f., Washington, 1949; and Abbott Market Research Report. The reason could not be discerned for the marked difference in proportion of proprietary prescriptions between Charters' 10.29 per cent about 1926 and Delgado's 25 per cent in 1931-32 (20% if considering the most-prescribed ingredients alone). Delgado's figure would be still higher if added to a portion of the further 25 per cent that were some mixture of official, proprietary and other nonofficial drugs.

82. Ruth, R. J.: The history of National Pharmacy Week, J. A. Ph. A. *20*:696, 1931; and Sonnedecker, G.: National Pharmacy Week—a pharmacist's vision fulfilled, Tile and Till *34*:38-41, 1948.

83. Abramson, Robert: A brief history of National Pharmacy Week, J. A. Ph. A. (Pract. Ed.) *17*:449, 1956. For the Truman letter, see *ibid.*: *9*:153, 1948.

84. American Social Hygiene Association, J. A. Ph. A. (Pract. Ed.) *1*:65-68, 1940; and committee reports in the Proceedings in following years. See also, Clarke, Walter: Pharmacy's role in the social hygiene program, *ibid.*, 5:16, 1944; also 9:295 and 348, 1948.

85. On the developing program and sample materials, see Henderson, Jean: Pharmacies become health information centers, J. A. Ph. A. (Pract. Ed.) 9:348 ff., 1948; and Fischelis, R. P.: *ibid.*, p. 721. See also, Fischelis, R. P.: The role of the pharmacist in the cancer program (mimeographed address), Public Health Cancer Assoc., New York, Oct. 24, 1949.

86. England, J. W.: *op. cit.*, p. 357.

87. *Ibid.*: p. 108.

88. J. A. Ph. A. *23*:1137, 1934.

89. Urdang, George: New light on the history of show globes, J. A. Ph. A. (Pract. Ed.) *10*:604-606, 640, 1949; and Griffenhagen, George: The show globe—a symbol of pharmacy *in* Doyle, P. A. (ed.): Readings in Pharmacy, pp. 111-117, New York, 1962.

90. Slavin, Morton: Will automation help pharmacists meet future challenges?, Am. Prof. Pharm. *29*:30, Feb. 1963.

91. 100 Years of Business Life, p. 32, Schieffelin & Co., New York, 1894.

92. Drugg. Circ. & Chem. Gaz. *10*:236, 1866; see also *12*:350, 1868.

93. Drugg. Circ. *51*:110, 1907.

94. Moxley, G. B.: Address, Proc. Natl. Wholesale Drugg. Assoc., p. 29, 1924.

95. Fisher, Albert: Facts, p. 19; How the Magic Pipeline Works (N.W.D.A. pamphlet), ed. 3, p. 12, New York, 1962. (The latter pamphlet has a useful glossary of business terms used in the drug field, particularly wholesaling.) For an analysis still significant, see Rorem and Fischelis: *op. cit.*, p. 133 et passim.

96. Statistical Abstracts of the United States, p. 846, Washington, 1961. On earlier figures and comparative margins, see Historical Statistics of the United States, Colonial Times to 1957, pp. 524 and 525, Washington, 1960. On postwar drop in profit, see Fisher, A. B.: Facts on . . . Service Wholesale Druggists, N.W.D.A. Bull. No. 49, p. 16, New York, 1954. On the changing marketing practices mentioned, see, e.g., Waterman, C. G. *in* Pharmaceutical Wholesalers Association Report of the Year 1960-61, p. 4; on the diagnosis concerning proportional distribution costs, see Werble, Wallace, The revolution in pharmaceutical wholesaling, *ibid.*, p. 27.

97. Sadtler, S. P.: Influence of pharmacists on the development and advance of modern chemistry, Am. J. Pharm. *93*:200, 1921; England, J. W.: The First Century, p. 31.

98. England, J. W.: *op. cit.*, p. 111.

99. *Ibid.*: p. 112.

100. *Ibid.*: p. 32.

101. *Ibid.*: p. 32.

102. *Ibid.*: p. 33.

103. Chemical industry's contribution to the nation, 1635-1935, Suppl. to Chem. Industries, p. 41, May, 1935.

104. Its original name was George K. Smith and Company. Successively, it became Smith and Shoemaker, Mahlon K. Smith and Company, and the Smith and Kline Company. The firm was incorporated under its present name, the Smith Kline & French Laboratories, in 1891.

105. In 1876, after John Uri Lloyd had entered into partnership, the H. M. Merrell Company changed its name to Merrell,

Thorp and Lloyd; in 1881 to Thorp and Lloyd Brothers; in 1885 to Lloyd Brothers and in 1924 to Lloyd Brothers Pharmacists, Inc. Under John Uri Lloyd the concern assumed a leading position in the field of plant preparations of every kind and, moreover, one of the valuable sources of progress in plant chemistry, colloidal chemistry and new pharmaceutical methods and devices. A list of the earliest "drug houses" still in existence, valuable if the meaning of some of the dates is understood, appears in Drug and Cosmetic Industry, *70*:29, Jan., 1952. (This includes additions and corrections to all previous lists published by Drug and Cosmetic Industry.)

106. Andrews, E. D.: The New York Shakers and their industries, N. Y. State Mus. Circ. *2*:5, 1930; Hoffman, G. N.: Mt. Lebanon medicine makers, the Shakers, Pharm. Era *53*:197, 1920.

107. For an interesting, excellent account, see Lee, C. O.: The Shakers as pioneers in the American herb and drug industry, Am. J. Pharm. *132*:178-193, 1960.

108. Pharm. Rec. *23*:141, 1905.

109. New Idea, *27*(No. 1):3, 1905; and Lakey, R. T.: Frederick Stearns, pharmacist, J. A. Ph. A. (Pract. Ed.) *9*:486-489, 1948.

110. Pharm. Rundschau *10*:276, 1892; England, J. W.: The First Century, p. 216; Remington, J. P.: E. R. Squibb, Am. J. Pharm. *73*:420, 1901. For a full-length biography see Blochman, L. G.: Doctor Squibb; The Life and Times of a Rugged Idealist, New York, 1958, 371 pp.

111. Smith, G. W.: The Squibb laboratory in 1863, J. Hist. Med. *13*:382-394, 1958.

112. Pharm. Rundschau *5*:250, 1887.

113. England, J. W.: The First Century, p. 107.

114. Pharm. Era *16*:941, 1896; Foote, P. A.: Tablets, Madison, Wis., Bull. of the Univ. of Wisconsin, Ser. No. 1566, Gen. Ser. No. 1340, Dec. 1928; Griffenhagen, G., and Sonnedecker, G.: A history of sugar-coated pills and tablets, J. A. Ph. A. (Pract. Ed.) *18*:486-488 and 553-555, 1957; Urdang, George: Compressed tablet, What's New (Abbott Labs.), p. 16, Fall 1943.

115. *Ibid.*: especially Foote, pp. 95 f., and Urdang, p. 16.

116. Facts about Pharmacy and Pharmaceuticals, New York, 1958, pp. 12 f.; Brown, Francis C.: The Pharmaceutical Industry, pp. 20 f. (republished separately, from Glover and Cornell: The Development of American Industries, New York, 1951).

117. Taylor, F. O.: 45 years of manufacturing pharmacy, J. A. Ph. A. *4*:468, 1915.

118. J. Chem. Ed. *8*:477, 1931.

119. Tile and Till *12*:30, 1927.

120. *Ibid.*: p. 50.

121. Mallinckrodt Chemical Works: Saint Louis Exhibition, 1904, p. 3.

122. Chemical industry's contribution, *op. cit.*, p. 139.

123. The discussion concerning Sterling Drug Incorporated is in its entirety based on, and partly literally taken from, The Sterling Story, published by the firm in 1947.

124. Dunn, C. W.: Pharmaceutical industry progress, Drug & Cosm. Ind. *72*:554, 1953.

125. Administered Prices: Hearings Before the Subcommittee on Antitrust and Monopoly of the Committee on the Judiciary, U. S. Senate, 86th Congress, 2nd Session, Part 19, Washington, D. C., 1960, p. 10,760 (F. L. Thomson quoting National Conference Board).

126. Smith, Austin, *ibid.*, p. 10,831; and Statistical Abstract of the United States, 1948, p. 840; cf., *ibid.*, 1961, p. 782 (for changing census classification, see also p. 776).

For access to further information on the American drug industry, see especially Southern, W. A.: Sources of drug market data, Drug & Cosm. Ind. *73*:328-9 and 417-21, 1953.

127. Facts about Pharmacy and Pharmaceuticals, pp. 12 f., New York, 1958.

128. Searle, J. G., *et al.*: The pharmaceutical industry, J. mondial Pharmacie, No. 3, p. 211, 1961.

129. Rorem and Fischelis, *op. cit.*, pp. 109-110.

130. *Ibid.*, p. 114.

131. *Ibid.*, p. 102.

132. *Ibid.*, p. 104.

133. Olsen, P. C.: Marketing drug products, Drug Trade News, p. 20, April 6, 1959; and Drug Topics, p. 75, April 8, 1963. Also Drug Topics, pp. 1 and 55, Sept. 27, 1948.

134. Statistical Abstract of the United States

1961, pp. 880 and 882; see also FDC Reports, *25*:16, April 22, 1963.

135. Pharmaceutical Manufacturers Association, Ethical Drug Industry Survey of Research and Development Expenditures 1960-61, p. 1, Washington, D. C., June 1961; Pharmaceutical Manufacturers Association Yearbook 1962-63, pp. 178 and 180, Washington, D. C., n.d.

136. de Haen, Paul: Review of Drugs, 1941-1961; Single Chemical Entities Introduced in the United States and Patent Status (multilith, Pharmaceutical Manufacturers Association), Washington, D. C., 1962; see especially the revision sheets issued February 28, 1963, p. iii. This report covers drugs "introduced primarily to the national market" (personal communication from H. L. Binkley [P.M.A.], August 30, 1962). Of drugs still on the market in 1962, it deals with those considered "major products, 1941-1948; [but] from 1949 through 1961, all products marketed . . ." (title page). See also Weikel, M. K., and Sonnedecker, Glenn: Emergence of Research as a Function of American Pharmaceutical Industry, Madison, Wis., publication pending.

137. FDC Reports, *25*:11, April 22, 1963; based on the studies of Paul de Haen of New York.

138. Thirty-seventh Annual Meeting, American Drug Manfucturers Association, Boca Raton, Florida, April 4-7, 1949, pp. 9-15, Baltimore, 1949.

17. THE AMERICAN PHARMACIST AND SOCIETY

1. Ward, James: In Webster's New International Dictionary of the English Language, Merriam-Webster, Springfield, Mass., 1931.

2. England, J. W.: The First Century of the Philadelphia College of Pharmacy, p. 348, Philadelphia, 1922.

3. *Ibid.*: p. 351.

4. *Ibid.*: p. 352.

5. *Ibid.*: p. 353; Urdang, George: The influence of the Quakers on Philadelphia institutions, Am. J. Pharm. *118*:81-88, 1946.

6. England, J. W.: *op. cit.*, p. 356.

7. Maisch, J. M.: G. H. E. Mühlenberg als Botaniker, Pharm. Rundschau 4:119, 1886.

8. Am. Prof. Pharm. *29*:58-64, 1963. For some other examples see Drug Topics, p. 40, Feb. 2, 1959; p. 15, March 16, 1959; p. 46, Aug. 17, 1959; p. 2, Sept. 28, 1959.

9. Lyman, R. A.: Dr. Roy Bird Cook, Am. J. Pharm. Ed. *2*:608, 1938.

10. Eli Lilly; man with a long view, The Lilly Review, pp. 5-12, May-June 1957; and Drug Trade News, p. 62, Oct. 3, 1960. Alongside the great industrialist may be placed an example of a community pharmacist, T. J. Gatchell of Buffalo, Wyoming. A community museum memorializes him because of his devotion to collecting memorabilia on the history of his county (more than 1,500 items) during a half century of practice there (Drug Topics, p. 6, March 31, 1958).

11. The types of service by pharmacists that have been needed are described by Shriver, R. S.: The pharmacist and the Peace Corps, J. A. Ph. A. n.s. *2*:353-354, 1962.

12. Information concerning pharmacists and their services in humanitarian work, either religious or secular, is invited for the historical record by the American Institute of the History of Pharmacy, whose address is: Pharmacy Building, Madison 6, Wisconsin. While no central registry has come to light, two of the pharmacist-missionaries—Henry C. Kammerer of Trenton, N. J. (about 1954) and James S. Palmgren of 532 Sheridan Road, Evanston, Ill.—served their colleagues well by compiling considerable information and the following names of American pharmacist-missionaries: Albert S. Bauman, Miss Frances Bell, Richard Blakney, Muriel Clemenger, H. S. Cliff, Mr. and Mrs. Ronald G. Coppola, Mrs. Max Gray, Miss Barbara Hartman, Larkin E. Harvey, Miss Betty K. Job, Henry Kammerer, Mrs. B. Koschade, Samson Huri Lal, C. O. Lee, Kennie M. Linn, William Wayne Logan, Donald Lutes, Curtis Matthews, Richard McLean, Harold E. McMillan, Robert A. McRuer, E. N. Meuser, James S. Palmgren, R. T. Roberts, Mr. Ronnesson(?), Miss Emmie Stevens, Raymond E. Watson, Norman Whipple and Miss J. S. Williams.

Other examples would be Lorraine Gribbens, who wrote from Borneo: Medicine vs. Ubat, Am. J. Pharm. Ed. *26*:475-480, 1962, and Jack Lesshafft, who left a community pharmacy in Louisville, Ky., to enter hospital administrative service in Africa (Drug Topics, p. 68, Jan. 28, 1963).

13. The project was conceived in 1958, by a physician. The American Pharmaceutical Association helped to raise funds. On the project, see Health mission to the world, J. A. Ph. A. (Pract. Ed.) *21*:764-765, 1960; on experiences of one of the pharmacists see Sherwood, M. F.: Letters from S. S. Hope, J. A. Ph. A. n.s. 2:708-710, 1962.

14. J. A. Ph. A. *16*:592, 1927.

15. N.A.R.D. J. *65*:564, 1945.

16. Costello, P. H.: Survey of pharmacy laws, p. 62, Proc. Natl. Assoc. Bds. Pharm., 1955.

17. Personal communication from American Pharmaceutical Association (G. Griffenhagen), June 26, 1961; see also A. Ph. A. Newsletter, p. 3, June 30, 1962, and Costello, *ibid.*, p. 67, 1961. For representative accounts of pharmacists as mayors see, e.g., Drug Topics, 1959: Aug. 17, p. 2; Aug. 31, p. 4; Sept. 14, p. 58; Oct. 26, p. 3; and Nov. 23, p. 4; and in Drug Topics, 1960: Feb. 15, p. 2, and Aug. 15, p. 2. A special issue was devoted to discussing the role of the pharmacist in political and civic life (J. A. Ph. A. n.s. 2(No. 7), July, 1962).

18. King, R. O.: The city that druggists run, Am. Drugg. 88:26, 90, Dec., 1933.

19. Griffenhagen, G. B.: Stepping stones in Golden State pharmacy, Pac. Drug Rev., 1950; a reprint was issued under the title "The Story of California Pharmacy" by the American Institute of the History of Pharmacy, Madison, Wis., 1950.

20. Ewe, George: David Henshaw—From druggist to secretary of the Navy, J. A. Ph A. *24*:858, 860, 1935; also see Cyclopaedia of American Biography.

21. On Carl Durham (b. 1892) see the feature "Nuclear pharmacist," New York Times, Feb. 20, 1957, and on Hubert Humphrey (b. 1911) see Time magazine, Feb. 1, 1960, pp. 13-16; both men are in Who's Who in America. Durham retired from Congress in 1960.

22. Wolfe, H. G.: James Cutbush—author, teacher, Apothecary General, Am. J. Pharm. Ed. *12*:89, 125, 1948.

23. Am. J. Pharm. 34:93, 1862.

24. Rittenhouse, H. N.: U. S. Army medical storekeepers, Am. J. Pharm. 37:87 ff.,

1865; Stevens, Hennel: The medical purveying department of the United States Army, Am. J. Pharm. 37:91 ff., 1865.

25. Fell, E. R.: The pharmaceutical department of the U. S. A. Hospital, Am. J. Pharm. 37:107, 1865.

26. Proc. A. Ph. A. *42*:vi, 1894.

27. Proc. A. Ph. A. *43*:75 ff., 1895.

28. Proc. A. Ph. A. *46*:72, 1898; *Ibid.*, *47*: 117 ff., 1899.

29. Proc. A. Ph. A. *50*:201, 1902.

31. Proc. A. Ph. A. *49*:94, 1901.

30. Proc. A. Ph. A. *48*:73, 1900.

32. Proc. A. Ph. A. *51*:111, 1903; Drugg. Circ. *46*:218, 1903.

33. J. A. Ph. A. *5*:1037, 1408, 1916.

34. J. A. Ph. A. *11*:764, 1922.

35. J. A. Ph. A. *13*:263, 1924.

36. J. A. Ph. A. *26*:1051, 1937.

37. For a good review especially of developments from the 1930's until after World War II, by the Chairman of the Joint Committee on Status of Pharmacists in Government Service, see: Einbeck, A. H.: Pharmacy in the army and navy, Merck Report, pp. 22-26, Jan., 1947.

37a. Committee on Pharmacists in Government Service, J. Am. Pharm. Assoc. n.s. 3:330, 1963.

38. Trygstad, V. O.: Utilization of pharmacists in Veterans Administration (mimeographed address, Pharmacy Section, Association of Military Surgeons of the United States), Nov. 11, 1953 (copy in Kremers Archive, University of Wisconsin). On Trygstad himself, see Am. J. Hosp. Pharm. *17*:376, 1960.

39. Promotions up to the grade corresponding to Captain in the Army were available at this time. See: Parker bill passed by Congress, Bulletin No. 5 (mimeograph, American Pharmaceutical Association), April 18, 1930 (copy in Kremers Archive, University of Wisconsin).

40. Archambault, G. F.: Your profession in the U. S. Public Health Service, J. A. Ph. A. (Pract. Ed.) 9:39-41, 1948; Archambault, G. F., Foster, T. A., and Kinsey, R. D.: Pharmacy in the U. S. Public Health Service . . . then and now, J. A. Ph. A. (Pract. Ed.) 9:345-347, 376-384, 1948.

41. In a personal communication, Mr. Archambault stated, "The utilization of pharmacists *per se* in the present U. S. Public Health Service program is due in main to the foresightedness of three individuals,

Dr. R. C. Williams, Assistant Surgeon General, Chief of the Bureau of Medical Services; Dr. Otis L. Anderson, Medical Director, Chief of the Division of Hospitals; and Dr. G. Halsey Hunt, Senior Surgeon, Assistant Chief of the Division of Hospitals."

42. Einbeck, Arthur (Chairman): Report of the [joint] Committee on the Status of Pharmacists in Government Service (mimeographed, American Pharmaceutical Association meeting), Boston, 1954 (copy in Kremers Archive, University of Wisconsin). On Foster, see Am. J. Hosp. Pharm. *17*:377 f., 1960; on Archambault, see Who's Who in America, the Election Bulletin, Am. Pharm. Assoc., 1961 (when he was elected President of the Association), and Am. J. Hosp. Pharm. *16*: 543, 1959.

43. Besides the Kremers Archive at the University of Wisconsin, the following sources of biographical information were consulted: on Power, Am. J. Chem. Ed. *31*: 258, 1954; on Giordano, Who's Who in America and Drug Topics, July 30, 1962, pp. 3 and 44; on Bransky, Am. J. Pharm. *132*:352, 1960; on Gasen, J. A. Ph. A. (Pract. Ed.) *6*:183, 1945.

44. Hutchins, Harold: Heroic druggists triumph over flood, Am. Drugg. *93*:24, 66, May, 1936.

45. See the civil defense issue of J. A. Ph. A. *21*: No. 10, 1960, particularly (Burney) p. 623 and (Dodge) p. 629.

46. Breese, Murray: John Uri Lloyd—rebel, Am. Drugg. *79*:106, Jan., 1929.

47. Drugg. Circ. *57*:105, 1913.

48. O. Henry, editorial in J. A. Ph. A. *20*:488, 1931.

49. Herman, E. P.: O. Henry, pharmacist, Modern Pharmacy, *34*(No. 4):7-10, 1949; Long, E. H.: O. Henry: His Life and Work, Philadelphia, 1949.

50. Readers interested in beginning a collection in the field of pharmaceutical literature may find of interest: Sonnedecker, G.: The pharmacist as a book collector, Am. J. Hosp. Pharm. *18*:24-30, 1961; a list of further readings and other aids for the book collector may be obtained on request to the American Institute of the History of Pharmacy, Pharmacy Bldg., Madison 6, Wis.

51. England, J. W.: The First Century, p. 243.

52. Schreiber, C. F.: William Alfred Speck,

in memoriam, Yale Univ. Lib. Gaz. *3*:55, No. 3, 1929.

53. On the "Lilly Rare Book Library" on the Bloomington campus, see Time magazine, pp. 54 f., April 13, 1959.

54. Urdang, George: Pharmacy's Part in Society, p. 82, Madison, Wis., 1946. On Breasted, see the essay in Doyle, P. A. (ed.): Readings in Pharmacy, New York, 1962, pp. 152-156.

55. For the apothecary as a figure in literature see the following, all of which are by Edward Kremers. Items are arranged in chronological sequence. 1. A preliminary bibliography, Pharm. Rev. *24*:1, 1906; 2. Du mein Jena, Pharm. Rev. *26*: 153, 1908; 3. Kussmaul, Jugenderinnerungen eines alten Arztes, Pharm. Rev. *26*:252, 1908; 4. Beschreibung aller Staende auf Erden, Pharm. Rev. *26*:342, 357, 1908; 5. The physician-apothecary, Midland Rev. *43*:447, 1910; 6. The drug seller of Paolo and Francesca, Midland Rev. *45*:5, 1911; 7. An American physician-apothecary of 1793, Pharm. Era *48*: 298, 1915; 8. Eine Zeitung aus dem 17. Jahrhundert, Deutsch-amerikanische Apo.-Z. *38*:115, 1917; 9. Kyritz-Pyritz, Deutsch-Amer. Apo.-Z. *39*:7, 1918; 10a. Zwei Söhne eines dänischen Apothekers, Deutsch-Amer. Apo.-Z. *39*:29, 1918; 10b. Two sons of a Danish apothecary, J. A. Ph. A. *7*:620, 1918; 11a. Fra Angelico, ein italienischer College, Deutsch-Amer. Apo.-Z. *39*:96, 1918; 11b. Fra Angelico, an Italian colleague, J. A. Ph. A. *8*:141, 1919; 12. Pharmazeutischer Humor: Der Neun und neunziger, N. Y. Apo.-Z. *40*:1, 15, 1919. The German text reprinted, also trans. into French, in "Der Mörser," *19*: 219, 230, 337, 1919; 13. The medico-pharmaceutical practitioners of Kingsley, Am. Drug. & Pharm. Rec. *67*:125, 1919; 14. Ein "Neues Heilmittel" aus dem Schwarzwald, N. Y. Apo.-Z. *40*:73, 1919; 15. Medizinisch-Pharmaceutisches am Hofe Ludwig des XIV. aus den Briefen der Lise-Lotte, N. Y. Apo.-Z. *43*:1, 15, 29, 1922; 16. Ein Rezept als Friedensstifter, N. Y. Apo.-Z. *43*:151, 1923; 17. Our presidents as pharmacists, Am. Drug., Feb., 1923, p. 12; 18. Herrn Wikings Meerfahrt, N. Y. Apo.-Z. *43*:17, 1923; 19. Aus der Hausapotheke, N. Y. Apo.-Z. *44*:85, 1923; 20. The House of Mirth, Am. Drug., Feb., 1926, p. 22; 21. Deserting pharmacy for journalism, Am. Drug.,

February, 1926, p. 22; 22. Apotheker-Pfuscher: Der Ameisler, N. Y. Apo.-Z. *46*:146, 1926; 23. Ein amerikanischer Sonderling, N. Y. Apo.-Z. *47*:57, 71, 85, 1926; 24. Apothecary M'Grady in "Handy Andy," J. A. Ph. A. *15*:1097, 1926; 25. Chef Ungelenk und sein Lehrling Bodo, N. Y. Apo.-Z. *47*:141, 1926; 26. Eine deutsche Apothekerin, N. Y. Apo.-Z. *48*:1, 1926; 27. Ein Ex-apotheker und dessen zwei Söhne aus Amerika, N. Y. Apo.-Z. *48*:141, 1928; 28. Upagupta, son of a "perfumer," J. A. Ph. A. *17*:366, 1928; 29. A New England physician-apothecary and his "infamous apprentice," Pharm. Era, Feb., 1928, p. 43; 30. Ein plebejisch, hanebüchener Poltron und Pecus, N. Y. Apo.-Z. *48*:155, 1928; 31. Apotheker-Pfuscher: Doktor Calmus, N. Y. Apo.-Z. *49*:15, 1928; 32. A charlatan of the Iowa frontier, Am. J. Pharm. *100*:294, 1928; 33. Ein moderner Confectionarius, N. Y. Apo.-Z. *49*:127, 1928; 34. Balzac's "druggist-perfumer," Am. J. Pharm. *101*:278, 1929; 35. The "Wunderdoctorin" of Lisa Wenger, Pharm. Era 1929, p. 107; 36. Ein pharmaceutischer Charletan auf dem Mississippi, N. Y. Apo.-Z. *50*:29, 43, 57, 1929; 37. Die Drogerie zum Goldenen Stern, N. Y. Apo.-Z. *50*:71, 1929; 38. Tom, the "Doctor's" apprentice, J. A. Ph. A. *19*:265, 1930; 39. An Italian diary of the Cinque Cento, Pharm. Era *68*:15, 1931. See also, Doyle, P. A.: Pharmacy and the American novel, Am. J. Hosp. Pharm. *19*:465-8, 1962.

56. A notable example was the series viewed by millions of Americans, "The Jones Family," which mirrored the spirit, the ambitions and the attitude toward life of a superior "average citizen." A pharmacist was the central figure. The pharmacist of course has served not only to portray middle-class virtues but also high-class humor, as in the short feature of W. C. Fields, "The Pharmacist."

18. CONTRIBUTIONS BY PHARMACISTS TO SCIENCE AND INDUSTRY

1. Sadtler, S. P.: Influence of pharmacists on the development and advance of modern chemistry, Am. J. Pharm. *93*:198, 1921.
2. Dictionary of National [British] Biography, London *14*:186, 1888.
3. Bouvet, Maurice: Histoire de la pharmacie en France, p. 368 ff., Paris, 1937.
4. André-Pontier, L.: Histoire de la pharmacie, p. 53, Paris, 1900. The note concerning Pasteur in Ferchl: Chemisch-pharmazeutisches Bio-und Bibliographicon, p. 396, Mittenwald, 1937, as an "apothecary's apprentice in Besançon," is erroneous. André-Pontier states that Pasteur, "who never was a pharmaceutical apprentice, visited with an apothecary of his town during his college time at Besançon, as frequently as possible, in order to become familiar with the chemical reactions."
5. Nordenskiöld, Erik: The History of Biology, p. 377, New York, London, 1928; Urdang, G.: Berzelius and Pharmacy, J. A. Ph. A. *37*:481-485, 1948.
6. Hoefer, Ferdinand: La chimie, p. 3, Paris, 1865.
7. Ferchl, F., and Süssenguth, A.: Kurzgeschichte der Chemie, pp. 57, 62, 70, Mittenwald, 1936. (English edition under the title "A Pictorial History of Chemistry," pp. 77, 79-81, London, 1939.)
8. *Ibid.*, p. 129 (in English edition, p. 146).
9. Bouvet, M.: *op. cit.*, p. 371.
10. Kopp, Hermann: Geschichte der Chemie, p. 69, reprint, Leipzig, 1931, 3.
11. *Ibid.*: p. 65.
12. Dann, G. E., Martin Heinrich Klaproth (1743-1817). Ein deutscher Apotheker und Chemiker, Berlin, 1958; and Ferchl and Süssenguth: *op. cit.*, p. 140 (in English edition, p. 152).
13. "The Forgotten Chemist," The Laboratory (Fisher Scientific Co., Pittsburgh), vol. 7, No. 2, p. 18.
14. Wallrabe, Gottfried: Zum Gedächtnis an Karl Gottfried Hagen, Pharm. Ztg. *74*:286, 1929.
15. Communications de l'Académie de Médecine de 1829 à 1833, quoted after Bouvet, M.: *op. cit.*, p. 380.
16. Bouvet, M.: *op. cit.*, p. 372.
17. Kopp, H.: *op. cit.*, 3, p. 368; Adlung and Urdang: *op. cit.*, p. 437.
18. Speter, Max: Liebig oder Soubeiran, Chem. Ztg. *55*:781, 1931.
19. Lieben, Fritz: *op. cit.*, p. 70.
20. Lieben, Fritz: Geschichte der physiologischen Chemie, p. 44, Leipzig, Wien, 1935.
21. Jöcher: Gelehrten Lexikon, Berlin, 1913.
22. The Laboratory, *loc. cit.*, p. 19.
23. Walden, Paul: Tobias Lowitz, ein vergessener Physiko-Chemiker, Diergart's Bei-

träge zur Geschichte der Chemie, Gedächtnisband für G. W. A. Kahlbaum, Leipzig, Wien, 1909, p. 533; Bloch, M.: Tobias Lowitz, in Bugge: Buch der grossen Chemiker, *1*, p. 362, Berlin, 1929.

24. Morton, A. A.: Laboratory Technique in Organic Chemistry, p. 202, New York, London, 1938.
25. *Ibid.*: pp. 38, 214.
26. Urdang, George: Pharmacy's Part in Society, p. 57, Madison, Wis., 1946.
27. Rosenthaler, Ludwig: Die Entwicklung der Pflanzenchemie von Du Clos bis Scheele, Ber. deutsch. pharm. Gesellsch. *14*:295, 1904.
28. Rosenthaler, L.: *op. cit.*
29. Zaunick, Rudolph: Albert Niemann, der Entdecker des Kokains, die Pharmazie *4*:475-477, 1949.
30. Mayer, F. F.: Assay of Alkaloids, Am. J. Pharm. *35*:20-29, 1863; Hoffmann, Fr.: Zur Geschichte des Mayerschen Alkaloid Reagenz und Ferdinand F. Mayer's, Pharm. Rund. *12*:125-131, 1894. Mayer's claims were not entirely unchallenged (Am. J. Pharm. *37*:5-16, 1865).
31. Pharm. J. & Pharm., London *117*:726, 1926.
32. Griffith, Ivor: Frederick Belding Power, Am. J. Pharm. *99*:252, 1927. See also the same author: A half century in plant chemistry, Am. J. Pharm. *96*:601, 1924.
32a. The comment and the examples concerning the remarkable contribution of French hospital pharmacists are based entirely on Berman, Alex: The scientific tradition in French hospital pharmacy, Am. J. Hosp. Pharm. *18*:116, 1961.
33. Lieben, Fr.: *op. cit.*, p. 395.
34. *Ibid.*: p. 340.
35. *Ibid.*: p. 42.
36. *Ibid.*: p. 597.
37. Binz, Arthur: Chemie, Technik und Weltgeschichte, Z. ang. Chemie *40*:450, 1927.
38. Kopp, H.: *op. cit.*, *4*, p. 227.
39. Kränzlein, G.: Zum hundertjährigen Gedächtnis der Arbeiten von F. F. Runge, Z. ang. Chemie *48*:1, 1935, p. 1.
40. *Ibid.*: p. 2; Urdang, G.: Der Anilinentdecker F. F. Runge, Pharm. Ztg. *80*:526. 1935.
41. Adlung and Urdang: *op. cit.*, p. 488.
42. The inventor of the caoutchouc synthesis Fritz Hofmann wrote the letter quoted in response to a request of Urdang, then editor of the Pharmazeutische Zeitung. It was published in Pharm. Ztg. *79*:999,

1934, under the title: Der Vater der Kautschuksynthese, Apotheker Fritz Hofmann. For biography, see: Schneider, Wolfgang: Fritz Hofmann, Pharm. Industrie *19*:38-41, 1957, and Zimmermann, Walther: Fritz Hofmann, Deutsch. Apoth. Ztg. *87*:1286-88, 1938.
43. Urdang, G.: Hermann Thoms, Pharm. Ztg. *76*:1351, 1931.
44. Adlung and Urdang, *op. cit.*, p. 166.
45. Koppen Julius: Zur Synthese des Adrenalins Pharm. Ztg. *79*:603, 1934.
46. Ritsert, E.: Über den Werdegang des Anästhesins, Pharm. Ztg. *70*:1006, 1925.
47. Urdang, George: Pharmacy's Part in Society, pp. 70, 71, Madison, Wis., 1946.
47a. Urdang, G.: Die deutsche Apotheke als Keimzelle der Deutschen pharmazeutischen Industrie, Die Vorträge der Hauptversammlung der Gesellschaft für Geschichte der Pharmazie in Wien, 1931, p. 93, Mittenwald, 1931; Urdang, G.: Retail pharmacy as the nucleus of the pharmaceutical industry, Bull. Hist. Med., Suppl. No. 3, pp. 325-346, 1944.
48. Dannemann, Friedrich: Vom Werden der naturwissenschaftlichen Probleme, p. 269, Leipzig, 1928.
49. Adlung and Urdang: *op. cit.*, p. 440.
50. Gilbert's Annalen *7*:525, 1801.
51. Ferchl, Fr. und Süssenguth, A.: *op. cit.*, p. 169 (in English edition, pp. 182-183).
52. Adlung and Urdang: *op. cit.*, p. 452.
53. *Ibid.*: p. 470.
54. Green, J. Reynolds: A History of Botany, 1860-1900, Oxford, p. 232.
55. André-Pontier, L.: Histoire de la pharmacie, p. 51, Paris, 1900.
56. Pharm. J. *146*:143, 1941.
57. Personal communication from Mr. Howard Bayles, Norwich, England; Chem. & Drug. *116*:255, 295, 1932.
58. Heimen, H.: Apotheker Pilâtre de Rozier, der erste Luftschiffer, Pharm. Ztg. *69*:1120, 1924.
59. Urdang, G.: Berühmte Berliner Apotheker, Pharm. Ztg. *77*:1239, 1932. See also, Seabra, P.: Oxidase in biology and in flying research, Med. Times, Dec., 1943; and Urdang, G.: Pharmacy and aviation, Bull. Hist. Med. *15*:324-326, 1944.
60. Urdang, G.: Pharmacy's Part in Society, *op. cit.*, p. 39. The book offers a more detailed and pictorially documented (47 illustrations) study of the subject dealt with in this chapter.

Appendix 1: Representative Drugs of the American Indians

Different lists of drugs have been published on the basis of studies on different tribes of North American aborigines. The following list represents Indian drugs considered by Corlett to be "of special interest or of some distinctive value" that once gave them a place in the white man's books of official drugs. (Abstracted from Corlett, W. T.: The Medicine-Man of the American Indian, New York, 1935, p. 318)*:

ANGELICA (*Angelica atropurpurea* L.)
ARBOR VITAE (*Tuja occidentalis* L.)
BALM OF GILEAD (*Populus candicans* Ait.)
BEARBERRY (*Arctostaphylos Uva-ursi* [L.] Spreng.)
BETH ROOT (*Trillium* species)
BLACKBERRY (*Rubus nigrobaccus* Bailey)
BLACK CHERRY (*Prunus serotina* Ehrh.)
BLACK COHOSH (*Cimicifuga racemosa* L.)
BLOODROOT (*Sanguinaria canadensis* L.)
BLUE COHOSH (*Caulophyllum thalictroides* [L.] Michaux.)
BLUE FLAG (*Iris versicolor* L.)
BLUE VERVAIN (*Verbena hastata* L.)
BONESET (*Eupatorium perfoliatum* L.)
BUTTERNUT (*Juglans cineria* L.)
CARDINAL FLOWER (*Lobelia cardinalis* L.)
CASCARA SAGRADA (*Rhamnus Purshiana* DC.)
CORN SMUT (*Ustilago maydis* Jul.)
CRANESBILL (*Geranium maculatum* L.)
CULVER'S ROOT (*Veronica virginica* L.)
DANDELION (*Taraxacum officinale* Weber)
DOGBANE (*Apocynum androsaemifolium* L.)
ELDERBERRY (*Sambucus canadensis* L.)
FLOWERING DOGWOOD (*Cornus florida* L.)
GINSENG (*Panax quinquefolium* L.)

GOLD THREAD (*Coptis trifolia* Salisb.)
GOLDEN RAGWORT (*Senecio aureus* L.)
GREEN HELLEBORE (*Veratrum viride* L.)
GUM PLANT (*Grindelia squarrosa* [Pursh] Dunal)
JACK-IN-THE-PULPIT (*Arisaema triphyllum* [L.] Schott)
JALAP (*Exogonium Jalapa* [Nutt.et Coxe] Baillon)
JIMSON WEED (*Datura meteloides* DC.)
JOINT FIR (*Ephedra antisyphilitica* C.A. Mey)
JUNIPER (*Juniperus communis* L.)
MANDRAKE (*Podophyllum peltatum* L.)
MULLEN (*Verbascum thapsus* L.)
NEW JERSEY TEA (*Ceanothus americanus* L.)
PARTRIDGE BERRY (*Mitchella repens* L.)
PASQUE FLOWER (*Pulsatilla patens* [L-] Mill.)
PEYOTE (*Lophophora Williamsii* [Lem.] Coult.)
PLEURISY ROOT (*Asclepias tuberosa* L.)
POKE ROOT (*Phytolacca americana* L.)
PRICKLY ASH (*Zanthoxylum americanum* Mill.)
PRINCE'S PINE (*Chimaphila umbellata* [L.] Nutt.)
PUFFBALL (*Lycoperdon gemmatun* Batsch)
PUMPKIN (*Cucurbita Pepo* L.)
PURPLE CONE FLOWER (*Echinacea angustifolia* DC.)
RASPBERRY (*Rubus occidentalis* L. and R. *Strigosus* Michx.)
RED CEDAR (*Juniperus virginiana* L.)
RED ELDERBERRY (*Sambucus racemosa* L.)
SENECA SNAKEROOT (*Polygala Senega* L.)
SLIPPERY ELM (*Ulmus fulva* Michx.)
SMOOTH SUMAC (*Rhus glabra* L.)
SOLOMON'S SEAL (*Polygonatum biflorum* [Walt] Ell.)
SOUR DOCK (*Rumex crispus* L.)
STAGHORN SUMAC (*Rhus typina* L.)
SWEET FLAG (*Acorus Calamus* L.)
TOBACCO (*Nicotiana quadrivalvis* Pursh.)
VIBURNUM—MAPLE-LEAVED (*Viburnum Acerifolium* L.)
VIRGINIA SNAKEROOT (*Aristolochia Serpentaria* L.)
WAHOO (*Euonymus atropurpurea* Jacq.)

* Among other lists, the one in the following report holds particular interest because of the scientific methods of compilation and of testing for physiologic activity of some drugs thus identified: Train, Percy, *et al.*: Contributions Toward a Flora of Nevada; No. 45—Medicinal Uses of Plants by Indian Tribes of Nevada, rev. ed., with summary of pharmacologic research, by W. Andrew Archer. Herbarium, U. S. National Arboretum, Washington 25, D. C., 1957.

WILD LICORICE (*Glycyrrhiza Pepidota* Pursh.)
WHITE OAK (*Quercus alba* L.)
WHITE PINE (*Pinus Strobus* L.)
WILD BERGAMOT (*Monarda fistulosa* L.)
WILD CHERRY (*Prunus Virginiana* L.)
WILD INDIGO (*Baptisin leucantha* T. and G.)

WILD MINT (*Mentha arvensis* L.)
WINTERGREEN (*Gaultheria procumbens* L.)
WITCH HAZEL (*Hamamelis virginiana* L.)
YARROW (*Achillea millefolium* L.)
YELLOW DOCK (*Rumex crispus* L.)
YERBA SANTA (*Eriodictyon glutinosum* Benth.)

Appendix 2: Founding of State Pharmaceutical Associations, U.S.A.

1867 Maine	1882 Nebraska
1869 California	1883 Maryland
1870 New Jersey	1883 Mississippi (reorganized)
1870 West Virginia	1883 Minnesota
1870 Vermont	1883 Michigan (reorganized)
1871 Mississippi	1883 Arkansas
1873 Tennessee	1885 North Dakota
1874 New Hampshire	1886 Tennessee (reorganized)
1874 Michigan	1886 South Dakota
1874 Rhode Island	1887 Delaware
1875 Georgia	1887 Florida
1876 South Carolina*	1887 Idaho
1876 Connecticut	1890 Washington
1877 Kentucky	1890 Oregon
1878 Pennsylvania	1890 Maine (reorganized)
1879 Texas	1890 Oklahoma Territory†
1879 New York	1890 Colorado
1879 Ohio	1891 Montana
1879 Missouri	1891 Mississippi (2nd reorganization)
1880 Iowa	1892 Utah
1880 Kansas	1893 New Mexico
1880 Wisconsin	1895 Indian Territory†
1880 North Carolina	1902 Mississippi (3rd reorganization)
1880 Illinois	1904 Florida (reorganized)
1881 West Virginia (reorganized)	1905 Idaho (reorganized)
1881 Alabama	1906 West Virginia (2nd reorganization)
1882 Virginia	1907 Oklahoma State†
1882 Louisiana	1910 Arizona
1882 Indiana	1915 Wyoming
1882 Massachusetts	1932 Nevada

* There is a notice in the Amer. J. Pharm, 44: 425, 1872, "That a pharmaceutical association in South Carolina is about being organized." However, there is no mention of the activity of such an association anywhere until March, 1876, the date of the incorporation.

† When, in 1907, the Territory of Oklahoma and the Indian Territory were formed into the State of Oklahoma, the respective pharmaceutical associations were merged into the Oklahoma Pharmaceutical Association.

Appendix 3:   Passage of State and Territory Pharmacy Laws, U. S. A.

"Pharmacy Law" here refers to the statutory establishment of some qualifications for the practice of pharmacy and to the limiting of that practice to such qualified practitioners. *In many states legislation pertaining to poisons, abortifacients and adulteration preceded the statutes listed by many years.*

The list below is the Kremers and Urdang list (ed. 2, p. 276) with corrections and additions from subsequent research by David L. Cowen. Concerted study of this statutory history would likely reveal the need for still further revision.

The date in square brackets is the year in which earlier legislation, still technically in effect, was superseded by a "modern" pharmacy law.

1808 Territory of Orleans (Louisiana)
1816 Louisiana, repealed 1852; new law, 1872
1817 South Carolina [1876]
1825 Georgia [1881]
1832 New York, for New York City; 1869 for State; 1871 for New York City; 1879 for Kings County; 1884 for Erie County; 1884 for all other counties; 1900 for State
1844 Mississippi, for Adams County; 1892 for State
1851 Kentucky, for Louisville; 1874 for State
1852 Alabama [1887]
1866 Pennsylvania, for Lycoming County; 1872 for Philadelphia; 1887 for State
1870 Maryland, for Baltimore; 1902 for State except Talbot County; 1906 for Talbot County; 1908 for State
1870 Rhode Island
1872 Florida
1872 California, for San Francisco; 1891 for State

The asterisks denote passage of the original statute by the territorial government.

1873 Ohio, for Cincinnati; 1884 for State
1873 Missouri, for St. Louis; 1881 for State
1875 New Hampshire
1876 Wisconsin, for Milwaukee; 1882 for State
1877 New Jersey
1877 Maine
1878 District of Columbia
1880 Iowa
1881 Connecticut
1881 Illinois
1881 North Carolina
1881 West Virginia
1883 Delaware
1885 Michigan
1885 Minnesota
1885 Massachusetts
1885 Kansas
1886 Virginia
1886 Wyoming*
1887 Idaho*
1887 Dakota Territory
1887 Nebraska
1887 Colorado
1889 New Mexico*
1889 Texas
1890 South Dakota
1891 North Dakota
1891 Arkansas
1891 Oregon
1891 Oklahoma Territory
1891 Washington
1892 Utah*
1893 Tennessee
1894 Vermont
1895 Montana
1899 Indiana
1901 Nevada
1902 Puerto Rico [1906]
1903 Arizona*
1903 Hawaii*
1904 Indian Territory
1909 Oklahoma
1913 Alaska*

Appendix 4:   Schools of Pharmacy in the United States*

INCLUDING SOME OF THE BETTER KNOWN EXTINCT SCHOOLS AND ARRANGED BY DATE OF ORGANIZATION

1821 Philadelphia College of Pharmacy and Science, Philadelphia, Pa. (called Philadelphia College of Pharmacy, 1822-1920.)

1829 Columbia University, New York, N. Y. (started as the College of Pharmacy of the City and County of New York, which became affiliated with Columbia University in 1904.)

1838 Tulane University of Louisiana, New Orleans, La.†

1840 University of Maryland, Baltimore, Md. (started as Maryland College of Pharmacy, which became a part of the state university in 1920.)

1859 University of Illinois, Chicago, Ill. (started as Chicago College of Pharmacy, which became affiliated with the University of Illinois in 1896.)

1865 St. Louis College of Pharmacy, St. Louis, Mo.

1865 Baldwin University, Berea, Ohio.†

1866 Medical College of the State of South Carolina. Charleston, S. C.‡ (a few occasional pharmacy graduates beginning 1867; separate pharmacy department 1882-84; reorganized as present School of Pharmacy 1894.)

1866 Medical College of Alabama, Birmingham, Ala.†

1867 Massachusetts College of Pharmacy (Between the founding of the College [association] in 1823 and the founding of the

present school, short lecture courses were given occasionally.)

1868 University of Michigan, Ann Arbor, Mich.‡

1868 Howard University, Washington, D. C.

1870 University of Kentucky, Louisville, Ky. (started as Louisville College of Pharmacy, which became a part of the University of Kentucky in 1947.)

1871 University of Cincinnati, Cincinnati, Ohio (started as the Cincinnati College of Pharmacy in 1850, which sometimes organized instructional discussion groups; the College's regular school, f. 1871, affiliated with the University in 1945.)

1872 University of California, San Francisco, Calif. (started as California College of Pharmacy, which became affiliated with the University of California in 1872, and a part of the latter in 1934.)

1872 George Washington University, Washington, D. C. (started as National College of Pharmacy, which became affiliated with the George Washington University in 1906; to be discontinued 1964.)

1873 Tennessee College of Pharmacy, Nashville, Tenn.†

1878 University of Pittsburgh, Pittsburgh, Pa. (started as Pittsburgh College of Pharmacy, which became affiliated with the University of Pittsburgh in 1896, and a part of the latter in 1947.)

1879 Vanderbilt University, Nashville, Tenn.†

1881 Union University, Albany College of Pharmacy, Albany, N. Y.

1882 Western Reserve University, Cleveland, Ohio.† (started as Cleveland School of Pharmacy, which became affiliated with Western Reserve University in 1908 and a part of the latter in 1918; discontinued in 1949.)

1882 Iowa College of Pharmacy, Des Moines, Iowa (affiliated with Drake University in 1886.)†

---

* Dates are intended to represent when organization was completed or instruction begun at the school in its *original* form (but consistent precision is difficult in a concise tabulation that involves so many mergers, suspensions and ambiguous records.)

† Discontinued school. A great many extinct schools are not listed.

‡ College (or school) of pharmacy established as part of state institution (universities or colleges) before 1900.

1883 University of Wisconsin, Madison, Wis.‡
1884 Purdue University, Lafayette, Ind.‡
1884 Ohio Northern University, Ada, Ohio (formerly Ohio Normal University.)
1885 University of Iowa, Iowa City, Iowa.‡
1885 Ohio State University, Columbus, Ohio.‡
1885 University of Kansas, Lawrence, Kansas.‡
1885 University of Kansas City, Kansas City, Mo. (started as Kansas City College of Pharmacy.)
1886 Northwestern University, Chicago, Ill.† (The College of Pharmacy was merged with the University of Illinois College of Pharmacy in 1917.)
1886 State University of New York at Buffalo (formerly University of Buffalo), Buffalo, N. Y.
1886 Minnesota Institute of Pharmacy, Minneapolis, Minn.†
1887 Scio College, Scio, Ohio.† (amalgamated with Pittsburgh College of Pharmacy in 1908.)
1888 South Dakota State College, Brookings, S. Dak.‡
1889 Walden University (Meharry Pharmaceutical College), Nashville, Tenn.†
1890 Detroit Institute of Technology, Detroit, Mich. (started as a Department of the Detroit College of Medicine; independent 1905 to 1907; then part of the Detroit Institute of Technology.)†
1890 Highland Park College; from 1920 to 1927, Des Moines University, Des Moines, Iowa.† (See also Drake University, 1927.)
1891 Brooklyn College of Pharmacy, Brooklyn, N. Y. (since 1929 affiliated with Long Island University.)
1891 Ohio Medical University, Columbus, Ohio.†
1891 College of Physicians and Surgeons, Atlanta, Ga.†
1891 Shaw University, Leonard Schools of Medicine and Pharmacy, Raleigh, N. C.†
1892 Valparaiso University, Valparaiso, Ind.† (started as Northern Indiana School of Pharmacy, a Department of the Normal School and Business Institute of Valparaiso, which became Valparaiso University in 1906.)
1892 Rutgers, The State University of New Jersey, College of Pharmacy located at

Newark, N.J. (started as New Jersey College of Pharmacy, which became a part of Rutgers University in 1927.)
1892 University of Minnesota, Minneapolis, Minn.‡
1892 Louisville College of Pharmacy for Women, Louisville, Ky.†
1893 Ferris Institute, Big Rapids, Mich.
1893 State University of Oklahoma, Norman, Okla.‡
1893 University College of Medicine, Richmond, Va. (absorbed 1913 by Med. Coll. Va.)
1893 University of Texas, Austin, Tex.‡
1894 University of Maine, Orono, Maine.†
1894 University of Washington, Seattle, Wash.‡
1895 Auburn University (formerly Alabama Polytechnic Institute), Auburn, Ala.‡
1896 Washington State University, Pullman, Wash.‡ (previously called State College of Washington, and, before 1905, The Agricultural College.)
1897 Medical College of Virginia, Richmond, Va. (From about 1876 on, medical students with certain pharmaceutical training were graduated in pharmacy. Absorbed in 1913 the pharmacy department of the University College of Medicine.)
1897 University of North Carolina, Chapel Hill, N. C.‡ (a pharmacy school existed from 1880 to 1886; revived in 1889, and again discontinued.)
1897 University of Notre Dame, Notre Dame, Ind.†
1898 Medico Chirurgical College of Philadelphia, Philadelphia, Pa.† (When, in 1916, the College and the University of Pennsylvania were consolidated, the department of pharmacy and chemistry of the College merged with the Philadelphia College of Pharmacy.)
1898 University of Tennessee, Memphis, Tenn.‡ (teaching started at Knoxville and came to Memphis in 1911.)
1898 College of Physicians and Surgeons, San Francisco, Calif.†
1898 Oregon State University [formerly College], Corvallis, Ore. (previously Oregon Agricultural College.)‡
1900 Marquette University, Milwaukee, Wis.† (founded as department of Wisconsin Medical College, with precursor in private tutorial school; affiliated with Marquette 1907.)
1900 Keokuk Medical College, Keokuk, Iowa.†
1900 Creighton University, Omaha, Nebr.

---

† Discontinued school.
‡ College (or school) of pharmacy established as part of state institution (universities or colleges) before 1900.

(started as a Department in the Fremont Normal School, which became a part of Creighton University in 1905.)

1900 Loyola University, New Orleans, La. (started as the New Orleans College of Pharmacy, which became affiliated with Loyola University, in 1913, and became part of the latter in 1919.)

1901 Baylor University, Dallas, Tex.† (originally part of the University of Dallas; taken over by Baylor University in 1905.)

1901 Temple University, Philadelphia, Pa.

1901 Illinois Medical College, Chicago, Ill.†

1902 North Dakota State University (formerly N. D. Agricultural College), Fargo, N. D. (organized as a Department of Chemistry and Pharmacy; a separate School of Pharmacy since 1919.)

1902 Tristate Normal School, Angola, Ind.†

1902 Rhode Island College of Pharmacy and Allied Sciences, Providence, R. I.;† see also 1957.

1903 Mercer University, Macon, Ga.†

1903 Southern College of Pharmacy, Atlanta, Ga.; now affiliated with Mercer University.

1903 University of Georgia, Athens, Ga.

1904 Butler University, Indianapolis, Ind. (started as Indianapolis College of Pharmacy, which became a part of Butler University in 1946.)

1904 University of Toledo, Toledo, Ohio.

1905 University of Southern California, Los Angeles, Calif. (the College became an integral part of the University in 1922.)

1907 Montana State University, Missoula, Mont.

1908 University of Mississippi, University, Miss.

1908 University of Nebraska, Lincoln, Nebr.

1908 North Pacific College of Oregon, Portland, Oreg.†

1911 University of the Philippines, Manila, P. I. (the Philippines received their independence in 1945.)

1911 University of Colorado, Boulder, Colo.

1911 Fordham University, New York, N. Y.

1913 University of Puerto Rico, Rio Piedras, P. R.

1914 West Virginia University, Morgantown, W. Va.

1918 The Idaho State College, Pocatello, Idaho (before 1947, University of Idaho, South Branch.)

1923 Wayne University, Detroit, Mich. (until 1933 named College of the City of Detroit.)

1923 University of Florida, Gainesville, Fla.

1924 University of South Carolina, Columbia, S. C. (Earlier attempts at establishing pharmaceutical instruction were active from 1866 to 1877 and from 1884 to 1891.)

1925 Duquesne University, Pittsburgh, Pa.

1925 University of Connecticut, New Haven, Conn. (started as Connecticut College of Pharmacy, which became a part of the University of Connecticut in 1941.)

1927 Northeastern University (established as Meriano School of Pharmacy; incorporated 1940 as Boston School of Pharmacy; in 1949 re-named New England College of Pharmacy; in 1962 absorbed by the University.)

1927 Xavier University, New Orleans, La.

1927 Drake University, Des Moines, Iowa (started as Des Moines College of Pharmacy, 1927-1939; then became a part of Drake University; see also: 1882: Iowa College of Pharmacy and 1890: Highland Park College.)

1929 St. John's University, Brooklyn, N. Y.

1932 Howard College, Birmingham, Ala.

1936 University of Grand Rapids, Grand Rapids, Mich.†

1939 Western Massachusetts School of Pharmacy, Willimansett, Mass.

1941 Southwestern State College, Weatherford, Okla. (formerly Southwestern Institute of Technology.)

1945 University of New Mexico, Albuquerque, N. Mex.

1945 College of the Ozarks, Clarksville, Ark.; see also 1951.

1946 University of Utah, Salt Lake City, Utah.

1946 University of Wyoming, Laramie, Wy.

1947 University of Arizona, Tucson, Ariz.

1947 University of Houston, Houston, Tex.

1949 Texas Southern University, Houston, Tex.

1951 University of Arkansas, Little Rock, Ark. (successor to College of Ozarks, f. 1945.)

1951 Florida A and M University, Tallahassee (called College until 1953.)

1955 University [formerly College] of the Pacific, Stockton, Calif.

1956 Northeast Louisiana State College, Monroe, La.

1957 University of Rhode Island, Kingston, R. I. (successor to Rhode Island College of Pharmacy, f. 1902.)

---

† Discontinued.

Appendix 5: International List of Pharmacy Museums

Compiled by George B. Griffenhagen

The artifacts of pharmacy provide a kind of historical information not otherwise available; in design and ornamentation they often rise to a level that gives artistic expression to a segment of everyday life. This accounts for the rather remarkable number of pharmacy museums and collections that have been placed on public display.

In the following bibliography we note the public and the outstanding private museum collections, representing mainly Europe and the Americas from the 16th through the 19th century. The arrangement is alphabetic by countries (and within the United States, alphabetic by states). References to published information are added wherever known. The list, which includes only collections open to public inspection and described in print, is intended as a guide for students, historians and travelers who may wish to see these survivals from pharmacy's past or to obtain information about them. It has not been practicable to list all collected pharmaceutico-historical artifacts, some of which may be found in nearly all historical museums and pharmacy schools and in many pharmacies.

The development of pharmacy museums and the various types of museums have been discussed by George Griffenhagen in his booklet, *Pharmacy Museums* (Madison, Wisconsin, 1956). Since this publication has gone out of print, its bibliographic guide has been revised and brought up to date as a supplement to the present volume.

AUSTRIA

For general references to pharmacy museum collections in Austria, see Ganzinger, Kurt, Apotheken-Altertümer in Österreich, Internationale Gesellschaft für Geschichte der Pharmazie, 1951.

Graz: Landesmuseum. Pharmacy restoration. Ganzinger, l.c.*

Innsbruck: Winkler Stadtapotheke. Private collection. Winkler's Stadtapotheke zu Innsbruck, Gesellschaft für Geschichte der Pharmazie, 1928; Chemist and Druggist *102*: 977, 1925; Apotheker-Kalender, 1935; Ganzinger, l.c.

Linz: Landesmuseum. Pharmacy restoration. Die Vorträge der Jubiläums Hauptversammlung in Salzburg, Internationale Gesellschaft für Geschichte der Pharmazie, 1951.

Salzburg: Hausapotheke des Benediktiner-Frauenstiftes Nonnberg. Österreichische Apotheker Zeitung 4:458, 1950; 9:759, 1955.

Vienna: Technisches Museum. Pharmacy restoration, alchemical laboratory. The Laboratory *21* (No. 1):2, 1951; Die Alte Apotheke, Paul Hartmann AG, Heidenheim/Brenz, 1954; Ganzinger, l.c.; Apotheker-Kalender 1956 (Sept. 1-10).

Vienna: Bildarchiv der Österreichischen National Bibliotek, Pharmacy manuscripts, illustrations, etc. Österreichische Apotheker Zeitung 9:759, 1955.

Vienna: St. Elisabeth Hospital, 18th century pharmacy. Zeckert, Otto: Kunst in Medizin und Pharmazie (Vienna, 1955, pp. 55-56); FIP Program, 1962, p. 126.

Vienna: Barmherzigen Brüder Apotheke, Zeckert, Otto: Kunst in Medicine und Pharmazie (Vienna, 1955, pp. 40-43).

BELGIUM

For general reference to pharmacy museum collections in Belgium, see Segers, E. G., and

---

* To conserve space, only the last name of an author and "l.c." (*loco citato*) appears in this Appendix when a publication, once previously cited in full, is referred to subsequently in connection with another museum here listed.

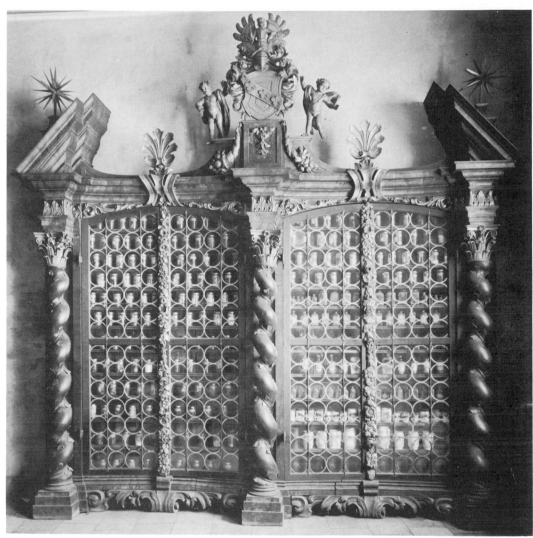

This unusually elegant drug cabinet, now prized as a museum piece, was used by the Star Pharmacy in the 18th century. The body of the cabinet (about 13 by 13 feet) has been marbled with gray oil-color. The serpentine columns are jet black, entwined by golden ivy. Heavily ornamented capitals and symbolic stars, above the elements of a pediment, glitter in gold. Above the central column, flanked by two cherubs, is the colorful coat of arms of the pharmacy's owner. (Photograph from the Germanischen Museum, Nuremberg, in Kremers Reference Files, Madison, Wis.)

Wittop Koning, D. A.: Apothicaireries anciennes en Benelux, Deventer, Holland, 1958; and various numbers of the Bulletin du Cercle Benelux d'Histoire de la Pharmacie.

Antwerp: Musée du Folklore. Pharmacy and laboratory restoration. Catalogue du Musée de la Vieille Boucherie, No. 815-17; Segers and Wittop Koning, l.c.

Assche: Hôpital d'Assche. Ancient pharmacy. Wittop-Koning, Delftse Apothekerspotten, Deventer, 1954; Segers and Wittop-Koning, l.c.

Bruges: St. Jans Hospital. Ancient pharmacy. van Eyck, Jef: Wat wee og over den Apotheker, 1944; Bulletin du Cercle Benelux d'Histoire de la Pharmacie No. 8, 15 (April

1954); Segers and Wittop-Koning, l.c.; Prescriber (Sept., 1956).

Brussels: Musée de Cinquantenaire. Pharmacy restoration. Chompret, J.: Les Faiences Francaises Primitives, Paris, 1946; Wittop-Koning, D. A.: Delftse Apothekerspotten, Deventer, 1954; Bulletin du Cercle Benelux d'Histoire de la Pharmacie No. 3, 19 (Aug. 1952); Pro Medico 13:17, 1936; Segers and Wittop-Koning, l.c.; Prescriber (Sept. 1956).

Doornik (Tournai): Musée de la Maison Tournaisienne. Pharmacy restoration. Segers and Wittop-Koning, l.c.

Ghent: Museum of Folklore. Pharmacy restoration. Pharmaceutisch Tijdschrift voor Belgie 28:42, 1951; Vandewiele, L. J.: Inventaris der Apothekerspotten van het Museum voor Folklore te Gent; Bulletin du Cercle Benelux d'Histoire de la Pharmacie No. 1, 6 (June 1951); Oostvlaamse Zanten, 49:1951; Segers and Wittop-Koning, l.c.

Louvain: Pharmaceutical Institute. University of Louvain, Couvreur collection. Bulletin du Cercle Benelux d'Histoire de la Pharmacie No. 3, 19 (Aug. 1952); Segers and Wittop-Koning, l.c.

Malines: Musée Ville de Malines. Pharmacy restoration. Van Doorselaer: L'Ancienne Industrie du Cuivre a'Malines, 4 vols.; Catalogue de l'Exposition, Brussels, 1954; Segers and Wittop-Koning, l.c.*

Orval: Pharmacie de l'Abbaye l'Orval. Ancient pharmacy. Pro Medico 6:88, 1929; Annales Merck, 13 (1935); Segers and Wittop-Koning, l.c.

BRAZIL

Rio de Janeiro: Pharmacy Museum, Brazilian Pharmaceutical Assoc. Alfonzo, R. G., The Journal (Michigan) 39:30 (May 1951).

CZECHOSLOVAKIA

Bratislava: Pharmacy museum. Zur Geschichte der Pharmazie 13, No. 2 (1962).

Brno: Pharmacy collection, at Augustinian monastery (accessible basement storage). Prague as the Pharmaceutical Museum of Charles University.

Prague: Technical museum. Alchemical laboratory restoration. Sarton, George: A Guide to the History of Science, Waltham, Mass., 1952.

DENMARK

For general references to pharmacy museum collections in Denmark, see Andersen, Dannesboe, Gammelt Dansk Apotheksinventar, Copenhagen, 1944, with English supplement entitled Antique Furniture from Danish Prescription Pharmacies.

Aarhaus: "Den gamle By." Pharmacy restoration. Andersen, l.c.; Købstadmuseet "Den Gamle By," Aarbog 16 (1942); 47 (1945); 31 (1949); Chem. & Drug. 167:274 (1957).

Copenhagen: Medicinsk-Histoirske Museum. Pharmacy restoration and collections. Københavns Universitets Medicinsk-Histoirske Museum, Annual Reports, 1952-54; Medicine Illustrated 3:134, 1949; München. med. Wchnschr. 81:1436, 1934; Anderson, l.c.; Medicinsk Forum 3:193, 1950; Archiv for Pharmaci og Chemi 102:653, 1945; 103:715, 1946.

Copenhagen: Nationalmuseet. Majolica. Andersen, l.c.

FINLAND

Helsinki: Pharmacy museum. Majolica and pharmacy material. Chem. & Drug. 102:964, 1925; Zur Geschichte der Pharmazie 10 (No. 4), 1958.

Helsinki: Stads museum. Pharmacy restoration, period 1700. Karsten, Walter, Farmacins Historia Finland, Helsingfors, 1933.

FRANCE

For general references to pharmacy museum collections in France, see Chem. & Drug. 72: 157, 1908; 102:964, 1925; Bulletin de la Société d'Histoire de la Pharmacie, 1913-1929; Rev. Histoire Pharm. 1930-1955; Am. Drug. 67:27, (Nov. 1919); Chompret, J.: Les Faiences Francaises Primitives, Paris, 1946 (includes a list of 79 hospital pharmacies possessing faience); Boussel, Patrice: Histoire Illustrée de la Pharmacie, Paris, 1949; "Apothicaireries de France," La Libre Pharmacie, Special No. (December 1961).

Angers: Hôtel-Dieu. Ancient pharmacy. Chem. & Drug. 102:968, 1925; Chompret, l.c.; La Libre Pharmacie, l.c.

Arles: Hospital. Ancient pharmacy. Chompret, l.c.

Bauge: Hôtel-Dieu. 17th century pharmacy. Chompret, l.c.; La Libre Pharmacie, l.c.

Bayeux: Public museum. Faience. Chem. & Drug. 102:968, 1925.

Bazas: Hôpital. Ancient pharmacy. Rev. Histoire Pharm. 41:178, 1953.

Besançon: Hôpital St. Jaques. Louis XIV pharmacy. Chem. & Drug. *102*:968, 1925; Chompret, l.c.; Boussel, l.c.; La Libre Pharmacie, l.c.

Carpentras: Hôtel-Dieu. 18th century pharmacy, Chompret, l.c.

Castres: Musée Goya. Faience. Rev. Histoire Pharm. *43*:184, 1955.

Chantilly: Hôtel-Dieu. Ancient pharmacy. Guides touristiques, through Guitard, E. H., personal correspondence, Dec. 7, 1955.

Dijon: Hospital. Ancient pharmacy. Chem. & Drug. *102*:968, 1925; La Libre Pharmacie, l.c.

Gayette: Hospital. Ancient pharmacy. Chompret, l.c.

Issoudun: Hôtel-Dieu. 17th century pharmacy. La Presse Medicale 57:32, 1949 (Jan. 5); Rev. Histoire Pharm. *38*:10, 1950; Robert, Louis: l'Ancienne Pharmacie de l'Hôpital d'Issoudun, 1950; Chompret, l.c.; La Libre Pharmacie, l.c.

Limoges: Musée de la porcelaine. Faience. Catalogues, through Guitard, E. H., personal correspondence, Dec. 7, 1955.

Louhans: Hôtel-Dieu. 17th century pharmacy. Chem. & Drug. *102*:968, 1925; Chompret, l.c.; La Libre Pharmacie, l.c.; Prescriber (Sept. 1956).

Lyon: Hôpital de la Charité. Ancient pharmacy. Chompret, l.c.; Bull. Soc. Histoire Pharm. No. 48, p. 129, 1925; La Libre Pharmacie, l.c.

Lyon: Bibliothéque et Musée d'Histoire de la Médecine, University of Lyon, Pharmacy material. Sarton, l.c.

Mans: Hôtel-Dieu. Ancient pharmacy. Bull. Soc. Histoire Pharm. No. 25, 159, 168, 1920.

Marseille: Hôpital de la Charité. Ancient pharmacy. Boussel, l.c.

Montpellier: Musée de la Société Archéologique. Faience. Chompret, l.c.

Nancy: Musée Historique Lorrain. 18th century pharmacy restoration, pharmacy material. Niklewski, Stefan: Biuletynu Farmaceutycznego 3:118, 1948.

Narbonne: Hospital. 16th century pharmacy. Chem. & Drug. *102*:968, 1925; Chompret, l.c.

Paris: Musée d'Histoire de la Pharmacie, 4 Avenue de l'Observatoire. Henri Fialon faience collection and other pharmacy material. Bull. Soc. Histoire Pharm. No. 14, p. 240, 1916; No. 16, p. 279, 1917; No. 18, p. 313, 1917; No. 20, p. 369, 1918; Am. Drug. 67:27, 1919 (Nov.); 69:46, 1921 (April), 74.12, 1920 (March); Chem. &

Drug. *102*:964, 1925; Rev. Histoire Pharm. 36:277, 1948; J. A. Pharm. A. (Pract.) *16*: 600, 1955.

Paris: Musée de l'Assistance Publique et de la Pharmacie Centrale des Hôpitaux. Faience. Chem. & Drug. 72:157, 1908; Am. Drug. 67:27, 1919 (Nov.); *102*:968, 1925; 74:10, 1926 (March); La Presse Médicale 57:19 (Jan. 5) 1949; Boussel, l.c.; Lothian, Agnes: "Pharmacy Jars," The Concise Encyclopedia of Antiques, Vol. II, Connoisseur, London, 1955.

Paris: Musée du Louvre. Faience. Bulletin de la Société d'Histoire de la Pharmacie, No. 56, p. 453, 1927; Am. Drug. 67:27, 1919 (Nov.); 72:12, 1924 (Sept.); 74:11, 1926 (March); Chem. & Drug. *102*:964, 1925; Chompret, l.c.

Paris: Musée de Sèvres. Faience. Bulletin de la Société d'Histoire de la Pharmacie, No. (1927); Chem. & Drug. *102*:964, 1925; Am. Drug. 75:15 (Feb.) 1927; Chompret, l.c.; Boussel, l.c.; Rev. Histoire Pharm. *41*:147, 1953.

Paris: Musée de Cluny. Faience. Chem. & Drug. 72:157, 1908; *102*:968, 1925; Am. Drug. 67:27, 1919 (Nov.); 72:13, 1924 (Sept.); Chompret, l.c.

Pont-Saint-Esprit: Grand Hospital. Ancient pharmacy. Chompret, l.c.

Rouen: Musée de l'Hôtel-Dieu. Ancient pharmacy. Rev. Histoire Pharm. *38*:91, 1950.

Rouen: Musée céramique. Faience. Catalogues, through Guitard, E. H., personal correspondence, Dec. 7, 1955.

Saint-Denis: Hôtel-Dieu. Ancient pharmacy. Bull. Soc. Histoire Pharm. No. 35, p. 65, 1922; No. 43, p. 377, 1924; Am. Drug. 74: 10, March, 1926.

Saint-Germain-en-Laye: Hospital. Ancient pharmacy. Savare, Paule, l'Apothicairerie Royale de Saint-Germain-en-Laye, Paris, n.d.; Boussel, l.c.; Chem. & Drug. *102*:968, 1925; Am. Drug. 74:12, March, 1926; Rev. Histoire Pharm. *34*:84, 1946; La Libre Pharmacie, l.c.

Saint-Malo: Hôtel-Dieu. Ancient pharmacy. Bull. Soc. Histoire Pharm. 97:122 (No. 24) 1919; 97:129 (No. 48) 1925; LeMarie, B., Contribution à l'Histoire de la Pharmacie dans la Bretagne Septentrionale, Rennes, 1946.

Tarascon: Hospital of St. Nicholas. Ancient pharmacy. Chem. & Drug. *102*:968, 1925.

Toulouse: Musée Paul-Dupuy. Bull. Soc. Histoire Pharm. No. 20, p. 392, 1918.

Tournus: Hôtel-Dieu. Ancient pharmacy.

Chem. & Drug. *102*:968, 1925; Bull. Soc. Histoire Pharm. No. 40, p. 277, 1923; La Libre Pharmacie, l.c.

Troyes: Hôtel-Dieu. 18th century pharmacy. Chompret, l.c.; Bull. Soc. Histoire Pharm. No. 43, p. 377, 1924; Pinsolle, S., Contribution à l'Histoire de la Pharmacie en Champagne, La Garenne, 1937; La Libre Pharmacie, l.c.

Versailles: Hôtel-Dieu. Ancient pharmacy. Am. Drug. *74*:11, March, 1926; Rev. Histoire Pharm. *26*:436, 1938.

Villefranche-Sur-Saune: 18th century pharmacy. La Libre Pharmacie, l.c.

Yssingeaux: Hospital. 16th century pharmacy. Chompret, l.c.

GERMANY

For general references to pharmacy museum collections in Germany, see Apotheker—Kalender (July 1, 1932) and subsequent editions; the Apotheker-Zeitung *41*:1276, 1926; Pharm. Zeitung *81*:1287, 1936; Gesch. Deutschen Apotheke, No. 6/7 (April/May) 1937; Hein, Wolfgang-Hagen, Apotheken-Kostbarkeiten in Bayern, 1954; "Oeffentliche und private pharmaziegeschichtliche Sammlungen in Deutschland", a series commencing in Zur Geschichte der Pharmazie (Beilage to the Deutschen Apotheker Zeitung), hereafter cited as "Gesch. Pharm.," No. 3, p. 21 (1955).

Aachen: Couven-Museum. Pharmacy museum. Felix Kuetgens, Das Couven-Museum in Aachen, Neuss, 1959.

Braunschweig: Vaterländisches Museum. Pharmacy restoration. Pharm. Zeitung *52*: 151 (1907); Gesch. Deutschen Apotheke, No. 6/7 (April/May) 1937.

Bremen: Focke-Museum. Pharmacy restoration. Gesch. Pharmazie, No. 3, p. 21, 1955.

Darmstadt: Hessisches Landes-Museum. Pharmacy restoration. Apotheker - Kalender (1925); Gesch. Deutschen Apotheke, No. 6/7 (April/May) 1937.

Eisenach: Thüringer Museum. Pharmacy material. Apotheker-Kalender (Dec., 1933); Pharm. Zeitung 79:1085, 1934; Fiek, Wolfgang: Die pharmaziegeschichtliche Sammlung im Thüringer Museum zu Eisenach, Gesellsch. Gesch. Pharmazie, Mittenwald, n.d.

Goslar: Goslarer Museum. Pharmacy and laboratory restoration. Gesch. Pharmazie, No. 3, p. 21, 1955.

Heidelberg: Heinrici and Ferchl collections,

among others. Gesch. Deutschen Apotheke No. 8, June, 1935; No. 9, July, 1935; No. 10, Aug., 1935; No. 11, Sept., 1935; No. 10/11, Aug./Sept., 1936; No. 2, Dec. 1937; No. 1/6, Jan./June, 1939; Deutsche Apotheker-Zeitung *91*:495, 1951; Neue Apotheken-Illustrierte No. 2, Feb., 1954; Die Alte Apotheke, Paul Hartmann AG, Heidenheim/ Brenz, 1954; Am. J. Pharm. Ed. *14*:577, 1950; J.A.Ph.A. (Pract. Ed.) *16*:600, 1955; Gesch. Pharm., vol. 9, No. 3, 1957; Deutsch. Apoth. Ztg. *95*:751, 1957; Schweiz. Apoth. Ztg. *95*:846, 1957; Führer durch das Deutsche Apothekenmuseum im Heidelberg (Frankfurt, 1959); Ibid., (ed. 2), (1962); Apotheker und Kunst, No. 7, p. 27, 1959; Pharm. Zeitung *105*:1421, 1960.

Heidelberg: Kurpfälzisches Museum. Pharmacy material. Pharm. Zeitung *91*:647, 1955; Deutsche Apotheker Zeitung *95*:547, 592, 1955.

Munich: Deutsches Museum. Pharmacy and laboratory restoration. Bol. Assoc. Brasil Pharm. *11*:25, 1930; Am. Drug. 87:44, Feb., 1933; Apotheker-Kalender (June 23-July 6, 1935); Gesch. Deutschen Apotheke, No. 6/7 (April/May) 1937; Hein, l.c.; Gesch. Pharm. vol. 9, No. 2, 1957.

Nuremberg: Germanisches Nationalmuseum. Pharmacy restoration. Peters, Hermann, Pharm. Zeitung *41*:183, 1896; *42*:765, 775, 783, 1897; Chem. & Drug. *112*:819, 1930; Apotheker-Kalender (1936); Deutsche Apotheken-Altertümer, Germanisches Nationalmuseum, Nurnberg, 1936.

Ulm: Gewerbemuseum. Pharmacy material. Apotheker-Kalender (1925); Gesch. Deutschen Apotheke, No. 6/7 (April/May) 1937.

Waldenbuch: Uhland-Apotheke, Schwäbisches Apothekenmuseum. Walter Dörr collection. Sammlung Walter Dörr, Stuttgart, 1933; Süddeutsche Apotheker Zeitung 89:949, 1949; Apotheker-Kalender (June 1933); Dörr, Walter: Das Schwäbische Apotheken-Museum zu Waldenbuch, Stuttgart, 1933; Kostbarkeiten aus der Apotheke, Paul Hartmann AG, Heidenheim/Brenz, 1954; J.A.Ph.A. (Pract. Ed.) *16*:629, 1955.

GREAT BRITAIN

For general reference to pharmacy museum collections in London, see Chem. & Drug. *159*: 584, 1953.

Leeds: Kirkstall Abbey House Museum. Taylor and Mason pharmacy (chemist shop) restoration. Chem. & Drug. *164*:189, 1955; J.A.Ph.A. (Pract. Ed.) *16*:540, 1955.

London: Wellcome Historical Medical Museum, 183-193 Euston Road. Extensive pharmacy material: Henry S. Wellcome collection. Historical Exhibition of Rare and Curious Objects Relating to Medicine, Chemistry, Pharmacy and Allied Sciences, Wellcome, London, n.d.; J.A.Ph.A. *16*:161, 1927; *20*:238, 1931; Am. Drug. *82*:30, Dec., 1930; Pharm. Zeitung 79:214, 1934; Underwood, E. A.: Catalogue of an Exhibition Illustrating the History of Pharmacy (May 4-Sept. 28, 1951), London, 1951; Chem. & Drug. *159*:584, 1953; *164*:338, 373, 1955; J.A.Ph.A. (Pract. Ed.) *16*:662, 1955; *21*:86, 1960; Pharm. J. (4th ser.) *183*:129, 116, 1959; Chem. & Drug. 72:27, 1959; Brit. Med. J. *2*:253, 1959; J.A.Ph.A. (Pract. Ed.) *21*:86, 1960.

London: Pharmaceutical Society of Great Britain Museum, 17 Bloomsbury Sq., Lambeth delft collection. Holmes, E. M., Catalogue of the Collections in the Museum of the Pharmaceutical Society of Great Britain (Materia Medica), London, 1878; Chem. & Drug. *159*:584, 1953.

London: Victoria and Albert Museum, South Kensington. Majolica. Rackham, Bernard: Catalogue of Italian Majolica, London, 1940; Chem. & Drug. *159*:584, 1953; J.A.Ph.A. (Pract. Ed.) *16*:540, 1955.

London: Society of Apothecaries, Blackfriar Lane. Lambeth delft. Ann. Roy. Coll. Surgeons England 7:497, 1950.

London: British Museum. Ancient pharmacy material. Chem. & Drug. *106*:797, 1927.

London: London Museum. Lambeth delft. Chem. & Drug. *128*:755, 1938.

Oxford: Museum of History of Science. Pharmacy material. Chem. & Drug. *126*:747, 1937; *161*:666, 1951.

York: Castle Museum. Pharmacy (chemist shop) restoration. Lewis, A. B.: The Parish of York Castle, A Description of the Museum 'Street,' York, 1949; J.A.Ph.A. (Pract. Ed.) *16*:540, 1955; Prescriber, Sept. 1956.

HUNGARY

Budapest: National Technical Art Museum. Pharmacy restoration. Chem. & Drug. *112*:818, 1930; *102*:978, 1925; Apotheker-Kalender (Feb. 4-6, 1932); Bull. Soc. Histoire Pharm. *20*:136, 1932. Present status unknown.

Budapest: Iprarmuveszeti Muzeum. Majolica. Acta pharm. Hungarica, vol. 132, June, 1955.

ITALY

Faenza: Musée Ceramique de Faience. Castiglioni, Arturo, La Farmacia Italiana del Quattrocento nella storia dell'arte ceramica, Faenza, 1922; Chompret, l.c. (much destroyed by war but collection being rebuilt).

Florence: Museo di Storia della Scienza. Pharmacy material. Catalogo Degli Strumenti del Museo di Storia della Scienza, Firenze, 1954.

Florence: Antica Farmacia del canto alle Rondini. Die Vorträge der Hauptversammlung der Gesellschaft für Geschichte der Pharmazie, Basel, May 17-20, 1934.

Naples: Museo Nazionale di Napoli. Ancient pharmacy material. Tergolina, Umberto, La Farmacia, Rome, 1939.

Parma: Museo Nazionale. Restoration of pharmacy of S. Giovanni Evangelista. La storica farmacia di S. Giovanni Evangelista, 1951; J. Hist. Med. & Allied Sciences *11*:227, 1956.

Pavia: Museo di Storia della Farmacia. La Chimica, No. 8, 1943; Scienza e Lavoro, No. 7, 1949; La Teriaca *10*:3, April, 1954.

Rome: Accademia di Storia dell'Arte Sanitaria. Pharmacy restoration. Apotheker-Kalender (Sept. 11-13, 1932); Il Farmacista *2*:347, 1948; Tergolina, l.c.

Rome: Instituto di Storia della Medicina dell'Universita di Roma. Pharmacy material, alchemical laboratory, Humana Studa, vol. 7, Series II, 1955; Rivista Ospedaliera, No. 9-10, 1955.

Venice: Pharmacie Santa Fosca (Farmacia Ponci 1730) Bull. Soc. Histoire Pharm., No. 40, p. 277, 1923.

THE NETHERLANDS

For museum collections in The Netherlands, see various numbers of the Bulletin du Cercle Benelux d'Histoire de la Pharmacie; Wittop-Koning, D. A., Nederlandse Vijzels, Deventer, 1953; Wittop-Koning, D. A., Delft Drug-Jars, Deventer, 1956; Segers, E. G., and Wittop-Koning, D. A., De oude apotheek in de Benelux, Deventer, Holland, 1958.

Amersfoort: Museum Flehite, Pharmacy restoration. Wittop-Koning, D. A., Delft Drug-Jars, Deventer, 1956; Segers and Wittop-Koning, l.c.

Amsterdam: Medisch Pharmaceutisch Museum, Koestraat. Pharmacy and laboratory restoration; pharmacy material. Pharmaceutisch Weekblad 39:764, 1902; Bull. Soc. Histoire Pharm. No. 30, p. 349, 1921; Apotheker-Kalender (1929); Pharmaceutisch Weekblad 88:354, 710, 1953; The Laboratory 23:56, Dec. 1953; Endeavor 13:128, July, 1954; J.A.Ph.A. (Pract. Ed.) 16:600, 1955; Bulletin du Cercle Benelux d'Histoire de la Pharmacie, No. 6, p. 14, Nov., 1953; Segers and Wittop-Koning, l.c.; Prescriber (Sept. 1956); Ned. Tijdschr. Geneesk., No. 13, 1955; Gesch. Pharm., vol. 9, No. 3, 1957.

Gouda: Museum Catherina Gasthuis. Pharmacy restoration. Wittop-Koning, D. A., Delft Drug-Jars, Deventer, 1956; Segers and Wittop-Koning, l.c.

Haarlem: Frans Hals Museum. Pharmacy restoration. Pharmaceutisch Weekblad 74:775, 1937; Segers and Wittop-Koning, l.c.

Leeuwarden: Fries Museum. Pharmacy restoration. Parmaceutisch Weekblad 75:729, 1938; Segers and Wittop-Koning, l.c.

Leiden: Rijksmuseum voor de Geschiedenis der Natuurwetenschapen. Pharmacy material. Pharmaceutisch Weekblad 82:185, 1947; J.A.Ph.A. (Pract. Ed.) 16:600, 1955.

Oldenzaal: Musée d'Antiquités. Pharmacy restoration. Pharmaceutisch Weekblad 77:273, 1940; Segers and Wittop-Koning, l.c.

Rotterdam: Museum Boymans. Majolica. Catalogus Oud-Aardewerk van 1250-1650 (1940).

NORWAY

Grimstad: Grimstad Bymuseum og Ibsenhuset. Restoration of pharmacy where Henrik Ibsen worked. Grimstad Bys Historie, pp. 624-26, 1926; Prescriber (Sept. 1956).

Oslo: Universitetets farmasøytiske Institutts museum. Pharmacy material. Jermstad, A.: Personal correspondence, Dec. 14, 1955.

Stavanger: Stavanger Museum. Hygeia pharmacy restoration. Jermstad, A.: Personal correspondence, Dec. 14, 1955.

PERU

Lima: Museo Maldonado de Farmacia, Laboratorios Maldonado, S.A. Angel Maldonado pharmacy collection. Museo Maldonado de Farmacia, Lima, 1951; Terreros, N.: personal corespondence, April 10, 1956.

POLAND

Crakow: Muzeum Historycznym Aptekarstwa

Polskiego. Pharmacy material. Farmacja Polska 8:111, 193, 229, 263, 315, 1952.

PUERTO RICO

Rio Piedras: Colegio de Farmacia, Universidad de Puerto Rico, Pharmacy Museum. Porcelain drug jars. Torres-Diaz, Luis. Breve Historia de la Farmacia en Puerto Rico, Amer. Inst. Hist. Pharm., Madison, Wisc., 1951.

ROMANIA

Bucharest: National Institute of the History of Medicine. Pharmacy material. Sigerist, H. E.: A History of Medicine, vol. I, Oxford Univ. Press, 1951.

Cluj: Institute of the History of Medicine and Pharmacy. Pharmacy material. Archeion 9:517, 1928; Gesch. Pharm., vol. 9, No. 4, 1957.

SPAIN

For general reference to pharmacy museum collections in Spain, see Folch Jou, D. Guillermo: Historia de la Farmacia, Madrid, 1951.

Madrid: Museo de Historia de la Farmacia Hispana, Faculty of Pharmacy. Pharmacy restoration, majolica. Bol. Soc. Españ. Historia Farmacia 2:171, 1951; Farmacia Nueva 16:543, 1951; 17:573, 1952; Rev. Farmaceut. Peruana 23:14, Sept., 1954; Chem. & Drug. 175:649, 1961.

Madrid: Museum of Military Pharmacy. Chem & Drug. 175:649, 1961.

Masnou (Barcelona): Museo Retrospectivo de Farmacia y Medicina, Laboratorios del Norte de España. Pharmacy restoration. Apotheker-Kalender (Aug. 1933); Museo Retrospectivo de Farmacia y Medicina, 1952; J.A.Ph.A. (Pract. Ed.) 16:504, 1955; Prescriber (Sept. 1956).

Santo Domingo de Silos: Monastery pharmacy. Anal. Real Academia Farmacia 6:40, 1940.

San Juan Evangelista de Burgos: Hospital. Ancient pharmacy. Jimeno y Jimeno, Pascual Domingo: La antigua y famosa botica del hospital de San Juan Evangelista de Burgos, Madrid, 1934.

Toledo: Tavera Hospital pharmacy. Chem. & Drug. 175:649, 1961.

SWEDEN

Stockholm: Farmacihistoriskt Museum. Svensk Farmaceutisk Tidskrift 57:449. 465, 1953; Gesch. Pharm. vol. 9, No. 4, 1957.
Stockholm: Nordiska Museum (Skansen). Pharmacy restoration, where Carl Wilhelm Scheele carried on early research. Kockum, Arnold, Nordiska Museets Farmaceutiska Afdelingen, Stockholm, 1916; Apotheker-Kalender (1929); J.A.Ph.A. *19*:103, 1017, 1930; Urdang, George: Pictorial Life History of the Apothecary Chemist, Carl Wilhelm Scheele, Am. Inst. Hist. Pharm., Madison, Wisc., 1944; Modern Pharmacy *39*:16, May, 1954.

SWITZERLAND

Basel: Schweizer Pharmazie-Historisches Museum, 3 Totengässlein. Outstanding collection, including two pharmacy restorations. Häfliger, Joseph Anton; Pharmazeutische Altertumskunde, B. Wepf & Cie., Basel, 1931; Schweiz. Apotheker Zeitung 65:439, 1927; 66:440, 1928; 67:401, 1929; 68:332, 1930; J.A.Ph.A. (Pract. Ed.) *16*:600, 1955; Prescriber (Sept., 1956).
Basel: Medizinhistorische Sammlung (Arturo Castiglioni collection), Roche; Antike Apotheken-Gefässe, Basel, n.d.; J.A.Ph.A. (Pract. Ed.) *16*:600, 1955.
Lausanne: University Museum. Burkhard Reber collection, formerly in Geneva. Deutsche Apotheker Zeitung 9:289, 297, 305, 315, 325, 1894; Therapeutische Monatshefte 20:419, 1906; Pharm. Rev. 25:161, 1907; Reber, B.: Considérations sur ma Collection d'Antiquités, Geneva, 1909; Bull. Soc. Histoire Pharm., No. 2, p. 17, 1913.
Zurich: Landesmuseum. Pharmacy restoration. Häfliger, l.c.; J.A.Ph.A. (Pract. Ed.) *16*:600, 1955.

TURKEY

Istanbul: Topkapi Seraglio Museum. Pharmacy material. Ünver, A. Süheyl: Kekimlik ve Eczcilik Tarihi Hakkinda, Istanbul, 1952.

U.S.S.R.

Moscow: Pharmaceutical museum. Pharm. J. *80*:487, 1935; J.A.Ph.A. 24:429, 1935. See also Fundárek, R.: Über pharmazeutische Museen in der USSR und in sozialistischen Staaten, Farmac. Obzor (CSSR) 33:264-265, 1962 (abstract, Pharmaz. Zhalle *101*: 737, 1962)

UNITED STATES

For general references to pharmacy museum collections in the United States, please see: Winters, S. R., Drug Stores of Colonial America, Travel *92*:22-24, 32, Oct. 1948; Winters, S. R., N.A.R.D. Journal 75:677-679, 700, May 4, 1953; Griffenhagen, G. B., Early American Pharmacies, Am. Pharm. Assoc., Washington, D.C., 1955.

CALIFORNIA

Anaheim: Disneyland. Upjohn drugstore restoration, period 1900. J.A.Ph.A. (Pract. Ed.) *16*:276, 1955; Drug Topics 99:52, Aug. 22, 1955; Louisiana Pharmacist *14*:6, Sept., 1955; Michigan Drug J. *43*:12, July, 1955.
Bakersfield: Kern County Pioneer Village, western-style drugstore restoration. J.A.Ph.A. (Pract. Ed.) *21*:489, 1960; A Journey Into the Past, Kern County Historical Society Official Museum Guidebook (1959).
Buena Park: Knott's Berry Farm Ghost Town. 12 foot store front of 1890 desert mining town drugstore. J.A.Ph.A. (Pract. Ed.) *14*:454, 1953; Early American Pharmacies, l.c.
Los Angeles: Southern California Pharmaceutical Association, 701 S. St. Andrews Pl. "Room of Memories," and early California drugstore restoration. Pacific Drug Rev. *63*: 84, Sept., 1951; J.A.Ph.A. (Pract. Ed.) *15*: 368, 1954; Early American Pharmacies, l.c.
Stockton: San Joaquin Pioneer Museum. E. S. Holden drugstore restoration, period 1900. J.A.Ph.A. (Pract. Ed.) *14*:454, 1953; Early American Pharmacies, l.c.

CONNECTICUT

Mystic: Mystic Seaport Marine Historical Association. Bringhurst pharmacy restoration from Wilmington, Del., and Karsh collection; founded 1793. Modern Pharmacy *31*:10, Sept., 1946; Northwestern Druggist 55:34, July, 1947; J.A.M.A. *152*:36, 1953; J.A.Ph.A. (Pract. Ed.) *14*:732, 1953; Early American Pharmacies, l.c.; Apothecary Shop (Mystic brochure) n.d.
New Haven: Yale Medical Historical Library, 333 Cedar Street. Edward Streeter collection and old apothecary shop. First Annual Report of the Historical Library, Yale

Univ. School of Medicine, June 30, 1941; Ciba Symposia 6:2083, 1945; J.A.Ph.A. (Pract. Ed.) 14:732, 1953; Early American Pharmacies, l.c.

Noroton (Darien): Milestone Village Apothecary Shop, private collection of Lurelle Guild. Tile and Till 19:102, 1933.

DELAWARE

Dover: Delaware State Museum, Pharmacy exhibit. Delaware State Museum News 3:1, Oct., 1953.

DISTRICT OF COLUMBIA

Washington: U.S. National Museum, Smithsonian Institution. Division of Medical Science. Pharmaceutical historical exhibits, national materia medica collection (commenced in 1881) and Old World Apothecary Shop. Pharm. Zeitung 75:19, 219, 487 & 735, 1930; J.A.Ph.A. 28:1055, 1939; 29:36, 41, 1940; Urdang, George, and Nitardy, F. W.: The Squibb Ancient Pharmacy, New York, E. R. Squibb & Sons, 1940; J.A.Ph.A. (Pract. Ed.) 6:184, 1945; 7:157, 227, 1946; Drug Topics 90:2, 97, July 8, 1946; Am. Druggist 115:82, Feb., 1947; Squibb News 1:14, May, 1950; Washington Star Pictorial Magazine, Feb. 14, 1954; for general review of pharmacy collections, see J.A.Ph.A. 19:1125, 1930; Meyer Druggist 75:8, June, 1955; Prescriptionist 2:37, Aug., 1955; Gesch. Pharm., vol. 10, No. 4, 1958.

Washington: American Institute of Pharmacy (headquarters of the American Pharmaceutical Association), 2215 Constitution Ave., N.W. Association memorabilia and pharmaceutical equipment. See numerous reports in J.A.Ph.A., 1930—to date; such as J.A.Ph.A. (Pract. Ed.) 1:393, 429, 1940.

ILLINOIS

Chicago: Chicago Historical Society, North Avenue at Clark Street. Early Chicago drugstore restoration, period 1850. J.A.Ph.A. (Pract. Ed.) 14:388, 1953; Early American Pharmacies, l.c.

Chicago: Museum of Science and Industry, 5th Street and South Lake Shore Drive. Philo Carpenter drugstore restoration, period 1900. J.A.Ph.A. 22:579, 593, 1933; J.A.Ph.A. (Pract. Ed.) 14:388, 1953; Early American Pharmacies, l.c.

Junction City: Master Prescription Shop apothecary restoration. J.A.Ph.A. n.s. 1:498, 1961.

INDIANA

Evansville: Physicians office and pharmacy. Evansville Museum of Arts and Science. Medical Evansville in the Nineteenth Century (Mead Johnson and Co., Evansville, n.d.); J.A.Ph.A. (Pract. Ed.) 21:488, 1960.

Indianapolis: Eli Lilly and Company, Restoration of Colonel Eli Lilly's first manufacturing laboratory founded 1876. Tile and Till 21:52, 1935; J.A.Ph.A. (Pract. Ed.) 16:402, 1955; Louisiana Pharmacist 14:6, Oct., 1955.

Mitchell: Spring Mill State Park. Spring Mill Village pharmacy restoration, period 1830-50. Saturday Evening Post, June 12, 1943; J.A.Ph.A. (Pract. Ed.) 15:172, 1954; Early American Pharmacies, l.c.

KANSAS

Lawrence: University of Kansas, School of Pharmacy. Restoration of B. W. Woodward drugstore, period 1870. Tile and Till 27:128, 1941.

KENTUCKY

Danville McDowell Apothecary Shop restoration. Courier-Journal Magazine, Sept. 13, 1959; J.A.Ph.A. (Pract. Ed.) 20:603, 1959.

LOUISIANA

New Orleans: La Pharmacie Française, 514 Chartres St. Museum housed in original building erected by Dulfilho, 1823. Restoration of pharmacy, period 1880, on ground floor. Drug Topics, vol. 94, No. 24, 1950; Am. J. Pharm. Ed. 15:126, 1951; N.A.R.D. Journal 76:36, April 5, 1954; J.A.Ph.A. (Pract. Ed.) 15:245, 1954; Early American Pharmacies, l.c.

MASSACHUSETTS

Salem: Essex Institute: Restoration of an old New England pharmacy, period 1830-50. J.A.Ph.A. (Pract. Ed.) 14:660, 1953; Early American Pharmacies, l.c.

MICHIGAN

Dearborn: Henry Ford Museum and Greenfield Village. Restoration of Phoenixville, Conn., pharmacy, period 1850. 1890 drugstore period room restoration in Museum. Greenfield Village Guide Book, 1951; J.A.Ph.A. (Pract. Ed.) 2:216, 1941; 15:172, 1954; Early American Pharmacies, l.c.

Grand Rapids: Public Museum. Pharmacy restoration. Drug Topics 99:34, Oct. 17, 1955.

Highland Park: Howard Mordue's "Apothecariana." J.A.Ph.A. (Pract. Ed.) *21*:489, 1960.

MINNESOTA

Minneapolis: College of Pharmacy, University of Minnesota Museum. J.A.Ph.A. *21*: 1162, 1932; Hobbies, vol. 59, Nov., 1954; Ivory Tower (U. Minnesota daily), April 1, 1957.

MISSOURI

Hannibal: Grant's Drug Store restored in building once occupied by Mark Twain. J.A.Ph.A. n.s. *1*:498, 1961; Hannibal, Mo., Chamber of Commerce (brochure), n.d.

MONTANA

Stevensville: St. Mary's Mission. Restoration of Rev. Anthony J. Ravalli's pharmacy, period 1845. J.A.Ph.A. (Pract. Ed.) *15*:678, 1954; Modern Pharmacy *11*:18, No. 4, 1955.

NEBRASKA

Minden: Harold Warp Pioneer Village Pharmacy restoration, period 1900. Antique Automobile *19*:43, Summer, 1955; J.A.Ph.A. (Pract. Ed.) *16*:662, 1955.

NEW JERSEY

New Brunswick: Kilmer Museum of Surgical Products, Johnson and Johnson, Inc. Johnson and Johnson Bull., vol. 12, Feb., May, Dec., 1953, and vol. 13, Oct., 1954.

NEW YORK

Albany: Albany College of Pharmacy. Restoration of Throop drugstore of Schoharie, N. Y., founded 1800. Tile and Till *24*:90, 1938; J.A.Ph.A. (Pract. Ed.) *15*:306, 1954; Early American Pharmacies, l.c.

Buffalo: Buffalo Historical Society. Prescription unit from Smith Drug Store, period 1881. J.A.Ph.A. (Pract. Ed.) *15*:505, 1954.

Cooperstown: Farmer's Museum, New York State Historical Association. Restoration of New York druggist's shop, period 1820-40. N. Y. State Pharmacist *28*:34, July, 1953; American Cyanamid Monthly News Bulletin *18*:12, Dec., 1953; J.A.Ph.A. (Pract. Ed.) *15*:124, 1954; Early American Pharmacies, l.c.

Monroe: Old Museum Village of Smith's Clove. Restoration of the Vernon drugstore, founded in Florida, N. Y., 1886. New York Herald Tribune, June 26, 1960; J.A.Ph.A.

(Pract. Ed.) *15*:306, 1954; Early American Pharmacies, l.c.

New York City: Columbia University College of Pharmacy. Restoration of an early New York drugstore. Merck Report 38:100, July, 1929; Columbia Alumni News, 35:5, April, 1944; Ballard, C. W.: A History of the College of Pharmacy, Columbia University, N. Y., 1954; J.A.Ph.A. (Pract. Ed.) *15*: 438, 1954; Early American Pharmacies, l.c.

New York City: J. Leon Lascoff and Son, Inc. Apothecaries, Lexington Ave. and 82nd St. Private museum. Coronet, Sept., 1947; Pharmacy International, Dec., 1952; J.A. Ph.A. (Pract. Ed.) *15*:744, 1954.

New York City: Schering Apothecary Restoration. Freedomland, U.S.A., J.A.Ph.A. (Pract. Ed.) *21*:488, 1960.

New York City: Smith, Miller and Patch Apothecary, 902 Broadway. J.A.Ph.A. (Pract. Ed.) *21*:489, 1960.

New York City: Museum of the City of New York. Restoration of John Carle drugstore period 1852. J.A.Ph.A. (Pract. Ed.) *15*:505, 1954.

New York City: New York Historical Society. Restoration of New York drugstore, period 1850-1900. This Week, Sept. 3, 1939; J.A.Ph.A. (Pract. Ed.) *15*:505, 1954.

New York City: Metropolitan Museum of Art. Majolica. Am. Prof. Pharm. *13*:163, 1947.

New York City: Mary Chess, Cosmetics, 601 Fifth Ave. 17th-century Florentine pharmacy fixtures. Drugg. Circ., vol. 29, June, 1935.

New York City: Hispanic Society of America Museum. Majolica. Frothingham, A. W.: Catalogue of Hispano-Moresque Pottery, New York, 1936; Notes Hispanic *1*:101, 1941.

Old Chatham: Shaker Museum. Restoration of Shaker medicine manufacturing plant, period 1850-70, originally located at Mount Lebanon, N. Y., J.A.Ph.A. (Pract. Ed.) *16*: 402, 1955.

Pearl River: Lederle Laboratories. Restoration in main entrance lobby of early American pharmacy. J.A.Ph.A. (Pract. Ed.) *15*:438, 1954; Early American Pharmacies, l.c.; Louisiana Pharmacist *14*:6, Oct., 1955; Hobbies, vol. 59, No. 8, Oct. 1954.

Rochester: Rochester Museum of Arts and Industries. Restoration of Benham Pharmacy, period 1865-75. J.A.Ph.A. (Pract. Ed.) *15*: 124, 1954; Early American Pharmacies, l.c.

NORTH CAROLINA

Chapel Hill: University of North Carolina School of Pharmacy Library and Museum. Pharmacy material. Carolina J. Pharmacy *36*:35, Jan. 1955; vol. 37, cover, Feb., 1956.

Greensboro: Greensboro Historical Museum. Restoration of Porter drugstore, in which William Sydney Porter (O. Henry) was apprenticed, 1876-81. Drug Topics *91* (No. 21):72, 1947; Rexall Ad-Vantages, vol. 34, 1948; J.A.Ph.A. (Pract. Ed.) *14*:752, 1953; Early American Pharmacies, l.c.

OHIO

Cincinnati: University of Cincinnati College of Medicine. Partial restoration of 15th century Italian pharmacy. Drug Topics *97*:28, Feb. 9, 1953.

Cleveland: Howard Dittrick Museum of Historical Medicine. Wall case and equipment from Smithknight drugstore, founded 1857, Bull. Hist. Med. *8*:1214, 1940; Northern Ohio Druggist *19*:14, Jan., 1941.

OKLAHOMA

Norman: University of Oklahoma, College of Pharmacy. Prescription desk, period 1885-90, and equipment. Drug Topics *98*:40, June 14, 1954.

PENNSYLVANIA

Bethlehem: The Apothecary (formerly Simon Rau) 420 South Main St. Partial restoration of Apotheke, founded 1743. Drugg. Circ. *71*: 1093, 1927; Am. J. Pharm. *111*:234, 1939; Merck's Report *41*:22, Jan. 1932; Tile and Till *25*:67, 1939; Dow Diamond *12*:6, Oct. 1949; Travel *91*:22, Oct. 1948; J.A.Ph.A. (Pract. Ed.) *14*:468, 1953; Drug Topics 99: 64, Feb. 21, 1955; Early American Pharmacies, l.c.; Moravian Historical Tours (brochure) Central Moravian Church, Bethlehem, n.d.

Philadelphia: Philadelphia College of Pharmacy and Science. Partial restoration of Glentworth pharmacy, founded 1812; and museum. Catalogue of the Historical Exhibition, Semi-Centennial Anniversary of the American Pharmaceutical Association, Philadelphia, Sept. 8-13, 1902; Am. J. Pharm. *98*:646, 1926; J.A.Ph.A. *25*:230, 1936; England, J. W.; The First Century of the Philadelphia College of Pharmacy, 1922; LaWall, C. H.; Four Thousand Years of Pharmacy, Garden City, 1927; Philadelphia Section of the Era Album, p. 100, 1908; J.A.Ph.A. (Pract. Ed.) *14*:468, 1953; Early American

Pharmacies, l.c. For general accounts of historical museum collections, see: Tile and Till *27*:28, March 1941; J.A.Ph.A. *22*:334, 1933; *23*:570, 1934.

Philadelphia: Franklin Institute. Pharmacy replica. The Museum News, Feb. 15, 1955.

RHODE ISLAND

Newport: Newport Historical Society. Original window from Charles Feke's pharmacy, founded 1796. The Rhode Islander, March 14, 1948; Modern Pharmacy *35*:19, Jan. 1950; Cosmopolitan, Nov. 1951; J.A.Ph.A. (Pract. Ed.) *14*:660, 1953.

SOUTH CAROLINA

Charleston: Charleston Museum. Restoration of Apothecaries' Hall, founded by Jacob De la Motta, 1820's. Bennett, John; Apothecaries' Hall, Charleston Museum, 1921; Merck's Report *40*:104, 1931; Ann. Med. His. *2*:259, 1940; Hoch, J. H.: The History of Pharmacy in South Carolina, Charleston, 1951; J.A.Ph.A. *12*:663, 1923 (Pract. Ed.); *14*:752, 1953; Early American Pharmacies, l.c.

TEXAS

Jefferson: Ye Olde Apothecary Shoppe, 312 Broadway. J.A.Ph.A. n.s. *1*:499, 1961.

UTAH

Salt Lake City: Pioneer Village Museum. Pharmacy restoration, 1860-80. J.A.Ph.A. (Pract. Ed.) *15*:505, 1954; U.Ph.A. Bulletin News *64*:4, Nov. 1955; *70*:2, May, 1961; J.A.Ph.A. n.s. *1*:499, 1961.

VERMONT

Burlington: Shelburne Museum, apothecary shop restoration. J.A.Ph.A. n.s. *1*:498, 1961.

VIRGINIA

Alexandria: Stabler-Leadbeater Apothecary Shop, 107 South Fairfax St. Restoration of original shop founded in 1792 and operated by same family for 141 years. Washington Herald, July 20, 1933; J.A.Ph.A. *22*:705, 1933; *23*:1137, 1934; J.A.Ph.A. (Pract. Ed.) *3*:216, 1942; *14*:322, 1953; Am. Drug. *117* (No. 5):75, 1948; Travel *91*:22, Oct. 1948; Early American Pharmacies, l.c.; Today's Health *39*:52, Feb. 1961.

Fredericksburg: Hugh Mercer Apothecary Shop, 1020 Caroline St. Restoration of original building operated as a pharmacy by General Hugh Mercer, 1761-77. Trenton

Sunday Times-Advertiser, March 20, 1932; Tile and Till *18*:31, 1932; J.A.Ph.A. (Pract. Ed.) *2*:61, 173, 1941; *3*:216, 1942; The Commonwealth *8*:15, April 1941; Waterman, J. M.: With Sword and Lancet, Richmond, Va., Garrett and Massie, 1941; Travel *91*: 22, 1948; Hygeia *26*:478, 1948; J.A.Ph.A. (Pract. Ed.) *14*:221, 1953; Builders *61*:7, Oct. 16, 1954; Early American Pharmacies, l.c.; J.A.Ph.A. (Pract. Ed.) *20*:649, 1959.

Richmond: Roy Apothecary Shop, Medical College of Virginia. Pharmacy restoration. Tile and Till *26*:52, May, 1940; The Virginia Pharmacist, Convention Number, May 5-12, 1940; The Commonwealth, vol. 7, April 1940. Disposition unknown.

Williamsburg: Colonial Williamsburg. Restoration of the Pasteur-Galt pharmacy, period 1760-76. Official Guide Book of Colonial Williamsburg, 1951; J.A.Ph.A. (Pract. Ed.) *11*:680, 1950; Midwestern Druggist *26*:22, Feb. 1950; Northwestern Druggist *59*:35, 1951; Am. Drug. *128*:18, July 20, 1953; Quarterly of Phi Beta Pi, vol. 50, Jan. 1954; Early American Pharmacies, l.c.

WISCONSIN

Madison: Wisconsin State Historical Society. Restoration of a pioneer Wisconsin drugstore, period 1848-98. The Pioneer Drug Store, Wisconsin State Historical Society, 1930; Pharm. Era *50*:45, 1917; Merck's Report *40*:14, Jan. 1931; Badger Pharmacist, special reprint, April, 1930; Tile and Till *19*:86, 1933; Northwestern Druggist *55*:28, 1947; Drug Topics *98*:24, Aug. 9, 1954; J.A.Ph.A. (Pract. Ed.) *15*:12, 1954; Early American Pharmacies, l.c.

Milwaukee: Milwaukee Public Museum. Restoration of a Milwaukee drugstore, period 1900. Am. Drug. *113*:84, April 1946; J.A.Ph.A. (Pract. Ed.) *15*:12, 1954; Early American Pharmacies, l.c.; Tile and Till *41*: 94, 1955.

YUGOSLAVIA

Dubrovnik (Ragusa): Franciscan pharmacy. Chem. & Drug. *124*:784, 1936; Pharm. Zeitung *87*:034, 1951; Pharmaceutical *113*: 339, 1951.

Sarajevo: Municipal Museum. "Old Jewish Pharmacy," Museum 8:79, 1955.

Split: Archeological Museum. Ancient pharmacy material. Farmaceutiski Glasnik *11*: 359, 1955.

Zagreb: Pharmacy Institute Museum. Pharmacy material. Farmaceutiski Glasnik *11*: 102, 269, 1955.

Appendix 6: Publications of the American Pharmaceutical Association

Because of the key position that publications of the American Pharmaceutical Association hold in the history of American pharmacy, the following chart has been prepared, with the cooperation of Professor George E. Osborne of the College of Pharmacy, University of Rhode Island, in relation to Chapter 15: "Establishing a Literature."

The National Formulary. Published approximately every 10 years from 1888 to 1940; every 5 years from 1940 to date; numbered by editions, e.g., "N.F. XI" (1960), not by revisions.

Bulletin of the National Formulary Committee. (Vols. 1 to 19, 1930-1951). Circulation at first irregular and restricted to Committee; took journal format with Vol. 7, 1938; continued under title *Drug Standards* from No. 5-&-6, Vol. 19 (1951) through Vol. 28 (1960), then absorbed into *Journal of Pharmaceutical Sciences.*

The Pharmaceutical Recipe Book. 1926, 1938 and 1943; now out of print.

Proceedings.* From 1852, when the American Pharmaceutical Association was established, a volume of *Proceedings* of the meetings was issued annually, except for 1861 when no meeting of the Association was held. A useful *General Index to Volumes One to Fifty of the Proceedings of the American Pharmaceutical Association, from 1852 to 1902 inclusive* appeared as a separate volume.

In 1912 the *Journal* and the *Year Book* took the place of the separate *Proceedings.* After each subsequent annual meeting the proceedings usually were printed in the following 3 issues of the Journal. The *Year Book* provided a place for Association data (such as the official roster, the constitution and by-laws, the treasurer's report, and a list of members, alphabetically and geographically), as well as the

---

* Based in part on J.A.Ph.A. (Sci. Ed.) 32:313, 1943.

ANNUAL	MONTHLY		SUPPLEMENTAL
1852　Proceedings of the A.Ph.A. through 1911	1906　Bulletin of the A.Ph.A. through 1911		
1912　Yearbook of the A.Ph.A. through 1934	1912　Journal of the A.Ph.A. (new vol. numbers) through 1939		1935　Pharmaceutical Abstracts (monthly in Scientific through Edition, but 1948　often bound separately)
	Scientific Edition (continuing vol. numbers)	Practical Pharmacy Edition (new vol. numbers)	
	1940 through 1960		occasional monographs
	Journal of Pharmaceutical Sciences (continuing vol. numbers) 50:1961 to date	P. P. Edition dropped from Journal title (New Series vol. numbering) 1:1961 to date	The A.Ph.A. Newsletter 1:1962, to date

abstracting service called "The Report of the Progress of Pharmacy."

The *Year Book* was discontinued with Volume 23, covering the calendar year 1934. Beginning with 1935 the annual "Report" was revamped as monthly "Pharmaceutical Abstracts," appearing as part of the *Journal*, but separately paged and indexed.

The proceedings later were published in one number of the *Journal* each year (rather than in three); and this number also included the Association data and list of members (which had appeared in the *Year Book*). In 1940 when the *Journal* began to be published in two editions, no proceedings number appeared, being combined with the proceedings for 1941. The Proceedings Numbers, which continued in the *Scientific Edition,* contained an abstract of the minutes of the various subdivisons of the Association and of its related organizations, and included addresses and reports (corresponding in part to the discontinued *Year Book*). Papers presented in the Sections have appeared, to the extent published by the Association, in other issues of the *Journal's* two editions.

The Proceedings Numbers were discontinued with the 1945 issue and have not been revived (except for an abortive attempt in 1950, a separate issue covering only the General Sessions and the House of Delegates). In the ensuing years the proceedings have been "published in narrative form" (news stories and principal addresses) in the *Journal* (Practical Pharmacy Edition prior to 1961).

Unpublished proceedings material has been classified into the Archive of the American Pharmaceutical Association (2215 Constitution Ave., N.W., Washington 7, D. C.), although much 20th-century material remains in storage. For a detailed topical outline, see: "Structure of the Archive of the American Pharmaceutical Association," *Pharmacy in History* 7:35-42, 1962. A roster of the officials and subdivisions of the Association continued to be published in the *Journal*, expanding into a "Directory" (Pract. Pharm. Ed. 5:187-193, 1944) that includes addresses of other American associations, publications, state boards, and schools of pharmacy, which (after a hiatus) appears annually in amplified form (*Journal* n.s. 1:19-38, 1961, et seq.).

Appendix 7:   Glossary

These pharmaco-historical notes are supplementary to topics of the text and do not provide an encyclopedic reference tool.

Abbott, Wallace Calvin (1857-1921), physician and founder of the Abbott Laboratories. See J. A. P. A. *10*:559, 1921.

Alexander Trallianus (525-605). The cognomen Trallianus refers to his native town of Tralles in Lydia. Living at Rome as a physician, he wrote in Greek a *Materia medica* in 12 volumes.

Allen, William (1770-1843), English pharmacist. He was not only a well-known chemist, but one of the leading English Quakers and a philanthropist of international importance. See E. C. Cripps: *Plough Court,* p. 25, London, 1927.

Almanach oder Taschenbuch für Scheidekuenstler und Apotheker (1780-1829), a very early serial publication used by pharmacists. Its title was changed in 1820 to *Trommsdorff's Almanach oder Taschenbuch für Chemiker und Apotheker,* and in 1822 to *Taschenbuch für Scheidekuenstler und Apotheker.*

Anderson, John F. (1873-   ), physician, from 1915 to 1942 director of the research and biological laboratories of E. R. Squibb's Sons. See *Who's Who in America, 20*:177; *American Men of Science,* ed. 8, p. 51, 1949.

Anepu, the apothecary of the Egyptian gods. He was considered the son of Isis and Osiris.

Animal drugs. Animal parts and excrements, and animal preparations, have always been used for medicinal purposes. Their bizarre use reached its climax in Joh. Jacob Wecker's *Antidotarium generale* (Basle, 1553) and in the *Neuvermehrte heylsame Dreckapotheke,* i.e., the newly augmented salutary dungpharmacy, by the German physician Franz Christian Paullini (1696 and reissued several times).

Antidotarium. See: **Pharmacopeia.**

Apollo. God of healing as well as of youth and beauty, of poetry and music, and of the wisdom of oracles. Gradually, he became identified with the sun god, Helios, and was considered the son of Zeus. Apollo was the first Greek deity to find a place in Roman religion, chiefly as a god of healing.

Apotheca. Latinized form of *Apotheke, q.v.* During Roman antiquity it was commonly applied to the storage room for wine. Galen differentiated between his *apotheca* or storeroom and his *iatron, q.v.,* the room in which he saw his patients. The Roman *apotheca librorum* corresponds to our library or storage room for books. In the Middle Ages the term was more or less restricted to storerooms for spices and drugs, and thus the German *Apotheke, q.v.,* and the French *apothicairerie, q.v.,* came into general use. The French equivalent was replaced by *pharmacie, q.v.,* toward the close of the 18th century.

Apothecarius, from Latin *apotheca, q.v.,* "storage room," and *-arius,* "pertaining to," literally the person in charge of a storage room. So far as pharmacy is concerned, it refers to the dealer in spices and drugs. See French *apothicaire,* English *apothecary,* German *Apotheker* (spelled variously in different Germanic countries and at different times).

Apothecary, anglicized form of *apothecarius, q.v.* In England the designation became restricted to a medicopharmaceutical practitioner after the middle of the 18th century.

Apothecary shop, outmoded English term for a pharmacy. See **Apotheca.**

Apotheke, the Germanized form of the Latin *apotheca, q.v.* During the Middle Ages the name was applied to the German apothecary's establishment. French *apothicairerie, q.v.* and *boutique, q.v.,* Italian *botica, q.v.,* Spanish *botega,* English "apothecary shop," *q.v.,* and "pharmacy," *q.v.* The word also occurs in several forms of book titles and in various combinations, e.g. *Hausapotheke* ("medicine chest"), *Militair-apotheke* ("regimental medicine chest"), and figuratively in *Seelenapotheke* ("medicine chest for the soul").

Apotheker. German form of *apothecarius, q.v.*

In Germany it is still the official designation of the pharmaceutical practitioner as opposed to the *Drogist, q.v.*

Apothicaire. French form of *apothecarius, q.v.* At the close of the 18th century the word was replaced officially by *pharmacien, q.v.*

Apothicairerie. Old French form for "pharmacy." See: *Apotheca.*

Apotteck. See: **Pharmacopeia.**

Apple, William S. (1918-), executive director of the American Pharmaceutical Association since 1959 (Assistant Secretary, 1958); noted for advocacy of progressive professionalization of community pharmacy and pharmaceutical reforms. At the University of Wisconsin, Apple helped to develop the field of pharmacy administration (1952-58); and he himself earned the first Ph.D. awarded there in that specialty. (*Who's Who in America.*)

Apprentice. See: **Personnel.**

Apuleius, Lucius or Pseudo-Apuleius, a late Roman medical author of uncertain identity (4th or 5th century A.D.).

Aquae aromaticae. In contrast to *aquae minerales* and other aqueous solutions (cf: **Spiritus aromatici),** aromatic waters (aromatic spirits) were aqueous distillates of aromatic plants. Compare *Eaux des plantes odorantes* with *Eaux des plantes inodorantes* (Baumé, *Elémens de pharmacie*). Rose water played an important role in Persian commerce as early as the 9th century. It was used not only as a perfume but also in the preparation of medicaments. Arnaldus de Villanova (died 1311) was important in in-

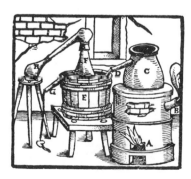

troducing products of distillation into European therapy. Distillation and the products obtained thereby became so important that a new type of medicopharmaceutical treatises, the *Destillierbücher* ("books on distillation"), made its appearance. For details see Gildemeister, Hoffmann and Kremers. *The Vola-*

tile Oils, 1:13, 1900. In modern pharmaceutical practice aromatic waters, for the most part, no longer are made by distillation, but by solution of volatile oils in water. For perfumery, however, such aromatic waters as rose water and orange flower water are still made by distillation.

Archambault, George F., Massachusetts pharmacist and lawyer; instructor, Massachusetts College of Pharmacy, 1931-1947; chief of Pharmacy Section, Division of Hospitals, U. S. Public Health Service since 1947.

Arny, Henry V. (1868-1943), completed his scientific education in Germany; editor, author, professor and dean at the New York College of Pharmacy, 1911 to 1936. See *New York State Pharmac. 10*:9, 1936.

Aromatarius, pl. *-i*, from Latin *aroma* ("spice"), and *-arius*, "pertaining to," i.e., dealer in spices.

Aromatic waters. See: *Aquae aromaticae.*

Asclepios, whose Egyptian antecedent was Imhotep, *q.v.* A culture hero considered to be a physician (Homer), he later became the Greek god of medicine and healing. The chief seat of his worship was Epidauros. In Greek mythology Asclepios is the son of Apollo. His sanctuaries not only were places of worship, but also centers of miracle-medicine. The Romans also worshiped him, frequently with his daughter Hygieia as the god of health, calling him Aesculapius or Asklepias. See Edelstein, Emma J., and Ludwig: *Asculepius, A Collection and Interpretation of the Testimonies,* Baltimore, 1947.

Assistant. See: **Personnel.**

Assistant pharmacist. See: **Titles.**

Assyria. During the era of its greatest expanse, ancient Assyria comprised the territory between the Euphrates and the mountain slopes east of the Tigris. At one time, i.e., during the reign of Ashurbanipal (668-626 B.C.) it extended to the Nile. Its history can be traced back to about 2300 B.C. Its civilization was borrowed almost wholly from Babylonia (*q.v.*).

Atkins, Henry (1558-1635), physician-in-ordinary to the English King James I, *q.v.* It was under the presidency of Atkins that the London College of Physicians issued the first *London Pharmacopoeia.* See *Dictionary (English) of National Biography, II*:220.

Attfield, John (1835-1911), English pharmacist, professor at the Pharmacy School of the Pharmaceutical Society of Great Britain and author of a textbook that was widely used in the United States as well as in England. See *Am. J. Pharm.* 78:102, 1906; Jos. P. Remington: *J. A. Ph. A. 1*:490, 1912.

Avenzoar, or Abū Marwān Ibn Zuhr (1113-1162). A Spanish-Arabic medical author called by Sarton "the most famous physician of his time, not only among Muslims, but in Christendom. See George Sarton: *Introduction to the History of Science,* vol. 2, pp. 231-234, Baltimore, 1931.

Avicenna, or Abū 'Ali al Husain ibn 'Abdallah ibn Sina (980-1037), the most famous and the most influential Persian-Arabic physician of the classical period of Arabian (or Greco-Arabic) medicine. See Tschirch: *Handbuch der Pharmakognosie, I,* Part 2, p. 602, Leipzig, 1910; George Sarton: *Introduction to the History of Science,* vol. 1, pp. 709-713, Baltimore, 1927. See also Soheil, M. A.: Avicenna, His Life and Work, London, 1957; and G. M. Wickens: Avicenna: Scientist and Philosopher, London, 1952.

Babylonia. In the time of her highest glory (6th century B.C.), Babylonia extended from the Euphrates valley into Asia Minor and Egypt. It was a center of the world's commerce and of the arts and sciences. Its language can be traced back to about 3500 B.C. See L. Delaporte: *Mesopotamia, the Babylon and Assyrian Civilization,* London, 1925.

Bache, Franklin (1792-1864), physician; professor of chemistry at the Philadelphia College of Pharmacy and later at Jefferson Medical College; co-author of the *United States Dispensatory.* See J. W. England: *First Century of the Philadelphia College of Pharmacy,* p. 399, Philadelphia, 1922.

Baitâr, Ibn al (1197-1248), Spanish-Arabic medical author, physician-in-ordinary to the ruler of Egypt. See Tschirch: *Handbuch der Pharmakognosie,* vol. 1, Part 2, p. 600, Leipzig, 1910; George Sarton: *Introduction to the History of Science,* vol. 2, part 2, pp. 663-664, Baltimore, 1931.

Balard, Antoine Jérome (1802-1876), French pharmacist. He discovered bromine (from the Greek *bromos* = "stench") in the salt brine of the Mediterranean (1826). Of his further discoveries, that of amyl nitrite (1834) is noteworthy. See *Am. J. Pharm.* 48:287, 1876.

Barton, Benjamin Smith (1776-1815), American botanist and professor at the University of Pennsylvania. See *Bull. Lloyd Lib., 1,* 1900.

Bartram, John (1699-1777), American botanist. At Kingsessing he founded the first

botanic garden in America. Linné termed him "the greatest natural botanist in the world." See *Am. J. Pharm.* 80:416, 1908; *Dictionary of American Biography, II,* p. 26.

Bartram, Moses (1732-1809), son of the famous botanist Bartram, *q.v.,* and pharmacist in Philadelphia. See Edward Kremers: "Two invoices of 1785," *J. A. Ph. A.* 20:691, 1931.

Bastedo, Walter A. (1874-1952), pharmacist, physician, professor of clinical medicine at Columbia University, president of the Pharmacopoeia Convention, 1930. See *J. A. Ph. A.* 20:199, 1931.

Bastin, Edson T. (1843-1897). Bastin started his career as a pharmacist in Chicago. Later he became a teacher of botany and of materia medica, first at the Northwestern College of Pharmacy and later at the Philadelphia College of Pharmacy. See *Proc. A. Ph. A.* 45:32, 1897; England: *First Century of the Philadelphia College of Pharmacy,* p. 413, Philadelphia, 1922.

Bate, George (1608-1669), physician-in-ordinary to the English Kings Charles I and Charles II and to the Lord Protector Cromwell. His formulae were published by a London apothecary, J. Shipton, under the title: *Bate's Dispensatory,* or *Pharmacopoeia Bateana.* See *Dictionary* (English) *Natl. Biog., III,* p. 390.

Bauhin, Caspar, professor of anatomy and botany at the University of Basle, Switzerland (1560-1624), one of the most learned botanists of all time. His book, *Prodromus theatri botanici,* in which he describes about 6,000 plants arranged according to a kind of natural system, represents the best dictionary of botanic nomenclature of his period.

Baumé, Antoine (1728-1804). Baumé is among the important French pharmacist-chemists of the 18th century, who simultaneously enriched pharmacy and chemistry. He introduced the hydrometer (Baumé's degrees), improved the process of distillation and gave in his *Elémens de pharmacie théorique et pratique* a comprehensive description of pharmaceutical apparatus and manipulation. He established the first laboratory for the manufacture of ammonium chloride and manufactured many other chemicals and galenics on a large scale.

Bayen, Pierre (1725-1798), French pharmacist. In 1774 Bayen published his observations on the "escape" of *"un fluide élastique"* (i.e., an air) when heating mercuric oxide. He is therefore supposed to have discovered oxygen before Scheele or Priestley, without, however, recognizing the importance of his discovery.

Beach, Wooster (1794-1868) founded the American "reformed school of medicine," which later on merged into the eclectic school. Beach's book, *The American Practice of Medicine,* was recognized all over the world as the standard work of the new movement. See A. Wilder: *History of Medicine,* p. 437, New Sharon, 1901; *Dictionary of American Biography, II,* p. 85.

Beal, James Hartley (1861-1945), pharmacist, lawyer, educator and writer. The personality and the ideas of J. H. Beal were of great influence on the development of American pharmacy. See J. A. Koch, American contemporaries, *Industrial and Engineering Chemistry,* News Edition *13*:352, 1935.

Becher, Johann Joachim (1635-1682), chemist, polyhistorian, author and, for some time, physician-in-ordinary to the elector of Bavaria. He was the first to determine the increase in weight after oxidation (calcination of lead). His mentioning of a principle of combustion inherent in all combustible substances laid the foundation of the phlogiston theory of Stahl, *q.v.*

Beck, John B. (1794-1851), physician in New York, professor of materia medica and botany in the New York College of Physicians and Surgeons and one of the earliest American historians of medicine.

Beckmann, Ernst Otto (1853-1923), pharmacist and professor of pharmaceutical chemistry at the University of Leipzig. His main work and merit lay in the field of physical chemistry. His apparatus for determination of the lowering of the freezing point and of the raising of the boiling point became indispensable tools in chemistry.

Bedford, Peter W. (1836-1892), New York pharmacist and (after 1873) professor at the New York College of Pharmacy; also editor of the *Pharm. Record.* See *Drug. Circ. 51*:82, 1907.

Behring, Emil von (1854-1917), German physician and academic teacher of hygiene in Marburg; inaugurator of serum therapy. See Sigerist: *The Great Doctors,* p. 372, New York, 1933; Garrison: *History of Medicine,* p. 84, Philadelphia, 1929.

Beissenhirtz, Friedrich Wilhelm (1779-1831), German pharmacist who helped found the *Apothekerverein im Noerdlichen Teutschland* and contributed many papers to the *Archiv* and to Trommsdorff's *Journal der Pharmacie.*

Bendiner, Samuel J., Hungarian-born pharmacist in New York (1839-1897). See *Proc. A. Ph. A. 45*:33, 1897.

Benger, Frederick Baden (1840-1903), English pharmacist and manufacturer. See *Pharm. J. 70*:145, 179, 1903.

Berendes, Julius. German pharmacist and pharmaceutical historian (1836-1914). Berendes' most important books are *Das Apothekenwesen,* especially devoted to German pharmacy, and *Die Pharmacie bei den alten Kulturvölkern* (pharmacy during antiquity). He also translated the *Materia medica* of Dioscorides and the *Seven Books of Paulus Aegineta,* from Latin and Greek texts into German. See Häfliger: Biographicon in Tschirch's *Handbuch der Pharmakognosie,* Leipzig, 1932; Adlung and Urdang: *Grundriss der Geschichte der deutschen Pharmazie,* Berlin, 1935.

Berzelius, Johann (Joens) Jacob (1779-1848), Swedish physician and one of the greatest chemists. He is the founder of the modern chemical nomenclature and was the first to observe and to describe isomorphism, polymorphism and allotrophy. An interesting controversy respecting nomenclature between Robert Hare of the University of Pennsylvania and Berzelius may be found in the *Am. J. Pharm. 9*:1, 1837. See Soederbaum: *Joens Jacob Berzelius,* biographical notes, English trans. by O. Larsell, Baltimore, 1934; George Urdang: Berzelius and pharmacy, *J. A. Ph. A. 37*:481-485, 1948.

Besler, Basilius, German pharmacist and botanist (1561-1629). His *Hortus Eystettensis* was one of the first botanic works to make use of copper etchings rather than woodcuts.

Bevan, Silvanus and Timothy, London wholesale druggist and apothecary. Silvanus Bevan (1691-1765) founded the establishment in 1715 and entered partnership with his brother Timothy between 1731-1736. This firm later became Allen and Howard; Allen, Hanburys and Barry; and, finally, Allen and Hanburys, Ltd., London. See E. C. Cripps, *Plough Court,* London, 1927; and D. Chapman-Huston and E. C. Cripps, *Through a City Archway,* London, 1954.

Bibliography. References have been given in the "Notes and References" to each chapter and in the text itself whenever it seemed appropriate to a survey volume for the general reader or student. To non-historians on the search for information about a specialized topic, mention of a few bibliographic guides may provide an entering wedge to expedite use of the library. Glenn Sonnedecker, J. H. Hoch, and W. Schneider: *Some Pharmaco-Historical Guidelines to the Literature*, Madison, Wis., 1959 (also in *Am. J. Pharm. Ed.* 23:143-172, 1959); *Index-Catalogue of the Library of the Surgeon-General's Office, U. S. Army*, 1880-1936 four series; E.-H. Guitard, *Manuel d'Histoire de la Littérature pharmaceutique*, Paris, 1942 (see also *Revue d'Histoire de la Pharmacie* for this and other rich bibliographic material); *Current Work in the History of Medicine* (quarterly since 1954); "Bibliography of the History of Medicine [and pharmacy] of the United States and Canada," in *Bulletin of the History of Medicine* annually since 1939; "Critical Bibliography" (including pharmacy) of *Isis* (87th in 1962); Glenn Sonnedecker and Alex Berman: *Some Bibliographic Aids for Historical Writers in Pharmacy*, Madison, Wis., 1958; David L. Cowen: *America's Pre-Pharmacopoeial Literature*, Madison, Wis., 1961; George Sarton: *Horus; A Guide to the History of Science*, Waltham, Mass., 1952; George Sarton: *Introduction to the History of Science*, Baltimore, 1927-1947; H. C. Bolton: *Chemical Bibliography*, Smithsonian Institution, Washington, D. C.; J. C. Poggendorff: *Biographischliterarisches Handwörterbuch zur Geschichte der exakten Wissenschaften*, Leipzig, 1863-; H. Schelenz: *Geschichte der Pharmazie*, Berlin, 1904; John Ferguson: *Bibliotheca chemica*, 1906; J. A. Häfliger: Biographikon, in Tschirch's *Handbuch der Pharmakognosie*, Leipzig, 1932; Adlung and Urdang: *Grundriss der Geschichte der deutschen Pharmazie*, Berlin, 1935; F. Ferchl: *Bio-und Bibliographikon*, Mittenwald, 1937.

Bigelow, Jacob (1787-1879), physician in Boston, professor of materia medica at Harvard, a great educational reformer and one of America's most learned botanists. See Kelly and Burrage: *American Medical Biographies,* p. 100, New York, 1920.

Biroth, Henry (1857-1912), German-born Chicago pharmacist, who was considered one of the leading pharmacists and chemists of the Northwest in his time. Biroth wrote on pharmaceutical and general subjects. See *J. A. Ph. A. 1*:776, 1912.

Bliven, Charles A. (1911-   ), first full-time Executive Secretary of the American Association of Colleges of Pharmacy, since 1961. He had taught at the U. of Nebraska (1936-

1938) and at George Washington U. (1940, and dean from 1947 to 1962) (Melvin R. Gibson in Am. J. Pharm. Edu. 23:499-502, 1959).

Bock, Hieronymus (1498-1554), German cleric, physician, and botanist. His *New Kreuterbuch* (1539) became well known, especially for its excellent illustrations.

Boë, François de le. See: **Sylvius.**

Boerhaave, Hermann (1668-1738). Dutch physician and academic teacher of medicine and of chemistry in Leyden. His medical writings were read all over the world, and his *Elementa chemiae* (Leyden, 1732) is considered the best book on the subject in the first half of the 18th century. F. Garrison: *History of Medicine*, p. 261, Philadelphia, 1929; Sigerist: *The Great Doctors*, p. 185, New York, 1933.

Boettger, Johann Friedrich (1682-1719), pharmacist and alchemist. In connection with E. Tschirnhaus, or at least assisted by the latter, he invented the process of production of European porcelain.

Bois, Jacques du (Latinized as Silvius or Sylvius; 1492-1552), French physician and academic teacher at the University of Paris. In his *Pharmacopoeae, libri tres* (1548), he first used the term "Pharmacopoe[i]a" as the title for a formulary.

Bond, Thomas (1712-1784), Philadelphia physician and one of the founders of the Pennsylvania Hospital. See *Dictionary of American Biography 2*, p. 433.

Boogaerdt (Bogart), Herman Meynders (or Myndertz) van den (1612-1648), Dutch-American surgeon. See John Shrady: *New York Med. Register 25*:231, 1887.

Botega. Spanish form of the Latin *apotheca, q.v.* See: ***Apotheke.***

Botica. Italian form of the Latin *apotheca, q.v.* See: ***Apotheke.***

Boutique. French form of the Latin *apotheca, q.v.* See: ***Apotheke*** and ***Apothicairerie.***

Bowditch, Henry I. (1808-1892), physician, author and one of the leading spirits of the antislavery movement before the Civil War. See *Dictionary of American Biography 2*:492, 1929.

Boyle, Robert (1627-1687), Irish-English aristocrat, one of the earliest eminent English chemists, a founder of the Royal Society of Great Britain and director of the East India Company. Boyle is one of the originators of analysis by precipitation. His general chemical knowledge was far ahead of his time. He formulated Boyle's Law and introduced the terms analysis, reaction and reagent into chemical language.

Boylston, Zabdiel (1679-1766), American-born medical practitioner, taught by his father, who likewise practiced medicine. Without academic study or a medical degree, he achieved a high reputation in his profession. See *Dictionary of American Biography, 2,* p. 535.

Braillier, Pierre (sixteenth century), French pharmacist. See L. André-Pontier: *Histoire de la pharmacie,* p. 210, Paris, 1900.

Brandes, Rudolph (1795-1842), German pharmacist. He initiated the *Apothekerverein im Noerdlichen Teutschland,* discovered delphinine and hyoscyamine (both in 1819), and wrote many books and essays.

Breasted, James Henry (1865-1935), the first American to specialize in ancient, especially Egyptian history. He became an international authority. His importance for pharmacy was two-fold. First, he started his career as a pharmacist, graduating from the Chicago College of Pharmacy (1886); and, secondly, he translated, annotated and published the Edwin Smith Papyrus. See John A. Wilson: James H. Breasted, National Academy of Sciences of the United States of America, *Biograph. Mem. XVIII,* p. 95, 1938; *Alumni Rec.,* University of Illinois, 1921, p. 346.

Bridges, Robert (1806-1882), physician and professor at the Philadelphia College of Pharmacy (1842 to 1879). See J. W. England: *First Century of the Philadelphia College of Pharmacy,* p. 401, Philadelphia, 1922.

Briggs, W. Paul (1903-), Commander U.S. N.R., 1942-1945; chief, Pharmacy Section, Bureau of Medicine and Surgery, U.S.N., 1948-51; chief, Pharmacy Service, Veterans Administration, 1946-1947; teacher and writer; Executive Director, American Foundation for Pharmaceutical Education, since 1951. Before entering government service, Briggs had served on the pharmacy faculty of George Washington University, 1927-46. *Am. Men of Science.*

Brockedon, William (1787-1854), a principal inventor of compressed tablets. See L. F. Kebler: The tablet industry. *J. A. Ph. A.* 3:820, 1914.

Brown, John (1735-1788), Scotch physician. See F. Garrison: *History of Medicine,* p. 314, Philadelphia, 1929; Sigerist: *Man and Medicine,* p. 43, New York, 1932.

Brown, William (1752-1792), Scotch-born American physician, graduated at Edinburgh, of high professional and social standing. He wrote the so-called Lititz pharmacopoeia. See L. C. Duncan: *Medical Men in the American Revolution,* p. 240; Carlisle, 1931; John Kebler: *J. A. Ph. A.* 16:1090, 1927; *Badger Pharmac.* Nos. 22-25, 1938; *Dictionary of American Biography, III,* p. 157.

Brown-Séquard, Charles-Edouard (1817-1894). A native of Mauritius, he was chiefly associated with French medicine. He was professor of the Collège de France (1878) and in the Harvard and the Paris medical faculties. See Garrison: *History of Medicine,* p. 553, Philadelphia, 1929.

Brunfels, Otto (1500-1534), German cleric, physician and botanist. He not only wrote his famous botanic work, first in Latin as a *herbarium,* then in German as a *Kreuterbuch,* but also many other treatises. Among them was a dictionary of synonyms and his

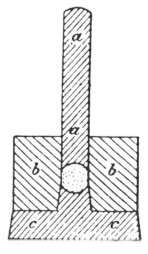

The earliest compressed-tablet machine, invented by an English watchmaker, William Brockedon (1843), was hand operated and simple. First, the upper die (a) was removed and the lower die (b, c) was filled with powder by means of a patented measuring instrument. Then the upper die was reinserted and struck sharply with a mallet, thereby compressing the powder. The upper die was then removed to extract the tablet, and the process was repeated. A century after this invention, compressed tablets had become the most popular form of medication (about ⅓ of all American prescriptions). (See Foote, P. A.: Tablets, Bull. Univ. Wis. No. 1566, Madison (1916?).)

Reformation de Apotecken, published after his death in 1536. His *Reformation* presents an account of pharmaceutical duties and served as a guide to both pharmacist and government.

Brunschwygk, Hieronymus (also spelled Brunschwig, Brunschwyk, etc.; 1430-1512), German surgeon. His books on the art of distillation initiated a new period of pharmaceutical art. In addition, Brunschwygk wrote a *Thesaurus pauperum* (literally "treasury of the poor"), a popular medicine book designed for self-treatment.

Buchner, Johannes Andreas (1783-1852), German pharmacist and professor of pharmacy, first at the University of Landshut, later at Munich. He discovered salicine in willow bark, solanine in potato plant, berberine in Berberis, aesculin in ashtree bark, nicotine in tobacco, and also acrolein. From 1815 to 1852, Buchner edited the *Repertorium der Pharmacie.*

Bulleyn (also Bullein), William (d. 1576), English physician, botanist and rector of Blaxhall, Suffolk. See *Dictionary* (English) *National Biography, VII,* p. 244.

Bullock, Charles (1826-1900), Philadelphia pharmacist. See *Drug. Circ. 51:*82, 1907; *Proc. A. Ph. A. 48:*38, 1900.

Burroughs, Silas Maineville (1850-1895), American pharmacist and, together with Henry Wellcome, *q.v.,* founder of the English pharmaceutic firm of Burroughs, Wellcome and Company. See *Am. J. Pharm. 67:* 433, 1895.

Cadet de Gassicourt, Charles Louis (1769-1821), French pharmacist. Of his books, *La chimie domestique* (8 volumes), *Pharmacie domestique* and his *Formulaire magistral et mémorial pharmaceutique* are noteworthy.

Carney, Charles T. (1832-1862), Boston pharmacist and teacher at the Massachusetts College of Pharmacy. See: *Drug. Circ. 51:*157, 1907.

Carpenter, Philo, Chicago's first pharmacist (about 1800-1850). See: *Bull. Pharm. 16:* 100, 1902.

Caspari, Charles J. (1850-1917), American pharmacist, professor at the Maryland College of Pharmacy and for 15 years general secretary of the American Pharmaceutical Association. See E. F. Kelly: *Am. J. Pharm. 89:*565, 1917.

Cassebeer, George A. (1817-1895), German-born and educated pharmacist of New York. See *Am. Drug. and Pharm. Rec. 27:*124, 1895.

Cataplasma, Greek *kataplassein,* to spread over.

Catelan, Laurent, pharmacist and lecturer at the University of Montpellier (16th and early 17th century). See J. A. Häfliger: *Das Apothekenwesen Basels,* p. 52, Mittenwald, 1938.

Catesby, Mark (1679-1749), English naturalist and artist, travelled 10 years in Southern North America and in the Bahama Islands, then wrote the books: *The Natural History of Carolina, Florida and the Bahama Islands,* and the *Hortus Britanniae Americanus.* See *Dictionary of American Biography, III,* p. 571.

Caventou, Joseph Bienaimé (1795-1877), French pharmacist and one of the earliest and most successful investigators of alkaloids. In collaboration with Pelletier, *q.v.,* he discovered strychnine (1818), brucine and, simultaneously with Meissner, veratrine (1819), quinine and cinchonine (1820). He coined the name chlorophyll (from Greek *chloros* = light green and *phyllon* = leaf) for the green pigment of plants. Among his many publications there was a textbook on pharmacy (*Traité élémentaire de pharmacie théorique*). See *Am. J. Pharm. 49:*384, 1877.

Chapman, William Barker (1813-1874), Ph.G. and M.D., pharmacist in Cincinnati and professor of pharmacy in the Cincinnati College of Pharmacy. See Sonnedecker, G.: A Philadelphia 'pharmaceutist' in the old West—William Barker Chapman, *Am. J. Pharm. 126:*91-97, 1954; also *Am. J. Pharm. 46:*544, 1874; *Drug. Circ. 51:*82, 1907.

Chaptal, Jean Antoine Claude, Count of Chanteloup (1756-1832), French physician and chemist. His major field was chemical technology.

Charas, Moise, French pharmacist (1618-1698). His *Pharmacopée royale galenique et chymique* (1672) passed through several editions in French, and was translated into English and Latin. Charas wrote several other treatises. One on treacle and the medical use of flesh of vipers and another on China bark and its preparation and employment received much attention.

Chiron. A centaur (half man, half horse) in Greek mythology, who knew all mysteries, among them those of the art of healing, which he taught to Asclepios, *q.v.*

Chemist. Origin of the term is not undisputed. The word is assumed to have as its root either the Arabic *Al-kimia* or the ancient name of the Egyptian country, *Kemi*, or the late Greek *chymeia*. "Chemist" as a designation for pharmaceutical practitioners is restricted primarily to the Anglo-Saxon world. Especially in the combination "chemist and druggist," (see: **Druggist**) it has become general since the early 19th century. After World War I, the chemists proper attempted to deprive pharmaceutical practitioners of their legal title. Attempts to introduce the designation "pharmacist" in Britain to replace "chemist" were not altogether successful. The designation "chemist's shop" for a pharmacy is common in England.

Chemist and Druggist. See: **Titles.**

China. On the early materia medica of the highly developed Chinese culture see especially the publications of Gottfried Schramm, e.g., in *Wissenschaft. Zeitschr. d. Karl-Marx Univ. Leipzig* (*Mathematisch-Naturwissensch. Reihe*), 6: Heft 5, pp. 481-503, and *Die Vorträge der Hauptversammlung der Internationalen Gesellschaft für Geschichte der Pharmazie*, Bd. 13, pp. 185-195, Eutin, 1958; A. Mosig and G. Schramm: *Der Arzneipflanzen und Drogenschatz Chinas and die Bedeutung des Pên-ts'ao kang-mu als Standardwerk der chinesischen Materia medica*, Berlin, 1955; also in H. Schelenz: *Geschichte der Pharmazie*, Berlin, 1904; I. Berendes: *Die Pharmazie bei den alten Kulturvölkern*, Halle, 1891; Tschirch: *Handbuch der Pharmakognosie*, Leipzig, 1910, *I*, Part 2.

On old Chinese medicine in general see Pierre Huard and Ming Wong: *La Médecine Chinoise au Cours des Siècles*, Paris, 1959; a comparable book in English, but without illustrations, is by Wang Yen Ming and Wu Lien Teh, *History of Chinese Medicine*, ed. 2, Shanghai, 1936; W. R. Morse, *Chinese Medicine*, New York, 1934; Wong Ch. and Wu, L.: *History of Chinese Medicine*, Chicago, 1936; K. L. Kaufman, a chronology of some events of pharmaceutical interest in ancient China and Japan, *J. A. Ph. A. 28:* 544, 1939; I. Cameron and K. K. Chen, The old and the new pharmacy in China, *Pharm. J. 114:*633, 1925; H. E. Hume: *The Chinese Way in Medicine*, Baltimore, 1940.

Christensen, Bernard V. (1885-1956), American educator and pharmacognosist from 1927; dean of pharmacy at U. of Florida (1933-39) and Ohio State U. (1939-55). At Ohio State Christensen initiated the first required 5-year undergraduate curriculum in U.S.A. pharmacy. He served pharmacy nationally in many official positions. (E. P. Guth in *Am. J. Pharm. Ed. 20:*649-651, 1956; and *Amer. Men of Science*, ed. 8, p. 429.)

Christensen, H. C. (1865-1947), Secretary of the National Association of Boards of Pharmacy. See *J. A. Ph. A. 19:*315, 1930.

Christison, Sir Robert (1797-1882), English physician. Besides his Dispensatory, which he wrote to replace Duncan's antiquated *New Edinburgh Dispensatory*, he published a *Treatise on on Poisons* which was well received. See *Pharm. J. 41:*659, 1882; *Dictionary of National* (English) *Biography, X*, p. 290.

Church, Benjamin (1734-1776), prominent American physician and the first medical director of the Revolutionary Army in 1775. He was found guilty of criminal correspondence with the enemy and was at first imprisoned. See L. C. Duncan: *Medical Men in the American Revolution*, p. 61, Carlisle, 1961; *Dictionary of American Biography, IV*, p. 100.

Circumforaneus, pl. *-i.* See **pharmacopolae circumforaneae.**

Clyster (also "ibis" or "enema") is a liquid injection into the lower intestine (from the Greek word *glyzein*, "wash off" or "out"). According to Pliny, the Egyptians learned the use of clysters from the bird called the "ibis," which was said to inject water into its bowel with its beak. Clysters were generally used during antiquity, as well as in modern times. See Friedenwald and Morrison: The history of enema, in *Bull. Hist. Med. 8:*68, 1940. Of special interest to modern pharmacy is the clyster fad in France immortalized by Molière in his *Le malade imaginaire*. For a sarcastic account of this chapter of French pharmaceutical history see Phillipe: *Histoire des apothicaires*, pp. 99 ff., 328, Paris, 1853; or Phillipe and Ludwig: *Geschichte der Apotheker*, pp. 119 ff., 923, Jena, 1855.

Coblentz, Virgil (1862-1932), American pharmacist, later professor at the New York College of Pharmacy and one of the American pharmaceutical teachers who supplemented their education at German universities. See *J. A. Ph. A. 21:*425, 1932.

Cochran, John (1731-1807), American physician of Scotch descent. He was the last medical director general of the Revolutionary Army. See L. C. Duncan: *Medical Men in the American Revolution*, p. 345, Carlisle, 1931; *Dictionary of American Biography, IV*, p. 251.

Codex. See **Pharmacopeia.**

Codigo. See **Pharmacopeia.**

Coggeshall, George D. (1809-1891), pharmacist in New York and one of the original members of the New York College of Pharmacy, as well as of the Am. Pharm. A. See J. W. England: *First Century of the Philadelphia College of Pharmacy*, p. 127, Philadelphia, 1922; *Proc. A. Ph. A.* 40:18, 1892.

Colden, Cadwallader (1688-1776), Scotch-born physician and botanist, who practiced medicine first in Philadelphia and later in New York. He collected some 100 American plants for Linné. See *Am. J. Pharm.* 80:419, 1908; *Pharm. Rundsch.* 4:121, 1886; *Dictionary of American Biography, IV*, p. 286.

Collyrium, Greek *kollyrion*, poultice or eye salve, used as a designation for medicated applications for the eyes, now usually eye-washes.

Compendium pharmaceuticum Le Coste. A formulary, compiled for the French forces in North America by Jean François Coste, chief physician of Rochambeau's French Expeditionary Forces in the American Revolution, printed in Newport in 1780. Republished in facsimile by John E. Lane in the *Bulletin of the Society of Medical History of Chicago* 45:214, 1930, and with a translation into English and annotations by Edward Kremers, in *Badger Pharmac.*, Madison, Wis., Nos. 27 to 30, 1940 (see Kremers, E.: *American Pharmaceutical Documents, 1643 to 1780*, Madison, Wis., 1944). For an account of Coste's life see John E. Lane: *Americana* 22:51, 1928, reprinted in *Military Surgeon* 63:219.

Composita, from the Latin *compositus* ("made up of parts") i.e., composite substance. In the system of humoral pathology, *q.v.*, in its Galenic form, *composita* are drugs with compound or composite effect, in contrast to *simplicia*, which exert only the simple effects of warmth or cold, moisture or dryness. Pharmaceutically speaking, however, composita were preparations and simplicia, *q.v.*, was the generic term for simple drugs used unmixed or for making the composita. It became customary to divide pharmacopeias into two groups, the one giving directions for making the composita, the other giving a list of simplicia. In the first official German pharmacopeia, the *Dispensatorium pharmacopolarum* of Valerius Cordus (1546), however, the simplicia were explained in connection with the formula for the preparation in which they are used; but there are separate indices, an *Index compositorium* and an *Index simplicium.*

Concordantia. See: **Pharmacopeia.**

Concordia. See: **Pharmacopeia.**

Confectio (nes). Lat. *conficio, -ere, feci, -fectum*, literally anything that is made. (Our word "factory," derived from *facio, facere, feci, factum*, implies a place where things are made.) In a more restricted sense, the term confectio designated certain preparations made by the pharmacist in his *officin* (from *opus*, "work," and *facere*, "to make"), particularly *confectiones* proper, *i.e.*, soft, semisolid or solid mixtures of powdered drugs with honey, syrup of sugared fruit juices. Modern English usage restricts the use of the word confection to candies and similar wares sold in a confectionery. See L. Winkler, *Dispensatorium des Valerius Cordus*, p. 13, Mittenwald, 1934. Compare *Electuary.*

Confectionarius, pl. *-i,* from *confectio,* "that which is prepared" (*con* and *facere*, "to make") and *-arius,* pertaining to a maker, in this case a maker of medicaments. The term appears in the **Law** of Frederick II of 1240, *q.v.* Cf. *Pharmakopoeos* and *Medicamentarius.*

Conservae. From Latin *con-servo, avi, atum.,* "to keep in existence, to preserve." One part of finely cut fresh flowers or herbs were mixed with two parts of sugar, the product representing sugary morsels or a sugary paste. Trommsdorff (See *"Konserven"* in his *Wörterbuch*) points out that they were subject to deterioration—the opposite of the property implied in the name! Hence, they were discontinued. Preparations resembling our candied fruits (and prepared the same way) were likewise called *Conservae* or, by the more specific term, *Condita.*

Constantinus Africanus (1020-1087), the first to translate on a large scale Greco-Arabic works (particularly Arabic works) based on Galen or the Hippocratean Corpus, into Latin. He is said to have been a North African Christian monk before coming to Salerno. See J. J. Walsh: *Old-Time Makers of Medicine*, p. 163, New York, 1911; Louis Figuier: *Vies des savants illustres du moyen age*, p. 103, Paris, 1867; George Sarton: *Introduction to the History of Science*, vol. 1, p. 769, Baltimore, 1927.

Cook, E. Fullerton (1879-1961) became chairman of the Committee of Revision of the U. S. Pharmacopeia in 1920 and served for three decades. He was the first U.S. chairman to take an active part in international drug standardization problems and helped to prepare the first *Pharmacopoeia Internationalis*. He was professor at the Philadelphia College of Pharmacy (from 1903), with which he remained associated for a lifetime. Author, and co-editor of *Remington's Practice of Pharmacy*. (*Am. J. Pharm. Ed.* 25: 478, 1961; and J. England: *First Century of the Philadelphia College of Pharmacy*, p. 421, Philadelphia, 1922.)

Cordus, Valerius (1515-1544), German physician whose *Dispensatorium* made his name famous. It was compiled at the suggestion of the apothecary Johannes Ralla, his uncle. In the laboratory of the pharmacy of Ralla, Cordus experimented with the distillation of ethereal oils. The results of these studies are not published in the *Dispensatorium Valerii Cordi* but in the writings which Conrad Gessner, *q.v.*, published after the death of the author. In one of these papers, *De artificiosis extractionibus*, the first known formula for the preparation of ether has been given. See Ludwig Winkler: *Dispensatorium des Valerius Cordus*, Gesellschaft für Geschichte der Pharmazie, Mittenwald, 1934.

Cosmas, (d. A.D. 303), Arabic-Christian martyr, who, together with his twin brother Damian, is said to have given medical and medicinal help gratuitously to all who needed it. After their martyrdom both brothers became the favorite patron saints of medicine and of pharmacy in all Christian countries. See Marie-Louise David-Danel: *Iconographie des Saints médecins Come et Damien*, Lille, 1958 (bibliography pp. 235-244); also below under **Saints.**

Costello, Patrick H. (1897-   ), pharmacist and authority on pharmacy law administration. He was Secretary of the National Association of Boards of Pharmacy, 1942-62, and previously had been Secretary of the North Dakota Board of Pharmacy, 1927-1942. Costello acquired his first pharmacy in 1919, and in the ensuing years has held many professional and civic positions. See: *Who's Who in America*.

Courtois, Bernard (1777-1838), French pharmacist, discovered (1811) iodine in the ashes of seadweeds. The name iodine (from the Greek iodes = "violet color," ion = "a violet") was given to the new element by Davy, because of its violet vapor.

Coxe, John Redman (1773-1864), American physician, professor at the University of Pennsylvania and author of the first dispensa-

tory to be published in the United States. See. *Am. J. Pharm.* 36:275, 1864; J. W. England: *First Century of the Philadelphia College of Pharmacy*, pp. 44, 60, Philadelphia, 1922.

Craigie, Andrew (1743-1819). Served in the "Army of the Patriots," during the American Revolutionary War, with the title "apothecary general" (given him January 1, 1777) and later as "apothecary" (October 6, 1780). After the war, he became a successful wholesale pharmacist. See L. F. Kebler: *J. A. Ph. A.* 17:63, 167, 1928; *Dictionary of American Biography, IV,* p. 497.

Croll, Oswald (1560-1609), German physician and one of the foremost followers of Paracelsus, *q.v.* His principal work, the *Basilica chymica*, contains numerous formulas for inorganic chemical remedies.

Culpeper, Nicholas (1616-1654), an English medical practitioner, who had been apprenticed to an apothecary. He wrote an amazing number of books on herbs and on materia medica in the short time of his life. He brought himself into notoriety by publishing (1649) his unauthorized English translation of the London College of Physicians' *Pharmacopoeia*. His herbal was reissued in revised editions under his name until the late 19th century. Together with Culpeper's *The English Physician*, it was widely used for self-treatment, not only in England but also in the North American colonies.

Cuming, Fortescue (1762-1828), Irish traveler, naturalist and writer. See *Dictionary of American Biography, IV,* p. 592; Thwaites: *Early Western Travels*, Cleveland, 1904-1907, vol. 4, "Cuming's Tour to the Western Country."

Curtman, Charles O. (1829-1896), German-born American pharmacist, during the Civil War director of the laboratories for manufacturing gunpowder and other products for the Confederate Army, professor of chemistry in the St. Louis College of Pharmacy, author of textbooks on analytic chemistry. See *Am. J. Pharm.* 68:351, 1896.

Cutbush, Edward (1772-1843), physician, chief surgeon of the United States Navy, after 1829 professor of chemistry at Geneva College, Geneva, N. Y. See Kelly and Burrage: *American Medical Biographies*, p. 272, 1920.

Cutbush, James (1788-1823), Philadelphia pharmacist and chemist. He was the first president of the Columbian Chemical Society, founded in 1811; and professor of chemistry in St. John's College, Philadelphia, and later at West Point. See *Dictionary of American Biography*, V, p. 10; H. George Wolfe: James Cutbush—author, teacher, apothecary general, *Am. J. Pharm. Ed. 12*: 89-125, 1948.

Cutler, Manasseh (1742-1823), American clergyman and botanist. See *Lloyd Libr.*, Reprod. Ser. No. 4, 1903; *Dictionary of American Biography*, V, p. 12.

Damian (d 303 A.D.), Arabic-Christian martyr and patron saint of medicine and particularly of pharmacy. See **Cosmas.**

Dargavel, John W. (1894-1961) was Executive Secretary of the National Association of Retail Druggists, 1933-61. He had been a practicing pharmacist in Minnesota from 1917 until called to the N.A.R.D. office in Chicago, and had served as Secretary of the Minnesota State Board of Pharmacy, 1923-34. As N.A.R.D. Secretary he gave pharmacy owners vigorous representation of their economic interests and worked relentlessly for Fair Trade Laws; also important was his role in the split between the N.A.R.D. and the A. Ph. A. during the 1950's. (*Drug Topics 23*:2 and 16, Oct., 1961; *Who's Who in America.*)

Davis, William (seventeenth century), apothecary in Boston. See *Bull. Mass. Coll. Pharm. III*:39, No. 4, 1914.

Dealers in drugs. During antiquity, and up to the European Middle Ages, the following designations of dealers in drugs were in use:—

In Greek literature the following terms are found: *migmatopoloi, myropoei, myrepsoi, pharmacopoeoi, pharmacolopoli* and *rhizotomoi.*

In Rome the following terms were used: *circumforaneae, pharmacopoei, pharmacotribae, pharmacotritae, pharmacopolae, pigmentarii, sellularii, seplasiarii* and *unguentarii.*

During the Middle Ages the following terms were coined: *apothecarius, aromatarius, herbarius* and its modifications, *speciarius* and *stationarius.*

Most of the modern designations are derived from two Greek words, *pharmakon* or *apotheke.* From the former, the French *pharmacien,* the English *pharmacist* and *pharmaceutist,* and the German *Pharmaceut* (*Pharmazeut*) are derived; from the latter, the French *apothicaire,* the English *apothecary* and the German *Apotheker;* also the corresponding terms, with slightly modified spelling, in other Germanic languages. With the advent of the iatrochemical school, the terms *chemist* and later *pharmaceutical chemist* came into use. Lastly should be mentioned the terms (usually referring to non-pharmacists): *druggist, q.v.,* the French *droguiste,* and the German *Droguist* and *Drogist.* Possibly the *Laboranten* and the *Olitätenhändler* (peddlers of medicaments in Germany) should not be omitted. For details look up each term; see also, Rudolf Schmitz: Über deutsche Apotheken des 13. Jahrhunderts; Ein Beitrag zur Etymologie des apoteca-apotecarius-Begriffs, Sudhoffs Archiv *45*:289-302, 1961, also Pharm. Ztg. *104*:871-872, 1959; M. Fialon: Histoire des mots "Pharmacien" et "Apothicaire," Bull. Soc. Hist. Pharm., Dec., 1920, No. 28, pp. 263-269; E.-H. Guitard: *ibid., 44*:383-384, 1956; T. D. Whittet: From apothecary to pharmacist: A study of changes of title, Chem. & Drugg., June 30, 1962, pp. 734-736; Oct. 6, 1962, pp. 385-386, et seq.; Wilkening: Zur Geschichte des Wortes "Pharmazie" und "Apotheker," Pharm. Ztg. *75*:225, 1930.

DeButts, Elisha (1773-1831), Irish-born physician, physiologist, a founder of the University of Maryland School of Medicine and professor of chemistry at the Maryland College of Medicine. See Kelly and Burrage: *American Medical Biographies,* p. 301, 1920.

Decoctio. From Latin decoctus, "boiled down," an aqueous potion prepared by boiling vegetable drugs with water; one of the earliest modes of administration.

Defectar. See: **Personnel.**

Defectarius. See: **Personnel.**

Degrees in American pharmacy for undergraduate or graduate studies, over the decades, have been: Bachelor of Pharmacy; Bachelor of Science (in Pharmacy); Doctor of Pharmacy; Doctor of Philosophy (with Pharmacy, Pharmacognosy, Pharmaceutical Chemistry, etc., as major); Graduate in Pharmacy; Master of Pharmacy; Master of Science (Pharmacy, etc.); Pharmaceutical Chemist.

Deities or deified persons to whom medicine, etc., is attributed.

1. Egyptian. Thoth, Osiris, Isis, Horus, Imhotep, Anepu (Anubis).

2. Greek: Apollo, Hephaistos, Herakles, Prometheus, Asklepios, Hygeia, Chiron.

For replacement of these pagan deities by Christian saints, see **Saints, Christian, as Patrons of Pharmacy.**

Demachy, Jean François (1728-1803), French pharmacist. Besides his *Manuel de pharmacien,* he wrote several books about industrial pharmaceutical and chemical technic, among them one concerning the preparation of liquors.

Derosne, Charles Louis (1780-1846), French pharmacist. As early as 1803, he prepared opium alkaloids, without, however, isolating the individual ones and recognizing their alkaline nature.

Dia-preparations. Preparations designated by putting the word *dia* before the main constituent of the compounded medicine or *confectio, q.v.* Thus one knew that the most important constituent of *Diasenna Nicolai* was senna.

Diehl, C. Lewis (1840-1917), German-born American pharmacist active in almost all branches of pharmacy: as owner of a pharmacy in Louisville; as professor of pharmacy at the Louisville College of Pharmacy; in pharmaceutical industry; and as a contributor to pharmaceutical literature. His reports on the progress of pharmacy in the *Proceedings* of the American Pharmaceutical Association offered an all-around survey of great value. See England: *First Century Philadelphia College of Pharmacy,* p. 217, Philadelphia, 1922; *J. A. Ph. A.* 6:423, 1917.

Digby (Digbi), Sir Kenelm (1603-1665). He was secretary of the navy under the English Kings Charles I and II, and left comprehensive collections of secret formulas which were published after his death. See A. C. Wootton: *Chronicles of Pharmacy,* London, 1910. *I,* p. 193; *Dictionary* (English) *National Biography, XV,* p. 60.

Dioscorides, Greek physician and botanist (first century A.D.), author of *"Perihylé,"* Latinized materia medica, which for 1500 years was one of the standard works on medicine, pharmacy and botany. See J. Berendes: *Des Pedanios Dioskurides aus Anazarbos Arzneimittellehre,* Stuttgart, 1902; Robert T. Gunther: *The Greek Herbal of Dioscorides,* New York, 1959 (English translation of the Materia Medica); A. C. Wootton: *Chronicles of Pharmacy,* London, 1910, *I,* p. 206; C. J. S. Thompson: *The Mystery and Art of the Apothecary,* London, 1929, p. 130; M. R. Cohen and I. E. Drabkin: *A Source Book in Greek Science,* New York, 1948.

Dispensary. The room or place where articles are dispensed. In pharmaceutical practice we refer to the dispensary of a hospital, a physician, a factory, etc. Contrast with

Medicine chest, or **Medicine cabinet.** However, it also finds nonpharmaceutical application, e.g., "milk dispensary," etc.

Dispensatorium. From *dispensare,* "to dispense." As a title for a book of formulas, etc. (directions for the making of preparations) it was employed before the designation "pharmacopeia" came into use. Thus we refer to the *Dispensatory of Valerius Cordus, q.v.,* or the *Nürnberg Pharmacopoeia.* The English dispensatories of the seventeenth century and later were for the most part commentaries on English translations of the London and other pharmacopeias, and expanded into more or less comprehensive reference books. Such commentaries, partly including the texts of the respective pharmacopeias, became common in the United States. See, e.g., *Coxe's Dispensatory,* the *United States Dispensatory,* the *American Dispensatory,* the *National Dispensatory.* Cf. **Pharmacopeia.**

Dispensatory. See *Dispensatorium.*

Dispenser. See **Personnel.**

Distillation apparatus. See Gildemeister-Hoffmann-Kremers: *The Volatile Oils,* pp. 51-82, Milwaukee, 1900; H. Schelenz: *zur Geschichte der pharmazeutisch chemischen Destilliergeräte,* Miltitz, 1911; R. J. Forbes: *Short History of the Art of Distillation,* Leiden, 1948.

Döbereiner, Johann Wolfgang (1780-1849), German pharmacist and professor of chemistry at Jena. He discovered the catalytic effect of platinum, and used it in converting alcohol into acetic acid (1821) and into acetaldehyde (1832). Finally, by the same means, he converted H_2SO_3 into H_2SO_4. He produced formic acid by treating manganese with acetic acid and prepared synthetically methyl alcohol. By his "theory of triads" (1829), based on his discovery that there are group of 3 elements in which the atomic weight of the one is the mean of those of the other two, Döbereiner created one of the forerunners of the periodic system.

Dohme, A. R. L. (b. 1867), a son of Charles Dohme, succeeded his uncle, Louis, as president of Sharp and Dohme until this firm and that of Mulford and Co. were merged (1911-1929). Author of numerous papers. See *Who's Who in America,* 21, p. 784; *American Men of Science,* ed. 8, p. 632, 1949.

Dohme, Charles E. (1843-1911), German-born American pharmacist and pharmaceutical manufacturer. See *Pharm. Era* 45:40, 1912; *J. A. Ph. A.* 1:82, 1912.

Doliber, Thomas (1836-1912), pharmacist in

Boston and president of the Mellin's Food Company. See *J. A. Ph. A. 1*:777, 1912.

Dorvault, François Laurent Marie (1815-1879), French pharmacist and writer on pharmaceutical subjects. He not only organized the *Pharmacie centrale de France,* but edited *L'officine, répertoire général de pharmacie practique,* which has been published in many editions as a standard French work on practical pharmacy.

Dow, Cora M. (b. 1871), Cincinnati pharmacist and entrepreneur who built a chain of pharmacies. See *Pharm. Era 43*:489, 1910.

Drogist, German for druggist, a merchant specializing in the sale of drugs not legally restricted to pharmacies and in the sale of spices, cosmetics, technical chemicals, paints, varnishes, etc. As a special group separate from pharmacy they estabished themselves in Germany in the second half of the 19th century. Also used in title for books and Journals (e.g., *Drogisten-Zeitung*).

Droguiste, French for druggist, a sort of third-class pharmaceutical practitioner discontinued in the 20th century.

Druce, George Claridge (1851-1932), considered the greatest British field botanist of his time. From a practicing pharmacist in Oxford, where he was mayor (1900), he developed into an influential member of Oxford University. His contributions to botanical literature were extensive. See *Chem. & Drugg. 116*:255, 1932.

Drug. French *drogue,* German *Droge.* In its restricted sense, the word has been used to designate so-called "crude" drugs of mineral, vegetable or animal origin, in contrast with galenic preparations or chemicals. In its wider sense, as defined in state and national laws, the term includes all preventive and therapeutic agents. Its derivation is in doubt. Formerly it was regarded as being derived from the Dutch verb *droog,* "to dry," i.e., a product of either vegetable or animal origin preserved by drying (German *Pflanzendrogen, Medizinaldrogen,* as contrasted with vegetables dried for culinary purposes). C. F. Seybold (*Zeitschr. für deutsche Wortforschung 10*:218, 1908) traces it back to the Arabic *dowa,* a remedy.

Druggist. (Derived from "drug," *q.v.*), "dealer in drugs." In its original usage in the Anglo-Saxon world the term referred to a wholesaler in drugs. In North America it gradually became the designation for the common type of pharmacist. As "chemist and druggist," the word became part (1868) of the official

designation of the English pharmaceutical practitioners, when an act of Parliament required all future "chemists and druggists" to pass examination and be registered.

Drugs, designations of dealers in. See: **Dealers in drugs.**

Dumas, Jean Baptiste (1800-1884), French chemist who started his career as a pharmaceutical apprentice and received the highest honors in science, as well as in the political life of his country. His determinations of the vapor densities of iodine, sulfur, phosphorus. mercury, etc., were important for theoretic chemistry. He determined the chemical formula for methyl alcohol, chloroform and iodoform, and laid the ground for modern structural formulas. He is considered one of the founders of physical chemistry and "one of those great chemical researchers . . . who served as landmarks" (A. W. v. Hofmann). He held the positions of Secretary of Agriculture and of Commerce in the French government (1849 to 1851) and was subsequently a senator. See *Am. J. Pharm. 56*:351, 1884.

Du Mez, Andrew G. (1885-1948) was active in a series of official and teaching positions and, after 1926, dean of the School of Pharmacy, University of Maryland. Of his numerous publications, the *Year Book* of the American Pharmaceutical Association, edited by him from 1921 to 1935, and after 1935 the *Pharmaceutical Abstracts,* made him especially well known. See *J. A. Ph. A. 28*: p. 67, 1939.

Duncan, Andrew (1744-1828), physician and professor at Edinburgh University. Besides his *New Dispensatory,* Duncan wrote several other books on medicine. See *Dictionary of (English) National Biography, XVI,* p. 161.

Dunning, Henry A. B. (1877-1962). A leader of the pharmaceutical manufacturing firm Hynson, Westcott and Dunning in Baltimore, one of the most ardent promoters of professional pharmacy in the United States, and a philanthropist. See *J. A. Ph. A. 13*:593, 1924; *18*:3, 1929; *Who's Who in America, 21,* p. 819.

Durand, Elias (1794-1873), French-born Philadelphia pharmacist. See England, *First Century of the Philadelphia College of Pharmacy,* p. 357, Philadelphia, 1922; *Am. J. Pharm. 45*:432, 509, 1873.

Dusseau, Michael, also called du Seau, a French pharmacist (16th century), whose early textbook for pharmaceutical apprentices was used in various editions for more than a century.

Dyott, T. W. (about 1775-1850), English-born pharmacist of Philadelphia. See *Bull. Pharm. 18:*237, 1904.

Ebers, Georg (1837-1898), German Egypt-tologist and novelist. He discovered and de-scribed the medicinally important papyrus named after him. See *Papyrus Ebers.*

Ebert, Albert Ethelbert (1840-1906), German-born pharmacist in Chicago; professor of pharmacy at the Chicago College of Pharmacy. He invented the sulfurous process for the manufacture of starch and glucose. His name is commemorated by the Ebert Prize for Scientific Research. See *Proc. A. Ph. A. 55:*iii, 1907; Drug. Circ. *51:*84, 1907.

Eger, George (1836-1900), German-born and educated American pharmacist. See *Proc. A. Ph. A. 49:*40, 1901.

Egypt. Ancient Egypt is of high importance in the history of medicine and pharmacy. Its culture, which immediately influenced the Greeks and, hence, European civilization, is usually considered within a framework of the following main approximate periods:

1. *Native Dynasties:*

A. The Old Empire: Dynasties 3 to 6, 2700 to 2200 B.C., with Memphis as capital. The Great Sphinx and the Pyramids date back to this period.

B. The Middle Empire: Dynasties 11 to 13, 2100 to 1788 B.C., with Thebes the prin-cipal upper Egyptian capital. (Domination by a Bedouin tribe, the so-called Hyksos from 1700 to about 1550.)

C. The New Empire: Dynasties 18 to 21, 1580 to 1090 B.C., during which Egyptian power and splendor were at their height. Thebes was the capital of the empire. To this period belongs the reign of Rameses II, who supposedly forced the Hebrews to labor at his extensive building enterprises.

2. *Foreign Rule:*

D. The Lybian Epoch: Dynasties 22 to 24, 945 to 712 B.C., the reign of the Ethi-opians and the Assyrians: Dynasties 23 to 25, 712 to 525 B.C., with a continuing decay of Egyptian civilization.

E. The Later Period: Dynasties 26 to 31, 525 to 332 B.C. Egypt was conquered by the Persians; as a Persian province, it fell into the hands of Alexander the Great in 332. Alex-andria became the center of Greek civiliza-tion amidst Egyptian decay. After the battle of Actium (31 B.C.) and the death of Queen

Cleopatra, Egypt became a Roman province. See J. H. Breasted: *A History of Egypt,* London, 1921.

Ehrlich, Paul (1854-1915), German physician and leader of the Institute for Experimental Therapy at Frankfurt-on-the-Main, founded as a means for his research. He was a pioneer in merging descriptive cellular pathology with experimental intracellular chemistry, and in testing and using the microchemical reaction of the tissues to dyestuffs. His best known research was the production of Sal-varsan (arsphenamine) which he carried out in collaboration with Hata. See Sigerist: *The Great Doctors,* p. 384, New York, 1933; Garrison: *History of Medicine,* p. 709, Phila-delphia, 1929; H. Loewe: Paul Ehrlich, Stuttgart, 1950.

Electuary. Latin *electuarium* and *electarium,* from *ecligma* (Greek *ek,* "out," and *leichein,* "to lick.") In classical Latin, "a medicine that melts in the mouth." A soft preparation made by mixing powders and other in-gredients with a sweet juice, honey, or a solution of sugar. Cf. **Confectiones.** For de-tails see "*Latwerge,*" in Trommsdorff's *Hand-wörterbuch.*

Elements, four. The four elements of the ancient world, i.e., earth, water, fire and air, were considered to have a mysterious rela-tion to the four humors of the human body (see **Humoral pathology**), blood being moist and warm like earth, phlegm moist and cold like water, yellow bile warm and dry like fire, and black bile cold and dry like air.

Elève. See **Personnel.**

Ellis, Charles (1800-1874), original member of the Philadelphia College of Pharmacy as well as of the American Pharmaceutical As-sociation, pharmacist in Philadelphia. See *Drug. Circ. 51:*84, 1907; J. W. England, *First Century of the Philadelphia College of Phar-macy,* p. 355, Philadelphia, 1922; *Proc. A. Ph. A. 55:*583, 1907.

Embalming was practiced by several peoples during antiquity, but was carried to perfec-tion by the Egyptians. See Tschirch and Reutter: *Über bei der Einbalsamierung der Leichen in Egypten and Carthago benutzte Harze, Archiv der Pharm. 250:*170, 1912; L. Reutter: *De l'embaumement chez les anciens, Bull. de l'institut national genevois,* Tome XLIII; and: *De l'embaumement avant et après Jésus-Christ,* Paris, 1912.

Encheiridion. See **Pharmacopeia.**

Enema. Greek *enjénai,* to send in. See **Clyster.**

Extra-Pharmacopoeia. An English formulary, supplementary to the *British Pharmacopoeia.*

Faraj Ibn Salim (thirteenth century); also called Fararius, Ferrarius or Faragut. Salernitan Jewish physician who was a master translator of Greco-Arabic medical treatises into Latin. See J. J. Walsh: *Old-Time Makers of Medicine*, p. 79, New York, 1911; George Sarton: *Introduction to the History of Science*, 2, part 2, pp. 833-834, Baltimore, 1931.

Farmacopen. See: **Pharmacopeia.**

Farmacopin. See: **Pharmocopeia.**

Farmacopoea. See: **Pharmacopeia.**

Farmakopo. See: **Pharmacopeia.**

Farr, John (1791-1847), English-born chemist and founder of the manufacturing firm later known as Powers and Weightman. See England: *First Century of the Philadelphia College of Pharmacy*, p. 33, Philadelphia, 1922.

Fée, Antoine Laurent Apollinaire (1789-1874), French pharmacist. He became professor of botany at the University of Strasburg (1833). Fée published his *Cours d'histoire naturelle pharmaceutique* in 1828; and his famous *Commentaires sur la botanique et la matière medicale de Pline* in 1853.

Fehling, Hermann von (1812-1885), German pharmacist and physiologic chemist. He developed the method for the determination of sugar and starch by means of an alkaline copper sulfate solution in the presence of alkali tartrates, which has been named after him. His discovery of paraldehyde is also noteworthy. See *Pharm. J.* 45:83, 153, 1885; *Am. J. Pharm.* 57:463, 1885.

Ferrand, Claude-Henry (1740-?), French *pharmacien-en-chef* with the French auxiliary corps in the American Revolutionary War. See A. Balland: *Les pharmaciens militaires Français*, p. 89, Paris, 1913.

Firmin, Giles, Jr. (1614 or 1615-1697), born in England, came to Boston first for a brief visit in 1632 and returned 1637, after having studied medicine in England. He is said to have delivered the first anatomic lectures to students in this country. Later on, he returned to England, where he entered the ministry.

Fischelis, Robert P. (1891-   ), pharmaceutical administrator, teacher, editor, writer, former executive secretary of the Board of Pharmacy of the State of New Jersey (1926-44); Secretary and General Manager, American Pharmaceutical Association (1945-1959); consultant to various governmental agencies, advisor to the American delegation to the International Health Conference of 1946, and member of executive committee, National Health Assembly 1948-49. A list of the many honors bestowed on him, and of the various capacities in which he has served American pharmacy, can be found in *American Men of Science*, ed. 8, p. 780, 1949; *Who's Who in America;* and *J. A. Ph. A.* (Pract. Ed.) 6:11-12, 1945.

Flückiger, Friedrich August (1828-1894). Swiss pharmacist and professor of pharmacy at the University of Strasburg. He was the first of modern pharmacognosists and wrote fundamental books on this subject. He also contributed important articles on the history of pharmacy. See Häfliger, *Fr. A. Flückiger, Gesellschaft für Geschichte der Pharmazie*, Mittenwald, 1928; New York *Pharm. Rund.* 10:107, 1892; F. Hoffmann: *Am. J. Pharm.* 67:65, 1895; *Pharm. J.* 54:538, 1894.

Foesius, Anutius (1528-1595), French physician living in Metz (Lorraine). His unlatinized name was Foès. His *Pharmacopoeia Mediomatrica* (Pharmacopeia of Metz) was widely used.

Formularium. See: **Pharmacopeia.**

Fourcroy, Antoine François, Count of (1755-1809), French physician and chemist. He was a teacher of Vauquelin, *q.v.*; with him he worked intimately. He analyzed many medicinal chemicals.

Fourneau, Ernest F. A. (1872-1949), French pharmacist who became one of the foremost representatives of chemotherapeutic research. Fourneau, who had been the owner of a pharmacy in Paris for years, was director of the pharmaceutical concern of Poulenc Frères (1901 to 1910) and (1911 to 1945) director of the chemotherapeutic laboratory of the Pasteur Institute for more than 30 years. See George Urdang: *Pharmacy's Part in Society*, pp. 70, 71, Madison, Wis., 1946.

Fowler, Thomas (1736-1801), English apothecary and physician. See Wootton: *Chronicles of Pharmacy, II*, p. 133, London, 1910.

Fownes, George (1815-1849), English professor and chemist. His *Manual of Elementary Chemistry* (1845) was widely used in America as well as England. See Ferchl: *Chemisch-Pharmazeutisches Bio-und Bibliographicon*, p. 162, Mittenwald, 1937.

Francke, Don E. (1910-   ), Director, Department of Scientific Services of the American Society of Hospital Pharmacists since 1963 and editor of the *American Journal of Hospital Pharmacy* since 1944. A hospital pharmacist of international distinction, Francke became the first American to be vice president of the International Pharmaceutical Federation (1958-   ). He directed the monumental Audit of Pharmaceutical Service in Hospitals (1956-59). He was formerly Director of Pharmacy Service at the University of Michigan Hospitals (1944-1963), and taught hospital pharmacy there (1948-63). See *Who's Who in America* and *American Men of Science*.

Frank, Adolf (1834-1916), German pharmacist and one of the most versatile inventors and organizers in industrial chemistry and technology.

Frederick II, a Hohenstaufen, German Emperor and King of Southern Italy and Sicily (1194-1250). See **Law for the separation of medicine and pharmacy,** of Frederick II. (*Note* that Frederick II, "The Great," of the House of Hohenzollern, King of Prussia, did not rule until 1712-1786.)

Fuchs, Leonhart (1501-1566), physician and botanist. He was the most learned of the contemporary authors of herbals, and, besides his *New Kreuterbuch* (1543), wrote many other treatises. His edition of the *Antidotarium* of the Byzantine physician Nicolaus Myrepsus, *q.v.,* with notes, is of special pharmaceutical interest. See *Annual Report of the Smithsonian Institution,* 1917; Eberhard Stübler: *Leonhart Fuchs, Leben und Werk,* Munich, 1928.

Fuller, Thomas (1654-1734), English physician and author of several books and pamphlets on medical subjects, including his *Pharmacopeia Extemporanea.* See *Dictionary of National* (English) *Biography, 20,* p. 320.

Gale, Edwin Oscar (1832-1913), Chicago pharmacist, historian and poet. See *J. A. Ph. A.* 2:283, 1913.

Gardiner, Silvester (1708-1786), American-born physician who studied medicine in London and Paris. He and Douglass, *q.v.,* were the first physicians to be adequately educated in England and then to practice in America, and both exerted a marked influence on American medicine. See Henry R. Viets: Some features of the history of medicine in Massachusetts, *Isis* 23:389, 1935; *Dictionary of American Biography, VII,* p. 139.

Gehlen, Adolph Ferdinand (1775-1815), German pharmacist and chemicopharmaceutical journalist. Having published chemical journals since 1803 and edited the *Neues Berliner Jahrbuch der Pharmacie,* 1805-1808, he founded in 1815 the *Repertorium für die Pharmacie,* which J. A. Buchner, *q.v.,* continued.

Geiger, Philipp Lorenz (1785-1836), German pharmacist and professor of pharmacy at the University of Heidelberg. In 1835 Geiger discovered coniine and, in cooperation with Hesse, isolated atropine, hyoscyamine, aconitine and daturine. From 1824 to 1836, he edited the *Magazin der Pharmazie.* Among his books the *Pharmacopoeia universalis* (started by him in 1835 and continued by Friedrich Mohr) was of greatest importance. See G. Urdang: Philipp Lorenz Geiger, *Pharmazeutische Zeitung* 74:1154, 1929.

Geoffroy, Etienne François (1672-1731), French pharmacist and member of a family which gave to the world a number of important scientists. His *Tractatus de materia medica seu de medicamentorum simplicium historia, virtute, et usu delectu* is considered the first book presenting pharmacognosy in a systematic way. With his chemical relationship tables (published first in 1718 in the *Memoirs of the Parisian Academy of Science*), Geoffroy laid the foundation of the theory of relationship between the chemical elements.

Gerard (Gerarde), John (1545-1612), English surgeon and botanist. Gerard's *Catalogus arborum, fructicum ac plantarum* (1596) and *The herball or general histoire of plantes* (1597) were highly regarded. The latter was issued in a second and enlarged edition (1633) by the English apothecary Thomas Johnson, *q.v.* See *Dictionary of* (English) *National Biography, XXI,* p. 221.

Gessner, Conrad (also publishing under the pseudonym Evonymus Philiatrus) (1516-1565), Swiss physician and botanist. His main work, *Historia plantarum,* was not published until 1751-1771, about 200 years after the death of the author. See Friedrich Dobler: *Conrad Gessner als Pharmazeut,* Zürich, 1955.

Ghina (or Ghini), Luca (1500-1556), Italian physician and botanist. He is assumed to be the inventor of the herbarium for the collecting of plants and for the preservation of the dried pressed mounts.

Glauber, Johann Rudolf (1604-1670). The work of Glauber was of an amazing extent and versatility. He taught the production of nitric acid by treating saltpetre with sulfuric acid; and of hydrochloric acid by treating sodium chloride with sulfuric acid. He produced sodium sulfate (Glauber's salt), ammonium sulfate, zinc chloride, potassium chloride, etc., and developed numerous methods and technics.

Glentworth, George (end of the eighteenth to middle of the 19th century). See England: *First Century of the Philadelphia College of Pharmacy,* pp. 56, 107, Philadelphia, 1922.

Glyn-Jones, Sir William (1869-1927), English chemist and pharmacist, manufacturer, lawyer and legislator. See *Chem. & Drug. 107*:365, 1927; *J. A. Ph. A. 13*:503, 1924; *16*:894, 1927.

Gmelin, Johann Friedrich (1784-1804), German chemist. In addition to many chemical treatises, pharmaceutical and chemical textbooks, etc., he wrote a history of chemistry. He was a member of the Gmelin family, which, descending from a pharmacist at Tübingen, through the generations gave men of importance to pharmacy as well as to the natural sciences in general. See Otto Raubenheimer: Gmelin, a German family of pharmacists, chemists, and botanists, *J. A. Ph. A. 19*:259, 1930.

Godfrey. See: **Hanckwitz.**

Goethe, Johann Wolfgang von (1749-1832), German poet of highest rank, whose ardent interest in science brought him into close contact with several pharmacists, who became his teachers in chemistry, botany, mineralogy and meteorology. For the relations of Goethe to pharmacists, see George Urdang: Goethe and pharmacy, Madison, Wis., 1949.

Goettling, Johann Friedrich August (1755-1809), German pharmacist and professor of chemistry and pharmacy at the University of Jena. He was one of the first chemists in Germany to repeat and confirm the investigations of Lavoisier, *q.v.*, and, therefore, to abandon the phlogiston theory. In 1780 he started publication of an annual under the title *Almanach oder Taschenbuch für Scheidekuenstler und Apotheker, q.v.,* the first periodical devoted primarily to the interests of pharmacy.

Grahame, Israel J. (1819-1899) was a pharmacist, first in Baltimore and later in Philadelphia. He was professor of pharmacy at the Maryland College of Pharmacy and, in Philadelphia, the principal of several educational institutions for women. His chief merit lies in his research work on percolation. See England: *First Century of the Philadelphia College of Pharmacy,* p. 115, Philadelphia, 1922; *Drug. Circ. 51*:85, 1907.

Grazzini, Antonio Francesco, called il Lasca (1503-1584), Italian pharmacist and poet, dramatist and novelist. Several of his books were still republished in the second half of the 19th century.

Gren, Friedrich Albert Carl (1760-1798), German pharmacist, physician and chemist. He isolated cholesterin from gallstones and wrote in his short life an amazing number of books and pamphlets.

Grew, Nehemiah (1628-1711), English physician. In 1695 he isolated sulfate of magnesium (epsom salt) from the water of Epsom Spring. Grew wrote botanic as well as chemical treatises.

Griffith, Ivor (1891-1961), American pharmacist, born in Wales, professor at the Philadelphia College of Pharmacy, and later President of the College (1912-1961); author of a number of books and articles of a literary as well as a professional nature; editor, *American Journal of Pharmacy* 1921-41. See *Drug Topics,* June 5, 1961, p. 16, and England: *First Century of the Philadelphia College of Pharmacy,* p. 443, Philadelphia, 1922.

Griffith, R. Eglesfield (1797-1850), Philadelphia physician, writer on medical and pharmaceutical subjects, for one year professor at the Philadelphia College of Pharmacy and (between 1831 and 1836) editor of the *Am. J. Pharm.* See *Am. J. Pharm. 22*:400, 1850.

Griffits, Samuel Powell (1759-1826), physician in Philadelphia, professor of materia medica at the University of Pensylvania. See Kelly and Burrage: *American Medical Biographies,* p. 468, New York, 1920.

Guthrie, Samuel (1782-1848), American physician who discovered chloroform at the same time (1831) as the French pharmacist Soubeiran, *q.v.,* and the German chemist Justus von Liebig, *q.v.* See The centenary of chloroform, *J. A. Ph. A. 20*:482, 1931.

Häfliger, Josef Anton (1873-1954), Swiss pharmacist, professor of pharmacy, including the history of pharmacy, at the University of Basle, creator of the pharmaceutico-historical museum which forms an annex to the Pharmaceutical Institute of the University of Basle, and author of numerous pharmaceutical-historical publications. See *Deutsche Apoth. Ztg. 94*:1180-81, 1954.

Hagen, Karl Gottfried (1749-1829), German pharmacist and professor of chemistry and physics at the University of Königsberg. He was one of the most eminent and progressive teachers of the sciences of pharmacy in his time. His textbooks dominated the field for many decades. See Gottfried Wallrabe: *Zum Gedächtnis an Karl Gottfried Hagen. Pharm. Zeit.* 74:285, 1929.

Hager, Hans Hermann Julius (1816-1897), German pharmacist who wrote commentaries on the German pharmacopeias appearing during his lifetime and, among other treatises, the two which became the most used reference books in the practice of pharmacy: his *Manuale pharmaceuticum* and his *Handbuch der pharmaceutischen Praxis.* The *pharmazeutische Zentralhalle (Centralhalle)* founded by Hager (1859) was for a long time one of the leading scientific pharmaceutical journals in Germany.

Hahnemann, Samuel Christian Friedrich (1755-1843), physician and chemist, creator of homeopathy. Of pharmaceutical interest is the fact that he wrote, besides books concerning his special medical theories, an excellent reference book (lexicon) on the art of the pharmacist, and also several chemical treatises. See Th. L. Bradford: *The Life and the Letters of Dr. Samuel Hahnemann,* Philadelphia, 1895, and Eveline Steinbichler: *Geschichte der homöopathischen Arzneibereitungslehre in Deutschland bis 1872* (Internationale Gesellschaft . . . Bd. 11) Eutin, 1957.

Hallberg, Carl Svante N. (1856-1910), Swedish-born American pharmacist, manufacturer, journalist, and professor of pharmacy in the Chicago College of Pharmacy. See England: *First Century of the Philadelphia College of Pharmacy,* p. 195, Philadelphia, 1922.

Hanbury, Daniel (1825-1875), English pharmacist and one of the most eminent modern pharmacognosists. His best-known work is the *Pharmacographia,* which he wrote in conjunction with Flückiger, *q.v.* See *Am. J. Pharm.* 47:238, 1875; E. C. Cripps, *Plough Court,* p. 67, London, 1927.

Hanckwitz, Ambrosius Gottfried (17th and early 18th centuries). German chemist who, in England, took the name Godfrey (anglicized second given name), instead of Hanckwitz. See C. J. S. Thompson, *The Mystery and the Art of the Apothecary,* p. 266, Philadelphia, 1929.

Hancock, John F. (1834-1909), Baltimore pharmacist. See *Drug. Circ.* 51:107, 183, 1007.

Hänle, Georg Friedrich (1763-1824). German pharmacist. In 1823 he founded the *Magazin der Pharmazie.*

Harrison, John (second half of the 18th and first half of the 19th century), Philadelphia pharmacist and manufacturer of chemicals. See England: *First Century of the Philadelphia College of Pharmacy,* p. 35, Philadelphia, 1922; S. P. Sadtler: *Am. J. Pharm.* 93: 201, 1921.

Hartshorne, Joseph (1779-1850). resident apprentice and apothecary in the Pennsylvania Hospital, later a physician in Philadelphia. See Kelly and Burrage: *American Medical Biographies,* p. 500, New York, 1920.

Hatcher, Robert A. (1868-1944), physician and pharmacist, professor of pharmacology and materia medica (1906, to 1935), at Cornell University Medical College; writer on materia medica. See *Who's Who in America, 20:* p. 1152.

Hausknecht. See: **Personnel.**

Hébert, Louis (about 1580-1627), French pharmacist and pioneer settler in Canada. See George Urdang: *Pharmacy's Part in Society,* pp. 50, 52, Madison, Wis., 1946.

Heberden, William (1710-1801), English physician whom Doctor Johnson called: "ultimus Romanorum, the last of our great physicians." His main importance to pharmacy lies in his fight against the drugs of old, the use of which was based on tradition and on outmoded beliefs, rather than on observed effects and/or scientific knowledge. His "Essay on Mithridatum and Theriaca" (1745) exploded a myth, almost 2,000 years old, about these panaceas. See F. H. Garrison: *History of Medicine,* pp. 358, 359, Philadelphia, 1929.

Hebrew medicine and pharmacy: See, e.g., Otto E. Ruhmer and Arthur G. Zupko: *Some Contributions by Jews to Pharmacy—a Historical Survey,* Madison, Wis., 1960; Harry Friedenwald, *The Jews and Medicine; Essays,* 2 vols., Baltimore, 1944; Solomon Kagan, *Jewish Medicine,* Boston, 1952; L. Glesinger, "Les Juifs et la pharmacie," *Revue Hist. Pharm.* 8:17, 1955; and Oswei Temkin: *Beiträge zur archaischen Medizin,* Kyklos, 1930, 3: pp. 90-135.

Hegeman, William (1817-1875), a New York pharmacist, as early as 1857 operated 4 New York drugstores; hence was one of the earliest forerunners of the chain-store system. See *Drug. Circ.* 51:85, 1907.

Helmont, Jean Baptist van (1577-1644), Flemish physician and academic teacher in

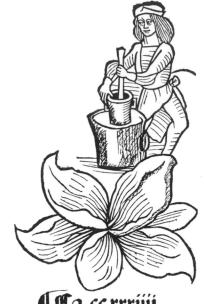

¶ Ca. cc xxxiiij.

Ndicus: Sera. li. aggre. cap. Mi
lech. auct: oyaf: Est de ipso dome
sticus z siluestris. Et domesticus e
sse q tinctores vtunt. Cuius foliu est simi
le folio plantaginis. nisi quia est magis

Typical woodcut and excerpt from an
herbal (*Hortus sanitatis*, 1491), concerning Indicus (indigo), which was then
used as a drug as well as a pharmaceutical coloring agent.

Leyden. He was a follower of Paracelsus,
and some historians consider him (not the
later De le Boe Sylvius) as the founder of
the Iatrochemical School. However, his
theories, like those of his master Paracelsus,
were mystifying; while Sylvius, *q.v.*, formulated his physiologicochemical ideas clearly
and understandably. Van Helmont made the
first attempt at a real analysis of urine. See
Garrison: *History of Medicine*, p. 261, Philadelphia, 1929; Sigerist: *The Great Doctors*,
p. 157, New York, 1933.

Hephaistos. The god of fire, and one of the
gods to whom healing power was attributed.
He was considered a son of Zeus and Hera,
and identified with their deity Vulcan by the
Romans.

Heracles. A deified hero, also called Hercules,
considered to be the son of Zeus and
Alcmene. He was worshiped chiefly as the
god of warlike strength and riches.

Herbal. Title of books of herbs, which often
also contained special sections on animals, on
parts of animals and on minerals used
medicinally. Thus they presented the simple
drugs not only of the vegetable but also of
the animal and the mineral kingdoms. The
best introduction to this genre of literature
in English is by Agnes Arber: *Herbals;
Their Origin and Evolution*, ed. 2, Cambridge 1953.

Herbalist, anglicized form of *herbarius*, *q.v.*,
a dealer in "herbs."

Herbarium. See *Herbarius*. A collection of
dried plants; also the title of books on
"herbs."

Herbarius, pl. *-i*, from Latin *herba* ("herb"),
and *-arius* ("pertaining to"), i.e., a dealer
in herbs. Compare French *herbaliste* and
herboriste, and English "herborist," also
"herbarium."

Herborist, anglicized form of *herbarius*, *q.v.*
A collector of "herbs."

Hermbstaedt, Sigismund (1760-1833), German pharmacist and professor of chemistry
at the University of Berlin. Hermbstaedt
made an attempt to give phytochemistry a
systematic basis in his *Kurze Anleitung zur
chemischen Zergliederung von Vegetabilien
nach physikalisch-chemischen Grundsätzen*
("Short directions for the chemical analysis
of vegetables according to physiochemical
principles"). He investigated many technologic problems and was one of the most
important chemical engineers of his time.

Hernandez, Francisco (1571-1677), wrote on
the animals, plants and minerals of Mexico.
See Tschirch; *Handbuch der Pharmakognosie*, ed. 2, *I*, Part 3, p. 1546, Leipzig, 1933.

Hewson, Thomas Tickell (1773-1848), English-born American physician. See: J. *Am.
Ph. A. 20*:680, 1931.

Hiera picra. Under this name, bitter-tasting
powders or *species* were in use fom antiquity
until about 1800. All contained aloes, except
the formula of Scribonius Largus, *q.v.*, which
contained colocynth in its place. These
powders or species were taken with honey in
the form of electuaries. See Wootton: *Chronicles cf Pharmacy, II*, p. 138, London, 1910.

Hildegard of Bingen (1098-1179), abbess
of a cloister at Bingen in Germany, author
of a materia medica, called "*physica,*" which
according to Tschirch may be considered the
first treatise on natural science in Germany.
See Tschirch: *Handbuch der Pharmakognosie, I*, Part 2, p. 667, Leipzig, 1910; Ger-
trude M. Engbring: Saint Hildegard, twelfth

century physician, *Bull. Hist. Med.* 8:770, 1940.

Hippocrates (fl. 400 B.C.), a Greek physician, known as the "father of medicine." To him has been attributed the first concept of humoral pathology, *q.v.*, which later on was systematized by Galen, *q.v.*; and, above all, the concept of the sick person as an entity, to be treated as such, instead of merely as the bearer of a particular sickness that had to be treated. This concept, and that of simplicity of medication in connection with adequate diet, has made his name a symbol for movements in medicine, now and again, extolling these principles. See W. S. Jones: *Hippocrates*, with an English translation, London, 1923-1931.

Hoffmann, Frederick (1832-1904), German pharmacist, who in more than 30 years of pharmaceutical activity in the United States as a pharmacist, editor, and as analytic chemist, was of the greatest influence in American pharmacy. See *Pharm. Rev. 14:1*, 1896; 23:1, 1905; *Am. J. Pharm. 78:144*, 1905.

Hoffmann, Friedrich (1660-1742), German physician and academic teacher in Halle, who was considered one of the greatest iatromechanists. In pharmacy his name survived in connection with "Hoffmann's drops," which he introduced into therapy. See Garrison: *History of Medicine*, p. 314, Philadelphia, 1929.

Horus. The Egyptian god of day, resembling the Greek god Apollo, and one of the gods to whom healing power was attributed. Represented as hawk-headed, he was considered the son of Isis and Osiris.

Humoral pathology, the theory that all diseases result from a disordered or abnormal condition of the fluids or humors of the body. As stated in the text, Galen divided the remedies to be used in order to counteract such conditions into three classes. The first class comprised those remedies developing only one of the elementary qualities—warmth, cold, moisture or dryness—drugs with "simple" effect. To the second class belonged those drugs which have, besides one main effect, a secondary effect. Thus their effect is "compound." The third class consisted of drugs with a specific effect, i.e., drugs efficient as "entities." These drugs were supposed to be efficient not because of one or the other "quality," but through their entire substance—hence "entities." They acted as purgatives, emetics, poisons, or antidotes.

Each medicine, and this applied to the drugs of all classes, could exercise its effect in four degrees. Typical of modes of administration is the direction given by Galen for the use of opium: Like all other narcotics, "opium" is, according to its temper, cold. It produces, therefore, in the body a considerable (in the highest degrees, an invincible) cold. Hence in order to soften its effects we have to combine it with heating remedies, the most recommendable of these being Castoreum. See Häuser: *Lehrbuch der Geschichte der Medizin, I,* p. 374, Jena., 1875; Ludwig Israelson: *Die Materia Medica des Claudis Galenos,* p. 12, 1894.

Hygeia. The Greek goddess of health, considered a daughter of Asklepios and often worshipped together with him. Her attributes, a bowl and sacred serpent, have become, in modern times, an international symbol of pharmacy.

Hynson, Henry P. (1855-1921), American pharmacist, one of the founders of the firm of Hynson, Westcott and Dunning, Baltimore, and professor in the Department of Pharmacy, University of Maryland.

Iatrochemistry. From the Greek *iatros* ("physician"). The doctrine based on a chemical concept of normal and pathologic conditions of the human body. Abnormal chemical conditions naturally were combated by chemical remedies. See **Sylvius.**

Iatron. From Greek *iatros* ("physician"), the room of the physician.

I-em-hetep. See: **Imhotep.**

Imhotep, originally written I-em-hetep, i.e., "He who cometh in peace," is also known as Imouthes and Imhotpou. He was an architect as well as a physician (about 3000 B.C.), and was deified as a god of medicine and healing about 2500 years after his death. According to Breasted, the Greeks recognized in him their own Asklepios, *q.v.* See Breasted: *A History of Egypt,* p. 113, London, 1921; K. Sethe: *Imhotep, der Asklepios der Aegypter,* Berlin, 1902; J. B. Hurry: *Imhotep, The Vizier and Physician of King Zozer,* Oxford, 1926.

Imhotpou. See: **Imhotep.**

Imouthes. See: **Imhotep.**

India. The name is derived from the river Indus. For ancient Indian medicine and drugs, see G. P. Srivastava: *History of Indian Pharmacy,* Vol. I, ed. 2, Calcutta, 1954; the chapters on "India" or "Indians" in H. Schelenz: *Geschichte der Pharmazie,* Berlin,

1904; T. Berendes: *Die Pharmazie bei den alten Kulturvolkern,* Halle, 1891; A. Tschirch: *Handbuch per Pharmakognosie, I,* part 2, Leipzig, 1910 and 1933; Henry R. Zimmer: *Hindu Medicine,* Baltimore, 1948. Furthermore, see F. R. Hoernle: *Studies in the Medicine of Ancient India,* Oxford, 1907; G. Piso: *De Indiae utriusque et medica libri XVI* (1658); Jacob Bontius: *De medica Indorum libri IV* (1718). In regard to modern Indian pharmacy, see George Cecil: Pharmacy in the Indian Native States, *Pharm. J.* 117:674, 1926; and The qualified chemist in India, *Chem. & Drug.* 105:693, 1926. In recent times two journals, "The Indian Pharmacist" (since 1945) and "The Indian Journal of Pharmacy" (since 1938), have been mirroring the modern development.

Isidorus Hispalensis (570-636), Bishop of Seville, the best known encyclopedist of the Middle Ages. See George Sarton: *Introduction to the History of Science, I*:471-472, Baltimore, 1927.

Isis. Egyptian goddess of fecundity and one of the divinities to whom healing power was attributed. She was considered sister and wife of Osiris and mother of Horus and Anubis (Anepu). Isis is sometimes represented as cowheaded. The word "Isis" has been used as the title of the journal of the History of Science Society, and was the title of the famous encyclopedic journal edited by the German naturalist, Lorenz Oken, from 1817 to 1848.

Ives, Eli (1779-1861), physician. See W. O. Richtmann: *J. A. Ph. A.* 20:681, 1931.

Jackson, James (1777-1867), physician in Boston and professor at the Boston Medical School. See Kelly and Burrage: *American Medical Biographies,* p. 599, New York, 1920.

Jackson, Samuel (1787-1872), physician, for some years a pharmacist, the first professor of materia medica and pharmacy in the Philadelphia College of Pharmacy; from 1827-1863, an instructor, after 1835 a full professor, at the University of Pennsylvania. See J. W. England: *First Century of the Philadelphia College of Pharmacy,* p. 396, Philadelphia, 1922; *Am. J. Pharm.* 44:329, 1872.

Jacobs, Joseph (1859-1929), owner of several drugstores in Atlanta, Ga., writer on pharmaceutical subjects and founder of the American Burns Club, an organization of the lovers of the Scottish poet Burns. See J. W. England: *First Century of the Philadelphia College of Pharmacy,* p. 242, Philadelphia, 1922; *Pharm. Era* 66:257, 1929; *J. A. Ph. A.* 18:1095, 1929.

Japan. The culture of ancient Japan was derived from China; hence, the known ancient Japanese medicine was Chinese. For details, see the chapters: "Japan" or "Japanese" in H. Schlenez, *Geschichte der Pharmazie;* T. Berendes, *Die Pharmazie bei den alten Kulturvölkern,* Halle, 1891; Tschirch, *Handbuch der Pharmakognosie, I:* Part 2, 1910. Furthermore, see Y. Fujikawa: *Japanese Medicine,* New York, 1934; Charles Rice: Japanese medicine and pharmacy, *New Rem.* 6:20, 1877; K. L. Kaufman, A chronology of some events of pharmaceutical interest in China and Japan, *J. A. Ph. A.* 28:544, 1939. An especially noteworthy book (in Japanese) is by the pharmacist-historian Tootaroo Simizu [or Shimizu], *History of Japanese Pharmacy,* Yokohama, 1960. Medicine and pharmacy in Japan are now Europeanized. The first pharmacopeia following occidental models appeared in 1887.

Jenner, Edward (1749-1823). English physician. With his inoculation he "transformed a local country tradition into a reliable prophylactic principle." See Garrison: *History of Medicine,* p. 374, Philadelphia, 1920; Sigerist: *The Great Doctors,* p. 258, New York, 1933.

Jephcott, Sir Harry (1891-   ). Starting as a practicing pharmacist, Jephcott became one of the leading British pharmaceutical manufacturers, The Glaxo Laboratories, of which he has been chairman and managing director. See *Pharm. J.* 156:395, 1946.

Johnson, Joseph (1776-1862), physician, wholesale druggist and author. Among his historical publications, *Traditions and Reminiscences chiefly of the American Revolution in the South* gained popularity. See *Dictionary of American Biography, X:* p. 108.

Johnson, Thomas (d. 1644), English apothecary, botanist and active royal partisan in the struggle between the English crown and Cromwell. See *Dictionary of* (English) *National Biography, XXX:* p. 44.

Josselyn, John (d. 1675), traveler and amateur scientist. See *Dictionary of* (English) *National Biography, XXX:* p. 208; *Dictionary of American Biography, X:* p. 219.

Journalism. The first pharmaceutical periodical to be classed with the journals (i.e., periodicals issued at more than annual intervals) was Trommsdorff's *Journal der Pharmacie* (1794). The first journal published in the French language appeared (1797) as the *Journal de le société des pharmaciens de Paris.* The first pharmaceutical journal in the English language did not appear in England but in the United States, the *Journal of the Philadelphia College of Pharmacy* (1825). The first Italian journal was the *Giornale di farmacia, chimica e scienze affini* (1824); the first Spanish journal, *El Restaurador Farmaceutica* (1844); the first Portuguese journal, the *Journal da Societada Pharmaceutica de Lisboa* (1840).

Most of the pharmaceutical journals have been published in these languages. English has been employed in British colonies, as well as in the mother country. German-language journals have appeared in Austria and Switzerland (also, for a time, in the United States and Russia). Spanish has been used in former Spanish colonies, and Portuguese in Brazil.

These journals have been devoted to pharmacy as a whole, or to special fields thereof. To a certain extent, the subject matter has been reflected in the titles: *journal* (English, French, German), *bulletin* (English, French; *bolletino,* Italian), *Annals* (German, *Annalen;* French, *Annales*), *Archives* (German and Danish; Italian, *Archivio*). Other titles are *Berichte, Magazin, Nachrichten, Zeitung,* etc.

A general bibliography was attempted (1913) by Eugène Guitard in his *Deux siècles de presse au service de pharmacie et cinquante ans de l'Union Pharmaceutique;* a concise bibliography of pharmaceutical journals up to 1894, using the German language (in the United States as well as in other countries) was prepared by F. Hoffmann, editor of the *Pharmazeutische Rundschau* (*12*:7-28). A more complete account will be found in Adlung and Urdang: *Grundriss der Geschichte der deutschen Pharmazie,* pp. 259-271. For American journals, see Minnie Meyer: "Pharmaceutical Journals of the United States," Master's Thesis, University of Wisconsin, 1933. A historical list of journals by states was published in the *J. A. Ph. A. 22*:424, 1933. The best key to currently published journals is the "World List of Pharmacy Periodicals," Theodora Andrews and Winifred Sewell, eds., *Am. J. Hosp. Pharm.* 20: 45-83, 1963 (and republished separately, 1963); see also, Henry C. Bolton: *A Cata-logue of Scientific and Technical Periodicals, 1665-1895,* ed. 2, Washington, D. C., 1897.

Kalefactor. See: **Personnel.**

Kebler, Lyman Fr. (1863-1955), chemist of most versatile activity, worked in governmental service, and in educational and industrial positions; and made contributions on chemical, food and medical subjects, and also on pharmaceutical history; with U.S.D.A. Bureau of Chemistry 1903-29 (chief, Drug division, 1907-23). See *Who's Who in America,* 1938, p. 1386; *American Men of Science,* ed. 8, p. 1317, 1949.

Kelly, Evander F. (1879-1944) was professor at the Maryland College of Pharmacy, active in manufacturing pharmacy, pharmaceutical author, and Secretary of the American Pharmaceutical Association from 1926 to 1944. See *J. A. Ph. A. 11*:3, 1922; *Ibid., Pract. Ed.* 5:322-326, 1944.

Kierstedt, Hans Taylor (1793-1882), pharmacist in New York. See *Proc. A. Ph. A. 30*:615, 661, 1882.

King, John (1813-1893), pioneer eclectic physician and pharmacologist. See H. A. Kelly and W. L. Burrage: *American Medical Biographies,* New York, 1920, p. 661; *Lloyd Libr., Bull.* No. 19, 4, 1912, p. 3.

Klaproth, Martin Heinrich (1743-1817), German pharmacist and one of the great chemists of his period. Most of his discoveries he made in the small laboratory of his own pharmacy. He is considered the father of modern analytic chemistry; he was the first to recognize with certainty the elementary character of uranium, titanium and zirconium in 1789; strontium and cerium, in 1803. He found fluorine in bones and potassium in feldspar, and was the first to separate barium and strontium. One of his biographers especially stressed the fact that Klaproth has never published anything other than his own investigations, and some new facts, and never repeated himself. When the University of Berlin was founded in 1809, he was made its first professor of chemistry. The first Prussian pharmacopeia (1799) bears, in its resolute adoption of the principles of modern chemistry, the impress of this great pharmacist. See Georg Edmund Dann: *Martin Heinrich Klaproth* (1743-1817), Berlin, 1958. George Urdang: M. H. Klaproth, *J. A. Ph. A.* Pract. Ed. 4:358-361, 1943.

Kraemer, Henry (1868-1924), pharmaceutical teacher and author, was especially known for his botanic and pharmacognostic research work. See J. W. England: *First Century of the Philadelphia College of Pharmacy,* p. 415, Philadelphia, 1922; *J. A. Ph. A. 13*:980, 1924.

Kremers, Edward (1865-1941), professor and director of the Course in Pharmacy, University of Wisconsin (1892 to 1935) editor, author, pharmaceutical historian. His example led the way to the modern reform of American pharmaceutical education. See *American Men of Science,* 1938, p. 803; *Who's Who in America,* 1938, p. 1457; George Urdang: Edward Kremers in *Am. J. Pharm. Ed. 11*:631-658, 1947.

Laborant. See: **Personnel.**

Laboranten. The German term has two meanings: (1) From the 17th to the 19th century, it designated the manufacturers and itinerant sellers—frequently the same persons—of the so-called *Olitäten, q.v.* (2) In more recent times, the term *Laboranten* has referred to people doing laboratory work requiring little or no scientific education.

Lagerist. See: **Personnel.**

Lasca, Il. See: **Grassini.**

Lascoff, J. Leon (1867-1943), Russian-born American pharmacist, by example and teaching, made promotion of American professional pharmacy his life task. Since 1947 a Lascoff honor plaque is given every year to a meritorious pharmacist by the American College of Apothecaries. See *J. A. Ph. A. 26*: 199, 1937.

Laufbursche. See: **Personnel.**

Lavoisier, Antoine Laurent (1743-1794), French chemist and victim of the French revolutionary tribunal. His fame rests on the recognition of oxygen (discovered almost simultaneously by Priestly, *q.v.*, and Scheele, *q.v.*) as the principle of combustion and on the experimental proof of the part played by oxygen in all chemical and biological changes (oxidation and reduction), thus disproving the phlogiston theory, *q.v.* See Douglas McKie: *Antoine Lavoisier,* Philadelphia, 1935; and Denis Duveen and Herbert Klickstein: A Bibliography of the Works of A. L. Lavoisier, 1743-1794, London, 1954.

Law for the separation of medicine and pharmacy. The medical edicts of Frederick II, issued in all probability between 1231 and 1241, had a far-reaching influence on pharmacy, as discussed in the text. A critical edition of Latin texts,* from collating various

manuscripts, has been prepared and given its proper historical setting and intepretation by the pharmacist-historians Wolfgang-Hagen Hein and Kurt Sappert, *Die Medizinalordnung Friedrich II; Eine pharmaziehistorische Studie* (Internationale Gesellschaft, Bd. 12), Eutin, 1957, pp. 48-57 for Latin text and German translation. To convey the general content of the two edicts holding most pharmaceutical interest, we quote a somewhat condensed English version (*Journal of the American Medical Association,* January, 1908; quoted according to J. T. Wash: *The Popes and Science,* p. 419-423).

"Title 46: Every physician given a license to practice must take an oath that he shall faithfully fulfill all the requirements of the law, and in addition, whenever it comes to his knowledge that any apothecary has for sale drugs that are of less than normal strength, he shall report him to the court. . . . He (the physician) must not enter into any business relations with the apothecary, nor must he take any of them under his protection nor incur any money obligations in their regard. Nor must any licensed physician keep an apothecary's shop himself. Apothecaries must conduct their business with a certificate from a physician,[1] according to the regulations and upon their own credit and responsibility, and they shall not be permitted to sell their products without having taken an oath that all their drugs have been prepared in the prescribed form, without any fraud. The apothecary may derive the following profits from his sales: Such extracts[2] and simples as he need not keep in stock for more than a year before they may be employed may be charged for at the rate of three tarrenes[3] an ounce. Other medicines, however, which in consequence of the special condition required for their preparation[4] or for any other reason the apothecary has to have in stock for more than a year, he may

---

* According to Sudhoff, the law was published in

Latin and, simultaneously, in Greek (*Mitt. zur Gesch. der Med.* 13 (1914), p. 180-182). This is important, not only because it allows a comparison of the two texts, but also because it is interesting proof of the fact that at that time Latin and Greek were spoken in the Kingdom of the Two Sicilies.

[1] A better translation, fitting better the sense of the Latin text, would be: "with the approval of the physicians."

[2] The Latin word *confectiones* cannot be translated by the word "extracts." It means *all* compounded preparations, in contrast to simple drugs.

[3] One *tarrene* equals about 30 cents.

[4] *Ex natura* means "because of their special nature." There is no reason for an interpretation like that given in the above translation.

charge for at the rate of six tarrenes an ounce. Stations for the preparation of medicines may not be located anywhere, but only in certain communities in the Kingdom, as we prescribe below.

"Title 47: In every province of our Kingdom which is under our legal authority, we decree that two prudent and trustworthy men, whose names must be sent to our court, shall be appointed and bound by a formal oath, under whose inspection electuaries and syrups and other medicines be prepared according to law and only be sold after such inspection. In Salerno in particular, we decree that this inspectorship shall be limited to those who have taken their degree as Masters in Physic. . . . We decree also that the growers of plants meant for medicinal purposes[5] shall be bound by a solemn oath that they shall prepare medicines conscientiously, according to the rules of their art, and as far as it is humanly possible that they shall prepare them in the presence of the inspectors. Violations of this law shall be punished by the confiscation of their movable goods. If the inspectors, however, to whose fidelity to duty the keeping of these regulations is committed shall allow any fraud in the matters that are entrusted to them, they shall be condemned to punishment by death."

LaWall, Charles H. (1871-1937). LaWall was active in almost all branches of pharmacy: in community practice and in pharmaceutical industry, as an analytic chemist and as a teacher, and in official governmental positions. In addition, he was a prolific writer on pharmaceutical subjects. His *Four Thousand Years of Pharmacy* represents the first attempt at a history of pharmacy written by an American and published in book form in America. See *J. A. Ph. A. 26*:1223, 1937; J. W. England: *First Century of the Philadelphia College of Pharmacy*, p. 420, Philadelphia, 1922.

---

[5] The translation is very dubious. The Latin word *conficientes* means, simply, "preparers." Alfred Bäumer translates it as "apothecary" (*Die Aerztegesetzgebung Kaiser Friedrichs II und ihre geschichtliche Grundlage*, Leipzig 1911). That seems to be dubious too, because the duties of the apothecaries, the *confectionarii*, are regulated above, without, however, mentioning the penalties. There is a third and probable possibility of interpretation. The "*confectionarius*" is the learned apothecary, without respect to the question whether he himself prepares medicines or not. *Conficiens* is anybody who actually prepares something, and *conficientes medicinas* are, therefore, all people who prepare medicines. Thus this term may be used to bring all kinds of preparers of medicines into the frame of the law, whether apothecaries or not.

LeCoste, Jean-François (1741-1819), Chief physician of the French Expeditionary Army in the American Revolution; author of a brief formulary in Latin for the use of the hospitals under his charge, which was published under the title *Compendium pharmaceuticum*," q.v.

LeFebvre, Nicaise (Nicolas), also called Lefèvre (1610-1674). French pharmacist and chemical author. His *Traité de chymie théorique et pratique*, the fifth edition of which was published under the title *Cours de chymie*, was considered the best chemical textbook of that period and was translated into several languages including English.

Lefèvre. See: **LeFebvre.**

Lehman, William (1779-1829), Philadelphia physician, M. D. of the University of Pennsylvania, active in scientific and political life. See J. W. England, *First Century of the Philadelphia College of Pharmacy*, p. 352, Philadelphia, 1922.

Lehr-Bube. See: **Personnel.**

Lehrbursche. See: **Personnel.**

Lehr-Junge. See: **Personnel.**

Lehrling. See: **Personnel.**

Lémery, Nicolas (1645-1715), French pharmacist who is considered the founder of modern phytochemistry. He taught the analysis of vegetable drugs by the extraction method. In accordance with the traditional classification of all natural objects into 3 kingdoms, he arranged the materia chemica into mineral, vegetable and animal categories. He was one of the most-translated authors of his time, and his principal books went through many editions. His *Cours de chymie* superseded the book of LeFebvre, q.v., and was for about a century the world's most-used chemistry text. Lémery's *Pharmacopée universel·* appeared in 1697.

Lespleigney, Thibault (1496-1567), French pharmacist and writer on pharmaceutical subjects. His *Promptuaire des medecines simples en rythme joyeuse* was reprinted (1898) by Paul Dorveaux.

Lewis, William (1714-1781), English physician and chemist. His *New Dispensatory*, containing the theory and the practice of pharmacy, and some of his books on technical chemistry, were translated into German. On the other hand, he translated the pharmaceutical treatise of the German pharmacist Caspar Neumann, q.v., into English. See Edward Kremers: William Lewis, *J. A. Ph. A. 20*:1204, 1931.

Libavius (Latinized form of Libau), Andreas (1540-1616), physician and one of the most eminent early chemists. See F. Ferchl: *Chemisch-Pharmazeutisches Bio- und Bibliographikon*, p. 313, Mittenwald, 1937.

Liebig, Justus von (1803-1873), German chemist, known especially because of his pioneer work in agricultural and in physiologic chemistry. He was connected with pharmacy by 10 months of pharmaceutical apprenticeship, by a later short activity as inspector of the pharmacies in the Grand Duchy of Hessen, and by collaboration with pharmaceutical chemists throughout his life. In the first laboratory at the University of Giessen, he introduced a type of experimental chemical instruction that became the model for modern chemical instruction the world over. See *Am. J. Pharm. 45*:240, 1873; J. Liebig, an autobiographic sketch, trans. by J. Campbell, *Annual Report* for 1891 of the Smithsonian Institution, p. 257; A. Hofman, The life-work of Liebig (Faraday lecture, 1875).

Liggett, Louis Kroh (1875-1946), American organizer of one of the largest drugstore chains in the world. See Samuel Merwin: *Rise and Fight Againe*, New York, 1935.

Lilly, Eli (1838-1898), pharmacist and founder of Eli Lilly and Company, in Indianapolis. See *Proc. A. Ph. A. 46*:48, 1898; *Tile and Till 12*: No. 2, 1926.

Lilly, Josiah K. (1862-1948), pharmacist and, in sequence, president and chairman of the board of Eli Lilly and Company. A graduate of the Philadelphia College of Pharmacy (1882), Josiah K. Lilly not only developed his plant into one of the world's greatest pharmaceutical concerns based on scientific research, but made it his task to foster, in fact as well as in idea, the concept of pharmacy as a unit comprised of research, manufacture, wholesaling, dispensing and teaching. For this reason he was given (1942) the highest honor American professional pharmacy grants, the Remington Medal. See *J. A. Ph. A. 9*:165, 1948; George Urdang: *Pharmacy's Part in Society*, p. 83, Madison, Wis., 1946.

Linstead, Hugh N. (1901-   ), distinguished British pharmacist and barrister; son of a pharmacist in Brighton. Secretary of the Pharmaceutical Society of Great Britain since 1926 (previously Asst. Sec.), President of the International Pharmaceutical Federation since 1954, Member of Parliament since 1942, and appointed to various governmental

bodies. Knighted by the Queen (1953), and decorated and honored by various governments and societies. See: *Who's Who* [British].

Lloyd, John Uri (1849-1936). One of the greatest and most versatile pharmacists that America has had. Lloyd was a scientific chemist, a pharmaceutical manufacturer, a teacher and an author of scientific literature as well as of novels; he excelled in all these fields. He was early connected with the Eclectic School of Medicine and played an important part in the development of plant chemistry and drug extraction. The Lloyd Library, initiated by him in Cincinnati, is one of the most comprehensive of its kind and contains not only modern books but also valuable publications out of the pharmaceutical past. See *Eclectic Med. J. 96*:178, 1936; *J. A. Ph. A. 25*:885, 1936.

Lohoch, from the Arabian *la aka*, "to lick." It was a thick liquid, being of a consistency between a syrup and an electuary.

Lonicerus, Adam (1528-1586), municipal physician in Frankfort-on-the-Main. His herbal (1557) continued through more than two centuries, the last (the 20th) edition being issued in 1783.

Loochs. See: *Lohoch.*

Lumen. See: **Pharmacopeia.**

Luminare. See: **Pharmacopeia.**

Lyekopis. See: **Pharmacopeia.**

Lyons, Albert B. (1841-1926), M.D., pharmacist, and professor of chemistry at Detroit College of Medicine, then editor of the *Pharmaceutical Era*, later government chemist and professor in Hawaii and, finally, manufacturing chemist. See *J. A. Ph. A. 15*:411, 1926; J. W. England: *First Century of the Philadelphia College of Pharmacy*, p. 218, Philadelphia, 1922.

Maben, Thomas (1855-1937), English pharmaceutical chemist and member of the English staff of the American pharmaceutical firm of Parke, Davis and Company. See *Chem. & Drug. 126*:675, 1927.

Macfarlan, John Fletcher (1790-1861), Scottish chemist, pharmacist and physician. A founding member of the Pharmaceutical Society of Great Britain, he also played an important part in medical association work. See *Pharm. J. 20*:488, 1861.

McIntyre, Ewen (1825-1913), New York pharmacist. See *J. A. Ph. A. 2*:282, 417, 552, 1913.

Maimonides or Abu 'Imran Mûsa ibn Maimon

(1135-1204). A Jewish-Spanish physician, who wrote in Arabic. See I. Muenz and H. T. Schnittkind: *Maimonides,* Boston, 1935; E. H. Rodin: Maimonides, *Calif. and West. Med. 44:*192, 1936; J. J. Wash: *Old-Time Makers of Medicine,* p. 90, New York, 1911; George Sarton: *Introduction to the History of Science, II,* part I, pp. 369-380, Baltimore, 1931. As for the so-called "Prayer of Maimonides," see David Reisman: *The Story of Medicine in the Middle Ages,* p. 64, New York, 1935.

Maisch, Henry C. C. (1865-1901), pharmacist, manufacturing chemist, oldest son of John M. Maisch, and one of the American pharmaceutical teachers who studied in Germany. See *Am. J. Pharm. 74:*458, 1902.

Maisch, John M. (1831-1893). Maisch entered pharmacy after his arrival in the United States as a German political refugee. He soon became prominent as a teacher, an author and above all as an editor of the *American Journal of Pharmacy,* and the first Permanent Secretary of the American Pharmaceutical Association (1865-1893). See Joseph P. Remington: J. M. Maisch, *Am. J. Pharm. 66:* 1, 1894; Joseph W. England: *First Century of the Philadelphia College of Pharmacy,* p. 405, Philadelphia, 1922; M. I. Wilbert: John Michael Maisch, an ideal pharmacist, *Am. J. Pharm. 75:*351, 1903. George Urdang: The fiftieth aniversary of the death of John Michael Maisch, *Am. J. Pharm. 110:*1-11, 1944.

Mallinckrodt, Edward (1845-1928), one of the founders and the chief organizer and leader of the firm of G. Mallinckrodt & Co., St. Louis. See *J. A. Ph. A. 17:*208, 1928.

Manlius de Bosco, Jacobus (16th century), Italian pharmacist and probably the first pharmaceutical author of a treatise in Italy; compiler of a book on materia medica.

Marggraf, Andreas Sigismund (1709-1782), German pharmacist and one of the greatest chemists of his time Marggraf differentiated between potassium and sodium compounds, identified magnesium, produced compounds of mercury and of silver with organic acids, was the first to prepare potassium cyanide, introduced numerous reagents and discovered sugar in various plants, particularly in the sugar beet. He reported this most important discovery in 1747. In his investigation he used the microscope, the employment of which in chemistry became customary.

Markoe, George F. H. (1840-1896), Boston pharmacist, pharmaceutical manufacturer and professor at the Massachusetts College of Pharmacy. See W. L. Scoville: *Am. J. Pharm. 68:*593, 1896.

Marshall, Charles (1744-1824), pharmacist in Philadelphia. He was the first president of the Philadelphia College of Pharmacy. See Joseph W. England: *First Century of the Philadelphia College of Pharmacy,* p. 348, Philadelphia, 1922; E. T. Ellis, *Am. J. Pharm. 75:*57, 1903.

Marshall, Christopher, Jr., pharmacist in Philadelphia (eighteenth century). He was the oldest son of Christopher Marshall, Sr., *q.v.,* and for a time, together with his brother, Charles, *q.v.,* owner of the Marshall pharmacy in Philadelphia. See E. T. Ellis: *Am. J. Pharm. 75:*57, 1903.

Marshall, Christopher, Sr. (1709-1797), Irish-born pharmacist in Philadelphia. See E. T. Ellis: The story of a very old Philadelphia drug store, *Am. J. Pharm. 75:*57, 1903.

Martius, Ernst Wilhelm (1756-1849), German pharmacist and professor of pharmacy at the University of Erlangen. He wrote one of the best-known German autobiographies, containing many interesting descriptions of pharmaceutical life.

Mathioli, Pietro Andrea (1501-1577), Italian physician and botanist in the service of the German Emperor Maximilian II. His revised and annotated edition of Dioscorides' *De materia medica* meant a revival of the work of the great Greek author. It went through many editions.

Mayerne, Theodore Turquet de (1573-1655), French-Swiss physician. Mayerne was forbidden to practice medicine in Paris because he was a Paracelsist and employed antimony in his practice. He went to England, where he became physician-in-ordinary to James I. He published several formulas for chemical remedies. See *Dictionary of National (English) Biography, 37:*150; George Urdang: *Pharmacopoeia Londinensis of 1618,* pp. 12, 18-21, 28, 55, 61-64, 72-73, Madison, Wis., 1944.

Mayo, Caswell A. (1862-1928), one of the best known American pharmaceutical journalists. See *J. A. Ph. A. 17:*209, 1928.

Meakim, John (1812-1863), pharmacist in New York and one of the original members of the American Pharmaceutical Association. See *Am. J. Pharm. 35:*574, 1863; *Proc. A. Ph. A. 12:*23, 1864.

Mease, James (1771-1846), physician, editor, author, one of the founders of the Philadelphia Athenaeum. See: *Dictionary of American Biography* 12:486.

Medicamentarius, pl. *-i.* from *medicamentum* (cf. the Greek *pharmakon*), "a remedy," and *-arius,* "pertaining to," i.e., a maker of remedies or medicaments.

Medici, a Florentine family of great power and wealth from the 14th to the 16th centuries. They furnished many rulers of Florence and two Popes. They were among the greatest bankers of the world and were noted for their patronage of art and literature. Because of the balls (pills) in their coat of arms, the Medici were erroneously said to have been pharmacists originally.

Medicine chest. The chest of an Egyptian princess (Berlin) is supposed to have been a medicine chest (possibly also a cosmetic chest). The *apotheca* found in Herculaneum was another such chest. The German language differentiates between *Hausapotheke,* "medicine chest" or "cupboard" for the home; *Reiseapotheke,* a medicine chest convenient while traveling; *Feldapotheke,* or "army chest," used by soldiers in the field. Such regimental chests were prepared at a central station during the American Revolutionary War, for regiments while in the field. (See George B. Griffenhagen: Drug Supplies in the American Revolution, Bulletin 225 [also as Paper 16 in Contributions from the Museum of History and Technology], Smithsonian Institution, Washington, D. C., 1961. Although pioneer physicians carried medical supplies in their saddle bags while on the road, in their surgeries they had small medicine chests.

Mercer, Hugh (1725-1777). Scotch-born American physician, who fought in the Revolutionary Army first as a colonel and then as a general, and died from wounds received on the battlefield. See *Dictionary of American Biography, XII,* p. 541; *J. A. Ph. A. 15:*425, 1926; and Waterman, Joseph M.: *With Sword and Lancet,* Richmond, Va., 1941.

Merck in Darmstadt, a German pharmaceutical firm, founded in the twenties of the 19th century, grew out of the "Engel-Apotheke" in Darmstadt, owned by the Merck family since 1668.

Mesuë, Johann, Jr. A pseudonym for writings of the 13th century. The books attributed to Mesuë Junior were: (1) The *Grabadin,* from the Arabic *al aqrâbâdhîn* ("compounded remedy"); (2) *Practica medicinarum par-*

ticularium or *Liber de appropriatis,* often designated a second part of the *Grabadin;* (3) *De medicinis laxativis* (*solutivis, purgatoriis*) or *De simplicibus* or *De consolatione simplicium* or *De medicamentorum purgantium simplicium delectu et castigatione.* See A. Tschirch: *Handbuch der Pharmakognosie,* Leipzig, 1910, *I,* part 2, p. 599; furthermore, George Sarton: *Introduction to the History of Science, II,* part II, p. 854, Baltimore, 1931 (in the subdivision dealing with Samuel Ben Jacob of Capua).

Mesuë, Johann, Sr. (777-857), a Christian physician who wrote in Arabic. See A. Tschirch: *Handbuch der Pharmakognosie,* Leipzig, 1910, *I,* part 2, p. 597; George Sarton: *Introduction to the History of Science, I,* p. 374, Baltimore, 1927.

Meune, Odo of (12th century), called also Odo Maydunensis, author of *Macer floridus,* a Latin poem about herbs. The name Macer goes back to the Roman poet Aemilius Macer, whom the author wished to honor.

Migmatopolos, pl. *-oi,* seller of mixtures, from the Greek migma (mixture), and polein (to sell).

Milhau, John (1795-1874), American pharmacist of French descent and of French pharmaceutical education. Milhau was one of the early leaders of the New York College of Pharmacy. "The passage of the U. S. drug law of 1848 is mainly due to his persistent and conscientious efforts." See *Am. J. Pharm. 47:*94, 1875; *Drug. Circ. 51:*89, 1907.

Minderer, Raymond (1570-1621), physician-in-ordinary to the German Emperor Mathias (1612-1619) and municipal physician in Augsburg. He edited the four earliest 17th-century editions of the *Pharmacopoeia Augustana* and tried to bridge the break between the Galenists, who wanted to restrict therapy to the old drugs known to Galen and his followers, and the Paracelsists, who recommended the employment of chemicals more or less exclusively. The *Medicina militaris,* published by Minderer in 1619, containing prescriptions for the most common diseases to which soldiers are subject, represents one of the earliest military pharmacopeias. See Theodor Husemann: introductory essays, in facsimile of the first edition of the *Pharmacopoeia Augustana,* Wisconsin State Historical Society, Madison, Wis., 1927.

Mitchill, Samuel L. (1764-1831), physician, chemist, author, editor and senator. See

Lyman F. Kebler: S. L. Mitchill, *J. A. Ph. A.* 26:908, 1937.

Mohr, Carl Friedrich (1806-1879). German pharmacist and inventor of pharmaceutical and chemical apparatus and technic. Many pieces of auxiliary apparatus used in volumetric analysis were invented by him. His balance for determining specific gravity became a universally used instrument. Among his many books, *Lehrbuch der pharmazeutischen Technik* is especially noteworthy. Upon it were based Redwood's book on *Practical Pharmacy*, in England, and an enlarged edition published by Procter, *q.v.,* in the United States.

Mohr, Charles (1824-1901), German-born American pharmaceutical manufacturer and botanist. He was one of the first, if not the first, forester agent of the U. S. Government. See: *Am. J. Pharm.* 74:459, 1902.

Moissan, Henri (1852-1907), French pharmacist, discoverer of fluorine and the first to prepare artificial diamonds, recipient of the Nobel prize in chemistry (1906). Before starting teaching at the *École supérière de pharmacie* in Paris, Moissan had been a pharmaceutical apprentice and a clerk, and had received his diploma as a *pharmacien de première classe.*

Molière, pen name of Jean Baptiste Poquelin (1622-1673). French dramatist, famous for his comedies. He often ridicules medical chicanery; *le Médecin malgré lui, le Malade imaginaire* and *l'Amour médecin* contain delightful caricatures of physicians and pharmacists.

Moore, J. B. (1832-1909), Philadelphia pharmacist and writer on pharmaceutical subjects. See England, *First Century of the Philadelphia College of Pharmacy*, p. 241, Philadelphia, 1922.

Moore, J. Faris (1826-1888), pharmacist in Baltimore and professor at the Maryland College of Pharmacy. See *Drug. Circ.* 51: 88, 1907; *Proc. A. Ph. A.* 36:34, 1888.

Morgan, John (1735-1789), American physician, founder of the first American school of medicine and the first influential advocate of the separation of American medicine from pharmacy. See M. I. Wilbert: John Morgan, *Am. J. Pharm.* 76:1, 1904; *Dictionary of American Biography, XIII*, p. 172.

Morsuli. Plural diminutive of *morsus*, a bite (German *Bissen*), from *mordeo*, to bite. According to Trommsdorff (*Wörterbuch*), *Morselen* or lozenges are hard confections prepared from spicy and other drugs and sugar. Certain *morsuli* are prepared for their taste as well as for their effect; others are prepared with medicaments, e.g., China *morsellen, Antimonialmorsellen. Wurmmorsellen.* (cf.: *Rotulae* and *Tabulae.*)

Motter, Murray Galt (1866-1926), physician, professor of physiology at Georgetown University, director of library service for the Public Health Service. See *J. A. Ph. A. 15:* 125, 1926.

Mühlenberg, Gotthilf Heinrich Ernst (1753-1815), American clergyman and botanist of German descent. Mühlenberg first identified about 100 species and varieties of American plants. See *Am. J. Pharm.* 80:420, 1908; *Pharm. Rund.* 4:119, 1886; *Dictionary of American Biography, XIII*, p. 308.

Mynsicht, Adrian van (real name Seumenicht) (1603-1683), was a German physician. In his book *Thesaurus et armamentarium medico-chymicum* he for the first time described the preparation of Tartarus emeticus.

Myrepsos, pl. *-oi,* maker of ointments, from the Greek *myron* ("ointment"). See also: *Myropoeos.*

Myropoeos, pl. *-oi,* makers of ointments, from the Greek *myron* ("ointment"). See also: *Myrepsos.*

Nees, von Esenbeck, Theodor Friedrich Ludwig (1787-1837), German pharmacist and professor of pharmacy and botany, first in Leyden and then in Bonn. He was the first to recommend flores koso as a remedy for tapeworm. Among his botanical books his *Plantae Officinales* received much attention.

Neumann, Caspar (1683-1737), German pharmacist who was one of the earliest scientific phytochemists. He objected to the pyrochemical method, which yields ashes as therapeutic products. He discovered thyme camphor (thymol) in 1719. An English translation of his lectures by William Lewis appeared (1760) under the title *The Chymical works of Gaspard Neumann Abridged and Methodized with Large Additions.*

Newcomb, Edwin Leigh (1882-1950), pharmacist, teacher, editor, administrator, one of the most influential leaders of American pharmacy of his period. While teaching at the College of Pharmacy of the University of Minnesota, he established one of the first North American medicinal plant gardens connected with a school of pharmacy. His broad knowledge and interest in pharmacognosy resulted in many contributions to the United States Pharmacopoeia and in the founding of the Plant Science Seminar (1923). In his capacity as Secretary (from 1927; later executive vice-president) of the National Wholesale Druggists' Association, he made this organization an important center for the endeavor to activate the concept of American pharmacy as a unit comprising all branches of the profession. The founding (1942) and early success of the American Foundation of Pharmaceutical Education was mainly due to the authoritative influence of E. L. Newcomb. See *J. A. Ph. A.* (Pract. Ed.) *11*:304-305, 1950.

Newton, Vandeveer L. (1809-1880), physician and, later on, editor of the *Druggists Circular.* See: *Drug. Circ. 51*:5, 1907.

Nicolaus Myrepsus or Alexandrinus (14th century), a physician living in Byzantium, author of a well-known antidotarium. The cognomen Alexandrinus means "the Alexandrian"; the cognomen *Myrepsus*, "ointment cook."

Nicolaus Praepositus (about 1500), a French physician who lived in Tours, wrote a well-known antidotarium. The cognomen *praepositus* indicates his position as presiding official, in this case dean.

Nicolaus Salernitanus. The presumed author of the oldest antidotarium or formulary associated with the name Nicolaus, an author-name of tangled and obscure literary tradition (note above). Probably formularies associated with the cognomen Nicolaus Salernitanus were based on the anonymous *Antidotarius magnus* (about 1087-1100), whose principal source, in turn, was the Salernitan work of Constantine the African, *q.v.* The name Nicolaus appears nowhere in the *Antidotarius magnus,* and did not become associated with this formulary tradition until after the 12th century. (See Lutz, Alfons: . . . Antidotarius magnus . . . , *Acta Pharmaciae Historica,* No. 1, 1959)

Occo, Adolf (or Adolph Occo III, to differentiate him from the two earlier Adolph Occos before him who also were physicians of Augsburg, Germany) (1524-1606). Occo III not only published treatises on medical subjects but also on philosophy, philology and numismatics. See introductory essays by Theodor Husemann, facsimile of the *Pharmacopoeia Augustana, 1565,* Madison, Wis., 1927.

Oerstedt, Hans Christian (1777-1851), eminent physicist, son of a Danish pharmacist, in whose pharmacy he passed through an apprenticeship. He even managed for a short time a pharmacy in Copenhagen. H. C. Oerstedt established the principles of electromagnetism and discovered piperine (1820). See Philippe and Ludwig: *Geschichte der Apotheken,* p. 707, Jena, 1855.

Officina. See: ***Officine*** and **Pharmacopeia.**

Officine. From Latin *opus,* "work" (still in common usage in music and literature) e.g., *magnum opus,* and *facere,* "to make" (cf. "factor" and "factory"). The room in which the pharmacist did his work. Later, when a separate laboratory and also a separate storeroom (German *Materialkammer*) were differentiated, the term *officine* was restricted to the dispensing (sales) room in which the pharmacist compounded his prescriptions. The Latin *officina* was Gallicized to *officine,* a designation introduced into English pharmaceutical literature by the Paris correspondent of the *Chemist and Druggist* of London. The German spelling is *Offizin.* Just as the Dutch *apothek* has been used as a title for a pharmaceutical treatise (e.g., pharmacopeia) so the French word has been used by Dorvault for his handbook *L'officine.*

This designation has been applied not only to the workshop of the pharmacist but also to printing offices, such as the world-famous printing establishment of Plantin and Morehus in Antwerp. On the titlepage of pharmacopeias there is frequently found the reference *ex officina,* followed by the name of the printer.

Oldberg, Oscar (1846-1913), Swedish-born American pharmacist. Oldberg was active and instrumental in various fields of pharmacy, as teacher, editor and author of several books. See *Am. J. Pharm. 85*:272, 1913; *J. Am. Ph. A.* 2:550, 1913.

Olitäten is a German term that designates popular proprietaries of secret composition, prepared since the 17th century, especially in small hamlets in the Silesian mountains and the mountainous parts of Saxony. The term *Olitäten* has been said to derive from the oily consistency of the first and the most popular of these medicines. The peddlers selling these preparations were called *Olitätenhändler.* See Adlung and Urdang: *Grundriss der Geschichte der deutschen Pharmazie,* pp. 122, 129, 174, Berlin, 1935.

Oreibasius Pergamenus (Oribasius) (325-

403), physician-in-ordinary to the Roman Emperor Julian the Apostate. The remnants of his work that came down to our time have been edited by Bussemaker and Daremberg in *Oeuvres d'Oribase* and translated into French (1851-1876). See A. Tschirch: *Handbuch der Pharmakognosie, I,* Part 2, p. 588, Leipzig, 1910.

Osiris. The Egyptian god of the underworld and judge of the dead; one of the gods to whom healing power was attributed. He was considered the brother and the husband of Isis, and the father of Horus and Anubis.

Painter, Emlen (1844-1890), pharmacist in San Francisco, and pharmaceutical manufacturer, later on, in New York; one of the founders of the California College of Pharmacy and a professor there. See *Pharm. Era* 4:21, 1890; *Druggist's Bull.* 4:36, 1800.

Papyrus. (1) The name of a tall sedge, *Cyperus papyrus,* which grows along the banks of the Nile. (2) The name applied to a paper-like material on which the ancient Egyptians painted their hieroglyphics. (3) The name applied to the manuscripts (pl. "papyri") thus prepared. See J. E. Mitchell: The Egyptian papyrus, past and present. *Scient. Am.* 1904, p. 484; D. A. Willy, *How Mud Chokes the Nile River,* p. 177, 1909.

Papyrus, Ebers. Bibliography: George Ebers: *Das hermetische Buch über die Arzeimittel der alten Aegypter in hieratischer Schrift,* Leipzig, 1875; H. Joachim: *Papyros Ebers,* translation into German, Berlin, 1890; Walter Wreszinski: *Der Papyrus Ebers, Um-Schrift Übersetzung und Kommentar,* Leipzig., 1913; B. Ebbel: *The Papyrus Ebers,* translated from W. Wreszinski's hieroglyphic transcript into English, Oxford, 1937.

Paracelsus, Aureolus Philippus (or with his original name, Theophrastus Bombastus of Hohenheim) (1493-1541). A Swiss-German physician whom William Osler (*The Evolution of Modern Medicine,* p. 135, New Haven, 1923) calls "the Luther of Medicine, the very incarnation of the spirit of revolt." His importance to pharmacy lies in his studies of drugs and of their effects which lead to the systematic introduction of metals into internal therapy and the dawn of pharmaceutical chemistry. See J. M. Stillman: *Paracelsus,* Chicago, 1920; Henry M. Pachter, *Paracelsus,* New York, 1951 (paperback, 1963); and especially Walter Pagel, *Paracelsus, An Introduction to Philosophical*

Medicine in the Era of the Renaissance, Basel, 1958.

Parke, H. C. (d. 1899), one of the founders of Parke, Davis and Company, Detroit. See *Am. J. Pharm.* 71:208, 1899.

Parke, Thomas (1749-1835), well-known Philadelphia medical practitioner. See J. A. Spalding: *Life of Dr. Lyman Spalding,* p. 354, Boston, 1916; and Joseph Parrish in ms. F909 of the Library of the College of Physicians of Philadelphia.

Parkinson, John (1567-1650), English apothecary and botanist, author of several treatises on botany. Parkinson was appointed apothecary to King James I, who honored the learned man with the title, *"Botanicus regius primarius."* See *Dictionary* (English) *National Biography, XLIII,* p. 315.

Parmentier, Jean Antoine Augustin (1737-1813), French pharmacist who introduced potatoes into France and popularized their use as food. He investigated milk and published a number of fundamental treatises about foodstuff chemistry.

Parrish, Edward (1822-1872), Philadelphia pharmacist and professor at the Philadelphia College of Pharmacy. See England: *First Century of the Philadelphia College of Pharmacy,* p. 404, Philadelphia, 1922; *Am. J. Pharm.* 45:225, 1873; G. Urdang: Edward Parrish, a Forgotten pharmaceutical reformer, *Am. J. Pharm. Ed. 14:*223-232, 1950.

Pasteur, Louis (1822-1897), French chemist and finally director of the Paris Pasteur Institute, founded to carry on his researches. His purely bacteriologic work was his most important contribution to science and to public welfare. His first investigation, his conversion of dextrotartaric acid into the inactive forms, and his discovery of the splitting of racemic acid into dextro- and levotartaric acid, laid the foundation for modern stereochemistry. See Garrison: *History of Medicine,* p. 575, Philadelphia, 1929; Sigerist: *The Great Doctors,* p. 360, New York, 1933.

Patin, Guy (1601-1672). French physician and head of the anti-Paracelsist group of the French medical world of that time, especially of the medical faculty of the University of Paris. See F. R. Packard: *Guy Patin and the Medical Profession in Paris in the Seventeenth Century,* New York, 1925.

Patrons of pharmacy. See: **Deities and Saints, Christian.**

Paullini, Christian Franz (1643-1712), German physician. Besides his famous *Dreckapotheke*, Paullini wrote numerous books on a multitude of subjects, containing "approximately 18,000 printed pages." See Leo Kauner: Christian Franz Paullini, *Med. Life* 41:231, 1934.

Pelletier, Joseph (1788-1842), French pharmacist and the first and most successful investigator in the field of alkaloids after Sertürner, *q.v.* He discovered, together with Caventou, *q.v.*, strychnine (1818), brucine (1819), quinine and cinchonine (1820), caffeine (simultaneously with Robiquet and Runge, in 1821). In cooperation with Dumas, *q.v.*, he discovered narceine, thebaine and pseudomorphine.

Pemberton, Henry (1694-1771), English physician, pupil of Boerhaave, author of several books on medicine, physics and chemistry; pharmacopeial work in England. See *Dictionary of National* (English) *Biography,* XLIV, p. 280.

Pereira, Jonathan (1804-1853), English apothecary, physician and finally professor of materia medica, at the School of Pharmacy of the Pharmaceutical Society of Great Britain. See *Am. J. Pharm.* 25:287, 1853.

Perkin, Sir William Henry (1838-1907). In 1856, he discovered aniline mauve in the course of attempts to prepare quinine artificially. This aniline dyestuff, although preceded by the emeraldine of F. Runge, *q.v.*, opened the way for the dyestuff industry, with all its sidelines. See H. Goodman: William Henry Perkin, *Med. Life* 42:151-162, 1935.

Persia. Ancient Persia had its period of highest development between 600 and 330 B.C. (Kyros to Darius III) and included the land southeast of the Caspian Sea, Mesopotamia, Asia Minor and Egypt. In regard to medicine and pharmacy in ancient Persia, see Tschirch's *Handbuch der Pharmagoknosie,* Leipzig, 1910, *I*: part 2; T. Berendes: *Die Pharmazie bei den alten Kulturvölkern,* Halle, 1891; H. Schelenz: *Geschichte der Pharmazie,* Berlin, 1904; C. Elgood: *Medicine in Persia,* New York, 1934. Concerning recent pharmaceutical practice in Persia, see George Cecil: How pharmacy is practiced in Persia (Iran), *Pharm. Era* 57:43, 1923. See especially, Sigerist, H. E.: A History of Medicine, Volume 2: Early Greek, Hindu and Persian Medicine, New York, 1961.

Personnel.

ENGLISH	GERMAN
Apprentice (French: Elève)	Lehrling Lehrbursche
	Lehr-Junge Lehr bube Tyro[1]
Assistant (French: Compagnon-apothicaire)	Assistent Geselle Subject[1] Adjunkt[1] Defectar[2] Defectuar[2]
Prescription clerk	(Latin: Defectuarius)
Dispenser Dispensing lady	Receptar Receptuar (Latin: Receptuarius)
Manager	
	Stoesser[3] Laborant[4] Kalefactor[5]
Relief clerk	Vertreter
	Lagerist[6]
Porter Janitor	Hausknecht
Errand boy	Laufbursche

[1] Designation common in Austria rather than in Germany.
[2] The person who attends to work in the laboratory, as opposed to the *Receptar.*
[3] One who comminutes drugs.
[4] A worker doing manual work in a laboratory.
[5] A person somewhat between the *Stoesser* and the *Laborant.*
[6] Person in charge of the stock.

Peters, Hermann (1847-1920), German pharmacist and historian of pharmacy. Of his many publications, the books *Der Arzt und die Heilkunde in der deutschen Vergangenheit* and *Aus pharmaceutischer Vorzeit* especially gained wide acknowledgment. The greatest part of the sketches in Volume I of *Aus pharmaceutischer Vorzeit* has been translated into English (with some changes and additions) and published by William Netter under the title *Pictorial History of Ancient Pharmacy.* See introduction to Peters: *Aus der Geschichte der Pflanzenwelt in Wort und Bild,* Gesellschaft Für Geschichte der Pharmazie, Mittenwald, 1929.

Pettenkofer, Max Joseph von (1818-1901), German pharmacist and professor of medicinal chemistry and hygiene at the University of Munich. He is considered the father of modern hygiene.

Pharmaceut. German for pharmacist, *q.v.*, also spelled **Pharmazeut.**

Pharmaceutical chemist. English title introduced by the Pharmacy Act of 1852. Former American degree introduced by the Pharmacy School of the University of Michigan in 1869.

Pharmacien. French for pharmacist, *q.v.*, which succeeded the term *apothicaire.* For some time there were two groups of *"pharmaciens,"* the *Pharmacien de première classe,* entitled to open a pharmacy without restriction, and the *Pharmacien de seconde classe,* allowed to operate a pharmacy only in the district in which he had passed his examination.

Pharmacist, from Greek *pharmakon* ("remedy") and *-ist* ("pertaining to"), a maker of or dealer in remedies. Cf. *Pharmacopoeus* and *Pharmacopolus.* See also French *Pharmacien* and German *Pharmaceut* or *Pharmazeut.* Cf. also **Pharmaceutical chemist.**

Pharmacopée. See: Pharmacopeia.

Pharmacopeia. From the Greek word *pharmakon* ("remedy") and *poiein* ("to make"). As the title for a formulary, it was first used by Jacques du Bois (Sylvius) in his *Pharmacopoeae, libri tres,* printed in Lyon in 1548, and by Bretschneider (called Placotomus) in his *Pharmacopoea in compendium reducta,* printed in Antwerp in 1560. The spelling varies in different countries: "pharmacopoeia, pharmacopoea, pharmacopea, pharmacopée, pharmaecopee, farmacopoea, farmacopen, farmacopee, farmacopoea, farmakop." Earlier treatises on the preparation of medicaments were also known under the following designations: "antidotarium, apotteck, codex, codigo, concordantia, concordia, dispensatorium, enchiridion, formularium, gyógyserkönyi, ljekopis, lumen, luminare, methodus, officina, ratio, receptarium, recettario."

The two earliest "pharmacopeias" mentioned were issued on private initiative, but since the early 18th century the designation "pharmacopeia" has been mostly restricted to treatises issued by governmental authority.

Pharmacopoeus, pl. *-i,* Latinized form of the Greek *pharmakopoeos, q.v.,* maker of remedies. Cf.: *medicamentarius.*

Pharmacopola. Latinized form of *pharmakopolos.* See also: *pharmacopolus.*

Pharmacopolae circumforaneae, itinerant venders of remedies, the Latinized form of the Greek *pharmakopoloi;* furthermore *circumforaneus* ("of or around the forum or market"). They traveled from market to market. Contrast *sellularii.* See also *sellularius* and *seplasiarius.*

Pharmacopolus, pl. *-i.* Latinized form of the Greek *pharmakopolos, q.v.* See also: **pharmacopola.**

Pharmacotribae, Pharmacotritae, drug grinders. They are said to have been employed by the *seplasiarii, q.v.* Cf.: *Rhizotomoi.*

Pharmacy. From Greek *pharmakon, q.v.* ("remedy"). (1) The art and science of the pharmacist; (2) his establishment (synonymous with apothecary shop). Cf. French *pharmacie,* German *Pharmazie* and *Pharmacie,* Italian *farmacia,* etc. Apparently an Egyptian prototype of the term is not to be seen in *ph-ar-maki,* as Schelenz and others supposed, but the etymology perhaps may stem from *phr(t)nhk3w* ("remedy of the sorcerer"). See Frans Jonckheere, *Le 'préparateur de remèdes'* . . . , Deutsche Akademie der Wissenschaften zu Berlin, Institut für Orientforschung, Veröffentlichung Nr. 29 (*Aegyptologische Studien*), 1955, p. 157 and f.n. 7.

Pharmakon. The Greek word from which many modern terms pertaining to pharmacy, *q.v.,* have been derived. The meaning of the Greek word developed from that of a charm or magic agency, exerted by means of plants with healing but often also with poisoning effect (Homer), to that of a remedy without any collateral significance. Often the designation was restricted to purgatives in a real as well as figurative sense. *Pharmacoi* was the name applied to two human scapegoats who, in early Athens, were driven out at the Thargelia feast (the feast of the first bread made of fresh grain), as a symbol of purifying of the city from all evil. These men were considered as personified *pharmakon,* in the meaning of "a purifying purgative," hence the name. In addition the word pharmakon could mean "dyestuff." See Walter Artelt: *Studien zur Geschichte der Begriffe 'Heilmittel' und 'Gift'* in *Studien zur Geschichte der Medizin,* Leipzig, 1937.

Pharmakopoeos, pl. *-oi,* "maker of remedies," from the Greek *pharmakon* ("remedy") and *poiein* ("to make"). Cf. also **pharmacopeia,** "a book that treats of the making of remedies," also, *Pharmacopolos.* See the French *pharmacien,* English **pharmacist** and **pharmaceutist,** German *Pharmaceut* or *Pharmazeut.*

Pharmakopolos, seller of remedies, "from the Greek *pharmakon* ("remedy") and *polein* ("to sell").

Pharmazeut. German for *pharmacist, q.v.* Also spelled **Pharmaceut.**

Philiatrus, Evonymus. See: **Gessner.**

Pigmentarius. pl. *-i,* from *pigmentum* ("paint," also used to designate ointment or pigmented paste and a plant juice); and *-arius,* meaning "pertaining to," i.e., makers of colored cosmetics. Gradually the Roman *pigmentarii* became rather high-class preparers of drugs and dealers in them.

Pill. Latin *pila* ("ball").

Platearius, Matthaeus (12th century), descendant of a well known Salernitan family of physicians and a renowned physician himself, who wrote the *Circa instans* and the annotated Salernitan *Antidotarius magnus.*

Pliny. (23-79 A.D.) Author of the most comprehensive known natural history in antiquity. See Pliny: *Natural History,* with an English translation by H. Rackham, London, 1938; John Bostock and T. H. Riley: *The Natural History of Pliny* (Bohn's Classical Library), London, 1855-57; M. E. Littré: *Histoire naturelle de Pline, avec la traduction en français,* Paris, 1877; K. C. Bailey, *The Elder Pliny's Chapters on Chemical Subjects,* London, 1929-32.

Potts, Jonathan (1745-1781). American physician, serving in the Revolutionary War as Deputy Director General and later on as head of the purchasing department for all medical supplies. See L. C. Duncan: *Medical Men in the American Revolution,* p. 184, Carlisle, 1931; *Dictionary of American Biography, XV,* p. 137.

Power, Frederick B. (1853-1927). The organizer and the first director of the school of pharmacy at the University of Wisconsin, scientific director of the Fritzsche Brothers laboratories in New Jersey (1892-1896), director of the Wellcome Research laboratories in London (1896-1914), and head of the phytochemical laboratory of the United States Department of Agriculture (1916-19). Power became one of the world's best-known research workers in the field of phytochemistry. Power was one of the American pharmacists who completed their professional education by studying at German universities. See J. W. England: *First Century of the Philadelphia College of Pharmacy,* p. 410, 1922; *Badger Pharmac.* 1936, No. 16; *J. A. Ph. A. 16:*380, 1927; *Am. J. Pharm. 96:*601, 1924 (containing a chronological record of Power's scientific contributions).

Powers, Justin L. (1895-   ), eminent pharmacist, author, and authority on drug standards. From 1940 to 1947, director developmental drug standards laboratory, American Pharmaceutical Association; chairman of the National Formulary Committee for 5 revisions (1940-60); active in work on international drug standardization since 1952; editor of the Scientific Edition of the *Journal of the American Pharmaceutical Association* and *Drug Standards* for two decades; consultant to National Cancer Institute since 1960; educator during most of period 1919-40. See *Who's Who in America* and *American Men of Science.*

Powers, Thomas H. (1812-1878), Philadelphia retail and wholesale pharmacist, became (1838) partner of John Farr in the business later known as Powers and Weightman. See J. W. England: *First Century of the Philadelphia College of Pharmacy,* p. 33, Philadelphia, 1922.

Prescott, Albert Benjamin (1832-1905). Without any drugstore practice, the physician Prescott became closely connected with American pharmacy and, as head of the University of Michigan School of pharmacy, one of its most progressive teachers. He was the author of several textbooks, and a member of the United States Pharmacopoeial Convention from 1880 to the time of his death. See Oscar Oldberg, A. B. Prescott, *Am. J. Pharm. 77:*251, 1905.

Procter, William, Jr. (1817-1874), one of the most eminent of American pharmacists. Procter was the 9th child of an English-born Quaker and entered pharmacy when the early death of his father forced him to devote himself to a calling. At the age of 20 he was graduated from the Philadelphia College of Pharmacy. Only 4 years later, he acted as secretary to the Committee on Revision of the U.S.P. In 1844 he opened a pharmacy, which he conducted for many years besides carrying on his comprehensive and successful work as experimenter, teacher and author. In 1846 he became a professor of pharmacy at the Philadelphia College of Pharmacy. From 1850 to 1871, he was the sole editor of the *American Journal of Pharmacy.* He published the first textbook on pharmacy by an American pharmacist for American students of pharmacy, which he adapted from a German-British text. No less than 550 original articles in the *American Journal of Pharmacy* bear witness to Procter's indefatigable industry. It was William Procter, Jr., who carried the idea of a national American pharmaceutical association to the Convention of Pharmaceutists and Druggists, held in New York on October 15 and 16, 1851. Thus the first step was taken toward its founding, which took place 1 year later in Philadelphia. See J. W. England: *First Century of the Philadelphia College of Pharmacy,* p. 402, Philadelphia, 1922.

Prometheus, a deified Titan who saved mankind from darkness by bringing fire from heaven. He was said to have embodied his medical knowledge in charms.

Proust, Joseph Louis (1754-1826), French pharmacist who discovered mannitol (1806) and leucin (1819), and found the element nickel in meteoric iron (1799). He furthermore stated the law of definite and constant proportions in chemical reactions.

Puckner, W. A. (1864-1932). Pharmacist, later professor at the Chicago College of Pharmacy, and consulting chemist. In 1907, he became director of the American Medical Association Chemical Laboratory. See *J. A. Ph. A.* 21:1115, 1932; *Indust. & Eng. Chem. News Ed.* 10:255, 1932.

Pulvis, pl. *pulveres.* In classical Latin, powder, dust distinguished from coarsely comminuted drugs or *species.* The finely comminuted drugs were designated *pulveres.* Powdering drugs facilitated their administration. Even today, mortar and pestle are the symbol of the art of the pharmacist. The early pharmacopeias designated a special class of preparations as powders. With the advance of iatrochemistry, the term was also applied to mineral preparations in powder form (e.g., Allgaroth powder). So far as vegetable preparations are concerned, it was applied to mixtures as well (e.g., *pulvis opii compositus*) and other mixtures containing inorganic chemicals (*Pulvis infantum = Pulvis Rhei compositus*), or organic chemicals (Tully's Powder — *pulvis morphinae compositus*).

Quercetanus. See: **Quesne,** Joseph du.

Quesne, Joseph du, Latinized Quercetanus (1544-1609), French physician and medical author. As a follower of Paracelsus, *q.v.,* he recommended chemicals as remedies, especially preparation of antimony and mercury, without, however, neglecting galenics. He is supposed to have been the first to employ calomel and sulfurated antimony.

Quincy, John (d. 1722). English apothecary, later a physician, and a very successful author on medical and pharmaceutical subjects. See: *Dictionary* (English) *National Biography, XLVI,* p. 112.

Quintessence. This term was used by Paracelsus for pharmaceutical preparations he considered to represent the most perfect extract of the essential contents of the raw material. His term derives from the 5th essence (Latin *quinta,* "five"), which the Pythagoreans added to the 4 elements of the ancient Greeks, thought to be a most subtle "ether," a kind of immaterial radiation of the material world.

Rafinesque, Constantine Smaltz (1783-1840), botanist of French descent residing in Philadelphia. He wrote several books on history, botany and science, and medical botany. See Alex Berman: C. S. Rafinesque (1783-1840): a challenge to the historian of pharmacy, *Am. J. Pharm. Ed.* 16:409-418, 1952; Alexander Wilder, *History of Medicine,* pp. 421-432, 438, 439, New Sharon, Maine, 1901.

Ratio. See: **Pharmacopeia.**

Raubenheimer, Otto (1867-1946), German-born Brooklyn pharmacist; a founding member of the *Gesellschaft für Geschichte der Pharmazie;* pharmaceutical historian, author, editor and teacher. See *New York Apoth. Ztg.* 47:2, Feb., 1927.

Receptar. See: **Personnel.**

Redwood, Theophilus (1806-1892). English pharmacist, editor of the *Pharmaceutical Journal,* and professor of chemistry and pharmacy to the Pharmaceutical Society of Great Britain. He edited, enlarged and translated Friedrich Mohr, *q.v., Lehrbuch der pharmaceutischen Technik.* See: *Am. J. Pharm.* 64:223, 1892.

Remington, Joseph P. (1847-1918), one of the most versatile and influential American pharmacists of his time. A graduate of the Philadelphia College of Pharmacy, he first engaged in manufacturing, and then in community pharmacy. He re-entered his alma mater, this time in a teaching position (1871), becoming its dean (1893). Remington was instrumental in the development of the American Pharmaceutical Association and of the *United States Pharmacopoeia* and was for years regarded by many as the outstanding representative of the American profession of pharmacy. In 1919, the New York branch of the American Pharmaceutical Association established the Remington Honor Medal, which is given annually for distinguished service to pharmacy in the United States. The recipients are chosen by majority vote of the living ex-presidents of the Association. See J. W. England: *First Century of the Philadelphia College of Pharmacy,* pp. 407, 408, Philadelphia, 1922.

Rhizotomos, pl. *-oi,* literally "root cutters," from the Greek *rhiza* ("root") and *temnein* ("to cut"). The name was also applied to collectors of indigenous drugs.

Rice, Charles, German-born American pharmacist (1841-1901), who was pharmacist at the Bellevue Hospital in New York, an excellent chemist, and a man of broadest cultural and scientific background. His phenomenal knowledge of languages gave him an opportunity to keep informed of progress in pharmacy all over the world and facilitated the reform of the *United States Pharmacopoeia,* effected under his chairmanship. See *Proc. A. Ph. A. 49:*45, 1901; John Uri Lloyd: Dr. Charles Rice, *J. A. Ph. A. 25:*1143, 1936. H. G. Wolfe: Charles Rice (1841-1901), an immigrant in pharmacy, *Am. J. Pharm. Ed. 14:*285-305, 1950.

Ricettario. See: **Pharmacopeia.**

Robiquet, Pierre Jean (1780-1840), French pharmacist who was one of the most successful phytochemists, he found asparagine simultaneously with Vauquelin (1805); narcotine (1817); caffeine in collaboration with Pelletier (simultaneously with Runge, 1821); alizarin in collaboration with Colin, 1826; amygdalin (1830); codeine (1832).

Rondelet, Guglielmo, French physician and academic teacher at the University of Montpellier, as well as practicing pharmacist (1507-1566). Besides his *Methodus de materia medicinali et compositione medicamentorum,* he wrote several books, of which *Liber de ponderibus* ("Book of Weights") lived to see several editions.

Rother, Reinhold (1843-1889), German-born American pharmacist, and writer on pharmaceutical subjects. See: *Am. J. Pharm. 61:*639, 1889.

Rotulae (Latin, rotula, a little wheel). Wheel-shaped lozenges. See: *morsuli.*

Rouelle, Guillaume François (1703-1770), French pharmacist and chemist. He was the teacher of Lavoisier and one of the most eminent and most diligent chemical authors of his time. He originated the chemical definition of the concept of "salt." See: **Chemistry, history of.**

Rouelle, Hilaire Marie (1718-1779), French pharmacist who was the younger brother of Guillaume François Rouelle, *q.v.,* and a chemist of high merit. He discovered urea (1773) and hippuric acid (1776); recognized the iron content of the blood; and found natural sulfide of hydrogen.

Rousseau, Georges Louis Claude (1724-1794), German pharmacist of French descent and professor of chemistry at the University of Ingolstadt. Lecturing in the laboratory connected with his pharmacy, he was one of the first teachers of chemistry before Liebig who accompanied his lectures with experiments and gave his students an opportunity for individual experimental work.

Ruddiman, Edsel A. (1864-1954), pharmaceutical teacher; from 1901 to 1914, United States food and drug inspector; research chemist; author. See: *Who's Who in America, 50:*2157, 1938; *American Men of Science,* ed. 8, p. 2131, 1949.

Ruelle, Jean de, Latinized Ruellius (1474-1537), French physician, canon and writer on botanic and medical subjects. His translation of Dioscorides' *Materia medica,* from the Greek original into Latin, appeared in 1540 with annotations by Euricius and Valerius Cordus (father and son). Among his further translations from Greek into Latin, that of Johannes Actuarius' book, *De compositione medicamentorum,* became especially noted.

Ruellius. See **Ruelle.**

Runge, Friedlieb Ferdinand (1794-1867), German pharmacist who discovered aniline, which he called "kyanol," in coal tar (1834). Simultaneously, he discovered carbolic acid, rosolic acid and other chemicals in the same substance. This was the beginning of coal-tar chemistry. Likewise, it was he who showed the way to produce dyestuffs with aniline as base. He discovered caffeine (1821). It is of interest to note that aniline had previously been prepared from indigo, first by means of dry distillation by Unverdorben, who called it "krystallin" (1826) and then by Fritzsche, who treated indigo with potassium hydroxide (1841). The designation "aniline" was coined by Fritzsche from the Spanish word *anil-indigo.* Synthetic aniline was prepared by Zinin, by reduction of nitrobenzene with ammonium sulfate (1841). Zinin called his product "benzidam." In 1843 A. W. Hofmann recognized that all these products were identical.

Rusby, Henry H. (1855-1940), M.D., botanist, professor at the New York College of Pharmacy, 1888-1920. See J. W. England: *First Century of the Philadelphia College of Pharmacy*, p. 219.

Ruth, Robert J. (1891-1931), pharmacist, teacher, organizer and leader in industrial pharmaceutical service, "father of American Pharmacy Week." See *J. A. Ph. A. 20*:725, 1931 and G. Sonnedecker, National Pharmacy Week, *Tile and Till 34*:38-41, 1948.

Sadtler, Samuel P. (1847-1924), professor of chemistry at Pennsylvania College, then at the University of Pennsylvania College, at the University of Pennsylvania, and the Philadelphia College of Pharmacy. See *Am. J. Pharm. 96*:134, 1934.

Saints, Christian, as patrons of pharmacy. In the early Middle Ages, the pagan deities associated with medicine and pharmacy, etc., were gradually replaced in the Christian countries by Christian saints, chosen as patrons by the local guilds of physicians and, in the 13th century, of apothecaries, spicers, etc. Most frequently, we meet Cosmas, *q.v.*, and Damian, *q.v.*, as patron saints of the healing arts. Then follow in frequency the Holy Virgin and Mary Magdalene, the latter because she oiled the feet of the Saviour with fragrant oil (a pharmaceutical preparation!). We know that in 1345 the English apothecaries were joined with the pepperers in the Fraternity of St. Anthony. Naturally, the custom of revering patron saints remained after the time of the Reformation primarily in the Catholic countries. M. Bouvet gives a comprehensive list of such patrons chosen by the apothecaries in the various parts of France. He names S. S. Nicolas, Luke, Michael, Marcus and Rochus, of course, in addition to Cosmas, Damian, the Holy Virgin, and Mary Magdalene. (M. Bouvet, *Histoire de la pharmacie en France*, p. 259-261, Paris, 1937.)

Salmon, William (1644-1713), English empiric, who wrote several books and pamphlets on medical and pharmaceutical subjects. See *Dictionary of National* (English) *Biography,* 50, p. 209; William Kirkby: A quack of the seventeenth century, *Pharm. J. 84*:255-262, 1910.

Santorio, Santorio, called Sanctorius (1561-1636), Italian physician and academic teacher at Padua. See Garrison: *History of Medicine,* p. 260, Philadelphia, 1929; Sigerist: *The Great Doctors,* p. 150, New York, 1933.

Savory, John (1800-1871), English apothecary. See *Pharm. J. 31*:319, 1871.

Sayre, Lucius E. (1848-1925), pharmacist in Philadelphia, later professor at the School of Pharmacy of Kansas State University. See *J. A. Ph. A. 8*:3, 1919; J. W. England: *First Century of the Philadelphia College of Pharmacy*, p. 260, Philadelphia, 1922.

Scammon, Frederick (1810-1864), physician and pharmacist, professor of botany of the University of Chicago. See *Alumni Record of the University of Illinois,* p. 431, 1921; *Am. J. Pharm. 36*:277, 1864.

Scheele, Carl Wilhelm (1742-1786), one of the greatest chemists of all time, who never left the pharmaceutical profession and made all his discoveries in the laboratories of the pharmacies in which he worked; in the last 11 years of his life, first as manager and then as owner of the pharmacy in the small town of Koeping (Sweden). Among inorganic acids, Scheele discovered arsenic (1771-1772), hydrofluoric (1771), molybdic (1778) and tungstic (1778); among organic acids, citric (1784), gallic (1770), lactic (1780), malic (1784), mucic (1780), oxalic (1770), pyrogallic (1770), tartaric (before 1768) and uric (1776). He identified baryta (1771-1774), chlorine (1774), glycerin (1783), manganese (1773), and milk-sugar (1780); he discovered oxygen (prior to 1773), hydrochloric acid gas (1770), ammonia (1770) and arsenetted hydrogen (1775); and he ascertained the chemical nature of sulfuretted hydrogen (1768). Among the new processes which he invented, those of special interest are for preparing phosphorus (1770), calomel (1774) and benzoic acid (1775). See George Urdang: *The Apothecary Chemist, Carl Wilhelm Scheele,* Madison, Wis., 1942.

Schelenz, Hermann (1848-1922), passed the *Staatsexamen* ("state board examination") as *Apotheker* (1873), then operated a pharmacy in Rendsburg, Schleswig (1875 to 1893). Frequent contributor to pharmaceutical journals, more particularly on historical subjects. Author of the following books: *Geschichte der Pharmazie* (1904); *Zur Geschichte der pharmazeutisch-chemischen Destilliergeräte* (1913); *Shakespeare und* *sein Wissen auf dem Gebiete der Arznei-und Volkskunde* (1914).

He was awarded an honorary M.D. by the University of Freiburg (1920), and he was made an honorary member of the American Pharmaceutical Association (1912). For a more detailed account of his life work, see *Pharm. Ztg.* 67:841, 1922; and, especially, Zimmermann, Walter: H. Schelenz' Lebenswerk, *Pharm. Monatshefte* 4:137, 1923. The last essay by Schelenz published before his death was "American apothecaries in literature," *Pharm. Zeit.* 67:371, 1922.

Schieffelin, Henry H., head of the New York wholesale drug firm W. H. Schieffelin and Company from 1814 to 1849 (at that time called H. H. Schieffelin and Company). See *One Hundred Years of Business Life, 1794-1894.* W. H. Schieffelin and Company, New York.

Schlotterbeck, Julius Otto (1865-1917), one of the American pharmaceutical teachers who studied at German or Swiss universities. He taught pharmacognosy at the University of Michigan, wrote a number of scientific papers, and later took up industrial work. See *Am. J. Pharm.* 89:336, 1917.

Schmidt, Ernst Albert (1845-1921), German pharmacist and professor of pharmacy at the University of Marburg. Schmidt specialized in alkaloid chemistry. His *Ausführliches Lehrbuch der pharmazeutischen Chemie,* highly regarded, has been edited again and again since Schmidt's death. He has, furthermore, the isolation of scopolamine to his credit.

Schoepf, Johann David (1752-1800), German physician and botanist. See H. Peters: Joh. David Schoepf, *Pharm. Rund.* 13:151, 1895.

Schulze, F., German military pharmacist (1914 to 1918). See Devin: *Die deutschen Militaerapotheker im Weltkriege,* Berlin, 1920.

Scoville, Wilbur L. (1865-1941), pharmaceutical teacher; from 1907-1934 research pharmacist with Parke, Davis and Comapny; after 1924, head of the analytic department of the firm; author and editor. See *American Men of Science,* p. 1263, 1938; *Who's Who in America, 20:* p. 2221.

Scribonius Largus (first century after Christ), Roman physician. The cognomen "Largus" is presumably derived from Latin *largiri,* meaning "the liberal giver." The formulary he wrote was printed in several editions between the 16th and the 18th centuries, under different and sometimes quite arbitrary titles.

Seaman, Valentine (1770-1817), New York physician and promoter of vaccination: co-author of the "pharmacopoeia" of the New York Hospital of 1816. See Kelly and Burrage: *American Medical Biographies,* p. 842, New York, 1920.

Sellularius, pl. *-i,* from Lat. *sellula,* "a little seat," and *-arius,* "pertaining to"; hence, people who had sedentary occupations or trades; stationary venders of remedies, as contrasted with ***pharmacopolae circumforaneae,*** *q.v.* They were also called *seplasiarii, q.v.*

Seplasiarius, from *seplasia,* a street in Capua where unguents (possibly also frankincense and other oriental drugs) were sold, and *-arius,* "pertaining to." Cf. *sellularius.*

Sertürner, Friedrich Wilhelm Adam (1783-1841), German pharmacist who became famous by his discovery of morphine as the *principium somniferum* ("somniferous principle") in opium. His first publications about "meconic acid, which also contained his discovery of the first alkaloid to be prepared in a pure state, appeared in 1805 and 1806 in Trommsdorff's *Journal der Pharmazie, q.v.* It is likely that morphine in a more or less pure state had been obtained before Sertürner by the French pharmacists Derosne and, especially, Seguin. However, the fact that Sertürner discovered the basic nature of the substance called by him morphium, made him the pioneer of alkaloidal chemistry. See Franz Kroemecke: *Fr. W. Sertürner,* Jena, 1925.

Sérullas, Georges Simon (1774-1832), French Pharmacist who discovered iodoform (1822) and produced several new compounds of bromide.

Seumenicht. See: **Mynsicht.**

Sharp, Alpheus Pireas (1824-1909), one of the founders of the firm of Sharp and Dohme, Baltimore. "Mr. Sharp read the first scientific paper before the American Pharmaceutical Association," and as an anniversary event "the identical paper was read again at the annual meeting held fifty years later." See *Am. Drug.* and *Pharm. Rec.* 54:352, 1909.

Sheppard, S. A. D. (1842-1915), Boston pharmacist and for 22 years treasurer of the American Pharmaceutical Association. He collected the "Sheppard Library" of about 2,500 volumes, among them about 300 pharmacopeias of different countries and periods, which he bequeathed to the Massachusetts College of Pharmacy. See *Bull. Pharm.* 22: 323, 1906; *J. A. Ph. A.* 4:1515, 1915.

Shoemaker, Robert (1817-1897), Philadelphia wholesale and retail pharmacist and pharmaceutical manufacturer. Shoemaker is believed to have been the first to manufacture glycerin in the United States (1848). See England: *First Century of the Philadelphia College of Pharmacy,* p. 106.

Show globes. There has been much conjecture about the origin of the peculiarly shaped bottles filled with colored liquids which have been used for a long time as a sign of pharmacy, especially in Anglo-Saxon countries. Attempts have been made to trace them back to antiquity. However, there is no mention of such use anywhere before the 17th century. C. J. S. Thompson thinks there is probably a connection between these display bottles and the carboys, use of which for transport and preservation of liquids became general at about the same time. (*The Mystery and Art of the Apothecary,* p. 251, Philadelphia, 1929.) It seems highly probable that the bottles filled with colored liquids originated in the early English chemists' shops, whose owners wanted to utilize the public attraction of the unusual bottle (apparatus) as well as of the mysterious products (represented by the colored liquids) obtained from the new art of chemistry. Later on, the druggists seized upon these signs, as well as the production or at least the sale of medical chemicals, until both groups merged into the united profession of chemist-and-druggist. See George Urdang: New light on the origin of show globes, *J. Am. Pharm.* (Pract. Ed.) *10*:604-6, 640; see also, George Griffenhagen, The Show Globe, *J. A. Ph. A.* (Pract. Ed.) *19*: 233-5, 1958 (and *Am. Drugg. 134*:9-11, No. 10, 1956); W. Schneider, in *Pharm. Industrie 17*:29, 1955.

Simon, Johann Franz (1807-1847), German pharmacist and physiologic chemist, supposed to have been the first to publish a modern, comprehensive collection of data pertaining exclusively to the "Chemistry of Man." See George Urdang: *Pharmacy's Part in Society,* p. 49, Madison, Wis., 1946.

Simon, William (1844-1916), German-born and pharmaceutically educated pharmacist, professor of chemistry at the Maryland College of Pharmacy (1872-1902) at the College of Physicians and Surgeons of Baltimore (1880-1916) and at the Baltimore College of Dental Surgery (1888 to 1916); author of a well-known textbook. See: *J. A. Ph. A.* 5: 886, 1916.

Simmons, Willard B. (1906-   ) has been Executive Secretary of the National Association of Retail Druggists since 1961, after serving on the Executive Commitee, 1953-61. His previous career was made in the practice of pharmacy at Texarkana, Texas (beginning at Bloomburg, 1925). He was prominent in organized civic and business endeavors of East Texas. (*N.A.R.D. Jour.,* pp. 16 and 74, Nov. 6, 1961.)

Simplicia, from the Latin *simplex* ("simple"), generic term for all those drugs not classified as *composita, q.v.* Lists of such simples were compiled very early. In the 11th century Contantinus Africanus wrote his treatise *De gradibus simplicium* and, in the 12th century, Matthaeus Platearius wrote his famous *Liber de simplici medicina dictus circa instans.* Later on such lists appeared in the pharmacopeias (after the 18th century chiefly under the title of materia medica). In general, only such drugs were listed as *simplicia* as had not passed a process of preparation beyond that of comminution or purification. However, this principle was not strictly followed. Thus the first U.S.P. (1820) mentions, on the one hand, prepared carbonate of lime (a purified simple drug), among the preparations, while on the other hand its materia medica presents "a catalogue of simple medicines together with some prepared medicines which are kept in the shop of the apothecary but not necessarily prepared by him."

Skoda, Josef (1805-1881), Bohemian physician and academic teacher in Vienna. He was the leading clinician of the so-called New Vienna School of medicine and the exponent of its therapeutic nihilism. See Garrison: *History of Medicine,* p. 431, Philadelphia, 1929; Sigerst: *The Great Doctors,* p. 297, New York, 1933.

Smith, Daniel B. (1792-1883), Philadelphia pharmacist, who was one of the founders of and leaders in the Philadelphia College of Pharmacy, and a man of high scientific and literary attainments. See England, *First Century of the Philadelphia College of Pharmacy,* p. 353, Philadelphia, 1922.

Smith, Peter (1753-1816), American preacher, farmer and medical practitioner, the so-called "Indian Doctor." See *Bull. Lloyd Libr.,* No. 2.

Soubeiran, Eugene (1797-1858), French pharmacist. Simultaneously with the American Samuel Guthrie, *q.v.,* and the German Justus v. Liebig, *q.v.,* he discovered chloroform (1831). The trichlormethane found by them was called "chloric ether" by Guthrie, "bi-chloric ether" by Soubeiran, and "trichloride of carbon" by Liebig. Dumas (1834) gave it the name of chloroform, from formyl (CH) and (tri) chloride.

Spagiric, from the Greek *span* (to separate) and *ageirein* (to combine). The term "spa-giric art" used by Paracelsus as a synonym for "chemistry" means, therefore, the art of separating and combining, or of analysis and synthesis.

Spalding, Lyman (1775-1821), physician, the "Father of the U. S. P." See *J. A. Ph. A. 6:* 675, 1917; James A. Spalding: *The Life of Dr. Lyman Spalding,* Boston, 1916.

Speciarius. See: *Species.*

Species. From the Latin verb *specio,* to look, to behold, changed in its meaning from the abstract sight to the thing seen. In late Latin, it was specialized to mean goods (wares generally, e.g., wine), but more particularly spices and drugs. Hence *speciarius* (pertaining to *species*), Italian *spetiali,* English *spicer,* French *épicier, speciaria* a female spice-dealer. In more modern pharmaceutical practice, the designation species was applied to mixtures of coarsely comminuted (cut or bruised) mixtures of parts of vegetable drugs, such as roots, barks, woods, leaves, flowers, stems, mosses and lichens, seeds and fruits. Occasionally, gums or gum resins were added (Trommsdorff, *Wörterbuch*) e.g., *species pectorales* or German *Brustthee,* and *species laxantes* or "laxative tea." The designation "tea," however, is also applied to unmixed vegetable drugs, e.g., senna tea (leaves), fennel tea (fruit), etc. In this sense, it is also applied to the tea par excellence, Chinese tea, the leaves (or tips of leaves) of *Thea chinensis;* also to its substitutes, e.g., New Jersey tea (leaves of *Ceanothus americanus*). (The word "species" is used in botany to designate a kind, as opposed to "genus.")

Speck, William Alfred (1864-1928), American-born pharmacist of German descent, until 1913 owner of a New York pharmacy inherited from his father. From then until his death, he was curator of the unique Goethe Collection created by him at Yale University. See Carl F. Schreiber: William Speck, in memoriam, *Yale University Library Gazette* 3:55, Jan., 1929.

Spiritus aromatici. Like the *aquae aromaticae, q.v.,* aromatic spirits were made by distillation of aromatic drugs with wine,

spirits or even stronger alcohol. Such a preparation was the *eau des Cannes,* which was later introduced into the pharmacopeias as *spiritus melissae compositus.* The term *spiritus* and *aqua* were used interchangeably. *Spiritus vini* was commonly known as *aqua vitae.* Today they are commonly prepared by the solution of volatile oils in alcohol.

Squibb, Edward R. (1819-1900). He was physician, manufacturer, chemist and, in his early days, apprentice and then clerk in a pharmacy from 1837 to 1842. Squibb belongs to the pioneers who became equally important to pharmacy and to medicine. See J. P. Remington: E. R. Squibb, *Am. J. Pharm.* 73:419, 1901.

Squire, Peter (1798-1884), English pharmacist. He was appointed chemist-in-ordinary in the court pharmacy of Queen Victoria and was one of the founders of the Pharmaceutical Society of Great Britain. See *Am. J. Pharm.* 56:400, 1884.

Stahl, Georg Ernst (1660-1734), Professor at the University of Halle, later physician-in-ordinary to the King of Prussia and formulator of the phlogiston theory. He developed the ideas of Becher, *q.v.,* to a complete system and coined the name "phlogiston" (from Greek *phlogizein,* "set on fire") for the substantive principle of combustion assumed by Becher. See Garrison: *History of Medicine,* p. 312, Philadelphia, 1929; Sigerist: *The Great Doctors,* p. 183, New York, 1933.

Starkey (Stirk), George (about 1620-1665), American physician and the only American alchemist of note. He wrote under his own name and under the pen name Eirenaeus Philoponus Philalethes. See George Lyman Kittredge: Dr. Robert Child, the Remonstrant, *Trans. Colonial Society of Massachusetts,* 1919, 21:1-146, 1920; *Isis* 9:440, 1927.

Stationarius, pl. *-i,* from Latin *statio* and *-arius,* "of or belonging to a post or station." Compare the older *sellularius.* The term, referring to pharmacist who owns one of the recognized pharmacies at a given locality, appears in the edict of Frederick II of 1231-1241.

Stearns, Frederick (1832-1907), pharmacist, first in Buffalo and then in Detroit; later on, founder of the pharmaceutical manufacturing house of Frederick Stearns and Company of Detroit. See *Drug Circ.* 51:244, 1907. Roland T. Lakey: Frederick Stearns, pharmacist, *J. A. Ph. A.* (Pract. Ed.) 9:487-489.

Stillé, Alfred (1813-1900), Philadelphia physician and professor of medicine at the University of Pennsylvania. His *Elements of General Pathology* (1848), was the first American book on the subject. See: *Dictionary of American Biography, XVIII*, p. 23.

Stirk, George. See: **Starkey, George.**

Stock, Fred J. (1908-   ). Starting as a practicing pharmacist (1928-41), Stock became Chief of the U. S. War Production Board, Drugs and Cosmetics Branch during World War II. In this capacity, he headed the War Production Board's drug program, including the overseeing of manufacture and distribution of penicillin, the sulfonamides, and antimalarials. Since the war Stock has been a Vice President of Chas. Pfizer & Co., Inc. (1945-51) and, since 1952, a Vice-President of Mathieson Chemical Corp. and then of its E. R. Squibb and Sons division. See *Who's Who in America.*

Stoesser. See: **Personnel.**

Subject. See: **Personnel.**

Swain, Robert L. (1887-1963), American pharmacist and lawyer, influential on American pharmacy as editor of *Drug Topics* (1939-1960) and through vigorous participation in the affairs of the American Pharmaceutical Association (e.g., Council, 1933-51 and 1953-59; President, 1933-34) and other organizations. Earlier in Maryland he served as editor of *The Maryland Pharmacist* (1925-1940), law enforcement official and professor (*J. A. Ph. A.* n.s. 3:1963, 153).

Sylvius. See: (1) **Boe, François de le;** (2) **Bois, Jacques du.**

Sylvius, Franciscus, or François **de le Boe Sylvius** (1614-1672). A Dutch follower of Paracelsus. He prepared the scientific foundation for the application of chemicals in therapy, preached by Paracelsus, and hence may be regarded as the real founder of the iatrochemical school. He introduced the word and the concept of fermentation; and by means of it he explained the chemical changes that take place within the human body. Not only was the food converted into blood under the influence of the saliva and of glandular secretion, but also the blood itself was transferred by certain "ferments," into a so-called "ether," a hypothetical substance which, according to this theory, is responsible for the life processes. The ultimate products of these changes were acids and alkalies, the proper relation of which in the body guaranteed health. Disturbances produced the so-called *acrimoniae*, which were either acid or alkaline, and were to be corrected by the administration of drugs of alkaline or acid character.

Symon, or Simon Januensis (d. 1303), an Italian medical author. The cognomen Januensis means from Genoa.

Tabernaemontanus. See **Theodor, Johann.** The word *tabernaemontanus* means "from Bergzabern," his birthplace.

Tabulae. Latin for "board or plank"; also "tablet," diminutive for "table." Comparable to our troches and lozenges.

Talbor, Robert, also called Talbot (1642-1681). Talbor started his career as an apprentice to the apothecary Dear in Cambridge, became a (self-styled) physician and, after having cured the English King Charles II with a decoction of cinchona bark, was appointed physician-in-ordinary to His Majesty. See C. J. S. Thompson: *The Mystery and Art of the Apothecary*, p. 232, Philadelphia, 1929; Wootton: *Chronicles of Pharmacy, II*, p. 97, London, 1910.

Taylor, Alfred B. (1824-1898), Philadelphia pharmacist. Taylor was the first treasurer of the American Pharmaceutical Association and active in the work of pharmacopeial revision. He was one of the early American pharmacists who combined practical pharmacy with scientific work. See *Proc. A. Ph. A.* 46:51, 1898; J. W. England: *First Century of the Philadelphia College of Pharmacy*, p. 207, Philadelphia, 1922.

Terra sigillata. Clay originating from certain districts of Europe, which was made up into round pastils weighing about ½ ounce. These were stamped with designs alluding to the places of their origin. Such earth tablets were given in dysenteries, internal ulcers · and hemorrhages; also in gonorrhea and in pestilential fevers. Externally they were applied to festering wounds. Their use through the ages rested mainly on their recommendation by Galen (*q.v.*). See Wootton: *Chronicles of Pharmacy, II*, p. 53, London, 1910.

Thacher, James (1754-1844), American physician. Besides his *American New Dispensatory*, he wrote some other books, among them an *American Medical Biography*. During his service in the Revolutionary Army, he kept a rather full journal, which is one of the most complete diaries of the war. See L. C. Duncan: *Medical Men in the American Revolution*, p. 262, Carlisle, 1931; *Dictionary of American Biography, XVIII*, p. 387.

Theodor, Johann (Jacob), called Tabernaemontanus (1510-1590), German pharmacist, physician, and botanist. The first part of his *New Vollkommentlich Kreuterbuch* ("New Perfect Herbal") was published in 1588 and the second part in 1613 after his death, by Caspar Bauhin, *q.v.*

Theophrasmus Bombastus of Hohenheim. See **Paracelsus.**

Theophrastus, Eresios (371-286 B.C.), pupil of the Greek philosopher Aristotle and one of the oldest botanists whose writings have come down to us. He has been called "the father of botany." See Tschirch: *Handbuch der Pharmakognosie, I,* Part 2, p. 545, Leipzig, 1910; George Sarton: *Introduction to the History of Science, I,* pp. 143, 144, Baltimore, 1927.

Theriac, also treacle. (Greek *theriake,* Latin *theriaca,* French *thériaque.*) The Greek term *theriake* was derived from *theriakós* (of wild or venomous beasts); hence, *theriaca* or *theriace* was an antidote, first primarily against the bite of serpents, then against poisons in general. Later it was regarded as a general panacea, although it retained its special reputation as an antidote. Nicander of Colophon, who lived during the second century B.C., is said to have been the first to recommend it. Its highest reputation was gained when prepared according to the supposed formula of Mithridates, King of Pontus in Asia Minor (132-63 B.C.) or according to the modified formulae of Democrates or Andromachus, physicians who lived in Rome during the first century. It was Andromachus who added the "flesh of serpents" to the ingredients of the panacea, and it was the formula of Andromachus which, through Galen, *q.v.*, gained recognition up to the eighteenth century, when the myth of the therapeutic value of theriaca was exploded by William Herberden, *q.v.* During certain periods and in certain countries the composition of theriaca was regarded as being of sufficient importance to have it made by the pharmacist under the supervision of representatives of the medical faculty. See J. Berendes, *Die Pharmacie bei den alten Kulturvoelkern,* p. 281, Halle, 1891; Peters and Netter, *Pictorial History of Ancient Pharmacy,* p. 115, Chicago, 1899; C. J. S. Thompson, *The Mystery and Art of the Apothecary,* p. 58, Philadelphia, 1929.

Thompson, William S. (1822-1894), pharmacist in Baltimore and editor of the *Journal* of the Maryland College of Pharmacy. See: *Proc. Am. Pharm. A.* 43:47, 1895.

Thoms, Hermann (1859-1931), German phar-

macist and professor of pharmaceutical chemistry at the University of Berlin. The exemplary Institute of Pharmacy at the University of Berlin was the fruit of his endeavor, and built according to his plans. See *Pharm. Rev.* 26:1, 1908. Thoms was the founder of the *Deutsche pharmazeutische Gesellschaft.* Of his discoveries the synthetic substitute for sugar, which he called "Dulcin," found widest recognition. See *Pharm. Ztg.* 76:1349, 1931.

Thomson, Samuel (1769-1843). Thomson founded the American botanic school of medical thought, which later on was merged into the eclectic school of medicine. See: *Lloyd Libr. Reprod. Ser.* No. 7; *Dictionary of American Biography, XVIII,* p. 488; and Alex Berman: *The Impact of the 19th Century Botanico-medical Movement on American Pharmacy and Medicine,* University of Wisconsin, Ph.D. dissertation, 1954.

Thoth. Egyptian god of wisdom, magic, and one of the gods to whom healing was attributed. He was represented with the head of Osiris or as *cynocephalus* (dog-headed), and identified with ph-ar-maki.

Tinctures. Earlier historians attributed the introduction of tinctures into pharmacy to a mysterious alchemist, Raymundus Lullus (1235-1315). Now it has been stated that most of the writings ascribed to him are not his work. However, there is no doubt of the mentioning of preparations of this type in what is now called the *Lullian Corpus,* i.e., pre-Paracelsian writings under the name of Lullus. On the other hand, it was the emphasis put on these liquid extracts of drugs by Paracelsus which was responsible for their introduction in the pharmacopeias and their common use.

The early tinctures, as they are found under this designation in the pharmacopeias of the 16th and even the 17th centuries, differ essentially from the products called tinctures in later times. Minerals, corals, rust (prepared by roasting of vitriol) together with orange peel, red rose petals, aloes, myrrh, crocus, etc., were digested with alcohol and the product called *tinctura coralliorum* or *martis e vitriolo* or *proprietatis.* A reddish alcoholic solution of roasted potassium carbonate was called *tinctura tartari.* Preparations like the usual tinctures of later times, i.e., alcoholic or hydroalcoholic solutions of the contents of vegetables or animal drugs produced by maceration are, in the seventeenth century, sometimes enumerated as *aquae cum spiritu vini.* In the language of alchemy, tincture, like elixir, was a term for the mysterious means of transmutation of base metals to gold or silver.

Trimble, Henry (1853-1898). He started his career as a pharmacist in Philadelphia and was (from 1883) professor of analytic chemistry at the Philadelphia College of Pharmacy, and editor (after 1894) of the *American Journal of Pharmacy.* See England: *First Century of the Philadelphia College of Pharmacy,* p. 412, Philadelphia, 1922.

Trommsdorff, Johannes Bartholomaeus (1770-1837), German pharmacist. Trommsdorff was a great teacher, devoting his life to the education of pharmacists and to the elevation of pharmacy. He founded a private school of pharmacy in Erfurt, which gained international fame and was the first of its kind, giving laboratory work, in the world. He wrote several textbooks on pharmacy and on chemistry, among them his *Handbuch der Apothekerkunst* (1790), the *Apothekerschule* (1804), the *Allgemeines pharmaceutisch-chemisches Wörterbuch oder die Apothekerkunst in ihrem ganzen Umfange,* in 5 volumes (1605-1813) and 2 supplements (1821 and 1822), and the *Handbuch der gesamten Chemie,* in 8 volumes (1800-1804). Furthermore, he was the first real pharmaceutical journalist, founding not only the first periodical devoted especially to scientific pharmacy and issued at more than annual intervals, *Trommdorff's Journal der Pharmacie, q.v.,* but trying to write in an interesting way. His research was devoted primarily to pharmaceutical preparations. See Otto Rosenhainer and Trommsdorff: *Trommsdorff's Lebensbild,* Jena, 1913; Curt T. Wimmer, *J. A. Ph. A.* 27:56, 1938.

Trommsdorff's Journal der Pharmacie (1794-1834). In 1817 the name was changed to *Neues Journal der Pharmacie für Ärzte, Apotheker und Chemiker.* Under this name, the journal was continued until its merger with the *Annalen der Pharmazie* in 1834, the latter journal a substantial contribution by pharmacy to chemistry, which later became *Liebig's Annalen.*

Troth, Henry (1794-1842), Philadelphia wholesale druggist and one of the most active founders of the Philadelphia College of Pharmacy. See England: *First Century of the Philadelphia College of Pharmacy,* p. 354, Philadelphia, 1922; *Am. J. Pharm.* 14:174, 1842.

Tschirch, Alexander (1856-1939). His chief work was the monumental *Handbuch der Pharmakognosie,* which not only supplies detailed accounts of the history of each drug but also contains a comprehensive *Pharmacohistoria.* For further details about his life-work see *Pharm. Zeit.* 83:1293, 1295, 1926. A bibliography, enumerating the publications of Tschirch to January 1, 1923, appeared in *Schweiz. Apoth. Zeit.* 60:730-742, 1922.

Turner, William (1515-1568), English physician and pioneer herbalist, and clergyman. He had a private botanic garden at Kew and is considered the father of English botany.

Unguentarius, pl. *-i,* from the Latin *unguentum* "ointment," and *-arius,* "pertaining to," i.e., "maker of ointments." Cf.: *myropoeos* and *myrepsos.*

Urdang: George (1882-1960), pharmacist, historian, journalist and teacher. Urdang arrived at Madison as a refugee from Hitlerian Germany (1939), to write the Kremers and Urdang *History of Pharmacy,* based on *Kremers', q.v.,* materials. Urdang was the first Director of the American Institute of the History of Pharmacy (1941-57) and later became Professor at the University of Wisconsin (history of pharmacy, 1947-52). In Germany he had been an editor of the *Pharmazeutische Zeitung,* helped to found the German Society for the History of Pharmacy (1926), and earlier in his career had practiced pharmacy in Rosenberg, Prussia (1910-19). See: *Pharmacy in History,* 5: Nos. 2 & 3, 1960 (especially H. George Wolfe's article), and G. Sonnedecker in *Isis* 51:562-564, 1960 and *Am. J. Pharm. Ed.* 24:536-539, 1960.

Vauquelin, Louis Nicolas (1763-1829), French pharmacist. He discovered chromium (1797) and asparagine simultaneously with Robiquet (1805); also, nicotine (1811), lecithin (1811) and cyanic acid (1818).

Vertreter. See **Personnel.**

Virey, Julien Joseph (1775-1846), French pharmacist, physician, professor of natural history and pharmacology, Virey was one of the founders and co-editor of the *Journal de Pharmacie, q.v.,* and a facile writer.

Wackenroder, Heinrich Wilhelm Ferdinand (1798-1854), German pharmacist and professor of pharmaceutical chemistry at the University of Jena. He discovered corydaline and carotine and worked intensively in the field of phytochemistry.

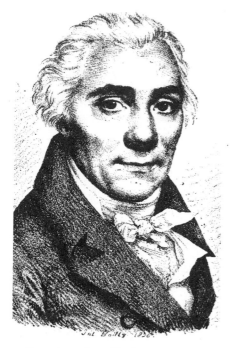

Born on a humble Normandy farm, L.-N. Vauquelin became a pharmacy owner in Paris, eventually reaching a scientific distinction that earned him the title of Chevalier of the Legion of Honor and his appointment by Napoleon as director of the school of pharmacy at Paris, and later as professor of chemistry at the Jardin des Plantes. (Drawing by J. Boilly, 1820; Collection L. Sergent; reproduced from Bull. Soc. Hist. Pharm. No. 65, 1929)

Wall, Otto A. (1847-1922), professor at the St. Louis College of Pharmacy and author of several books. See *J. A. Ph. A. 11*:226, 1922.

Warner, William R. (1836-1901), American pharmacist and manufacturer. See *Am. J. Pharm. 73*:414, 1901.

Warren, John C. (1778-1856), physician, founder of the Massachusetts General Hospital and responsible for the introduction of ether anesthesia. See Kelly and Burrage: *American Medical Biographies,* p. 1196, New York, 1920.

Wayne, Edward S. (1818-1885), pharmacist in Cincinnati and professor at the Cincinnati College of Pharmacy. See *Drug. Circ. 51*:93, 1907; *Am. J. Pharm. 58*:54, 1886.

Wedel, Georg Wolfgang (1645-1729), German physician and chemist. He wrote many essays on the constituents and the use of vegetable drugs.

Weightman, William (1813-1904), English-born chemist. In 1878, he became executive head of the firm of Powers and Weightman. See J. W. England: *First Century of the Philadelphia College of Pharmacy,* p. 33, Philadelphia, 1922.

Weights and measures. In general the old systems are built up on the division of a certain unit by 12, the so-called duodecimal system, while the modern system, the decimal system, provides a division by ten.

The Babylonians, Assyrians, Egyptians, Hebrews, Greeks and Romans had their own weights and measures. A general and comparative survey of the weights used for pharmaceutical purposes from the Babylonian period to the present time is given by Ludwig Winkler under the title *Das Apothekergewicht,* in *Pharm. Monatshefte,* 1924, No. 6. An article, "Weights and Measures in History," *Chem. & Drug. 110*:817, 1929, contains 84 photographs of weights and balances which have been used from ancient times to the present, with an explanatory text referring especially to medicine and pharmacy. Further details may be found in such books and articles as William Ridgeway: *The Origin of Metallic Currency and Weight Standards,* Cambridge, 1892; Ch. Rice: On the origin of our pharmaceutical signs for weights and measures, *New Remedies 6*:212, 1877; H. Sigerist: Masse und Gewichte in den medizinischen Texten des frühen Mittelalters, *Kyklos* (Leipzig) *3*:439, 1930; George Sarton: The first explanation of decimal fractions and measures by S. Stevin, *Isis 23*:153, 1935; Oscar Oldberg: Metrology, Parts 4, 5, 6, *Pharm. Era 13*:198, 1895, and The development of our systems of weights and measures, *Pharm. Era 14*:713, 1895; Geerto Snyder: *Wägen und Waagen,* Ingelheim am Rhein, n.d. [1957]; Bruno Kisch: *Gewichte-und-Waagemacher im Alten Köln (16.-19. Jahrh.),* Köln, 1962? (author is Curator of outstanding Edward Clark Streeter Collection of Weights and Measures, Yale University); Hans J. Albert: *Mass und Gewicht; Geschichtliche und tabellarische Darstellungen von d. Anfängen bis zur Gegenwart,* Berlin, 1957; Augustín M. Merck: *Antigua Metrologia Farmacéutica,* Valencia, 1960; Paul Walden: *Mass, Zahl und Gewicht in der Chemie der Vergangenheit. Ein Kapitel aus der Vorgeschichte des sogenannten quantitativen Zeitalters der Chemie,*

Stuttgart, 1931; K. M. C. Zevenboom and D. A. Wittop Koning: *Nederlandse Gewichten Stelsels, Ijkwezen, Vormen, Makers en Merken*, Leiden, 1953; and M. Geoffroy: *Dictionnaire des Poids et Mesures*, Baugé, 1907.

Wellcome, Sir Henry Solomon (1853-1936), American pharmacist and founder of the English firm of Burroughs Wellcome and Company. Sir Henry Wellcome was a scientific pharmacist as well as an anthropologist, an archaeologist, a writer, a philanthropist, and a collector of all items of historical pharmaceutical and medical interest. See *J. A. Ph. A.* 23:285, 1934; 25:734, 888, 1936.

Westrumb, Johann Friedrich (1751-1819), German pharmacist. He published many papers, especially on technical chemistry, and analyzed many mineral waters.

Whelpley, Henry Milton (1861-1926), pharmacist, anthropologist and archaeologist. Professor and dean of the St. Louis College of Pharmacy from 1904, active in a number of offices of the American Pharmaceutical Association. See *J. A. Ph. A.* 15:523, 1926.

Wiegand, Thomas S. (1825-1909), Philadelphia pharmacist and pharmaceutical author, for many years registrar at the Philadelphia College of Pharmacy. See *Am. J. Pharm. 81:* 502, 1909.

Wiegleb, Johann Christian (1732-1800), German pharmacist. An opponent of alchemy, he was at the same time one of the last and most zealous defenders of the phlogiston theory. Among his numerous publications was a chemical instructor in the form of letters, an attempt at popularizing chemical knowledge and a precursor of the famous *Chemical Letters*, published half a century later by Liebig.

Wilbert, Martin I. (1865-1916). For 17 years a pharmacist at the German Hospital in Philadelphia and, later on (1908-1916) Assistant in the Division of Pharmacology of the Hygienic Laboratory, United States Public Health Service. Wilbert was a voluminous writer on pharmaceutico-historical subjects. For a number of years he edited *Comments and Criticisms on the U. S. P.* See John K. Thum: *Am. J. Pharm.* 89:49, 1917.

Wilder, Hans M. (1831-1901), Iceland-born American pharmacist and pharmaceutical author. See *Am. J. Pharm.* 73:411, 1901.

Willdenow, Carl Ludwig (1765-1812), German pharmacist, director (after 1801) of the Botanic Garden and (after 1810) professor of botany at the University of Berlin. He was one of the best known botanists of his time.

Williamson, Peter (1795-1886), wholesale druggist and one of the founders of the Philadelphia College of Pharmacy. See England: *First Century of the Philadelphia College of Pharmacy*, p. 351, Philadelphia, 1922.

Winthrop, John (1588-1649), governor of Massachusetts Colony. He became important to pharmacy by the list of drugs sent to him from England and used by him in his attempts at caring for the sick in his colony. See *Dictionary of American Biography, XX*, p. 408. See: Whitfield J. Bell, Jr.: *Early American Science; Needs and Opportunities for Study*, p. 78, Williamsburg, Va., 1955.

Winthrop, John, Jr. (1606-1676), governor of Connecticut Colony, one of the earliest preparers of chemicals on North American soil. See *Dictionary of American Biography, XX*, p. 411. See: Whitfield J. Bell, Jr.: *Early American Science; Needs and Opportunities for Study*, p. 78, Williamsburg, Va., 1955.

Wöhler, Friedrich (1800-1882), German chemist. His artificial preparation of urea in 1828 broke down the supposedly impassable barrier between inorganic and organic chemistry. He first isolated several elements or improved the process of isolation of them, such as potassium, beryllium, aluminum, titanium, boron. Without being a pharmacist himself, as a teacher of students of pharmacy and, for some time, as inspector of the pharmacies of Hannover, he kept in contact with pharmacy. See *Am. J. Pharm.* 54:591, 1882.

Wood, George B. (1797-1879), physician, professor at the Philadelphia College of Pharmacy and later at the Medical Department of the University of Pennsylvania. Wood was for several decades the decisive factor in the revisions of the U. S. P. and, in collaboration with Franklin Bache, editor of the *U S Dispensatory*. See England: *First Century of the Philadelphia College of Pharmacy*, p. 397, Philadelphia, 1922.

Wood, Horatio C. (1841-1920), physician, author and professor at the University of Pennsylvania. See *Am. J. Pharm.* 92:136, 1920; *Dictionary of American Biography, XX*, p. 459.

Wood, Horatio C., Jr. (1874-   ), physician, professor at the University of Pennsylvania and, since 1921, at the Philadelphia College of Pharmacy. See *First Century of the Philadelphia College of Pharmacy*. First Supplement, p. 102, Philadelphia, 1934.

Wulling, Frederick J. (1866-1947). Professor and dean of the College of Pharmacy, University of Minnesota, 1892-1936, author of numerous pharmaceutical papers, etc., one of the foremost agitators for and promoters of the betterment and broadening of American pharmaceutical education. See *J. A. Ph. A.* 23:177, 1934; *Pharmacy Forward*, selections from F. J. Wulling's diary, autobiography, speeches and reports, edited and published by his son, Emerson G. Wulling, La Crosse, Wis., 1948.

Ximenez, Francisco (late 16th to early 17th century), Dominican monk and botanist. See Tschirch, *Handbuch der Pharmakognosie*, ed. 2, *I*, Part 3, p. 1346, Leipzig, 1933.

Yaple, Florence (1865-1912), one of the outstanding American woman pharmacists. Miss Yaple was closely connected with the Philadelphia College of Pharmacy and participated, for many years, in the work of editing and managing the American Journal of Pharmacy. See *Am. J. Pharm.* 84:481, 1912.

Yearbooks. The annual report is a special type of pharmaceutical serial. Indeed, the very first pharmaceutical periodical, the *Almanach, oder Taschenbuch für Scheidekünstler und Apotheker.* (1780) was an annual of this sort. See also the *Berlinisches Jahrbuch* (1795). With the specialization in pharmaceutical journalism, there developed an annual publication exclusively for supplying, in convenient form, abstracts of original articles published in any and all journals, no matter in what country or language.

Youngken, Heber W. (1885-1963), American botanist and pharmacognosist, professor at the Massachusetts College of Pharmacy, and author. His son, Heber, Jr., in turn, became one of the important pharmacognosists of his generation and then dean of the College of Pharmacy at the University of Rhode Island. See England: *First Century of the Philadelphia College of Pharmacy,* p. 418, Philadelphia, 1922.

Zwelffer, Johann (1618-1668), at first pharmacist in Palatine (Germany), later physician in Vienna. His *Animadversiones in Pharmacopoeam Augustanam* (1652) are, if we disregard ironic comments in Nicholas Culpeper's translation of the London *Pharmacopoeia* (1649), the first known commentary on a pharmacopeia. He was also the author of a *Pharmacopoea-regia seu dispensatorium novum et absolutissimum, adnexa spagyrica-muntissa.*

Index

Asterisks indicate pages in glossary.